THE
MERCK
MANUAL
OF
HEALTH & AGING

THE
MERCK
MANUAL
OF
HEALTH & AGING

MARK H. BEERS, MD
EDITOR-IN-CHIEF

THOMAS V. JONES, MD, MPH
EDITOR

MICHAEL BERKWITS, MD, JUSTIN L. KAPLAN, MD,
and ROBERT PORTER, MD
ASSISTANT EDITORS

BALLANTINE BOOKS • NEW YORK

Merck Editorial and Production Staff

Executive Editor	**Keryn A.G. Lane**
Senior Staff Writer	**Susan T. Schindler**
Senior Staff Editors	**Debra G. Share**
	Susan C. Short
Production Editor	**Melody Sadighi**
Textbook Operations Manager	**Diane C. Zenker**
Manager, Electronic Publications	**Barbara Amelia Nace**
Project Manager	**Diane Cosner-Bobrin**
Executive Assistant	**Jean Perry**
Administrative Assistant	**Marcia Yarbrough**
Designer	**Lorraine B. Kilmer**
Illustrator	**Michael Reingold**
Indexer	**Susan Thomas, PhD**
Publisher	**Gary Zelko**
Advertising and Promotions Supervisor	**Pamela J. Barnes-Paul**
Subsidiary Rights Coordinator	**Jeanne Nilsen**

2006 Ballantine Books Mass Market Edition

Published in the United States by Ballantine Books, an imprint of The Random House Publishing Group, a division of Random House, Inc., New York.

Originally published in hardcover in the United States by Merck & Co., Inc., in 2004.

ISBN: 0-345-48275-1

This edition published by arrangement with Merck & Co., Inc., West Point, PA.

Printed in the United States of America

www.ballantinebooks.com

OPM   9   8   7   6

PREFACE

Many people are able to take good health for granted for much of their lives. When they occasionally become ill, the health care system seems well suited to meet their needs. But as people age, everything changes. The need to prevent illness becomes more pressing, illnesses become more common, and the need for health care seems to be a routine part of life. The health care system may seem complex, impersonal, and difficult to manage, as though it were created for someone else. Explanations and useful information are often difficult to find.

The Merck Manual of Health & Aging was written to help people navigate the health care system and find useful information on health and disease. Whether you are in the best of health and hope to stay that way, are ill and hope to get better, or are in persistently poor health and facing the reality of living with disease, *The Merck Manual of Health & Aging* gives you and those who care about you the information needed. Its goal is to explain when others will not or cannot. The vast experience of The Merck Manuals, which are relied upon worldwide by millions of health care practitioners and members of the general public, has gone into creating this new book. The contributors, consultants, and editorial board members—recognized experts in the field of caring for older people—bring their knowledge, experience, and good judgment to this book. You can rely on the accuracy and honesty of this book.

Because care of older people is complex and involves the expertise of many different health care practitioners, this book covers a wide variety of information. Included is how the body ages, how the health care system does and should care for older people, how to strengthen and improve relationships with health care practitioners, and how to cope with disease.

The book provides in-depth information about most of the disorders that affect older people and about differences in how disorders may affect older people.

Knowledge is power, and today knowledge is essential. The more information you have, the better you are able to work with your doctors, nurses, social workers, and other health care practitioners. *The Merck Manual of Health & Aging* is a supplement to, not a substitute for, professional health care. It provides you with what you need and want to know in a way that other books cannot. Use the information to better understand what is happening to your body, to ensure that you are getting the best care, and to make the best decisions about health care. If you are fortunate enough to never need this information, we hope that it will still fascinate you with the wonder of the human body.

Mark H. Beers, MD, and Thomas V. Jones, MD, MPH

SPECIAL NOTE

The authors, reviewers, editors, and publisher have made extensive efforts to ensure that the information is accurate and conforms to the standards accepted at the time of publication. However, you are advised to discuss information obtained in this book with a doctor, pharmacist, nurse, or other health care practitioner.

COMMITTED TO PROVIDING MEDICAL INFORMATION: MERCK AND THE MERCK MANUALS

In 1899, the American drug manufacturer Merck & Co. first published a small 192-page book titled *Merck's Manual of the Materia Medica*. It was meant as an aid to physicians and pharmacists, reminding doctors that "Memory is treacherous." Compact in size, easy to use, comprehensive, and inexpensive, *The Merck Manual* (as it was later known) became a favorite of those involved in medical care and others in need of a medical reference. Even Albert Schweitzer carried a copy to Africa in 1913, and Admiral Byrd carried a copy to the South Pole in 1929.

By the 1980s, the book had become the world's largest selling medical text and was translated into more than a dozen languages. While the name of the parent company has changed somewhat over the years, the book's name has remained constant, known officially as *The Merck Manual of Diagnosis and Therapy* but usually referred to as *The Merck Manual* and sometimes "The Merck." Throughout the book's modern history, Merck & Co., Inc. has published it on a not-for-profit basis, keeping its price low so that as many people as possible can own and use a copy.

In 1990, the editors of *The Merck Manual* introduced *The Merck Manual of Geriatrics*. This new book quickly became the best-selling textbook of geriatric care, providing specific and comprehensive information on the care of older people. Now in its 3rd edition, *The Merck Manual of Geriatrics* is published in five languages. The creation and continued publication of this book reflect Merck's commitment to the world's aging population and the company's desire to improve geriatric care globally.

In 1997, *The Merck Manual of Medical Information—Home Edition* was published. In this revolutionary book, the editors translated the complex medical information in *The Merck Manual* into plain language, producing a book meant for all those people interested in medical care who did not have a medical degree. The book received critical acclaim and sold over 2 million copies. The *Second Home Edition* was released in 2003 and continues Merck's commitment to providing comprehensive, understandable medical information to all people at low cost.

The Merck Manual of Health & Aging continues Merck's commitment to education and geriatric care, providing information on aging and the care of older people in words understandable by the lay public.

Merck also supports the community of chemists and others with the need to know about chemical compounds with *The Merck Index*. First published in 1889, this publication actually predates *The Merck Manual* and is the most widely used text of its kind. *The Merck Veterinary Manual* was first published in 1955. It provides information on the health care of animals and is the preeminent text in its field.

Merck & Co., Inc. is one of the world's largest pharmaceutical companies. Merck is committed to bringing out the best in medicine and, as part of that effort, continues to proudly provide all of The Merck Manuals on a not-for-profit basis as a service to the community. Additionally, *The Merck Manual, The Merck Manual of Medical Information—Second Home Edition, The Merck Manual of Geriatrics, The Merck Manual of Health & Aging,* and *The Merck Veterinary Manual* are available free on Merck's Internet site at www.merck.com.

A GUIDE FOR READERS

The Merck Manual of Health & Aging is organized into 4 sections and 66 chapters. Understanding this organization will help readers navigate the book. Topics of general interest may be quickly located by looking in the Table of Contents or the Index. When looking for a specific topic, the Index is especially likely to be helpful.

Sections

The first section, "Fundamentals of Aging," covers three topics that set the stage: why aging occurs, how aging affects specific parts of the body, and how aging is changing the United States and world population.

The second section, "Caring for Self and Others," shines a light on topics that help people become more active in caring for themselves or a loved one. Topics include preventive care, healthy nutrition, appropriate use of drugs, and the wide array of diagnostic tests and complementary and alternative therapies. Also included are topics about obtaining and organizing care, including communicating with doctors and other health care practitioners, a review of the continuity of health care in different settings, caregiving, and palliative and end-of-life care.

The third section, "Medical Conditions," focuses on how disorders are different in older adults rather than discussing all aspects of disease. Some of the disorders discussed occur nearly exclusively in older adults; others occur more commonly in older adults. Still others occur in all age groups but are different in older adults.

The fourth section, "Social, Legal, and Ethical Issues," addresses several challenging, practical concerns relating to health and health care, including coping with change, driving, intimacy in relationships, mistreatment, legal and ethical issues, and the many ways of paying for health care.

Chapters

Some chapters in "Medical Conditions" describe a single disorder or condition, such as delirium or falls. Others describe related disorders, such as mouth and dental disorders or heart valve disorders. In either case, the discussion usually begins with a brief definition. The information that follows is typically organized under causes, symptoms, diagnosis, prevention, treatment, and outlook.

Additional Information

In some chapters, a more in-depth and sometimes more technical explanation of a topic is identified by the heading "additional detail." Some readers will want to read this material to better understand a disorder; others may wish to skip it.

Cross-References

Throughout the book are cross-references that identify other important or related discussions of a subject. Cross-references are identified within the text by numbered footnotes. Corresponding numbers are at the bottom of the page, along with the page number or numbers where more information can be found. Some cross-references guide the reader to an illustration, sidebar, or table elsewhere.

Medical Terms

Medical terms are often provided, usually in parentheses after the common term.

Diagnostic Tests

Diagnostic tests are mentioned throughout the book. In addition, chapter 10 explains several commonly used tests, including information about what a person is likely to experience when undergoing a test.

Illustrations, Sidebars, Tables

The many illustrations, sidebars, and tables help explain material in the text or give additional, related information.

Drug Information

Individual drugs are always referred to by their generic name, rather than by their brand or trade names. The first appendix contains two tables of drug names. The first table lists drugs mentioned in the book along with some of their corresponding trade names. The second table provides trade names with corresponding generic names.

Scattered throughout the book are many drug tables, identified by an Rx symbol. These drug tables provide additional information about a class or group of drugs.

Doses can be affected by age, sex, weight, height, the presence of more than one disorder, and the use of other drugs. Therefore, drug doses are not provided.

Essays

Twenty-five essays are scattered throughout the book. The authors share their personal views and insights about aging and its effects on something they love. A few of the authors are famous; most are not.

Resources for Help and Information

The second appendix lists many organizations that can provide additional information about a disorder or help locate various support services. Information about how to contact these organizations is provided.

CONTENTS

Section 1: FUNDAMENTALS OF AGING

Section 2: CARING FOR SELF AND OTHERS

Contents

Section 4: SOCIAL, LEGAL, AND ETHICAL ISSUES

EDITOR-IN-CHIEF

Mark H. Beers, MD
Executive Director of Geriatrics and Clinical Literature, Merck & Co., Inc.
and Clinical Professor of Medicine, Drexel University

EDITOR

Thomas V. Jones, MD, MPH
Merck & Co., Inc. and Clinical Associate Professor of Medicine,
Temple University School of Medicine

ASSISTANT EDITORS

Michael Berkwits, MD
Merck & Co., Inc. and Adjunct Assistant Professor of Medicine,
University of Pennsylvania School of Medicine

Justin L. Kaplan, MD
Merck & Co., Inc. and Clinical Associate Professor of Emergency Medicine,
Thomas Jefferson University

Robert Porter, MD
Merck & Co., Inc. and Clinical Assistant Professor of Emergency Medicine,
Thomas Jefferson University

M. Boyd Gillespie, MD
Assistant Professor, Department of
Otolaryngology–Head and Neck Surgery,
Medical Univeristy of South Carolina

Dev R. Gupta, MD
Chief, Department of Neurology,
Hackensack University Medical Center;
Assistant Professor of Neurology, New
Jersey Medical School

Robert L. Krugman, MD
Chairman, Department of Radiology,
Hackensack University Medical Center

Charles Riccobono, MD
Clinical Associate Professor of Medicine,
University of Medicine and Dentistry of
New Jersey; Vice Chairman, Department
of Internal Medicine and Chief, Division
of Digestive Disease and Nutrition,
Department of Internal Medicine,
Hackensack University Medical Center

Perry Charles Ritota, MD, PA
Director, Division of Reconstructive
Surgery, Department of Plastic Surgery,
Hackensack University Medical Center

Clark A. Rosen, MD, FACS
Associate Professor, Department of
Otolaryngology, University of Pittsburgh
School of Medicine and Director,
University of Pittsburgh Voice Center

Louis Evan Teichholz, MD
Chief, Department of Cardiology,
Hackensack University Medical Center;
Professor of Medicine, University of
Medicine and Dentistry of New Jersey—
New Jersey Medical School

Richard A. Watson, MD
Professor, Division of Urology,
Department of Surgery, University of
Medicine and Dentistry of New Jersey—
New Jersey Medical School; Chief of
Ambulatory Urology, Department of
Urology, Hackensack University Medical
Center

Acknowledgments

We thank Andrew J. Fletcher, MB, BChir, Sandra J. Masse, and Jonathan S. Simmons,
who assisted with initial editing of this book.

CONTRIBUTORS

Elias Abrutyn, MD
Professor of Medicine & Public Health
and Associate Provost and Associate Dean
for Faculty Affairs and Interim Chief,
Division of Infectious Diseases, Drexel
University College of Medicine
Urinary Tract Infections

Cathy A. Alessi, MD
Associate Professor, School of Medicine,
University of California–Los Angeles;
Geriatric Research, Education and Clinical
Center; Veterans Administration Greater
Los Angeles Healthcare System
Sleep

Neil B. Alexander, MD
Professor, Division of Geriatric Medicine,
University of Michigan; Associate
Director for Research, VA Ann Arbor
Health Care System GRECC
Falls

Mary Ann Anderson, PhD, RN
Associate Professor, University of Illinois
at Chicago, College of Nursing, Quad
Cities Regional Program
Continuity of Care

Nir Barzilai, MD
Director, Institute for Aging Research,
Albert Einstein College of Medicine
Diabetes Mellitus

Dan G. Blazer, MD, MPH, PhD
J. P. Gibbons Professor, Department of
Psychiatry and Behavioral Sciences, Duke
University Medical Center
Mental Health Disorders

Marjorie A. Bowman, MD
Professor and Chair, Department of
Family Practice and Community
Medicine, University of Pennsylvania
School of Medicine
*Communicating With Health Care
Practitioners*

Susan B. Bressler, MD
Professor of Ophthalmology, Johns
Hopkins University School of
Medicine; Wilmer Eye Institute
Eye Disorders

**Marquette L. Cannon-Babb,
PharmD**
Professor and Assistant Dean, Temple
University School of Pharmacy;
Certification in Geriatric Pharmacy
Drug Names: Generic and Trade

Emily Chai, MD
Assistant Professor, Brookdale
Department of Geriatrics and Adult
Development, Mount Sinai School of
Medicine
Complementary or Alternative Medicine

Barry S. Collet, DPM, MPH
Chief, Podiatry Department, Hebrew
Rehabilitation Center for Aged
Foot Disorders

David S. Cooper, MD
Professor, Department of Medicine, Johns
Hopkins University School of Medicine;
Director, Division of Endocrinology, Sinai
Hospital of Baltimore
Thyroid Disorders

Jill Crandall, MD
Assistant Professor, Division of
Endocrinology, Albert Einstein College
of Medicine
Diabetes Mellitus

Daniel F. Danzl, MD
Professor and Chair, Department of
Emergency Medicine, University of
Louisville
Hypothermia and Hyperthermia

G. Willy Davila, MD
Chairman, Department of Gynecology and
Head, Section of Urogynecology and
Reconstructive Pelvic Surgery, Cleveland
Clinic Florida
Female Genital and Sexual Disorders

Nancy Neveloff Dubler, LLB
Professor of Epidemiology & Population
Health, Albert Einstein College of
Medicine; Director, Division of Bioethics,
Montefiore Medical Center
Understanding Legal and Ethical Issues

Jonathan M. Evans, MD, MPH
Chief, Section of Geriatric Medicine,
University of Virginia
*Temporal Arteritis and Polymyalgia
Rheumatica*

Daniel Fischberg, MD, PhD
Assistant Professor, Departments of
Geriatrics and Medicine, Mount Sinai
School of Medicine
Palliative and End-of-Life Care

Jerome L. Fleg, MD
Medical Officer, Clinical Trials Scientific
Research Group, National Heart, Lung,
and Blood Institute
Abnormal Heart Rhythms

Joseph Francis, MD, MPH
Vice President for Education and
Academic Affairs, St. Vincent Hospitals
and Health Services
Confusion; Delirium

Michael L. Freedman, MD
The Diane and Arthur Belfer Professor
of Geriatric Medicine; Professor and
Director, Division of Geriatrics and The
Diane and Arthur Belfer Geriatric Center,
New York University School of Medicine
Blood Disorders

Eugene P. Frenkel, MD
Professor of Internal Medicine and
Radiology, Patsy R. and Raymond D.
Nasher Distinguished Chair in Cancer
Research, and A. Kenneth Pye
Professorship in Cancer Research,
University of Texas Southwestern Medical
School at Dallas
Finding and Living With Cancer; Cancers

Sandor A. Friedman, MD
Professor, Department of Medicine, State
University of New York at Downstate
Medical Center; Attending Physician and
Chief, Vascular Clinic, Jacobi Medical
Center
Blood Vessel Disorders

Tobin N. Gerhart, MD
Assistant Clinical Professor, Department
of Orthopaedic Surgery, Harvard Medical
School
Fractures

Barbara A. Gilchrest, MD
Professor and Chairman, Department of
Dermatology, Boston University School
of Medicine; Chief, Department of
Dermatology, Boston Medical Center
Skin Disorders

F. Michael Gloth, III, MD
Associate Professor, Division of Geriatric
Medicine and Gerontology, Johns Hopkins
University School of Medicine; President,
Victory Springs Senior Health Associates
Pain

Larry B. Goldstein, MD
Professor, Division of Medicine
(Neurology), Duke University Medical
Center; Director, Duke Center for
Cerebrovascular Disease and Durham VA
Medical Center
Stroke

Jack M. Guralnik, MD, PhD
Chief, Epidemiology and Demography
Section, Laboratory of Epidemiology,
Demography and Biometry, Intramural
Research Program, National Institute on
Aging
The Aging of America

Richard J. Havlik, MD, MPH
Chief, Laboratory of Epidemiology,
Demography and Biometry, Intramural
Research Program, National Institute on
Aging
The Aging of America

Helen M. Hoenig, MD, MPH
Associate Professor of Medicine, Duke
University Medical Center; Chief,
Physical Medicine & Rehabilitation
Service, Durham VA Medical Center
Rehabilitation

Larry E. Johnson, MD, PhD
Associate Professor, Departments of
Geriatrics and Family and Preventive
Medicine, University of Arkansas for
Medical Sciences; Medical Director,
Geriatrics and Extended Care, Central
Arkansas Veterans Healthcare System
*Maintaining Good Nutrition; Nutritional
Disorders; Water and Electrolyte Balance*

Fran E. Kaiser, MD
Clinical Professor, Division of Geriatric
Medicine, University of Texas
Southwestern Medical Center; Adjunct
Professor, Department of Internal
Medicine, Division of Geriatric Medicine,
Saint Louis University School of
Medicine; Executive Medical Director,
Merck & Co., Inc.
Intimacy

Paul R. Katz, MD
Professor, Department of Medicine,
University of Rochester School of
Medicine; Medical Director, Monroe
Community Hospital
Long-Term Care

Philip O. Katz, MD
Chairman, Division of Gastroenterology,
Albert Einstein Medical Center
Swallowing and Reflux Disorders

Young S. Kim, MD
Assistant Professor, Division of Infectious
Diseases, Drexel University College of
Medicine
Urinary Tract Infections

Mark Lachs, MD, MPH
Professor of Medicine, Weill Medical
College of Cornell University
Mistreatment

Lewis A. Lipsitz, MD
Professor and Director, Harvard Division
on Aging, Harvard Medical School; Usen
Co-Director, Research and Training
Institute, Hebrew Rehabilitation Center
for Aged; Chief of Gerontology, Beth
Israel Deaconess Medical Center
Dizziness and Fainting

Elan D. Louis, MD, MS
Associate Professor of Neurology, G. H.
Sergievsky Center and Department of
Neurology, College of Physicians and
Surgeons, Columbia University
Nerve Disorders; Movement Disorders

Edward R. Marcantonio, MD
Assistant Professor, Department of
Medicine, Harvard Medical School;
Director of Research, Division of General
Medicine, Beth Israel Deaconess Medical
Center
Dementia

Charles V. Mobbs, PhD
Associate Professor, Department of
Neurobiology and Geriatrics, Mount Sinai
School of Medicine
Age-Old Questions

Mark Monane, MD, MS
Adjunct Associate Professor, Ernest Mario
School of Pharmacy, Rutgers, The State
University of New Jersey; Principal,
Equity Research, Needham & Company
Drugs and Aging

R. Sean Morrison, MD
Hermann Merkin Professor of Palliative
Care and Associate Professor, Brookdale
Department of Geriatrics and Adult
Development, Mount Sinai School of
Medicine
Palliative and End-of-Life Care

Marvin Moser, MD
Clinical Professor, Department of
Medicine (Cardiology), Yale University
School of Medicine
High Blood Pressure

Michael P. O'Leary, MD
Associate Professor, Department of
Surgery, Harvard Medical School; Senior
Surgeon, Department of Urology, Brigham
& Women's Hospital
Male Genital and Sexual Disorders

J. David Osguthorpe, MD
Professor, Department of Otolaryngology,
Medical University of South Carolina
Nose and Throat Disorders

Sharon K. Ostwald, PhD, RN
Isla Carroll Turner Chair of
Gerontological Nursing; Professor and
Director, Center on Aging, University of
Texas Health Science Center at Houston
Caregiving

Catherine M. Otto, MD
Professor of Medicine, Division of
Cardiology, University of Washington
Medical Center
Heart Valve Disorders

Joseph G. Ouslander, MD
Professor and Director, Division of
Geriatric Medicine and Gerontology,
Emory University
Urinary Incontinence

James T. Pacala, MD, MS
Associate Professor, Distinguished
University Teaching Professor,
Department of Family Practice and
Community Health, University of
Minnesota
Preventive Medical Care

Robert M. Palmer, MD
Head, Section of Geriatric Medicine,
Cleveland Clinic Foundation; Associate
Clinical Professor, Case Western Reserve
University
Hospital Care

Cynthia X. Pan, MD
Assistant Professor, Brookdale
Department of Geriatrics and Adult
Development and Director of Education,
Hertzberg Palliative Care Institute, Mount
Sinai School of Medicine
Complementary or Alternative Medicine

Contributors

Joel D. Posner, MD
Audrey Meyer Mars Professor of Gerontologic Research, Professor of Medicine and Public Health, Drexel University College of Medicine
Exercise

Lawrence G. Raisz, MD
Professor, Department of Medicine, UConn Health Center and Director, UConn Center for Osteoporosis
Osteoporosis

Shobita Rajagopalan, MD
Associate Professor, Division of Infectious Disease, Charles R. Drew University of Medicine and Science and King-Drew Medical Center
Pneumonia and Influenza

Sheldon Retchin, MD, MSPH
Professor of Internal Medicine, Virginia Commonwealth University
Driving

Michael W. Rich, MD
Associate Professor of Medicine, Washington University School of Medicine; Director, Cardiac Rapid Evaluation Unit, Barnes-Jewish Hospital
Coronary Artery Disease; Heart Failure

Eric W. Sargent, MD, FACS
Michigan Ear Institute, Farmington Hills, Michigan
Hearing and the Ear

Edna P. Schwab, MD
Assistant Professor, Division of Geriatrics, Geriatric Fellowship Program Director, Hospital of the University of Pennsylvania; Acting Chief of Geriatrics, Philadelphia VA Medical Center
Arthritis

Jonathan A. Ship, DMD
Professor, Department of Oral Medicine and Director, Bluestone Center for Clinical Research, New York University College of Dentistry
Mouth and Dental Disorders

Knight Steel, MD
UMDNJ Endowed Professor of Geriatrics, New Jersey Medical School; Chief, Division of Geriatrics, Hackensack University Medical Center
Understanding Medical Tests

David Sutin, MD
Clinical Assistant Professor, Department of Medicine, New York University Medical Center; Chief, Geriatric Clinic, Bellevue Hospital
Blood Disorders

Peter B. Terry, MD, MA
Professor, Departments of Pulmonary Medicine and Critical Care, Johns Hopkins University School of Medicine
Chronic Obstructive Pulmonary Disease

David R. Thomas, MD
Professor of Medicine, Departments of Internal Medicine and Geriatrics, Saint Louis University Health Sciences Center
Undergoing Surgery

Kara K. Urnes, MD
Cardiology Fellow, Division of Cardiology, University of Washington
Heart Valve Disorders

Arnold Wald, MD
Professor, Division of Gastroenterology, Hepatology, and Nutrition, University of Pittsburgh Medical Center
Bowel Movement Disorders

Terrie Wetle, PhD
Associate Dean of Medicine for Public Health and Public Policy and Professor, Community Health, Brown Medical School
Coping With Change; Paying for Health Care

Heidi Wierman, MD
Geriatrician, Maine Medical Center
How the Body Ages

T. Franklin Williams, MD
Professor of Medicine (Emeritus), University of Rochester School of Medicine; Scientific Director, American Federation for Aging Research, 1991–2002; Director, National Institute on Aging, National Institutes of Health, 1983–91
How the Body Ages

ESSAYISTS

THE RESULT OF LIVING WITH YOUR "CHILD-SELF"—
THE REVOLTING-PETER-PAN-THAT FANS THINK
IS "EVER-SO-PRECIOUS", INHABITING THE EVER-
SO-LUCKY-KIDDIE-BOOK-ARTIST.
<u>QUESTION</u>
WHO -<u>SERIOUSLY</u>!- WOULD WANT TO
LIVE WITH AN ANCIENT PSYCHO-KIDSELF!
UGH!

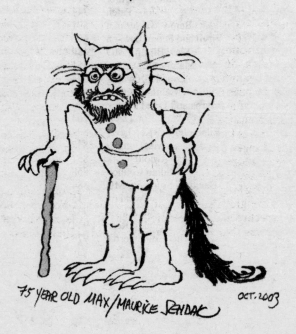

75 YEAR OLD MAX/MAURICE SENDAK   OCT. 2003

FUNDAMENTALS OF AGING

Aging in the 21st century is a story of success, but it is also a story with subplots of concern and peril. One of the best tools people can use when facing concerns and perils is information. Information about aging abounds. Much is known, for example, about how lifestyle and societal practices influence how long and how well people live. But the question of what actually causes people to age is but one of many "Age-Old Questions About Aging" that remain unanswered.

Much is known about "How the Body Ages"—that is, the changes that can occur with aging itself, apart from the influence of disorders and other factors.

In many countries of the world, more and more people are living longer. "Aging of America" sheds some light on how the growing group of older people looks from the perspective of a whole nation or society: who is old, what resources they have, where they live, and how healthy they are.

1

Age-Old Questions

Aging begins the moment a person is born. A baby develops and matures into an adult. Then, at some point, the aging process changes. The person begins a decline in function that ultimately leads to death—what people usually think of as aging or growing old. The technical term for this decline in function that ends in death is "senescence."

Science can provide information about changes in the body that lead to aging and death. Science can determine how some of the changes occur. But two basic mysteries remain: whether aging and dying have a purpose and, if so, what that purpose is. Throughout history, people have responded to these mysteries by searching for a "fountain of youth" that will prolong the time spent as vigorous, healthy young adults. And the search continues as researchers look for ways to slow or reverse the aging process.

Some progress has been made in the search. During the last century, life expectancy for people in the United States has greatly increased. As a result, what people consider to be old age has changed dramatically. Improvements in life expectancy occurred in two stages. First, death during childhood has become less likely, largely because sanitation has improved and because vaccines and treatments for childhood diseases, such as antibiotics, were developed. Second, disease and disability have become less likely to develop or have been postponed in older people because health care and approaches to prevention have improved. In spite of these improvements, even the healthiest and luckiest people do not live beyond about age 130.

LOOKING FOR THE FOUNTAIN OF YOUTH

Books about how to stay young and live longer abound. Almost everyone is interested in living a long life and looking and feeling young. No Ponce de Leons are traveling to new lands on a search for a magic fountain to restore their youth. However, researchers are looking at genes, cells, hormones, eating patterns, and other factors for clues about what causes aging and how to prevent or slow it.

Research has identified three strategies that may help people live longer: exercising, following certain types of diets, and eating fewer calories.

People who exercise are healthier than those who do not. Exercise has many established health benefits: improving and maintaining the ability to function, maintaining a healthy weight, and helping prevent or postpone disorders such as coronary artery disease and diabetes.

People who eat a low-fat diet that includes lots of fruits and vegetables are healthier than people who eat more fat and starch. Also, people who live in Mediterranean countries and consume the so-called Mediterranean diet seem to live longer. This diet is generally thought to be healthier than northern European and American diets because it consists of more grains, fruits, vegetables, legumes, nuts, and fish and less red meat. In addition, the main fat consumed is olive oil. Olive oil contains many vitamins and consists mainly of mono-unsaturated fat rather than saturated fat. Monounsaturated fats do not increase cholesterol the way saturated fats do.

A low-calorie diet over a lifetime may lead to longer life because it reduces the number of certain damaging substances in the body. These substances, called free radicals, are by-products of the normal activity of cells. The damage done to cells by free radicals is thought to contribute to aging and to disorders such as coronary artery disease and cancer. But no studies to test this theory have been done in people.

These three strategies would require a change in lifestyle for most people. Consequently, many people look for other, less demanding ways to prevent or slow aging. For example, they may look for other ways to manage free radicals. Substances called antioxidants can neutralize free radicals and thus help prevent damage to cells. Vitamins C and E are antioxidants. So some people take large amounts of these vitamins as supplements in the hope of slowing the aging process. Other antioxidants, such as beta-carotene (a form of vitamin A), are also sometimes taken as supplements. In theory, the use of antioxidants to prevent aging makes sense. However, no studies have shown that antioxidants prevent or slow aging.

Levels of some hormones decrease as people age. Another way people try to delay or slow aging is to take supplements of these hormones. Examples are testosterone, estrogen, DHEA (dehydroepiandrosterone), human growth hormone, and melatonin. But whether hormonal supplements have any effect on aging is unknown. Furthermore, some of these supplements have known risks.

Some people believe that Eastern practices, such as yoga, tai chi, and qigong, can prolong life. These practices are based on the principle that health involves the whole person (physical, emotional, mental, and spiritual) and balance within the body. The practices may include relaxation, breathing techniques, diet, and meditation as well as exercise. They are safe for older people and probably improve their health. But whether these practices prolong life is difficult to prove.

WHEN DOES A PERSON BECOME OLD?

The traditional designation for old age—65 years—has no basis in biology. Many people are vigorous and active at 65. Others are sick and inactive at 40. Rather, the basis for choosing age 65 is in history. Age 65 was chosen as the age for retirement in Germany, the first nation to establish a retirement program. (In 1889, Bismarck, Germany's Chancellor, first chose age 70, but in 1916, the age was lowered to 65.)

The question as to when a person becomes old can be answered in different ways. Chronologic age is based solely on the passage of time. It is a person's age in years. Chronologic age has limited significance in terms of health. Nonetheless, the likelihood of developing a health problem increases as people age. Because chronologic age helps predict many health problems, it has some legal and financial uses. It is also used to determine eligibility for some programs for older people.

Biological age refers to changes in the body that commonly occur as people age. For example, vision and hearing typically worsen as people age. Because these changes affect some people more than others, some people are biologically old at 40, and others are biologically young at 60 and even older.

Psychologic age is based on how people act and feel. For example, an 80-year-old who works, plans, looks forward to future events, and participates in many activities is considered psychologically young. Such a person is commonly described as "being young at heart."

People often wonder whether what they are experiencing as they age is normal or abnormal. Although people age somewhat differently, many changes occur in almost everyone and are thus considered "normal." However, a more accurate description of these changes is "usual." Usual aging refers to what happens to most people, including disorders that are common among older people. Usual aging does not necessarily mean that the changes are unavoidable or desirable.

Usual aging was once thought to include such unavoidable changes as muscle weakness, slowed movement, loss of balance, and memory loss. Research has shown that many of these common, "normal" changes result from an unhealthy lifestyle or from disorders that can be prevented or treated and reversed, rather than from aging itself. So the question to ask may be whether changes can be avoided rather than whether they are "normal." This question leads to the concept of healthy aging.

Healthy aging refers to a postponement of or reduction in the undesired effects of aging. The goals of healthy aging are maintaining physical and mental health, avoiding disorders, and remaining active and independent. For most people, maintaining general good health requires more effort as they age. Certain healthy habits have been shown to reduce the risk of developing several disorders that commonly occur as people age. These habits include following a nutritious diet, exercising regularly, and staying mentally active. Developing these habits is an important part of healthy aging. The sooner a person develops them, the better. However, it is never too late to begin.[1] In this way, people can have some control over what happens to them as they age.

WHY DOES THE BODY CHANGE?

The body changes with aging because changes occur in individual cells and in whole organs. These changes result in changes in function, in appearance, and thus in the experience of aging.

Aging Cells

As cells age, they function less well. Eventually, they must die, as a normal part of the body's functioning.

Cells may die because they do not divide normally or because they are damaged. Cells may be damaged by harmful substances in the environment, such as radiation, sunlight, and

1. see page 33

chemotherapy drugs. Cells may also be damaged by certain by-products of their own normal activities. These by-products, called free radicals, are given off when cells produce energy.

Many cells die because the genes they contain program a process that, when triggered, results in death of the cell. This programmed death, called apoptosis, is a kind of cell suicide. Reasons for cell suicide include replacing old cells with new ones and eliminating excess cells.

Also, cells die because they can divide only a limited number of times. This limit is also programmed by genes. When a cell can no longer divide, it grows larger, exists for a while, then dies. The mechanism that limits cell division involves a structure called a telomere. Telomeres are used to move the cell's genetic material in preparation for cell division. Every time a cell divides, the telomeres shorten a bit. Eventually, the telomeres become so short that the cell can no longer divide. The telomeres of cancer cells, unlike those of normal cells, do not shorten each time the cell divides. Consequently, cancer cells can divide forever.

Aging Organs

How well organs function depends on how well the cells within them function. Older cells function less well. Also, in some organs, cells die and are not replaced, so the number of cells decreases. The number of cells in the testes, ovaries, liver, and kidneys decreases markedly as the body ages. When the number of cells becomes too low, an organ cannot function normally. Thus, most organs function less well as people age. However, not all organs lose a large number of cells. The brain is one example. Healthy older people do not lose many brain cells. Substantial losses occur mainly in people who have had strokes or who have Alzheimer's disease or Parkinson's disease.

A decline in one organ's function, whether due to a disorder or to aging itself, can affect the function of another. For example, if atherosclerosis narrows blood vessels to the kidneys, the kidneys function less well because blood flow to them is decreased.

WHY DOES FUNCTION DECLINE?

For most people most of the time, the decline in organ function does not affect the body's ability to function during normal daily activities. People usually notice the decline in organ function only when very demanding tasks are attempted or when a disorder develops. For example, the amount of blood pumped by the heart during vigorous exercise decreases as people age. Older people may notice this change only when they play tennis or jog, not when they take a walk. They may notice changes in brain function only when they try to learn new information, such as a new language.

A noticeable decline in function is more likely to result from factors other than aging itself. The most common culprit is a disorder. A disorder may cause pain or confusion, make movement more difficult, rob a person of energy, or lead to depression.

The psychologic, sociologic, and financial situation of older people affects their behavior. Their behavior, in turn, affects their ability to function. Fear or worry may cause older people to become less active. If older people are less active, their ability to function tends to decline. Older people may fear being hurt or embarrassed, so they withdraw from their favorite activities and stay home. Older people with balance problems may fear that they might fall and break a bone. Older people with urinary incontinence may worry that they could have a wetting accident. Not having a partner with whom to share experiences or not having adequate funds may also stop people from participating in activities. People who participate in meaningful activities tend to remain healthy and live longer, as do people who have social support (married men in particular), adequate funds (those in a higher socioeconomic bracket), and a higher educational level.

Taking preventive measures can help older people remain healthy, active, and able to function.[1] Older people can develop healthy habits and continue to participate in activities. Learning to recognize situations and tendencies (such as fear) that can lead to further problems can help. Having a positive attitude toward aging—expecting life to continue to be full, hopeful, and worthwhile—can also help.

If older people remain fit and well, they do not lose their ability to remember, learn, think, and reason. They can remain physically active and capable. They can adapt to change. They

1. see page 33

can resist most disorders. When they develop a disorder, they can tolerate and respond to medical and surgical treatments and usually recover.

2

How the Body Ages

As the years pass, most people experience changes in the way their body functions. Some changes are obvious. For example, before age 50, most people begin to have trouble seeing objects that are up close. Other changes are hardly noticeable. For example, few people are aware that the kidneys may become less able to filter waste products out of the blood, because the kidneys usually continue to filter the blood well enough to avoid problems. Most people learn that their kidneys have aged only if a disorder develops.

Predicting how a particular person will age is hard, because each person ages at a different pace. In addition, how well a person takes care of the body influences how the person ages. Nonetheless, some changes are almost universal. Knowing what changes may be expected can help a person adjust to aging.

EYES

A change in vision is often the most undeniable sign of aging. Between the ages of 40 and 50, most people notice that seeing objects closer than 2 feet becomes difficult. This change in vision, called presbyopia, occurs because the lens in the eye stiffens. Normally, the lens changes its shape to help the eye focus. When the lens stiffens, the eye cannot easily focus on objects that are close.

Many people try to ignore presbyopia for as long as they can.

But ultimately, almost everyone with presbyopia ends up wearing reading glasses. People who need glasses to see distant objects may need to wear bifocals or glasses with variable-focus lenses.

As people continue to age, vision changes in other ways. Seeing in dim light becomes more difficult. This change occurs because the lens tends to become denser. Light passes through the lens to the retina at the back of the eye. A denser lens means that less light enters the eye. Also, the retina, which contains the cells that sense light, becomes less sensitive. So for reading, brighter light is needed. On average, 60-year-olds need 3 times more light to read than 20-year-olds.

With aging, the pupil of the eye reacts more slowly to changes in light. Light enters the eye through the pupil, which widens or narrows to let more or less light in. Consequently, older people may be unable to see when they first enter a dark room. Or they may be temporarily blinded when they enter a brightly lit area. This effect is particularly bothersome when a person enters or leaves a dark movie theater or drives in or out of a dark tunnel. Older eyes are less able to adjust partly because the muscles that widen and narrow the pupils tend to weaken as people age. Older people may also become more sensitive to glare (bright light that shines directly or is reflected into the eyes). However, increased sensitivity to glare is usually due to an eye disorder, such as cataracts.

Colors are perceived differently as people age. This change occurs partly because the lens tends to yellow slightly with aging. Yellowing affects how colors at the blue-violet end of the light spectrum are seen. Blues tend to lose their vividness and look more like gray. This change is insignificant for most people. However, older people may have trouble reading black letters printed on a blue background or reading blue letters. At the other end of the spectrum, reds tend to appear more vivid.

The ability to see differences in shades and tones and to see fine details decreases. This change probably occurs because the number of nerve cells that transmit visual signals from the eyes to the brain decreases. This change affects the way depth is perceived, and judging distances becomes more difficult.

Older people may see more tiny black specks moving across

ORGANS AFFECTED BY AGING

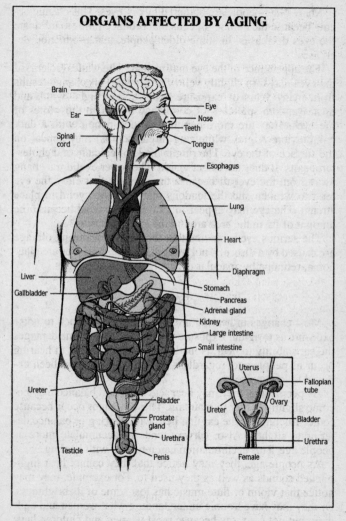

their field of vision. These specks, called floaters, are bits of fluid within the eye that have solidified. Floaters do not significantly interfere with vision. Unless they suddenly increase in number, they are not a cause of concern.

Many older people are bothered by dry eyes. This change occurs because the number of cells that produce fluids to lubricate the eyes decreases. In some older people, tear production decreases.

The appearance of the eye may change. The whites (sclera) of the eyes may turn slightly yellow or brown. This change results from many years of exposure to ultraviolet light, wind, and dust. Random splotches of color may appear in the whites of the eyes. They are more common among people with a dark complexion. A gray-white ring (arcus senilis) may appear on the surface of the eye. The ring is made of calcium and cholesterol salts. It does not affect vision. The lower eyelid may hang away from the eyeball because the muscles that close the eye tend to weaken and the tendons that hold the eyelid in place stretch. The eye may appear to sink into the head because the amount of fat in the area around the eye decreases.

The serious eye problems that tend to occur during old age are caused by a disorder, not by aging itself. Examples are glaucoma, retinopathy, macular degeneration, and cataracts.[1]

EARS

Most changes in hearing are probably due as much to noise exposure as to aging. Exposure to loud noise over time damages the ear's ability to hear. Nonetheless, some changes in hearing occur as people age, regardless of whether they have been exposed to loud noise.

As people age, they may hear less well, and balance may become slightly harder to maintain. These changes occur because some structures in the ear that help with hearing or balance deteriorate slightly. Also, earwax tends to accumulate more as people age. This accumulation can interfere with hearing.

As people age, they may notice that they cannot hear high-pitched sounds as well as they used to. For example, they may notice that violin or flute music has lost some of its brightness. Or they may have trouble understanding what women and children, but not men, say because most women and children have higher-pitched voices than men.

Perhaps more disturbing for older people is that other people

1. see page 511

seem to always be mumbling. Even when other people speak more loudly, the words are still hard to comprehend. This experience also results from difficulty hearing high-pitched sounds. Most consonants, such as c, k, p, s, and t, are closed, quick, high-pitched sounds. Vowels are open, longer, and lower-pitched sounds. So older people hear vowels much better than consonants. Consonants are the sounds that help people identify words. For example, when a person hears mainly vowels, "Tell me exactly what you want to keep" sounds like "Ell me exaly wha you wan oo ee." The sentence sounds as if the person speaking is not pronouncing the words clearly, and the meaning is lost. Speaking loudly does not help because it tends to accentuate the vowels, not the consonants.

Many older people have more trouble hearing in loud places or in groups because there is more background noise. Hearing aids can help people with hearing loss hear better.[1]

MOUTH AND NOSE

Generally, when people are in their 50s, the abilities to taste and smell start to gradually diminish. The abilities to taste with the tongue and to smell with the nose are both needed to enjoy the full range of flavors in food. The tongue can identify only basic tastes: sweet, sour, bitter, and salt. More subtle and complex flavors (raspberry, for example) require the sense of smell as well.

As people age, the number and the sensitivity of taste buds on the tongue decrease. These changes tend to reduce the ability to taste sweet and salt more than the ability to taste bitter and sour. The ability to smell declines slightly. Strong smells remain easy to detect, but more subtle smells become more difficult to notice and identify. As a result, many foods tend to taste bitter, and foods with subtle smells may taste bland.

Older people may notice that their mouth feels dry more often. As people age, less saliva is produced. However, dry mouth may result from a disorder or the use of certain drugs. Dry mouth further reduces the ability to taste and smell the aromas of food.

All of these changes contribute to a loss of taste. To compen-

1. see page 539

sate, older people may add more spices, including salt, to their food. If too much salt is used, certain health problems, such as high blood pressure, can result.

As people age, the gums recede slightly. Consequently, the lower parts of the teeth are exposed to food particles and bacteria. Also, tooth enamel tends to wear away. These changes make the teeth more susceptible to decay and cavities (caries), which make tooth loss more likely.[1]

SKIN

As people age, the skin tends to become thinner, less elastic, drier, and finely wrinkled. However, exposure to sunlight over the years contributes to wrinkling and to making the skin rough and blotchy. The effects of exposure to sunlight can be seen when skin that is normally exposed to sunlight, such as that on the face, is compared with skin that is usually covered, such as that on the buttocks. People who have avoided exposure to sunlight often look much younger than their actual age.

The layer of fat under the skin thins and is replaced by more fibrous tissue. The fat layer acts as a cushion for the skin, helping protect and support it. The fat layer also helps conserve body heat. As this layer thins, the skin is torn more easily, wrinkles are more likely to develop, and tolerance for cold decreases.

The number of nerve endings in the skin decreases. As a result, sensation, including sensitivity to pain, may be reduced, and injuries may be more likely. The number of sweat glands and blood vessels also decreases, and blood flow in the deep layers of the skin decreases. Normally, heat is moved from the inner parts of the body through blood vessels to the surface of the body. When blood flow decreases, less heat leaves the body, and the body cannot cool itself as well. Thus, older people are more likely to develop disorders due to overheating, such as heatstroke. Also, the skin tends to heal more slowly when blood flow is decreased.

The number of pigment-producing cells (melanocytes) de-

1. see page 559

creases. Thus, the skin has less protection against ultraviolet (UV) radiation, such as that from sunlight.

BONES AND JOINTS

As people age, bones tend to become less dense. Thus, bones become weaker and more likely to break. In women, loss of bone density speeds up after menopause.

Bones become less dense partly because the amount of calcium they contain decreases. Part of the reason is that less calcium is absorbed in the digestive tract and levels of vitamin D (which helps the body use calcium) decrease slightly. Calcium is the main mineral that gives bones strength. Certain bones are weakened more than others. Those most affected include the end of the thighbone (femur) at the hip, the ends of the arm bones (radius and ulna) at the wrist, and the bones of the spine (vertebrae).

In the center of bones is bone marrow, where most blood cells are produced. As people age, the amount of bone marrow decreases. Therefore, fewer blood cells are produced. Even with this decrease, the bone marrow can usually produce enough blood cells throughout life. Problems may occur when the need for blood cells is greatly increased—for example, when anemia or an infection develops or bleeding occurs. In such cases, bone marrow is less able to increase its production of blood cells in response to the body's needs.

As people age, the cartilage that lines the joints tends to thin. The surfaces of a joint may not slide over each other as well as they used to, and the joint may be slightly more susceptible to injury. Repeated injury or the lifelong use of joints often leads to osteoarthritis, which is one of the most common disorders of later life.[1]

Ligaments, which bind joints together, tend to become less elastic as people age, making joints feel tight or stiff. This change results from chemical changes in the proteins that make up the ligaments. Consequently, most people become less flexible as they age. Ligaments tend to tear more easily, and when they tear, they heal more slowly.

1. see page 585

MUSCLES AND BODY FAT

As people age, the amount of muscle tissue (muscle mass) and muscle strength tend to decrease. This process is called sarcopenia (which literally means loss of flesh). Loss of muscle mass begins around age 30 and continues throughout life. Muscle mass decreases because the number of muscle fibers decreases. This change may occur because the levels of growth hormone and testosterone, which stimulate muscle development, decrease with aging. Also, muscles cannot contract as quickly in old age.

Most older people retain enough muscle mass and strength to perform all necessary tasks. Many older people remain strong athletes. They compete in sports and enjoy vigorous physical activity. However, even the fittest may notice some decline as they age.

Regular exercise can partially overcome or at least significantly delay the loss of muscle mass and strength. With regular exercise, even people who have never exercised can increase muscle mass and strength. Conversely, physical inactivity, especially bed rest during an illness, can greatly worsen the loss. During periods of inactivity, older people lose muscle mass and strength much more quickly than younger people do. Thus, after 1 day of bed rest, older people may need about 2 weeks of progressively becoming more active to get back to the level of muscle strength they had before bed rest.

As people age, the amount of body fat tends to increase. Too much body fat can increase the risk of health problems. A healthy diet and exercise can help older people keep body fat from increasing too much.

BRAIN AND NERVOUS SYSTEM

As people age, the number of nerve cells in the brain decreases only slightly. Several things help compensate for this decline. As cells are lost, new connections are made between the remaining nerve cells. New nerve cells may form in some areas of the brain, even during old age. In addition, the brain has more cells than it needs to perform most activities—a characteristic called redundancy.

The substances and structures involved in sending messages

in the brain change. The levels of some chemical messengers (neurotransmitters) and enzymes decrease, and others increase. The number of some types of receptors on nerve cells decreases, and the number of others increases. (Receptors are structures on the nerve cells that neurotransmitters attach to, causing a specific action in the cells.)

Because of these changes, the brain may function slightly less well. Older people may react and do tasks somewhat more slowly. Some mental functions may be subtly reduced. They include vocabulary, short-term memory, the ability to learn new material, and the ability to recall words.

After about age 60, the number of cells in the spinal cord begins to decrease. As a result, older people may notice a decrease in sensation.

As people age, nerves may conduct signals more slowly. Usually, this change is so minimal that people do not notice it. Also, the nervous system's response to injury is reduced. Nerves may repair themselves more slowly and incompletely in older people than in younger people. Therefore, older people are more vulnerable to injury and disorders.

HEART AND BLOOD VESSELS

As people age, the heart and blood vessels change in many ways. The walls of the heart become stiffer, and the heart fills with blood more slowly.

The walls of the arteries become thicker and less elastic. The arteries become less able to respond to changes in the amount of blood pumped through them. Thus, blood pressure is higher in older people than in younger people.

Despite these changes, a normal older heart functions well. At rest, the differences between young and old hearts are trivial. The differences become apparent only when more work is required of the heart, as occurs when a person exercises vigorously or becomes sick. An older heart cannot increase how fast it beats as quickly or as much as a younger heart. Regular exercise can reduce many of the effects of aging on the heart and blood vessels.

MUSCLES OF BREATHING AND THE LUNGS

As people age, the muscles used in breathing, such as the diaphragm, tend to weaken. Also, slightly less oxygen is absorbed from air that is breathed in. In people who do not smoke or have a lung disorder, the muscles of breathing and the lungs continue to function well enough to meet the needs of the body during ordinary daily activities. But these changes may make exercising vigorously (for example, running or biking energetically) more difficult. Older people may also have more difficulty breathing at high altitudes.

The lungs become less able to fight infection, in part because the cells that sweep debris out of the airways are less able to do so. Cough, which also helps clear the lungs, tends to be weaker.

DIGESTIVE SYSTEM

Aging affects the digestive system in several ways. But these changes have little effect on function. The muscles of the esophagus contract less forcefully, but movement of food through the esophagus is not affected. Food is emptied from the stomach more slowly, and the stomach cannot hold as much food because it is less elastic. But in most people, these changes are too slight to be noticed.

Certain changes in the digestive system cause problems in some people. The digestive tract may produce less lactase, an enzyme the body needs to digest milk. As a result, older people are more likely to develop intolerance of dairy products (lactose intolerance). People with lactose intolerance may feel bloated or have gas or diarrhea after they consume milk products. In the large intestine, materials move through a little more slowly. In some people, this slowing may contribute to constipation.

The liver also changes. It tends to become smaller (because the number of cells decreases), and less blood flows through it. Certain enzymes produced in the liver work less efficiently. These enzymes help the body process drugs and some other substances. As a result, the liver may be slightly less able to help rid the body of drugs and other substances. And the effects of drugs—intended and unintended—last longer.

KIDNEYS AND URINARY TRACT

As people age, the kidneys tend to become smaller (because the number of cells decreases), and less blood flows through them. Beginning at about age 30, the kidneys begin to filter blood less well. As years pass, they may remove waste products from the blood less well. They may also excrete too much water, making dehydration more likely. Nonetheless, they almost always function well enough to meet the body's needs.

The urinary tract changes in several ways that may make controlling urination more difficult. The maximum volume of urine that the bladder can hold decreases. Older people may be less able to delay urination after they first sense a need to urinate. The bladder muscles may contract sporadically, apart from any need to urinate. The bladder muscles weaken. As a result, more urine is left in the bladder after urination is finished. These changes are one reason that urinary incontinence (the uncontrollable loss of urine) becomes more common as people age.

As women age, the urethra (which carries urine out of the body) shortens and its lining becomes thinner. The muscle that controls the passage of urine through the urethra (urinary sphincter) is less able to close tightly and prevent leakage. These changes may result from the decrease in the estrogen level that occurs with menopause.

As men age, the prostate gland tends to enlarge. In many men, it enlarges enough to partly block the passage of urine.[1]

REPRODUCTIVE ORGANS

The effects of aging on the reproductive system are more obvious in women than in men. In women, most of these effects are related to menopause, when the levels of female hormones (particularly estrogen) decrease, menstrual periods end permanently, and pregnancy is no longer possible. The decrease in female hormone levels causes the ovaries and uterus to shrink. The tissues of the vagina become thinner, drier, and less elastic (a condition called atrophic vaginitis). The breasts become less firm and more fibrous, and they tend to sag.

Some of the changes that begin at menopause may interfere

1. see page 886

with sexual activity.[1] However, for most women, aging does not significantly affect sexual activity.

In men, the changes in the reproductive system are less dramatic. Most men remain fertile until death, even though testosterone levels decrease, resulting in fewer sperm and a decreased sex drive (libido). Most men can continue to have erections and reach orgasm throughout life. However, erections may not last as long or may be slightly less rigid. In addition, the time needed to achieve a second erection may increase markedly. Erectile dysfunction (impotence) becomes more common as men age.

ENDOCRINE SYSTEM

The endocrine system consists of several glands and organs that produce hormones. Hormones act as messengers to help regulate and coordinate activities throughout the body. As people age, the levels and activity of some hormones (in addition to sex hormones) decrease. For example, the level of growth hormone decreases, causing changes in muscles such as a decrease in muscle mass. The level of aldosterone, a hormone produced by the adrenal glands, also decreases. This decrease may contribute to the tendency of older people to become dehydrated more easily.

Most hormonal changes do not affect how the body functions. However, during certain circumstances, the body's functions may be affected. For example, after eating a large meal, insulin released from the pancreas is not used as efficiently as usual. Insulin helps control the level of sugar in the blood. When insulin is used less efficiently, the level of sugar in the blood rises slightly higher than usual, and the level takes longer to return to normal. This change may have no noticeable effect. But in some people, it can be an early warning of diabetes.

IMMUNE SYSTEM

As people age, the immune system becomes less effective. But the change is so slight that most people do not notice it. Most people notice that the body is less able to fight infections

1. see page 871

only when infections linger or become severe. People who are infected with tuberculosis during early adulthood may have no symptoms until old age. Then, symptoms develop because the immune system is weaker.

The immune system may be less able to distinguish the body's own cells from foreign substances that invade the body. Consequently, disorders in which the immune system attacks some of the body's own cells (autoimmune disorders) become more common.

The cells of the immune system destroy cancer cells, bacteria, and other foreign substances more slowly. This slowdown may be one reason that cancer is more common among older people. Also, vaccines tend to be less protective in older people. These changes in the immune system may help explain why some infections, such as pneumonia and influenza, are more common among older people and result in death more often.

Changes in the immune system may have one beneficial effect. Allergy symptoms may become less severe.

3

The Aging of America

America is growing old. During the early days of our nationhood and for more than a century thereafter, the population consisted mostly of children and young and middle-aged adults. The percentage of people over 65 was small. In the 21st century, however, that percentage has increased dramatically. Since 1900, when average life expectancy was 47 years, the percentage of older Americans has more than tripled.

There are now more than 35 million Americans (about 12% of the U.S. population) over 65. As the baby boomers (the generation of Americans born between the late 1940s and the early 1960s) age, this number will nearly double by 2030.

People over 85 (the oldest old) are the fastest growing seg-

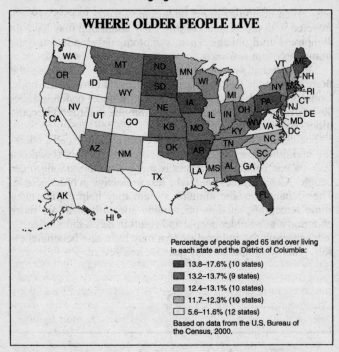

WHERE OLDER PEOPLE LIVE

Percentage of people aged 65 and over living in each state and the District of Columbia:

- 13.8–17.6% (10 states)
- 13.2–13.7% (9 states)
- 12.4–13.1% (10 states)
- 11.7–12.3% (10 states)
- 5.6–11.6% (12 states)

Based on data from the U.S. Bureau of the Census, 2000.

ment of the U.S. population. About 1.5% of Americans are 85 or over. The number of Americans 100 years or older is expected to swell from 1 out of 5,578 in the year 2000 to 1 out of 472 in the year 2050.

Women have a longer life expectancy than men, so as the U.S. population ages, there is a greater proportion of women. Among people 65 or over in the year 2000, there were 70 men for every 100 women. Among people 85 or over, there were 41 men for every 100 women.

Like the total U.S. population, the older U.S. population is more racially and ethnically diverse than in the past. This diversity is due in part to immigration and in part to increased life expectancy among minority groups. In 1999, minority groups represented about 16% of the population of people over 65; in 2030 that percentage is expected to rise to about 25%.

Within the United States, the distribution of older adults is not uniform. Florida has the highest percentage of people 65 or over (17.6%), followed by Pennsylvania (15.6%) and West Virginia (15.3%).

FINANCES

Not long ago, older Americans typically were poor. Once people stopped working, their fixed income from Social Security or a pension was rarely adequate to support them comfortably. Today, a greater number of older Americans have funds and investments that provide them with financial security. Nevertheless, about 11% of Americans 65 or over have incomes below the poverty line, despite the fact that for a person 65 or over living alone, the threshold for being classified by the government as living in poverty is stricter than it is for younger people. A person 65 or over living alone is not considered impoverished unless annual income is less than $7,990, compared with $8,667 for a person under 65. Some older people have limited resources but have assets, particularly homes, that prevent them from meeting the strict definition of poverty. Fluctuations in interest rates tend to hit older people hardest because of their reliance on what is often called investment income. High inflation rates hit older people hard as well, because their incomes do not usually adjust upward as prices increase.

Even with homes and investments, many older Americans may not have incomes that are sufficient to meet all of their needs. They may be unwilling or unable to sell their home, or they may be faced with increased expenses, such as for prescription drugs or in-home assistance. The complicated issues involving real estate and other investments and the need to plan for longer retirement periods have made careful financial planning and preparation an essential part of growing old.

The aging of the population has put a burden on the country's ability to pay for the services needed by older people. The proportion of the population 65 or over is increasing as the proportion of the population made up of adults under 65 is decreasing. The situation is similar or worse in most developed nations.

Many provided services involve medical care, but many others, including Social Security, do not. As the proportion of older to younger people increases, less financial and social support will be available for older people. This imbalance occurs be-

THE AGING POPULATION

In 1995, there were 21 people 65 or over for every 100 people aged 18 to 64. Between 2030 and 2040, there will be 35 people 65 or over for every 100 people aged 18 to 64.

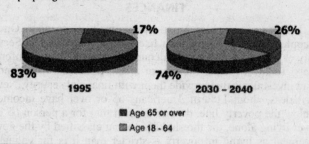

■ Age 65 or over
▨ Age 18 - 64

cause after retirement people pay less in taxes due to decreased earnings, while the proportion of workers available to pay more into the system decreases.

LIVING ARRANGEMENTS

Most people 65 or over continue to live in the community, and even among people 85 or over, more than 78% of women and 88% of men continue to do so. By age 65, one third of women live alone; by age 75, more than half do so. Because women tend to live longer than men, fewer older men live alone. Some older people are able to remain in their homes because of help from relatives or outside services.

In the past, older Americans typically moved in with younger relatives if they became impaired. Nursing homes served few older people, mostly those who had no family to care for them. The situation has changed dramatically. Older people who are no longer able to live alone can now choose among several levels of care, including retirement facilities, assisted living communities, and nursing homes.[1] Currently, about 1.8 million Americans reside in nursing homes. About 15% of nursing home residents are in a nursing home for a relatively short pe-

1. see page 190

iod of time while they recover from an illness or accident. The
emainder will spend the rest of their lives in the nursing home.

DISABILITY AND DISEASE

Older people tend to have more disease and disability than
younger adults. Most of the diseases are chronic, and older people often have many diseases at the same time. Disease and disability can greatly limit independence and increase the need for
support. How well a person functions is determined by the abil-
ty to perform essential self-care activities (usually called activi-
ies of daily living), such as eating, dressing, bathing, transferring
between bed and chair, and using the toilet. How well a person
functions is also determined by the ability to perform additional
mportant activities (usually called instrumental activities of
daily living), such as preparing meals, performing housework,
aking drugs as instructed, going on errands, managing finances,
and using a telephone.

MOST COMMONLY REPORTED CHRONIC CONDITIONS IN PEOPLE 65 AND OVER IN 1996

Condition	%*
Arthritis	50
High blood pressure	36
Heart disease	32
Hearing loss	29
Problems of bones, ligaments, and tendons	17
Cataracts	17
Chronic sinusitis	15
Diabetes	10
Tinnitus (ringing in the ears)	9
Vision loss	8

*Percentages add up to more than 100 because older people often have
more than one condition.

From Adams PF, Hendershot GE, and Marano MA. Current estimates from
the National Health Interview Survey, 1996. National Center for Health Statistics. *Vital Health Statistics* 10(200). 1999.

One of the goals of care is to help keep older people indepen dent and functioning well for as long as possible. In a perfec world, most people would remain fully functional and indepen dent until just before their death, when they would get sick and die without a prolonged period during which they have a poor level of function.

Fortunately, progress is being made toward this goal. Only £ to 8% of people 65 or over who live in their own home need as sistance with one or more self-care activities, and this percent age has decreased slightly over the past decade. Even among people 85 or over, one half of women and two thirds of men are able to live at home without needing assistance with self-care activities.

Chronic conditions that cause disability include those tha also commonly cause death (for example, heart disease, stroke chronic obstructive pulmonary disease, diabetes). Other chronic conditions are unlikely to cause death but affect how well peo ple are able to function (for example, arthritis, osteoporosis vision and hearing loss). Women tend to have more nonfata chronic conditions than men. However, the chronic condition. of men are more likely to be fatal.

CAUSES OF DEATH

In the United States, about 70% of all deaths occur after age 65. In 1999, the greatest percentages of deaths in this age group were due to heart disease, stroke, and cancer. However, because many older people have more than one chronic illness, the tru cause of death is often uncertain, especially for people over 85

Even as enormous strides are made in the treatment of dis ease, one thing remains true: eventually every person must die of something. So, as improvements in health care have helped decrease deaths due to heart disease and stroke, deaths due to cancer have increased. If, in turn, a way to decrease cance deaths is found, some other cause of death will take its place Humans have a maximum life span, and even the best health care cannot overcome this biological imperative.

Although life expectancy in the United States is not the high est in the world (this distinction is held by Japan), American reaching old age live longer than older people in many othe countries. For women who reach age 80, life expectancy is 9.

years, which is higher than life expectancy in Japan, Sweden, France, and England. Life expectancy is higher for older men in the United States as well.

LEADING CAUSES OF DEATH AMONG PEOPLE 65 AND OVER IN 1999

Cause of Death	%*
Heart disease	34
Cancer	22
Stroke and related diseases	8
Chronic obstructive pulmonary disease and related diseases	6
Influenza and pneumonia	3
Diabetes mellitus	3
Alzheimer's disease	2
Kidney failure	2
Blood infections	1
Accidents (excluding motor vehicle accidents)	1
Motor vehicle accidents	Less than 1
All other causes	17
All causes	100

*Percentages have been rounded to the nearest tenth.
From Anderson, RN. Deaths: Leading causes for 1999. National Vital Statistics Reports 49(11). Hyattsville, Maryland: National Center for Health Statistics. 2001.

When the current generation of older people was young, most people died in the privacy of their own home, usually cared for by family. If an illness developed slowly, a doctor probably came to visit often. If an illness developed suddenly, a doctor may not have seen the person until just before or just after death.

Today, most older Americans die in a hospital or nursing home. If an illness worsens at a slow pace, an older person living at home is likely to be admitted to a hospital several days or weeks before death. Those who get ill rapidly are typically sent to an emergency room, where treatment is given briefly before death. Even people residing in nursing homes are sometimes transferred to a hospital when they get sick enough that the medical staff fears they will die. Yet, despite the statistics on what does happen, surveys show that many older people would rather not die in a hospital, preferring, if possible, to die at home surrounded by loved ones.[1] The thought of dying away from home is disturbing to many. It also adds greatly to the cost of medical care. Dying in a hospital is expensive.

Of total Medicare expenditures for a given year, more than 25% are for services provided during a person's last year of life, with much of this amount spent in the last 60 days. Medicare expenditures are 7 times higher for those who are in the last year of their life than for those who are not.

Older Americans now have several mechanisms to help ensure that they die where and in the manner they most prefer. Americans can choose to be hospitalized or not, to have aggressive treatment or not, to undergo resuscitation attempts or not, and to be fed artificially or not. An advance directive document called a living will[2] allows people to make their wishes known regarding medical care and heroic resuscitation attempts. A different document called a durable power of attorney for health care[3] allows people to choose someone to make decisions for them in such matters if they become unable to make those decisions themselves. Completing and updating such documents have become essential parts of aging.

WORLDWIDE AGING

The world's population is aging at a remarkable rate. Much of this is due to a decrease in birth rates and an increase in life expectancy over the last 20 years. In Europe, the percentage of people 60 or over is expected to increase by about one third from 1996 to 2025, depending on the country. In some developing countries, the percentage of people 60 or over is expected to increase 200% in the same time period. By 2025, it is expected that in Italy and Japan nearly one third of the population will be

1. see page 211
2. see page 954
3. see page 955

60 or over. China and India, which are both developing countries, have the largest total populations, so they have and will continue to have the largest number of older people. By 2020, the world's population is expected to include more than 1 billion people 60 or over, and most will be in developing, rather than in developed, countries.

I owe it all to Adolph Hitler and Dr. Sam Levit. The former inspired me that "living well is the best revenge." The latter taught me "better living through chemistry."

During the Second World War, I had been in concentration camps. Afterward—never being sure what perils would arise in the future—I resolved to live every day as hedonistically as possible . . . to live every day as if it were my last one.

Admittedly, for the first few years I overdid it. I ate too much (always the best food available). I drank too much (always the best wine available). I did too many things that they tell me I shouldn't do.

Inevitably this life style took its toll. That's when I went to see Dr. Sam. When I explained what I was doing and my unwillingness to change, he told me that medicines were available to correct all imbalances caused by my excesses. He prescribed a handful of capsules and tablets. To this day, every day, I swallow about 15 pills in the morning and then go about my business.

Check-ups, at 6-month intervals, allow adjustment of these medications. Now my blood pressure is perfect, my cholesterol (good + bad) is perfect, my triglycerides and uric acid levels are where they should be, etc., etc.

Of course Ellen, my young companion, attributes this flawless health to the fact that I eat mostly fresh food (prepared food and junk food simply don't taste good) and that I drink a hefty amount of Bordeaux wine. Of course, some say that genes might have something to do with it. No matter, I intend to continue the same way for at least another quarter century.

Walter Rich

CARING FOR SELF AND OTHERS

The need for good, unbiased health care information runs deep, whether people are seeking to become more active in caring for themselves or others. Prevention, healthy nutrition, appropriate use of drugs, and the wide array of diagnostic tests and complementary and alternative therapies are topics at the forefront of caring for self.

Communicating effectively with health care practitioners goes hand-in-hand with caring for self or others. The variety of practitioners to communicate with is vast: doctors, nurses, therapists, social workers, pharmacists. And communications take place in many sites: doctor's office, hospital, rehabilitation facility, nursing home. Navigating a complex health system that has so many types of practitioners and sites of care can be exceedingly difficult and is often frustrating. Interacting with health care practitioners and ensuring continuity of care can be improved by effective communication, which begins with being well informed.

Critically important for most people, also, are strategies for caregiving. Knowing what kind of care loved ones need and how to provide it is never easy. Finally, palliative and end-of-life care is a delicate issue that nearly everyone faces.

4

Preventive Medical Care

Traditional medical care focuses on improving health by identifying and treating health problems that have already produced symptoms or complications. In contrast, preventive medical care focuses on preventing health problems from occurring. Preventive care also focuses on diagnosing problems before symptoms or complications arise, when the chances of recovery are greatest.

Pessimists might see an effort to prevent health problems in older people as an attempt to "close the barn door after the horse is already out." These pessimists think preventive measures are pointless once a person has reached old age. Although beginning at an early age is best, it is probably never too late to start on the road to prevention.

Choosing and establishing a relationship with a primary care doctor is an important step toward preventive medical care. A primary care doctor can provide much of the preventive medical care a person might need and, when necessary, make referrals and coordinate care with other health care practitioners.[1]

GOALS OF PREVENTION

The general goal of prevention is to reduce a person's likelihood of becoming ill or disabled or of dying prematurely. Some factors that increase risk are beyond a person's control, such as age, sex, and family history. But other factors, such as a person's lifestyle and physical and social environment, can be altered. And, risk can be reduced through good medical care.

1. see page 94

Preventive medical care is not a case of "one size fits all"; specific goals are developed by and for each person.

Specific goals usually depend on a person's overall health. For example, a healthy older person who can function independently may focus on preventing disease. A person with several mild chronic diseases who remains independent may focus more on preventing or slowing decline in function and avoiding frailty. A frail person with several advanced chronic diseases who has become mostly dependent on others may focus on preventing accidents and complications that could lead to complete dependence or death.

Specific goals also depend on a person's risk factors for developing health problems, sometimes referred to as a risk profile. Information in a risk profile includes many considerations, including whether the person is sedentary, smokes cigarettes, drinks alcohol, gets a lot of sun exposure, has balance problems, has friends and relatives who check in on him, drives without a seat belt, and eats well-balanced meals. Working from this profile, health care practitioners can develop goals and help a person make any necessary changes.

Setting specific goals also depends on how much proof there is that making a change will be helpful. Quitting smoking, for example, is undoubtedly beneficial at any age. Screening for prostate cancer, on the other hand, is of questionable benefit and even controversial in older men, because its role in preventing complications and death is less certain. If effectiveness of a preventive health measure is in doubt, a frank discussion with the doctor is important.

Finally, some lifestyle changes prompted by prevention goals are easier to make and more acceptable than others. Many smokers, for example, are resistant to quitting smoking. The same people, however, may not find it burdensome to begin wearing a seat belt while driving. Some people are unwilling to make even the smallest change, such as walking briskly a few minutes a day, even if they know it will help prevent disease. Others are willing to comply with major changes, such as following highly restrictive diets, when they learn that such changes can help prevent life-threatening or disabling diseases.

TOOLS OF PREVENTION

People working to reach their prevention goals have three major tools from which to choose. One tool is establishing a healthy lifestyle, which includes wearing a seat belt, eating a healthy diet, getting some physical exercise, wearing sunscreen, and not smoking. Another tool is getting vaccinated to prevent infectious diseases such as influenza and pneumococcal pneumonia. A third tool is participating in screening efforts so that diseases such as high blood pressure and cancer are detected early.

Healthy Lifestyle

Lifestyle and disease are clearly linked. The three leading causes of death in the United States—heart disease, cancer, and stroke—are more likely to occur in people who make poor lifestyle choices, especially eating a diet high in saturated fats, trans fatty acids, and cholesterol (such a diet increases the risk of having high cholesterol levels in the blood); not exercising regularly; and smoking. By having informative discussions with doctors and other health care practitioners, older people can make good decisions and establish healthy habits.

Some people believe that adopting a healthier lifestyle would take all the fun out of life. Others fear the cost of putting a healthier lifestyle into practice. Establishing a healthy lifestyle, however, need not lead to drudgery and unmanageable costs. Taking responsibility for one's own health can prove to be exciting, rewarding, and affordable.

Healthy eating habits can help older people prevent or control diseases such as high blood pressure, heart disease, diabetes, osteoporosis, and certain cancers. A diet that includes plenty of vegetables, fruits, and whole-grain cereals and breads is recommended, in part because such a diet is high in fiber.[1] Cutting down on harmful types of fat (saturated fats and trans fatty acids) by eating fish, skinless poultry, and very lean meat and by choosing low-fat dairy foods is recommended as well. Limiting salt and increasing the intake of calcium are considered to be part of a healthy diet. Limiting calories to maintain an ideal body weight is also recommended.

1. see also page 41

Physical activity and exercise can play an important role in preventing obesity, high blood pressure, heart disease, stroke, diabetes, some types of cancer, and other health problems, including such vexing problems as constipation. The best routine includes moderate physical activity for 30 minutes or more on all or most days of the week. People who can devote only 10 minutes at a time to physical activity may still reap benefits if they repeat the activity several times throughout the day. Walking is one simple, effective exercise that many older people enjoy. Certain types of exercise can also target specific problems. For example, stretching improves flexibility. Weight lifting helps protect against muscle weakness and osteoporosis by strengthening muscles and increasing bone density. Dancing and tai chi may preserve or even enhance balance, which in turn helps prevent falls.

Quitting smoking is important to a healthy lifestyle. Older people who quit smoking experience many benefits, so it is never too late to quit. A doctor can offer encouragement and advice on ways to avoid situations and circumstances that contribute to a person's tendency to smoke. Further, a doctor can provide information and recommendations on the use of nicotine replacement products, bupropion (a drug that helps reduce cravings), and other tools.

Safe sex practices remain important during later adulthood. Older people who have more than one sex partner can greatly reduce their risk of contracting a sexually transmitted disease by using a latex condom every time they have sex.

Limiting alcohol use is important to a healthy lifestyle as well. Small amounts of alcohol may have some health benefits. However, aging changes the way the body handles and reacts to alcohol. Older people who drink alcohol need to be aware that more than one drink a day may increase their risk of injuries and other health problems.

Injury prevention plays a major role in maintaining a healthy lifestyle. Older people can lower their risk of injury by taking the following precautions:

• Wearing a seat belt regularly, whether as a driver or as a passenger.
• Not driving when taking drugs that cause sedation or at night if night vision is poor.

• Installing smoke and carbon monoxide detectors. Testing and maintaining smoke and carbon monoxide detectors regularly is also important, as is installing fire extinguishers.

• Setting the maximum temperature on a home hot water heater to 130° F or below.

• Cleaning up cluttered areas in the home, removing loose rugs and long phone and electrical cords, maintaining adequate lighting, and adding handrails and traction surfaces (such as strips or mats) to stairways and bathtubs.

Understanding drug therapy is also important. A primary care doctor and pharmacist can provide information on all prescription and nonprescription drugs. Knowing the brand and generic name of all drugs they take; each drug's purpose; the length of time each drug is to be taken; and what activities, foods, drinks, and other drugs are to be avoided while taking each drug can help older people avoid problems. All drugs need to be reviewed with the doctor periodically.

Vaccines

Vaccinations are not just for children; they provide an important defense against certain infectious diseases that affect older people as well.

Influenza (often called flu) is a common viral infection that is potentially dangerous; it can lead to pneumonia and, in many cases, death. Receiving the influenza vaccine is an effective and safe way for people 65 and over to prevent influenza. People who are severely allergic to eggs or egg products, however, cannot receive the influenza vaccine. An influenza vaccine is needed every autumn because of frequent changes in the influenza virus and because protection does not last longer than 1 year.

Pneumococcal pneumonia (a bacterial lung infection) is the most common pneumonia among older people living in their own homes. The pneumococcal pneumonia vaccine is safe, and it may prevent many of the most common types of pneumococcal pneumonia. If pneumococcal pneumonia does occur in someone who has been vaccinated, the infection tends to be less severe. The vaccine also helps prevent pneumococcal infections in other parts of the body, such as the blood. The vaccine is recommended at least one time for everyone 65 and over. Some older people need to be revaccinated a few years later. People who are unsure of whether they ever received the pneumococcal vaccine should be vaccinated.

The tetanus vaccine is safe and effective for preventing tetanus. Tetanus vaccine is often combined with diphtheria vaccine. An older person who has never been vaccinated for tetanus should receive two injections of a combined tetanus and diphtheria vaccine given 1 month apart. For a person who has had an initial series of tetanus and diphtheria vaccine injections, many authorities recommend a tetanus booster or a tetanus and diphtheria booster every 10 years. Others suggest that a single revaccination at age 65 is sufficient.

Screening

Experts agree on the importance of screening for certain health problems that commonly affect older people. These health problems, when detected early, can be cured or, if not curable, treated to help prevent symptoms and complications from developing.

Screening for high blood pressure (hypertension), followed by treatment when needed, helps lower the risk of heart attack, stroke, and kidney failure. Older people should have their blood pressure checked at least once a year. A top reading (systolic blood pressure) less than 140 and a bottom reading (diastolic blood pressure) less than 90 are desirable.

Screening for abnormal cholesterol levels (especially high LDL, the "bad" cholesterol, and low HDL, the "good" cholesterol) and high triglyceride levels is important in young and old people. Screening, followed by treatment when needed, helps to decrease the risk of heart attack, stroke, and peripheral vascular disease. Levels that are often recommended as desirable are LDL less than 130 mg/dL (less than 100 mg/dL for people with certain diseases, such as diabetes or atherosclerosis), HDL greater than 40 mg/dL, and triglycerides less than 150 mg/dL.

Screening for low bone density (specifically osteopenia or osteoporosis, depending on how low the density has become) is recommended for all women 65 and over. Some experts advise repeating the test every 2 to 3 years. Dual-energy x-ray absorptiometry (DEXA) is the most commonly used method for screening, although other tests are available. When low bone

POTENTIALLY USEFUL TESTS FOR DISEASE PREVENTION*

Disorder to Be Detected or Prevented	Test	How Often	Comment
High blood sugar levels (diabetes and its complications)	Measurement of sugar (glucose) levels in the blood	Yearly, beginning in young adulthood	Some experts recommend screening only those people who are at high risk of developing diabetes, especially obese people.
Prostate cancer	Rectal examination	Yearly, beginning at age 40	The effectiveness of rectal examinations and measurement of PSA levels for preventing death due to prostate cancer is unproved.
	Measurement of prostate-specific antigen (PSA) levels in the blood	Yearly	
Skin and mouth (oral) cancer	A full-body examination of the skin by a doctor, as well as an examination of the mouth by a dentist or doctor, is recommended by many experts	Yearly	Skin and (oral) cancers found at an early stage are much more likely to be curable. However, the effectiveness of examination of the skin and the mouth for preventing deaths due to cancer is unproved.

Table continues on the following page.

Disorder to Be Detected or Prevented	Test	How Often	Comment
Dementia, delirium	Testing for mental abilities (such as memory) by asking certain questions	Yearly, beginning at age 50	Testing may become more important if early treatment of dementia is shown to change outcomes.
Low thyroid hormone levels (hypo-thyroidism)	Measurement of thyroid-stimulating hormone levels in the blood	Yearly, beginning at age 65	Some experts recommend screening only women.

*The importance of these tests is controversial.

density is identified through screening, the risk of fractures can be reduced if osteopenia or osteoporosis is treated.

Vision or hearing loss can interfere with a person's ability to perform everyday activities, which can affect quality of life. Annual vision and hearing tests are recommended.

Screening for depression is recommended for adults of all ages. Screening usually involves responding to a set of certain questions. Experts have not agreed on the frequency with which screening should be repeated. Screening followed by treatment can improve quality of life and decrease the risk of suicide.

Breast cancer found at an early stage is more likely to be curable. A screening mammogram every year or every other year is recommended for women over 50.

Because colorectal cancer is more likely to be curable at an early stage, screening is advised beginning at age 50. However, experts disagree on the best way in which to screen for colorectal cancer and on how often screening should be done. Almost all experts recommend checking a person's stool for small amounts of blood every year. Additionally, most experts recommend that the person undergo a sigmoidoscopy (an examination of the last part of the large intestine with the use of a short flexible viewing tube) every 5 years or a colonoscopy (an examination of the entire large intestine with the use of a longer flexible viewing tube) every 10 years.

Screening for cervical cancer involves the Papanicolaou (Pap) test. Women who have never had a Pap test before reaching age 65 are advised to have two Pap tests 1 year apart. Some experts believe that if both tests are interpreted as normal, further testing is unnecessary. Doctors often recommend discontinuing Pap testing in women who have had normal Pap test results during the 10 years before turning 65.

5

Maintaining Good Nutrition

Good nutrition is necessary for keeping the body functioning normally, maintaining a healthy weight, and preventing disease. If disease develops, good nutrition helps minimize the effects. People never outlive the need for good nutrition.

Good nutrition involves consuming a variety of foods in appropriate amounts. No one food provides all the substances the body needs (nutrients) for good health: protein, carbohydrates, fats, vitamins, minerals, fiber, and many others. Consuming enough water is also important.[1] Water is necessary for all of the body's functions, including moving nutrients into cells and removing waste products from cells.

For older people, following standard nutritional recommendations, such as those of the standard daily food pyramid and recommended dietary allowances (RDAs), may not always be wise. Older people who try to follow these recommendations may gradually gain weight or develop a nutritional deficiency.[2] Research has not determined the best diet for older people. Changes in diet, based on the way the body changes as it ages, may be beneficial. A different daily food pyramid has been developed with these changes in mind.

1. see page 249
2. see page 231

A DAILY FOOD PYRAMID FOR OLDER PEOPLE

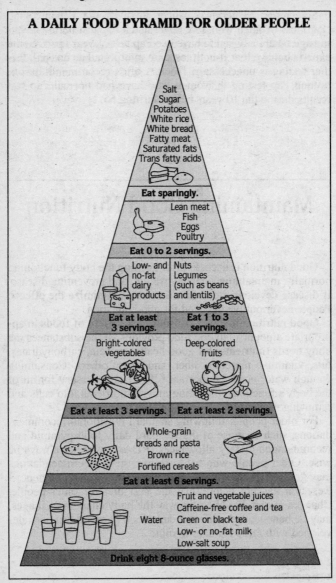

Salt
Sugar
Potatoes
White rice
White bread
Fatty meat
Saturated fats
Trans fatty acids

Eat sparingly.

Lean meat
Fish
Eggs
Poultry

Eat 0 to 2 servings.

Low- and no-fat dairy products	Nuts Legumes (such as beans and lentils)
Eat at least 3 servings.	**Eat 1 to 3 servings.**
Bright-colored vegetables	Deep-colored fruits
Eat at least 3 servings.	**Eat at least 2 servings.**

Whole-grain breads and pasta
Brown rice
Fortified cereals

Eat at least 6 servings.

Water

Fruit and vegetable juices
Caffeine-free coffee and tea
Green or black tea
Low- or no-fat milk
Low-salt soup

Drink eight 8-ounce glasses.

How Aging Affects Nutritional Needs

Calories: Older people tend to be less active and to use less energy. As people age, body fat tends to increase, and muscle tissue tends to decrease. Muscle tissue burns more calories than fat. So the aging body burns fewer calories, and weight may be gained. Therefore, older people may need to consume fewer calories to avoid gaining too much weight. However, if older people remain physically active, they may need as many calories as they did when younger. Calories are the measure of how much energy foods contain. All of the calories needed by the body come from carbohydrates (sugars and starches), fats, and proteins. Fats have about twice as many calories per gram as carbohydrates and proteins.

When people need to consume fewer calories, getting all the nutrients they need—particularly vitamins and minerals—is more difficult. They should choose foods that are rich in nutrients but not high in calories. Whole-grain cereals and whole-grain breads that are fortified with vitamins, such as folic acid (folate), are good choices. Fruits and vegetables that are deeply colored (such as strawberries, peaches, broccoli, spinach, and squash) tend to contain more nutrients than those that are less deeply colored.

Some foods that are high in sugar or fat (and thus high in calories) do not contain many vitamins and minerals. These foods are sometimes called empty-calorie foods. Examples are candy bars, doughnuts, cookies, and certain fried foods. Some fried foods contain many nutrients. But frying adds calories, and the nutrient it adds the most of is saturated fat. People should limit the amount of empty-calorie and fried foods they eat. Alcoholic beverages also contain many calories and few nutrients.

Carbohydrates: Older people should follow the standard nutritional recommendations for carbohydrates. Some foods contain complex carbohydrates. Examples are whole-grain cereals, breads, and pasta as well as peas, beans, brown rice, and many vegetables. Other foods contain simple or refined carbohydrates. Examples are ice cream, candy, syrups, jellies, and sodas. White rice, white bread, and other foods made with white flour also contain simple or refined carbohydrates. Foods containing complex carbohydrates are better choices because they are digested more slowly and are less likely to be converted to fat. These foods also tend to contain more fiber, vitamins, and minerals. A diet high in simple or refined carbohydrates increases the risk of obesity and diabetes.

Fats: The most important consideration is what type of fat is consumed. People of all ages should consume less saturated fat and less partially hydrogenated fat (trans fatty acids).[1] These fats should provide no more than 10% of daily calories. Saturated fats are found in meat, butter, and whole-milk dairy products. Trans fatty acids are found in margarine, shortening, and many processed foods, such as cookies, crackers, doughnuts, and chips.

When possible, monounsaturated fats and polyunsaturated fats, particularly omega-3 fats, should be substituted for saturated fats and trans fatty acids. These fats may help protect the heart. Monounsaturated fats are found in avocado, olive, and peanut oils and in peanut butter. Polyunsaturated fats are found in canola, soybean, and many other liquid vegetable oils. Omega-3 fats are found in flaxseed and in certain fish, such as mackerel, salmon, and albacore tuna.

Some experts also recommend limiting the amount of total fat to no more than 30% of daily calories. When reducing the amount of fat in the diet, people must be careful about what foods they eat instead. Replacing fatty foods with foods that contain simple or refined carbohydrates can also cause weight gain.

Protein: As people age, they tend to lose muscle, because the level and activity of some hormones decrease and because they exercise less. Muscle may also be lost if older people do not consume enough protein.

Lean meat is a good source of protein. But for some older people, certain types of meat are hard to chew. Meat may also be expensive. Protein sources that are easier to chew and may be less expensive include fish, poultry, dairy products, and eggs. Peanut butter, beans, soy products, and nuts are also good sources of protein. These foods can provide enough protein for people who choose not to eat animal products.

Fiber: As people age, food moves more slowly through the digestive tract. Part of the reason is that older people become less physically active and drink less fluids. Eating enough fiber

1. see table on page 628

can help counter this slowing. Fiber, sometimes called roughage, provides bulk to stool. The increased bulk helps food move through the digestive tract. Fiber also helps prevent constipation and diverticular disease.

Fiber has other benefits. Some types of fiber slow the body's absorption of sugar and cholesterol after a meal. Fiber-rich foods are low in calories and tend to produce a feeling of fullness. So they can help people eat fewer calories. Good sources of fiber are high-fiber breakfast cereals (such as bran cereals), whole-grain breads and pastas, brown rice, and whole fruits and vegetables (with skins, if possible). Prunes, apples, and pears are good sources of fiber. Meat and dairy foods do not contain fiber.

About 20 to 30 grams of fiber should be consumed daily. An average serving of fruit, vegetable, or cereal contains 2 to 4 grams of fiber. Consequently, older people should eat 8 to 12 servings of these foods daily. Fiber supplements, such as psyllium, are also available. But getting fiber from foods is preferable.

Vitamins and minerals: As people age, some vitamins and minerals become more important. Consuming enough calcium (which is used to build bones) and vitamin D (which helps the body absorb calcium) is important. Fortified milk is a good source of both calcium and vitamin D. Other sources of calcium include other dairy products and juices fortified with calcium. Dark green vegetables such as turnip greens and collard greens contain calcium, but calcium in vegetables may be harder for the body to use. Older people often need to take supplements of calcium and vitamin D, because getting enough from the diet is difficult.

Older people absorb and store some vitamins and minerals differently. For example, many people cannot absorb vitamin B_{12} from food well. So people who consume the recommended daily amount of vitamin B_{12} in foods may not get enough of it into the body. Taking vitamin B_{12} supplements may be necessary.

Getting enough vitamins and minerals from foods is usually preferable to getting them from supplements. Foods, unlike supplements, contain other substances necessary for good health. However, always eating a healthy, well-balanced diet is difficult. So taking a multivitamin that contains the recommended daily allowances for vitamins and minerals, in addition to trying to eat a healthy diet, is a good idea.

Water: Older people are more likely to become dehydrated for many reasons.[1] Consequently, older people need to make a conscious effort to drink enough fluids rather than wait until they feel thirsty. Water, fruit or vegetable juices, and caffeine-free coffee and tea are good choices. Alcoholic beverages and caffeinated coffee, tea, and sodas may make people urinate more, so they are less advisable.

How Disorders and Drugs Change Nutritional Needs

Disorders or drugs may change the body's nutritional needs or change the body's ability to meet those needs.[2] They can decrease appetite or interfere with the absorption of nutrients.

Diuretics (used to treat high blood pressure) cause the body to excrete more water, increasing the risk of dehydration. So a person taking a diuretic, particularly during hot weather, may need to drink more fluids.

People with certain disorders sometimes need to follow a special diet. For example, a low-fat diet may be recommended for people who have had a heart attack or stroke. A low-salt diet may be recommended for people who have high blood pressure or heart failure. A low-protein diet may be recommended for people who have a kidney disorder. However, older people who follow such diets may be forced to give up foods they enjoy and to eat less of foods that contain nutrients they need. As a result, they may lose weight or develop a nutritional deficiency. They may need to take supplements. For some people (particularly very frail older people), limiting fat, salt, or protein may not be appropriate.

Screening for Adequate Nutrition

Many health care practitioners routinely check older people to determine whether their nutrition is adequate.[3] Often, a careful description of what a person eats helps most. So practitioners may ask what the person typically eats in a day and how active the person is. Questions related to shopping for, prepar-

1. see page 249
2. see page 232
3. see also page 236

ing, and eating foods are also important. Problems with these tasks can result in nutritional deficiencies. Practitioners may ask about the person's mood. Feeling depressed, anxious, or stressed can affect what a person eats. A blood or urine sample may be taken, so that levels of nutrients may be measured.

Weight and height are measured. From these measurements, the body mass index (BMI) can be calculated. BMI is a single number that adjusts weight for height. It indicates whether a person is underweight, normal weight, overweight, or obese.

Estimating how much fat and muscle a person has (body composition) can help determine whether nutrition is adequate. In a test called bioelectric impedance analysis, the resistance of body tissues to the flow of a very low-voltage electrical current is measured. (The voltage is so low that it cannot be felt.) Body fat and bone resist the flow much more than does muscle tissue. By measuring the resistance to the current, health care practitioners can estimate the percentage of body fat. This test takes only about 1 minute. A simple but less accurate way to estimate body composition involves two measurements. A health care practitioner measures around a person's arm, leg, or waist. Then the thickness of fat under the skin, usually at the back of the upper arm, is measured with a caliper. But the most accurate way to estimate body composition is immersion in a water-filled tank, an expensive and cumbersome method rarely used for older people.

BODY MASS INDEX: ADJUSTING WEIGHT FOR HEIGHT

By itself, weight is not a measure of whether a person is healthy. Height must also be considered. For example, 200 pounds is a healthier weight for a person who is 6 feet tall than for a person who is only 5 feet tall. To adjust a person's weight for height, a health care practitioner uses the body mass index (BMI). BMI is calculated by dividing weight (in kilograms) by height (in meters squared).

Underweight:	Less than 19
Normal weight:	19 to 25
Overweight:	More than 25 but less than 30
Obese:	
Moderate	30 to 40
Severe	More than 40

Weight (pounds)

Height	100	110	120	130	140	150	160	170	180	190	200	210	220	230	240	250	260
4'10"	21	23	25	27	29	31	33	36	38	40	42	44	46	48	50	52	54
4'11"	20	22	24	26	28	30	32	34	36	38	40	42	45	47	49	51	53
5'0"	20	21	23	25	27	29	31	33	35	37	39	41	43	45	47	49	51
5'1"	19	21	23	25	26	28	30	32	34	36	38	40	42	43	45	47	49
5'2"	18	20	22	24	26	27	29	31	33	35	37	38	40	43	44	46	48
5'3"	18	19	21	23	25	27	28	30	32	34	35	37	39	41	43	44	46
5'4"	17	19	21	22	24	26	27	29	31	33	34	36	38	39	41	43	45
5'5"	17	18	20	22	23	25	27	28	30	32	33	35	37	38	40	42	43
5'6"	16	18	19	21	23	24	26	27	29	31	32	34	36	37	39	40	42
5'7"	16	17	19	20	22	23	25	27	28	30	31	33	31	36	38	39	41
5'8"	15	17	18	20	21	23	24	26	27	29	30	32	33	35	36	38	40
5'9"	15	16	18	19	21	22	24	25	27	28	30	31	32	34	35	37	38
5'10"	14	16	17	19	20	22	23	24	26	27	29	30	32	33	34	36	37
5'11"	14	15	17	18	20	21	22	24	25	26	28	29	31	32	33	35	36
6'0"	13	15	16	18	19	20	22	23	24	26	27	28	30	31	33	34	35
6'1"	13	15	16	17	18	20	21	22	24	25	26	28	29	30	32	33	34
6'2"	12	14	15	17	18	19	21	22	23	24	26	27	28	30	31	32	33
6'3"	12	14	15	16	17	19	20	21	22	24	25	26	27	29	30	31	33
6'4"	12	13	15	16	17	18	19	21	22	23	24	26	27	28	29	30	32
6'5"	12	13	14	15	17	18	19	20	21	23	24	25	26	27	29	30	31
6'6"	12	13	14	15	16	17	19	20	21	22	23	24	25	27	28	29	30

Reading Food Labels

To eat a healthy diet, people need to know what they are eating. Reading food labels can help people make good choices. Food labels define a serving and state how many servings are in a container.

Labels are required to provide the number of calories and the amounts of certain nutrients in each serving.

Labels list the amounts for fat, cholesterol, salt (sodium), and

HOW MUCH IS A SERVING?

Food Group	Serving Size
Breads, fortified cereals, rice, and pasta	1/2 bagel or English muffin 1 dinner roll, slice of bread, or small muffin 2 or 3 graham crackers 1/2 cup cooked cereal 1 ounce of cold cereal 1/2 cup cooked rice or noodles
Vegetables	2 spears broccoli 1 cup leafy greens 1/2 cup green beans, carrots, or corn 3/4 cup vegetable juice
Fruits	1 orange or banana 5 prunes 1/2 cup strawberries, fruit cocktail, or applesauce 3/4 cup fruit juice
Milk, yogurt, and cheese	1 cup milk, yogurt, pudding, or milkshake 1/2 cup ice cream 1 1/2 ounces Swiss cheese 2 ounces American cheese 1/2 cup cottage cheese
Meats, poultry, fish, eggs, dry beans, and nuts	2 ounces of cooked lean meat (the size a deck of cards) 2 ounces of meatloaf 1 chicken leg or thigh 2 fish sticks 3 ounces of tuna 1 egg 1/2 cup baked beans 1/3 cup nuts 2 tablespoons peanut butter
Fiber	1 banana 1 apple or pear with the skin or medium sweet potato 1 cup broccoli 1/3 cup bran cereal 3/4 cup bran flake cereal

carbohydrates (including fiber and sugars) by weight (in grams or milligrams) and as a percentage. The amount for protein is given only by weight. The percentage indicates what proportion of the total recommended daily amount of a nutrient is provided in a serving. The percentages are based on a diet of 2,000 calories a day. So they vary somewhat depending on how many calories are consumed each day.

Food labels list the amount of total and saturated fat and the number of calories supplied by fat in the food. Listing the amounts of cholesterol and salt (sodium) helps people, especially those with certain disorders, control how much salt and cholesterol they consume.

Food labels must list vitamins A and C and the minerals calcium and iron. Other vitamins and minerals are often listed.

The ingredients of a food are listed in order of weight. The ingredient with the greatest weight is listed first. Whether the food contains trans fatty acids can usually be checked by reading this list. They are usually described as hydrogenated oils or partially hydrogenated oils.

6

Drugs and Aging

When people get older, they tend to use more drugs. On average, an older person takes four or five prescription drugs plus two nonprescription (over-the-counter) drugs each day.

Most drugs used by older people are taken for years. Such drugs are usually used to control chronic disorders, such as high blood pressure, diabetes, and arthritis. Or these drugs may be used to prevent or relieve symptoms caused by such disorders. Other drugs may be taken for a short time to treat such problems as infections, pain after surgery, and constipation.

Benefits and Risks

Drugs are an important part of medical care for older people. They can prevent, control, or cure disease. They can also control many of the symptoms caused by disease. Without drugs, many older people would die or function less well.

Many of the improvements in the health and function of older people during the past several decades can be attributed to drugs. Vaccines prevent many infectious diseases (such as influenza and pneumonia) that once killed many older people. Antibiotics are effective in treating pneumonia—once known as the killer of older people—and many other serious infections. Drugs to control high blood pressure help prevent strokes and heart attacks. Drugs to control blood sugar levels enable millions of people with diabetes to lead normal lives. Drugs to control pain and other symptoms enable millions of people with arthritis to continue to function.

On the other hand, drugs can have effects that are not intended or desired (side effects). Some side effects are merely bothersome. But others are harmful. Starting in late middle age, the risk of having side effects from drugs increases. Older people are more than twice as likely to have side effects from drugs as younger people are. Furthermore, in older people, side effects are more likely to be severe, to worsen the quality of life, and to require visits to the doctor or hospital stays.

Certain drugs and types of drugs are particularly likely to cause problems in older people. Such a drug can often be replaced with a safer drug that is just as effective. For example, the effects of some drugs used to treat insomnia or anxiety, such as chlordiazepoxide, diazepam, and flurazepam, last too long. As a result, these drugs may make older people become unsteady or confused. The effects of other drugs used to treat insomnia or anxiety, such as lorazepam, oxazepam, and temazepam, usually do not last as long. Thus, these drugs are less likely to make older people unsteady or confused. Knowing which drugs are particularly likely to cause problems in older people helps avoid side effects. Older people who are taking these drugs can ask their doctor about changing to a different drug.

Reasons for Increased Risk

Drugs are more likely to cause problems in older people for three main reasons. The aging body processes drugs differently, certain drugs affect the aging body differently, and older people take more drugs and have more disorders.

How the aging body processes drugs: Changes due to aging itself affect how the body processes drugs. For example, the amount of water in the body decreases and the percentage of body fat increases. These changes are important because some drugs dissolve in water and others dissolve in fat. Drugs that dissolve in fat tend to accumulate in the body because there is relatively more fat to store them.

Changes in the kidneys and liver also affect how the aging body processes drugs. The liver chemically alters (metabolizes) many drugs. It activates some drugs, inactivates others, and prepares many drugs to be eliminated from the body. Most drugs are eliminated from the body by the kidneys in urine. As people age, the liver is less able to alter certain drugs, and the kidneys are less able to eliminate drugs.

SOME DRUGS PARTICULARLY LIKELY TO CAUSE PROBLEMS IN OLDER PEOPLE

Drug	Use	Problem
Amitriptyline	To treat depression	Amitriptyline has strong anticholinergic effects*. It also causes excessive drowsiness.
Antihistamines that have anticholinergic effects (such as chlorpheniramine, cyproheptadine, diphenhydramine, hydroxyzine, promethazine, and tripelennamine)	To relieve allergy symptoms, to aid sleep, or to relieve cold symptoms	All nonprescription and prescription antihistamines have strong anticholinergic effects*.
Antipsychotic drugs (such as chlorpromazine, haloperidol, thioridazine, and thiothixene)	To treat loss of contact with reality (psychosis), or with some controversy, to treat behavioral disturbances in	Antipsychotic drugs can cause drowsiness, movement disorders (that resemble Parkinson's disease), and uncontrollable facial twitches. These

Drug	Use	Problem
	people with dementia	drugs also have anticholinergic effects*. Antipsychotic drugs should be used only when a psychotic disorder is present.
Antispasmodic drugs (drugs that reduce or stop muscle spasms in the digestive tract, such as belladonna alkaloids, clidinium, dicyclomine, hyoscyamine, and propantheline)	To relieve abdominal cramps and pain	These drugs have strong anticholinergic effects*. Their usefulness—especially at the low doses tolerated by older people—is questionable.
Barbiturates (such as phenobarbital and secobarbital)	To calm, to relieve anxiety, or to aid sleep	Barbiturates have more side effects than other drugs used to treat anxiety and insomnia. They also interact with many other drugs. Generally, older people should take barbiturates only as treatment for a seizure disorder.
Benzodiazepines that have long-lasting effects (chlordiazepoxide, diazepam, and flurazepam)	To calm, to relieve anxiety, or to aid sleep	The effects of these drugs last a very long time (often more than several days) in older people. These drugs can cause prolonged drowsiness and loss of balance when a person is walking. Thus, the risk of falls and fractures is increased.
Chlorpropamide	To treat diabetes	This drug's effects last a long time. In older

Table continues on the following page.

Drug	Use	Problem
		people, chlor-propamide can lower blood sugar levels (causing hypoglycemia) for several hours. This drug can also lower the sodium level in the blood (causing hyponatremia). A low sodium level can lead to changes in personality, confusion, and sluggishness (lethargy).
Cimetidine	To treat heartburn, indigestion, or ulcers	Typical doses of cimetidine, a histamine-2 (H_2) blocker, may produce side effects, especially confusion.
Digoxin	To treat heart failure or abnormal heart rhythms (arrhythmias)	As people age, the kidneys are less able to excrete digoxin. Large doses of the drug can more easily reach harmful (toxic) levels. Side effects may include loss of appetite, nausea, and confusion.
Disopyramide	To treat abnormal heart rhythms	Disopyramide has strong anticholinergic effects*. It may cause heart failure in older people.
Doxepin	To treat depression	Doxepin has strong anticholinergic effects*. It also causes excessive drowsiness.
Famotidine	To treat heartburn, indigestion, or ulcers	To some extent, high doses of famotidine, an H_2 blocker, may

Drug	Use	Problem
		produce side effects, especially confusion.
Indomethacin	To relieve pain	Of all nonsteroidal anti-inflammatory drugs (NSAIDs), indomethacin affects the brain the most. It can cause confusion or dizziness.
Iron supplements	To provide supplemental iron	Doses higher than 325 milligrams daily do not greatly improve the absorption of iron and are much more likely to cause constipation.
Meperidine	To relieve pain	Meperidine, an opioid, often causes confusion. Like all opioids, it may cause constipation, retention of urine, drowsiness, and confusion. When taken by mouth, meperidine is not very effective.
Meprobamate	To calm, to relieve anxiety, or to aid sleep	This drug is very likely to make people become dependent on it. It also causes excessive drowsiness.
Methyldopa	To lower high blood pressure	Methyldopa may slow the heart rate and worsen depression.
Muscle relaxants (such as carisoprodol, chlorzoxazone, cyclobenzaprine,	To relieve muscle spasms	Most muscle relaxants have anticholinergic effects*. They also cause drowsiness and weakness. The

Table continues on the following page.

Drug	Use	Problem
metaxalone, and methocarbamol)		usefulness of all muscle relaxants at the low doses tolerated by older people is questionable.
Nizatidine	To treat heartburn, indigestion, or ulcers	To some extent, high doses of nizatidine, an H_2 blocker, may produce side effects, especially confusion.
Pentazocine	To relieve pain	Pentazocine, an opioid, is more likely to cause confusion and hallucinations than other opioids. Like all opioids, it may cause constipation, retention of urine, drowsiness, and confusion.
Propoxyphene	To relieve pain	Propoxyphene, an opioid, provides no more pain relief than acetaminophen. Like all opioids, it may cause constipation, retention of urine, drowsiness, and confusion.
Ranitidine	To treat heartburn, indigestion, or ulcers	To some extent, high doses of ranitidine, an H_2 blocker, may produce side effects, especially confusion.
Reserpine	To lower high blood pressure	Reserpine can cause dizziness when a person stands up, depression, drowsiness, and erectile dysfunction (impotence).

Drug	Use	Problem
Trimethobenzamide	To relieve nausea	This drug can cause abnormal movements of the arms, legs, and other parts of the body. It is one of the least effective drugs for relieving nausea.

*Anticholinergic effects include confusion, blurred vision, constipation, dry mouth, light-headedness, difficulty starting and continuing to urinate, and loss of bladder control.

All of these changes tend to make certain drugs (but not all) stay in an older person's body much longer than they would in a younger person's body. As a result, the drug's effects continue for a longer time and may be stronger. The risk of side effects may also increase. For these reasons, older people often need to take smaller doses of certain drugs or sometimes fewer doses a day.

How drugs affect the aging body: As people age, the body changes in ways that affect how the body responds to drugs. As a result, older people are more sensitive to many drugs and less sensitive to a few. A drug's intended effect may be stronger. For example, sleep aids may make older people sleepier and more likely to become confused than they would younger people. Some drugs that lower blood pressure tend to lower the pressure much more dramatically in older people than in younger people. Increased sensitivity to a drug's effects also means that side effects are more likely to occur and that they may be more severe.

Older people are particularly sensitive to a group of drugs that have anticholinergic effects. Anticholinergic effects include confusion, blurred vision, constipation, dry mouth, light-headedness, difficulty starting and continuing to urinate, and loss of bladder control (urinary incontinence). Sometimes anticholinergic effects are desirable. For example, one anticholinergic effect is to make the bladder less active. Drugs with this effect can be used to treat certain types of incontinence. When anticholinergic effects are undesirable, another drug can sometimes be used instead. If another drug cannot be used, health care practitioners monitor the person for undesirable effects.

WHAT ARE ANTICHOLINERGIC EFFECTS?

Anticholinergic effects are caused by drugs that block the action of acetylcholine. Acetylcholine is a neurotransmitter—a chemical messenger that helps nerve cells communicate.

Acetylcholine helps with memory, learning, and concentration. It also helps control the functioning of the heart, blood vessels, airways, and organs of the urinary and digestive tracts. So drugs with anticholinergic effects can disrupt the normal functioning of these organs. Anticholinergic effects include confusion, blurred vision, constipation, dry mouth, light-headedness, difficulty starting and continuing to urinate, and loss of bladder control. Most of these effects are undesirable.

Older people are more likely to experience anticholinergic effects, because as people age, the body produces less acetylcholine. Also, cells in many parts of the body (such as the digestive tract) have fewer sites where acetylcholine can attach to them. Thus, the acetylcholine produced is less likely to have an effect, and the effect of anticholinergic drugs is greater.

Drugs with anticholinergic effects include many commonly used drugs: some antidepressants (used to treat depression), some antipsychotic drugs (used to treat loss of contact with reality, or psychosis), and many antihistamines (contained in nonprescription sleep aids, cold remedies, and allergy drugs).

More drugs, more disorders: The more drugs taken, the more likely drug interactions are to occur. Drug interactions are problems that occur because one drug affects another drug or a disorder other than the one being treated. When two or more drugs, including nonprescription drugs, are taken about the same time, one drug can interfere with how the other drug works, leading to side effects. Taking dietary supplements (such as vitamins, minerals, or medicinal herbs[1]) or consuming food about the same time a drug is taken can cause similar problems.

Also when many drugs are taken, the schedule for taking them can be hard to follow. If the schedule is not followed, side effects are more likely to occur or the drugs may be less effective.

When two or more disorders are present, a drug taken to treat one disorder may worsen another disorder. For example, a nonprescription sleep aid that contains diphenhydramine can make urinating more difficult for men who have a prostate disorder.

1. see table on pages 66 to 72

This drug can also worsen vision in people who have glaucoma and worsen confusion in people who have dementia.

Maximizing Benefits, Reducing Risks

Older people and the people who care for them can do many things to maximize the benefits and reduce the risks that may result from taking drugs.

Information about the drugs and disorders being treated is vital:

• Learn why each drug is taken and what its effects are supposed to be.
• Learn what side effects each drug may have.
• Learn how to take each drug, including what time of day it should be taken, whether it can be taken at the same time as other drugs, and when to stop taking the drug.
• Learn what to do if a dose is missed.
• Write down information about how to take the drug or ask the doctor, nurse, or pharmacist to write it down (because such information can easily be forgotten).
• Keep a list of all drugs being taken.
• Keep a list of all disorders present.

To work, drugs must be used properly:

• Take drugs as instructed.
• Use memory aids if needed to take drugs as instructed.
• Before stopping a drug, consult the doctor about any problems caused by taking the drug—for example, if side effects occur, if the drug does not seem to work, or if purchasing the drug is burdensome.
• Discard any unused drug from a previous prescription, unless instructed not to do so by a doctor, nurse, or pharmacist.
• Do not take another person's drug, even if that person's problem seems similar.
• Check the expiration date on drugs.

Working closely with a doctor and pharmacist can help:

• Get all prescriptions from the same pharmacy, preferably one that provides comprehensive services (including checking for possible drug interactions) and that maintains a complete drug profile for each person.

• Periodically discuss the list of drugs being taken and the list of disorders with the doctor, nurse, or pharmacist.

• Review the list of drugs with the doctor, nurse, or pharmacist every time any drug is changed (doctors and pharmacists can check for interactions between drugs).

• Make sure the doctor and pharmacist know about all nonprescription drugs and supplements being taken, including vitamins, minerals, and medicinal herbs.

• Consult the doctor before taking any new drugs, including nonprescription drugs and supplements, such as medicinal herbs.

• Report to the doctor or pharmacist any symptoms that might be related to the use of a drug.

• If the schedule of taking drugs is too complex to follow, ask the doctor about simplifying it.

• If seeing more than one doctor, make sure each doctor knows all the drugs being taken.

Drugs should be labeled and packaged in a way that makes them easy to use:

• Ask the pharmacist to print the labels in large print and check to make sure they can be read.

• Ask the pharmacist to package the drugs in containers that are easy to hold and to open.

Any questions about or problems with a drug should be discussed with the doctor or pharmacist. Taking drugs as instructed is essential for avoiding problems and promoting good health.

Remembering to Take Drugs

To benefit from taking drugs, people must remember not only to take the drugs but also to take them at the right time and in the right way. When many drugs are taken, the schedule for taking them can be complex. For example, drugs may have to be taken at different times throughout the day to avoid interactions. Some drugs may have to be taken with food. Other drugs have to be taken when no food is in the stomach. The more complex the schedule, the more likely a person is to make mistakes following it.

If an older person has memory problems, following a complex schedule is even harder. Such a person usually needs help, often from family members. The doctor can be asked about simplifying the schedule. Often, doses can be rescheduled to make taking the drugs more convenient or reduce the total number of daily doses.

Memory aids can help older people remember to take their drugs. For example, using a drug can be associated with a specific daily task, such as a meal.

A pharmacist can provide containers that help people take drugs as instructed. Daily doses for 1 or 2 weeks may be packaged in a plastic pack marked with the days, so that people can keep track of doses taken by noting the empty spaces. More elaborate containers with a computerized reminder system are available. These containers beep or flash at dosing time. Another alternative is a paging service with a beeper. This service is available from subscriber-based telecommunications companies.

Nonprescription Drugs

Nonprescription drugs have many beneficial effects in older people and are commonly used. However, the fact that these drugs are nonprescription is no guarantee that they are safe. Some nonprescription (over-the-counter) drugs can cause problems in older people. The package insert of nonprescription drugs typically includes a warning for older people. However, the warnings often do not make a strong enough impression, and the print may be small, making them hard to read. Also, nonprescription drugs, like prescription drugs, may have undesirable side effects as well as benefits.

Antihistamines that have anticholinergic effects (such as diphenhydramine and chlorpheniramine) can cause problems. For example, these antihistamines may worsen some disorders common among older people, such as closed-angle glaucoma and an enlarged prostate gland. They may cause light-headedness or unsteadiness, leading to falls and broken bones. They may also cause dry mouth, blurred vision, constipation, and confusion. Antihistamines are contained in many nighttime pain relief formulas, cough and cold remedies, allergy drugs, and sleep aids. When an antihistamine is needed, one without anticholinergic effects (such as loratadine) is preferable.

Older people who take aspirin or other nonsteroidal antiinflammatory drugs (NSAIDs) may develop ulcers and bleeding ulcers. Older people may be more susceptible to side effects of antacids. Antacids that contain aluminum are more likely to cause constipation. Antacids that contain magnesium are more likely to cause diarrhea.

7

Complementary or Alternative Medicine

Alternative medicine is so named because it may be used instead of conventional medicine. It may also be used with conventional medicine and thus is sometimes called complementary medicine. Much of complementary and alternative medicine is rooted in ancient cultures, such as Chinese, Indian, Tibetan, African, and Native American cultures.

Alternative medicine differs from conventional Western medicine in its basic approach. Conventional Western medicine generally defines "health" as the absence of disease. The focus is on treating disease and its symptoms. As a result, only one part of the person (the affected part) is treated. In contrast, many alternative therapies define "health" as balance within the body. Imbalance is thought to cause disease. The focus is on treating the whole person (physically, emotionally, mentally, and spiritually), so that balance can be restored. When balance is restored, the body can heal itself.

In alternative medicine, health is also thought to be influenced by a person's experiences, environment, diet, and rela-

WHAT MAKES MEDICINE "ALTERNATIVE"?

What makes medicine alternative is hard to nail down. For many people, alternative medicine means therapies that are not a part of conventional Western medicine. That is, alternative medicine is not usually taught in medical schools or prescribed by Western doctors. But there is a problem with this understanding: What is accepted as part of conventional Western medicine is changing all the time. More alternative therapies are being studied. If they are shown to be safe and effective, they will be accepted into the mainstream of conventional Western medicine. For example, in

the past, most doctors considered chiropractic to be quackery. But now, many doctors refer their patients to chiropractors, and some insurance plans cover the costs.

In the United States, there are some therapies almost everyone considers alternative. Examples are certain dietary supplements (such as medicinal herbs and vitamins in large doses), acupuncture, and magnet therapy. Other therapies, although not quite conventional, are not usually considered alternative. They include massage, relaxation techniques, exercise, changes in diet, prayer, and spiritual healing.

tionships with other people. This type of approach is called holistic. Consequently, many alternative medicine practitioners find out as much as they can about a person before they make a diagnosis or propose a treatment for a health problem.

The Appeal

Alternative medicine is becoming more popular, especially with older people. Between 2 and 4 out of 10 older people use alternative therapies. Popular therapies include dietary supplements, chiropractic, acupuncture, and homeopathy. Most commonly, older people use alternative therapies to prevent or treat back problems, to treat arthritis, or to relieve pain (especially chronic pain). Another common use is to improve general health. Sometimes older people use alternative therapies to treat specific problems, such as coronary artery disease, memory loss, problems with vision, osteoporosis, wrinkles, prostate enlargement, depression, or anxiety.

Why do so many older people use alternative therapies? Many older people turn to alternative therapies when conventional therapies cannot cure or even relieve a chronic disorder, such as arthritis, cancer, or low back pain. Some older people think conventional therapy has too many side effects or is too expensive. Some use an alternative therapy because they do not have to go to a doctor or hospital to get it. Thus, they may feel they have more control over their health. Also, some people prefer the longer appointment times and extra attention given by some alternative medicine practitioners.

Some older people may like the emphasis on the whole person and on health rather than disease. Or they may believe that alternative therapies are more natural, safer, or healthier than conventional therapies. Some people come from cultural and religious traditions that discourage the use of conventional therapies. Other people use an alternative therapy because friends and caregivers who have tried it recommend it. Still others use an alternative therapy because they hear about it on television or the radio or read about it in advertisements.

The Problems

In spite of the increasing acceptance and use of alternative therapies, there are reasons for caution. Most important, there is little information about effectiveness and safety. Unlike drugs, most alternative therapies are just beginning to be studied scientifically. Even less is known about their use in older people.

For a few alternative therapies, evidence supports their effectiveness. For other therapies, evidence suggests that they are not effective. However, for most alternative therapies that have been studied, the evidence is inconclusive. That is, the evidence is conflicting, or the studies were not designed well enough to provide the needed information.

The safety of alternative therapies is also a concern. An alternative therapy, especially when used for a long time, may have side effects. An alternative therapy used for one disorder may worsen another disorder. Because older people tend to have more than one disorder, the risk of such problems is even higher.

An alternative therapy, especially a dietary supplement, may interact with a conventional drug (prescription or nonprescription).[1] An interaction occurs when a drug and a supplement are taken about the same time, and one of them interferes with how the other works. A supplement may increase or decrease the effect of a conventional drug. Sometimes serious problems result. For example, ginkgo biloba can increase the effect of certain

1. see table on pages 66 to 72

drugs taken to prevent blood clots (anticoagulants, or so-called blood thinners), such as warfarin. As a result, bleeding is more likely to occur. Ginkgo can make anticonvulsants (taken to prevent seizures) less effective. As a result, seizures may be more likely to occur. Interactions between drugs and dietary supplements have been studied, but more study is needed. Supplements may also interact with foods.

More than 50% of older people who use alternative therapies do not tell their doctor. Discussing an alternative therapy with a doctor before using it is best. But people who are already using one should tell their doctor. Doing so may help prevent interactions between a prescribed drug and a dietary supplement. It may also prevent older people from using a therapy that is unsafe. Older people should be cautious when using an alternative therapy because their response may be different from that of younger people. As the body ages, it processes substances, such as drugs, differently.[1]

Dietary supplements are of particular concern. No government agency checks to make sure that a product contains what it says it contains and nothing else. No agency checks that all products with the same name contain the same ingredients in the same amounts. Thus, people have no way of knowing exactly how much of a substance they are taking. A person may get less, more, or, in some cases, none of the active ingredient supposed to be in a product. Products that differ in content may differ in effectiveness. Also, an alternative product may contain substances not listed on the package. Thus, people do not know all of the substances they are taking. A product may contain a potentially harmful substance, such as one that can cause an allergic reaction.

DIETARY SUPPLEMENTS

"Dietary supplement" refers to any product (besides tobacco) that contains a vitamin, a mineral, a medicinal herb, an amino acid, an enzyme, or a hormone and that is intended to supplement the normal diet. Dietary supplements are taken as capsules, tablets, or liquids. In the United States, the Food and Drug Administration (FDA) does not closely regulate dietary

1. see page 52

supplements. Thus, the claims that dietary supplements help maintain or restore health and are safe may or may not be true. "Nutraceutical," a similar term, refers to any food or supplement that is thought to have a health benefit.

TAKING MEDICINAL HERBS AND DRUGS TOGETHER: SOME POSSIBLE INTERACTIONS

Medicinal Herb	Affected Drugs	Interaction*
Chamomile	Drugs that can prevent blood from clotting (anticoagulants), such as warfarin	Theoretically, chamomile may increase the effect of anticoagulants, making bleeding more likely to occur. No cases of bleeding have been reported.
	Drugs used to calm or produce drowsiness (sedatives), such as phenobarbital (a barbiturate)	Chamomile may increase the effect of sedatives, resulting in excessive or prolonged drowsiness.
	Iron supplements	Theoretically, chamomile may reduce the amount of iron absorbed by the body. This effect has not been reported.
Echinacea	Drugs that can suppress the immune system (immuno-suppressants), such as corticosteroids, anabolic steroids, methotrexate, and cyclosporine	By stimulating the immune system, echinacea may cancel out the effects of immunosuppressants. Echinacea, if taken for more than 8 weeks without a break, may suppress the immune system.
Feverfew	Anticoagulants, such as warfarin, and drugs that make platelets less likely to clump and form blood clots (antiplatelet drugs), such as aspirin	Feverfew may increase the effect of anticoagulants and antiplatelet drugs, making bleeding more likely to occur.

Medicinal Herb	Affected Drugs	Interaction*
	Iron supplements	Theoretically, feverfew may reduce the amount of iron absorbed by the body. This effect has not been reported.
Garlic	Anticoagulants, such as warfarin, and antiplatelet drugs, such as aspirin	Garlic may make platelets less likely to clump and form blood clots. So it may increase the effect of anticoagulants and antiplatelet drugs, making bleeding more likely to occur.
	Drugs that decrease the blood sugar level (antihyperglycemic drugs), such as chlorpropamide and insulin	Garlic may increase the effects of antihyperglycemic drugs, causing the blood sugar level to become too low (a condition called hypoglycemia). However, whether garlic lowers the blood sugar level is unclear.
Ginger	Anticoagulants, such as warfarin, and antiplatelet drugs, such as aspirin	Ginger may increase the effect of anticoagulants and antiplatelet drugs, making bleeding more likely to occur.
	Drugs that reduce stomach acid production, such as sucralfate, H_2 blockers (including cimetidine, famotidine, nizatidine, and ranitidine), and proton pump inhibitors (including lansoprazole, omeprazole, and pantoprazole)	Theoretically, ginger may neutralize the effect of these drugs because it may increase stomach acid production.

Table continues on the following page.

Medicinal Herb	Affected Drugs	Interaction*
	Antihyperglycemic drugs, such as sulfonylureas and insulin	Ginger may increase the effects of anti-hyperglycemic drugs, causing the blood sugar level to become too low.
	Drugs used to treat heart disorders	Theoretically, ginger may directly stimulate the heart and thus interfere with the effects of these drugs.
Ginkgo	Anticoagulants, such as warfarin, and antiplatelet drugs, such as aspirin	Ginkgo makes platelets less likely to clump. So it may increase the effect of anticoagulants or antiplatelet drugs, making bleeding more likely to occur.
	One type of antidepressant called monoamine oxidase inhibitors (MAOIs), such as phenelzine	Theoretically, ginkgo may increase the effect of these antidepressants.
	Drugs taken to treat seizure disorders (anticonvulsants), such as phenytoin	Some components of ginkgo may cause seizures. So ginkgo may make anticonvulsants less effective in preventing seizures.
Ginseng	Anticoagulants, such as warfarin, and antiplatelet drugs, such as aspirin	Ginseng increases the effect of anticoagulants and antiplatelet drugs, possibly making bleeding more likely to occur.
	Antipsychotics, such as chlorpromazine, haloperidol, and risperidone	Ginseng may make people restless, hyperactive, or agitated and thus cancel out the effects of antipsychotics.
	Antihyperglycemic drugs, such as glipizide	Ginseng may decrease the blood sugar level. So it may increase the effects

Medicinal Herb	Affected Drugs	Interaction*
		of antihyperglycemic drugs, possibly causing the blood sugar level to become too low.
	Digoxin	Siberian ginseng may cause the level of digoxin in the blood to be measured as high when it is not; no harmful effects result.
	One type of antidepressant (MAOIs), such as phenelzine	Ginseng can cause headaches, tremors, and manic episodes when it is taken with MAOIs.
Goldenseal	Anticoagulants, such as warfarin and heparin	Goldenseal may make anticoagulants less effective, possibly increasing the risk of blood clots.
	Diuretics	Goldenseal can increase the amount of water excreted in urine. So it may increase the effect of diuretics, causing dehydration.
	Drugs used to lower blood pressure (antihypertensives)	Goldenseal may make antihypertensives less effective in controlling blood pressure.
	Certain drugs that reduce stomach acid production (H_2 blockers, such as cimetidine, nizatidine, and ranitidine, and proton pump inhibitors, such as lansoprazole, omeprazole, and pantoprazole)	Goldenseal may increase stomach acid production and thus cancel out the effects of these drugs.

Table continues on the following page.

Medicinal Herb	Affected Drugs	Interaction*
Horse chestnut	Anticoagulants, such as warfarin and heparin, and antiplatelet drugs, such as aspirin	Theoretically, horse chestnut may increase the effect of anticoagulants and antiplatelet drugs, possibly making bleeding more likely to occur.
Kava	Sedatives, antianxiety drugs, antihistamines, and drugs used to treat loss of contact with reality (antipsychotic drugs)	Kava may increase the effect of sedatives and other drugs that produce drowsiness, resulting in excessive drowsiness.
	Muscle relaxants, such as carisoprodol, cyclobenzaprine, and diazepam	Components of kava act on the brain to relax muscles. When taken with other muscle relaxants, kava can result in slowed breathing.
	Alcohol	Alcohol may increase the sedating effect of kava.
Licorice	Digoxin	Licorice can decrease the level of potassium, which makes people more sensitive to digoxin. Then digoxin is more likely to have harmful effects (digoxin toxicity).
	Diuretics	When licorice is taken with certain diuretics, the potassium level may become too low. (Certain diuretics cause the body to excrete more potassium as they cause more urine to be excreted.) A low potassium level can have dangerous results.
	Corticosteroids	Licorice may increase the effects of corticosteroids,

Medicinal Herb	Affected Drugs	Interaction*
		making side effects more likely.
Saw palmetto	Estrogen therapy	Theoretically, saw palmetto may make the side effects of estrogen worse. This effect has not been reported.
St. John's wort	Cyclosporine (an immunosuppressant)	St. John's wort may reduce the blood level of cyclosporine, making it less effective, with potentially dangerous results. For example, an organ transplant may be more likely to be rejected.
	Digoxin	St. John's wort may reduce blood levels of digoxin, making it less effective, with potentially dangerous results.
	Protease inhibitors (used to treat HIV infection), such as indinavir and ritonavir	St. John's wort may reduce blood levels of these drugs, making them less effective.
	One type of antidepressant (selective serotonin reuptake inhibitors—SSRIs), such as fluoxetine, paroxetine, and sertraline	St. John's wort may increase the effects of these drugs, causing a group of symptoms (dizziness, lethargy, confusion, and very high blood pressure), called serotonin syndrome. Emergency treatment is usually necessary.
	Theophylline	St. John's wort decreases the blood level of theophylline, making it less effective as treatment for asthma.

Table continues on the following page.

Medicinal Herb	Affected Drugs	Interaction*
	Warfarin	St. John's wort may reduce the blood level of warfarin, making it less effective and increasing the risk of blood clots.
Valerian	Sedatives, including barbiturates (such as phenobarbital) and benzodiazepines (such as diazepam)	Valerian may increase the effects of sedatives, causing excessive drowsiness.

*Most of the drug-herb interactions listed have been reported. A few have not been reported and are theoretical. But in almost all cases, there is not enough evidence to prove that the interaction caused the side effect(s).

Medicinal herbs are one type of dietary supplement. They are derived from plants. Many herbs have been used to prevent disease and improve health for centuries. The herbs most commonly used by older people include ginkgo, garlic, and saw palmetto.

Some supplements contain hormones or enzymes that the body produces less of as it ages. People hope that such supplements will slow aging, increase energy, or prevent disorders that are common in old age. However, why the body produces less of these substances is not known. So replacing them may not be beneficial and may be harmful. No supplement has been shown to slow or reverse aging.

Acetyl-L Carnitine

Acetyl-L carnitine is a form of carnitine, an amino acid produced in the body. Carnitine is involved in heart function, brain function, the body's processing (metabolism) of fats, and energy production.

Medicinal claims: Acetyl-L carnitine supplements are used to increase energy and exercise performance, relieve chronic fatigue, prevent weight gain, improve heart or brain function, help persistent leg ulcers heal, and prevent aging. Acetyl-L carnitine has also been used to treat people who have dementia (including Alzheimer's disease), depression, or coronary artery disease.

At present, there is not enough evidence to determine whether this supplement is beneficial or harmful in treating older people with Alzheimer's disease. No evidence supports other claims. Acetyl-L carnitine supplements are approved to treat people with a deficiency in carnitine.

Possible problems: Acetyl-L carnitine may cause body odor, skin rashes, and digestive disturbances (such as nausea, vomiting, diarrhea, and abdominal cramps). People with chronic liver disease should not use this supplement.

Use of D-carnitine, another form of carnitine, can result in severe weakness and loss of muscle tissue. So checking the label of carnitine supplements is particularly important.

Chamomile

Chamomile is a perennial herb with a daisylike flower. The flower is dried and used as tea or in extracts.

Medicinal claims: Chamomile has been used to calm, relax, and help with sleep. Chamomile extract applied in a compress is used to soothe irritated skin. Various substances in chamomile reduce inflammation and fever. Chamomile is sometimes used to relieve stomach cramps and indigestion. It is also claimed to help gastric ulcers heal.

Studies in animals suggest that substances in chamomile inhibit the growth of the bacteria involved in stomach ulcers (*Helicobacter pylori*). However, no studies in people support the claim that it can prevent or treat ulcers.

Possible problems: Chamomile may interact with several drugs, iron supplements, and alcohol. Some people are allergic to the pollen in chamomile products. These people may have a severe allergic (anaphylactic) reaction if they take chamomile by mouth. If they apply chamomile to the skin, they may develop a skin rash.

Chondroitin

Chondroitin is a component of cartilage, bone, and blood vessels. As a supplement, it is derived from cow or shark cartilage or is made synthetically. It is often combined with glucosamine, which also occurs in cartilage.

Medicinal claims: Chondroitin supplements have been shown to relieve the pain of one type of arthritis, osteoarthritis. Whether chondroitin protects cartilage or prevents the progression of osteoarthritis is not clear.

Possible problems: Chondroitin supplements appear to be

relatively safe. They may cause some mild digestive disturbances, such as abdominal pain and nausea. Supplements derived from cartilage may cause an allergic reaction. Chondroitin may interact with drugs taken to prevent blood clots (including anticoagulants and aspirin).

Coenzyme Q_{10}

Coenzyme Q_{10} (ubiquinone) is a protein produced by the body. It is used to produce energy in cells. It also acts as an antioxidant. That is, it protects cells from free radicals. Free radicals, which are by-products of normal cell activity, can damage cells.

Medicinal claims: Coenzyme Q_{10} is claimed to help the heart and immune system function better, to control diabetes, and to lower blood pressure. Coenzyme Q_{10} is added to skin care products to minimize and prevent wrinkles.

A few studies suggest that coenzyme Q_{10} is likely to benefit people with heart disorders, especially those with heart failure. However, in other studies, no benefit was seen. Some evidence suggests that coenzyme Q_{10} protects the heart from the harmful effects of certain chemotherapy drugs used to treat cancer. Some advocates suggest that coenzyme Q_{10} is useful in treating cancer because of its antioxidant effects. But the evidence supporting this claim is inconclusive.

Possible problems: Side effects include mild insomnia, rashes, an increase in levels of liver enzymes, and digestive disturbances (including loss of appetite, heartburn, nausea, and diarrhea). Coenzyme Q_{10} may interact with the anticoagulant warfarin, drugs taken by mouth to treat diabetes (such as glyburide and tolazamide[1]), and certain drugs used to lower cholesterol (statins, such as atorvastatin, fluvastatin, pravastatin, and simvastatin[2]).

Creatine

Creatine is an amino acid made in the liver and stored in muscles. It is a readily available source of energy in the body. Certain foods, such as milk, steak, and some fish, contain creatine.

Medicinal claims: Creatine supplements are used to help

1. see table on page 482
2. see table on page 630

people exercise better, increase muscle mass, and decrease fatigue. In some studies, creatine helped muscles perform better during brief, high-intensity exercise.

Possible problems: Creatine can cause nausea, diarrhea, and dehydration, which may lead to kidney problems. How taking creatine continuously for a long time affects the body is unknown. Creatine has no known interaction with other drugs.

Dehydroepiandrosterone

Dehydroepiandrosterone (DHEA) is a steroid hormone produced by the adrenal glands. It is converted into sex hormones, such as estrogen and testosterone. The effects of DHEA on the body may be similar to those of testosterone. In times of stress, the adrenal glands produce DHEA to maintain hormonal balance in the body.

Medicinal claims: DHEA supplements are claimed to improve memory, mood, energy, sense of well-being, and the ability to function under stress. They are thought to stimulate the immune system. Many athletes claim that DHEA supplements build muscles. Other claims include deepening nightly sleep, lowering cholesterol levels, decreasing body fat, and slowing down or reversing the effects of aging. Some advocates think DHEA supplements may help people with Parkinson's disease or Alzheimer's disease function better. These supplements have been used to treat people who have depression (because DHEA levels may be low).

Whether DHEA builds muscle or enhances athletic performance in people with normal adrenal glands and DHEA levels is unclear. There is no reliable evidence that DHEA supplements slow aging or help people who have Parkinson's disease, Alzheimer's disease, or depression.

Possible problems: Use of DHEA supplements may result in breast enlargement in men and hairiness in women. These supplements may also lead to hair loss, a decrease in the level of high-density lipoprotein (HDL) cholesterol (the "good" cholesterol), an increase in the blood sugar level in people with diabetes, and liver problems. When DHEA is used for a long time or in large amounts, it may stimulate the growth of certain prostate and breast cancers. However, none of these effects have been substantiated. For most people, the risks of using DHEA supplements probably outweigh any possible benefits.

Echinacea

Echinacea, also called purple coneflower, is a perennial herb. Various parts of the plant are used medicinally.

Medicinal claims: Several substances in echinacea may stimulate the immune system. Echinacea has been used to help prevent and treat viral infections in the upper respiratory tract, such as the common cold. Applied as a cream or an ointment, echinacea has been used to speed the healing of wounds.

Some evidence suggests that echinacea can reduce the duration of colds, the severity of symptoms, and the frequency and number of recurrences. However, these studies were not designed well enough to provide conclusive results. In a recent well-designed study, echinacea did not prevent or shorten the duration of colds.

Possible problems: Side effects appear to be rare. However, allergic reactions can occur and may be serious. Echinacea should not be taken for more than 8 weeks without a break because daily use for a long time may suppress the immune system. Because echinacea stimulates the immune system, it may cancel out the effects of immunosuppressants (used to treat arthritis and to prevent rejection of organ transplants).

Feverfew

Feverfew is a perennial herb with a daisylike flower. The content of different feverfew products may vary.

Medicinal claims: Feverfew has been used to prevent migraine headaches and treat arthritis. It may reduce inflammation and fever. Feverfew makes blood less likely to clot. Because of this effect, the herb is claimed to reduce the risk of heart attack and stroke.

Some evidence suggests that feverfew is slightly effective in reducing the number and severity of migraines. Feverfew has not been shown to relieve the symptoms of arthritis or to help treat any other disorder.

Possible problems: Feverfew may cause mouth ulcers and skin inflammation (dermatitis). Taste may be altered, and heart rate may be increased. After people stop taking feverfew, they may feel nervous and have headaches, insomnia, and joint pain and stiffness. Feverfew may interact with many drugs.

Garlic

Garlic is a perennial plant, long used in cooking and in medicine. The active component of garlic is allicin. Allicin gives garlic its strong odor and medicinal properties. It is released when garlic is crushed or chewed. Heat and acid can destroy the enzymes that release allicin.

Medicinal claims: Garlic makes blood less likely to clot. Advocates suggest that garlic may thus improve circulation and reduce the risk of heart attack and stroke. Garlic stops microorganisms (such as bacteria) from reproducing. Thus, it has been used as an antiseptic and antibacterial. Garlic has also been used to prevent or treat respiratory infections (such as bronchitis), urinary tract infections, sinusitis, fungal infections, and the common cold. In large doses, garlic is claimed to reduce blood pressure, overactivity of the intestine, and the blood sugar level (slightly).

Advocates suggest that garlic reduces the risk of atherosclerosis and, in people who have atherosclerosis, the buildup of plaque. These claims are based on garlic's effect on high cholesterol levels (a risk factor for atherosclerosis). However, garlic only slightly lowers the levels of total cholesterol and low-density lipoprotein (LDL) cholesterol—the "bad" cholesterol.[1]

Some evidence suggests that garlic may be useful in treating mild high blood pressure (hypertension), but the effect is small. Whether garlic lowers the blood sugar level is unclear. Garlic may reduce the risk of certain types of cancer. However, more studies are needed to substantiate this and the many other claims. Nevertheless, using garlic with other measures to lower cholesterol (including exercise, weight loss, and cholesterol-lowering drugs) may be helpful.

Possible problems: Garlic usually has no harmful effects other than making the breath or body smell like garlic. However, consuming large amounts can cause nausea and burning in the mouth, esophagus, and stomach. Consuming large amounts may also increase the risk of bleeding. Garlic may interact with several drugs.

1. see table on page 625

Ginger

Ginger is a perennial plant, long used in cooking and in medicine. The root of this herb contains substances called gingerols, which give ginger its flavor and odor.

Medicinal claims: Ginger appears to soothe the stomach, relieve intestinal cramps, and reduce inflammation and pain. Ginger has been used to prevent nausea, vomiting, motion sickness, and dizziness (including vertigo).

In studies of how well ginger prevents motion sickness and nausea, the results were inconclusive.

Possible problems: Ginger is usually not harmful. However, some people experience a disagreeable taste in the mouth or a burning sensation when they eat it. Ironically, ginger may increase stomach acid production and cause digestive disturbances. Consuming large amounts of ginger can make the brain function more slowly and cause irregular heart rhythms. Ginger may interact with several drugs.

Ginkgo

The ginkgo is a large tree, often planted for ornamental purposes. As a supplement, ginkgo is derived from the tree's fan-shaped leaves. Ginkgo is available as tea or in extracts.

Medicinal claims: Ginkgo appears to make blood less likely to clot and expands (dilates) blood vessels, thereby improving blood flow. Ginkgo has been used to improve blood flow to the brain and in the lower legs. It is sometimes used to treat dizziness, headaches, noise in the ears (tinnitus), memory loss, concentration problems, and depression. It also is claimed to prevent damage to the kidneys caused by the immunosuppressant cyclosporine.

The active components of ginkgo may prevent the airways from narrowing (constricting). Thus, ginkgo is sometimes used to treat asthma and bronchitis.

In some studies, when people with reduced blood flow in the legs (peripheral arterial disease) took ginkgo, they could walk farther without pain. In some studies, ginkgo stabilized or improved mental and social function in people with mild to moderate dementia, including Alzheimer's disease. In another study, ginkgo improved mental function in healthy older people. But other studies show no benefit. Ginkgo appears to reduce the loudness of tinnitus. The effectiveness of ginkgo in treating other disorders requires further study.

Possible problems: Ginkgo supplements usually have no side effects except mild digestive disturbances and headaches. These effects usually disappear as people continue to take ginkgo. Ginkgo can increase the risk of bleeding. Ginkgo may interact with several drugs.

Ginseng

Ginseng is usually derived from two different species of plant: American and Asian ginseng. American ginseng has milder effects than Asian ginseng. Ginseng is available in many forms, such as fresh and dried roots, extracts, solutions, capsules, tablets, cosmetics, sodas, and teas.

Siberian ginseng is not really ginseng and contains different active components, but it is used in similar ways.

Ginseng products vary considerably in quality. Many contain little or no active ingredient.

Medicinal claims: Ginseng is claimed to enhance physical (including sexual) and mental performance. It is also claimed to increase energy, prevent fatigue, help the body cope with stress, and slow aging. Other claims include reducing the blood sugar level and increasing the level of high-density lipoprotein (HDL) cholesterol—the "good" cholesterol.

In one study of people with diabetes, ginseng reduced the blood sugar level, and people who took ginseng reported that their mood improved and energy increased. In another study, people who took ginseng reported that their quality of life improved. In one study, people who took ginseng appeared to have fewer cases of cancer. However, the results of these studies are inconclusive. Most of ginseng's claims, including improvement of athletic or sexual performance, have not been proved.

Possible problems: Ginseng has a reasonably good safety record. The most common side effects are nervousness and excitability, which usually decrease after the first few days. The ability to concentrate may be decreased, and the blood sugar level may decrease to an abnormally low level (causing hypoglycemia). Occasionally, serious side effects occur. They include asthma attacks, increased blood pressure, palpitations, insomnia, diarrhea, and, in postmenopausal women, vaginal bleeding. In one study, ginseng appeared to stimulate the growth of breast cancer cells. Ginseng may interact with many drugs. If older people are taking several drugs, taking ginseng is not advisable.

Glucosamine

Glucosamine is a component of cartilage. It stimulates cells to rebuild cartilage and helps lubricate joints. As a supplement, it is derived from crab shells or is made synthetically. It is often combined with chondroitin, another component of cartilage.

The contents of glucosamine products vary considerably. Some glucosamine products do not contain any glucosamine.

Medicinal claims: Glucosamine supplements are claimed to relieve pain and increase the range of motion in people with arthritis. Some evidence supports these claims. In one study, the combination of glucosamine, chondroitin, and manganese decreased pain in the knee due to osteoarthritis. A large, well-designed study of the effects of glucosamine (and chondroitin) is under way. It will provide more conclusive evidence. Whether taking glucosamine supplements helps to rebuild cartilage is unclear.

Possible problems: Glucosamine supplements appear to be relatively safe. They may cause some mild digestive disturbances, such as heartburn or nausea. There is some concern that glucosamine derived from crab shells may cause a reaction in people with a shellfish allergy. Glucosamine may affect the blood sugar level, so people with diabetes should talk with their doctor before they take glucosamine.

Goldenseal

Goldenseal is an endangered plant, related to the buttercup. Its active components are hydrastine and berberine.

Medicinal claims: Goldenseal has been used as an antiseptic wash for mouth sores, inflamed and sore eyes, and irritated skin and as a douche for vaginal infections. It has been combined with echinacea as a cold remedy. Goldenseal has also been used as a remedy for indigestion and diarrhea.

The effectiveness of goldenseal as a cold remedy has not been proved. Some evidence suggests that berberine, isolated from goldenseal, may reduce the severity and duration of diarrhea due to a bacterial infection. Berberine may also inhibit the growth of parasites in the intestines. However, goldenseal is not recommended to relieve diarrhea because its other components may irritate the digestive tract.

Possible problems: Goldenseal has many side effects, including digestive disturbances, confusion, contractions of the uterus, and worsening of high blood pressure. Large amounts of goldenseal can cause seizures, respiratory failure, and death. It may affect the contraction of the heart. Goldenseal may interact with several drugs. People who have heart disorders or problems with blood clotting should not take goldenseal.

Horse Chestnut

The horse chestnut is a tree. Supplements are made from the seed. They are available as a tablet, a capsule, or an ointment. The active component is aescin.

Medicinal claims: Horse chestnut supplements have been used to treat chronic venous insufficiency, varicose veins, and hemorrhoids. In these disorders, blood vessels are damaged, allowing fluids to leak from blood vessels into the tissues. The result is swelling. Horse chestnut supplements are thought to strengthen the walls of small blood vessels and thus help prevent leakage. Swelling may then be reduced. Horse chestnut supplements have also been used to relieve swelling after injuries. They are claimed to help prevent bruising, which is common among older people because aging causes blood vessels to become more fragile.

Evidence suggests that horse chestnut supplements relieve leg swelling and pain in people with chronic venous insufficiency. No evidence supports the other claims.

Possible problems: When taken off the tree, seeds of the horse chestnut are poisonous. So people should use only commercial preparations, which are detoxified. Horse chestnut supplements are relatively safe. But because these supplements are used to treat symptoms that may indicate a serious disorder, talking with a doctor before starting to take them is always recommended.

Horse chestnut supplements may irritate the stomach, cause itching, or cause the blood sugar level to decrease to an abnormally low level (causing hypoglycemia). Large doses may cause kidney or liver disorders, so people who already have one of these disorders should not take these supplements. Rarely, horse chestnut supplements cause an allergic reaction.

Human Growth Hormone

Human growth hormone is produced by the pituitary gland, which is located at the base of the brain. This hormone is essential for growth and affects how the body uses energy (metabolism). Production of human growth hormone is greatest during adolescence, then progressively decreases after age 30.

Human growth hormone is available only by prescription and must be injected. Some products that are available without a prescription are claimed to contain substances that stimulate the body's production of human growth hormone. A few are claimed to contain small amounts of the hormone itself. These products are available as a powder, tablet, or liquid taken by mouth, as a topical gel, and as a mouth or nasal spray. These products are highly unlikely to have any effect at all. Also, human growth hormone taken by mouth cannot be used by the body because it passes through the digestive tract without being absorbed. Human growth hormone applied to the skin or used as a spray cannot be absorbed by the body.

Medicinal claims: Human growth hormone is claimed to reverse the effects of aging, reduce body fat, help the heart and immune system function better, lower blood pressure and cholesterol levels, strengthen bones, improve physical (including sexual) performance, and increase energy.

Evidence supports some of the claims for human growth hormone when it is given as an injection. But the effects of long-term use are unknown.

Certain uses of a synthetic form of human growth hormone given by injection have been established. It is approved for use by children whose growth has been stunted. It is also used to reverse muscle wasting (atrophy) in people with AIDS and to treat people who have a deficiency of human growth hormone.

As the body ages, it produces less human growth hormone. Some theories suggest that this decrease may contribute to frailty during old age. As a result, several studies have focused on whether human growth hormone replacement can reverse the aging process by increasing muscle (lean body mass), physical strength, and mobility and thus improve quality of life. Results of these studies have been disappointing, showing no improvements.

Possible problems: Human growth hormone given by injection can cause a high blood sugar level (hyperglycemia), temporary fluid retention, high blood pressure, headaches, carpal tunnel syndrome, mild pain in joints, and excessive growth (acromegaly). It can also cause the thyroid gland to function less well.

Kava

Kava is a shrub that grows in the South Pacific. As a supplement, kava is derived from the dried rhizome (underground stem or root) of the shrub.

Medicinal claims: Kava has been used mainly to relieve anxiety. It has also been used to treat insomnia, restlessness, stress, seizure disorders, and depression.

Evidence suggests that kava, given for a short time, is effective in relieving anxiety and helping with sleep.

Possible problems: The safety of kava is uncertain, especially if used for a long time. Kava may cause serious side effects, including severe liver damage and liver failure. Such effects appear to be rare. Nonetheless, people with liver disorders should not take kava. In a few people, kava causes nausea, headaches, dizziness, or a rash. Kava can also cause drowsiness. After taking it, people should not drive a car or do other activities requiring alertness. People with Parkinson's disease should not take kava, because it may worsen symptoms. Kava may interact with several drugs and with alcohol.

Licorice

Licorice is a perennial shrub. As a supplement, licorice is derived from the root of the shrub. Natural licorice has a very sweet taste. It is used as flavoring in foods, beverages, and tobacco.

Medicinal claims: Licorice is used to suppress coughs, soothe a sore throat, decrease inflammation, and relieve stomach upset. Applied externally, it is thought to soothe irritated skin. Licorice has not been proved to have any of these effects.

Possible problems: Licorice causes people to retain fluids. Frequently taking large amounts of licorice can result in headaches, fatigue, high blood pressure (hypertension), and substantial changes in sodium or potassium levels. People are advised to take licorice no longer than 4 to 6 weeks.

Licorice should not be taken with diuretics (used to reduce

the volume of fluid in the body) or digoxin (used to treat heart failure).

Melatonin

Melatonin is a hormone produced by the pineal gland, which is located in the middle of the brain. Melatonin regulates the sleep-wake cycle. As a supplement, melatonin is derived from animal brains or is made synthetically.

Medicinal claims: Melatonin supplements have been used to treat insomnia and help reduce the effects of jet lag. People who are traveling across time zones may benefit from melatonin given on the day or night of departure and for two or three nights after arrival. Melatonin is claimed to help the immune system function better, to prevent cancer, and to help people live longer.

Evidence suggests that melatonin supplements may help prevent or reduce the effects of jet lag in people who are traveling across several time zones. A few studies suggest that these supplements are effective for treating insomnia, but other studies found no benefit. There is no evidence that melatonin can prevent cancer or help people live longer.

Possible problems: Drowsiness may occur 30 minutes after taking melatonin and lasts about 1 hour. Whether melatonin is safe when used for a long time is unknown. Theoretically, a viral infection or prion disease (such as Creutzfeldt-Jakob disease, the human equivalent of mad cow disease) could result from taking melatonin derived from animal brains but not from taking synthetic forms of melatonin. Thus, synthetic forms are a wiser choice than natural forms. Headaches and temporary depression have been reported. In people who are depressed, melatonin may worsen symptoms. The use of melatonin should be supervised by a doctor because it may interact with several drugs.

Saw Palmetto

Saw palmetto is a tree that grows in the southeastern United States. Saw palmetto supplements are derived from the dried berries of the tree. They are available as tea, tablets, capsules, and a liquid extract.

Medicinal claims: Saw palmetto blocks the actions of testosterone, which stimulates growth of the prostate gland. Saw palmetto has been used to treat benign enlargement of the prostate gland (benign prostatic hyperplasia). Other claims include increasing sperm production, increasing breast size, and improving sexual performance.

Evidence suggests that saw palmetto can relieve the symptoms of an enlarged prostate gland, such as the frequent urge to urinate and decreased urine flow. Other claims have not been proved.

Possible problems: Side effects are rare and usually mild. They include headaches and diarrhea.

St. John's Wort

St. John's wort is a plant that grows wild in many areas of the world. The reddish substance in the plant's yellow flowers contains hypericin, which is the main active component. Supplements are available as capsules, liquids, skin lotions, and tea.

Medicinal claims: St. John's wort is used mainly to treat depression. This herb can act like a monoamine oxidase inhibitor (MAOI), an antidepressant. However, St. John's wort, when used as directed, does not seem to have the same side effects or interactions with certain foods. St. John's wort is also used to reduce inflammation and fight infection. It has been used to treat HIV infection, vitiligo (loss of normal skin pigment in patches), burns, insect bites, cancer, bronchitis, and kidney disorders. It has also been used to help wounds heal.

In many studies, St. John's wort relieved symptoms in people with mild to moderate depression. Some of these studies included older people. However, in one large, well-designed study, St. John's wort was no more effective than placebo (a pill with no active ingredients) in relieving symptoms in people with moderate depression. St. John's wort has not been shown to be effective in treating HIV infection or vitiligo.

Possible problems: When used as directed, St. John's wort can make the skin very sensitive to sunlight. St. John's wort interacts with many drugs.

Valerian

Valerian is a pink-flowered perennial plant. Valerian supplements are derived from the plant's dried root. Valerian is used to flavor foods and beverages, such as root beer.

Medicinal claims: Valerian appears to have a calming effect.

Thus, it is used as a sedative and sleep aid. Some evidence suggests that valerian can improve sleep quality and shorten the time needed to fall asleep.

Possible problems: Valerian occasionally causes headaches, excitability, uneasiness, and heart palpitations. After taking it, people should not drive a car or engage in other activities requiring alertness. Valerian may interact with drugs used to calm or produce drowsiness (sedatives).

CHIROPRACTIC

Chiropractic is a philosophy that is believed to restore balance in the body and thus enable the body to heal itself. According to this philosophy, balance is achieved by keeping open the lines of communication within the body—the nerves. Chiropractic was developed as a therapy in the late nineteenth century.

Communication begins in the mind, travels down the spinal cord, and reaches all parts of the body through the nerves. The nerves emerge from the spinal cord through openings between the bones of the spine (vertebrae). If vertebrae are out of line (misaligned), they may interfere with communication through the nerves, and a problem can result. The problem may affect any part of the body, depending on the location of the misalignment (subluxation). By correcting the misalignment, chiropractic enables communication through the nerves to occur normally and helps the body restore balance and maintain health.

To locate misalignments, chiropractors may use their hands to feel along the spine. Many chiropractors take x-rays to determine where the problem is and to make sure that no bones are fractured before therapy is begun. To correct misalignments, chiropractors use their hands to apply pressure to the spine in a specific direction and location. Several different techniques and approaches can be used. Chiropractic does not use drugs or surgery. When done correctly, the therapy is painless.

Chiropractic is licensed in all 50 states. Medicare and many private insurance companies cover it.

Medicinal claims: Chiropractic has been used to relieve back pain (especially low back pain), neck pain, other muscle pain, and headaches. Chiropractic is claimed to relieve the symptoms of many other disorders, including asthma, sinusitis, constipation, and migraines.

Studies support the effectiveness of chiropractic for short-term relief of low back pain. This therapy may help relieve headaches and neck pain. However, continuing treatment longer than a few weeks does not appear to produce additional benefits. And whether chiropractic is effective for persistent (chronic) back pain is not clear. No reliable evidence supports its use for problems that are not related to muscles.

Possible problems: Chiropractic rarely causes serious problems. However, increased pain, ruptured disks, paralysis, and strokes have been reported. Back pain may result if a nerve root (the part of the nerve located near the spine) is damaged. Because chiropractic provides only short-term relief of pain, people may become dependent on chiropractors for continued treatments.

ACUPUNCTURE

In acupuncture, hair-thin needles are inserted into specific points of the body. Practitioners of acupuncture believe the needles stimulate these points and thus unblock the pathways of the body's energy flow (qi). Stimulation at the appropriate points restores balance in the body. Blockage of energy flow is considered to be the cause of pain and disease.

Acupuncture originated in China more than 2,000 years ago. In the United States, a few doctors, including some neurologists, anesthesiologists, and specialists in physical medicine, are trained in acupuncture.

After insertion, the needles may be twirled rapidly and intermittently for a few minutes, or a low electrical current may be applied through the needles. Acupuncture is usually painless. Pain is more likely to be felt if the person moves or if the needle is improperly placed. Some people feel energized after treatment. Others feel relaxed.

Medicinal claims: Acupuncture has been used to relieve pain and to prevent nausea and vomiting. It has also been used to treat carpal tunnel syndrome, arthritis, asthma, and bronchitis and to help with rehabilitation after a stroke. It is claimed to help people stop smoking, drinking alcohol, and using illicit drugs.

Evidence indicates that acupuncture releases various chemical messengers in the brain (neurotransmitters) that act as natural pain relievers. There is also evidence that acupuncture can relieve low back pain and pain after surgery or dental procedures. Acupuncture may relieve myofascial pain (pain that occurs in muscles, tendons, and ligaments), as occurs in fibromyalgia. However, whether acupuncture relieves chronic pain (as occurs in arthritis) is unclear. Acupuncture may be effective in helping treat drug or alcohol addiction, carpal tunnel syndrome, arthritis, asthma, and headaches and in helping with rehabilitation after a stroke. There is no evidence that acupuncture helps people stop smoking.

Possible problems: If done correctly, acupuncture causes few problems. Infections are rare, because most practitioners use sterile needles. If the needles are not inserted correctly, an organ may be punctured. Some people faint. Sometimes symptoms worsen after treatment. People should choose practitioners who are well trained and licensed.

MAGNET THERAPY

In magnet (bioelectromagnetic) therapy, magnets are placed on or near certain points of the body (the same ones used in acupuncture) or on the area to be treated.

The use of magnets is based on the fact that the body produces electrical currents. These currents are thought to create internal magnetic (energy) fields that extend outside the body. Magnets are used to correct imbalances in these magnetic fields. Imbalances are thought to cause disease.

Magnets are available as bracelets, necklaces, rings, straps, patches, shoe inserts, mattress pads, pillows, and individual magnets. The type of magnet needed depends on which area of the body needs to be treated. For example, the wrist can be treated by wearing a bracelet.

Medicinal claims: Magnet therapy has been used to treat joint and muscle pain, such as that in the back, neck, shoulders, or hands. It has also been used to treat headaches and kidney disorders. Magnet therapy is claimed to reduce inflammation, restore energy, improve sleep, increase blood flow, and help tissues (such as bones) heal and nerves regenerate. Other claims include treatment of diabetes, multiple sclerosis, high or low blood pressure, and pneumonia.

There is not enough evidence to determine whether magnet therapy is useful in relieving pain. However, this therapy is fairly safe.

Possible problems: Magnet therapy is not known to cause any problems. However, before starting magnet therapy, people who have a pacemaker, work with high-voltage machines or cables, are allergic to metals, or use an insulin pump should consult a doctor.

HOMEOPATHY

Homeopathy is based on the principle that "like cures like." In homeopathy, a person is given small amounts of a substance that, if taken in large amounts, is thought to cause the same symptoms the person has. According to homeopathy, symptoms result from the body's attempt to heal itself. Thus, small amounts of a substance that causes symptoms can be used to stimulate the person's body to heal itself.

The remedies used in homeopathy are very dilute. The more dilute a remedy is, the stronger it is thought to be. Some remedies are so dilute that modern technology cannot detect the active substance. The active substance may come from plants or animals or may be a mineral. Examples are belladonna (from the deadly nightshade plant), venom (from pit vipers), calcium carbonate (from oyster shells), and the minerals sulfur and arsenic. Sometimes dilutions of drugs such as penicillin or streptomycin are used. Alcohol is usually used to dilute the substance.

The Food and Drug Administration (FDA) considers homeopathic products drugs, but it does not regulate them as drugs. For example, they are not tested for strength. They are considered so weak that their use poses little risk to the user. Homeopathic products claimed to treat serious disorders (such as cancer) may be available only by prescription from homeopathic practitioners. Only products used for minor disorders (such as colds or headaches) are available without a prescription (over-the-counter).

To determine what remedy is appropriate, homeopathic practitioners evaluate the person's mental, emotional, and physical condition and consider the person's history, personality, and lifestyle. For example, a person may be asked about food preferences and sleep habits. A well-trained, preferably licensed practitioner should be sought.

Medicinal claims: Homeopathy has been used to treat many disorders. The claims of homeopathy are hard to evaluate. Most studies have been small and poorly designed. No well-designed studies have shown that homeopathy is effective as treatment for any specific disorder.

Possible problems: Homeopathic remedies are thought to be relatively safe because they are so dilute. Allergic reactions may occur. Depending on the strength of a homeopathic remedy, the remedy may interact with other drugs.

"One good thing about growing old," someone one time told me, "is not having to worry about one's future any more."

This seems to have been true for me. "Let someone else worry about the loose leg on the sofa," I tell myself. "Or finding a painter for the kitchen cabinet." My former sense of urgency is gone.

There are many changes to be made in life styles with aging. Much of my time today is spent in looking for lost things. Glasses. My wallet. The name of some person whose name begins with "M" I need to speak with. It continues to elude me. But later, when it is no longer needed, the name will return.

Travel presents another problem. A trip today entails the confirmation of an aisle seat on the plane. This is followed by a frantic search for my 1990 driver's license that will be necessary for identification when getting on. Once at the airport, however, seated in a wheelchair and rolling past long lines of people and passing through closed gates without challenge, old age travel takes an upward swing.

Meetings, appointments, and ringing telephones diminish with growing older, and it is therefore a good idea to take along some piece of what your life has been before. I took writing. Editors change and new writers come and go, but this doesn't mean one can no longer write. Writing can be done on a bus or in a hospital or in bed. When something interesting comes my way I always start by taking notes, so that, even today, I sleep always with a pad and pencil handy in case the right word may be waiting for me in the dark.

The fact that I am 90 sometimes seems inconceivable. My youngest son should be 6, as youngest sons so often are, not 60. A young man with a familiar name whom I speak to at a cocktail party turns out not to be the son, but the grandson, of a person I had one time known. This often leads me to a feeling of being out of date. I have no fax or e-mail. I don't know how to "have a nice one," and www.abcdefg.com is a mystery to me.

Dying has always seemed as normal to me as being born. With aging, however, the dying has taken on a more concrete form. There is what to give to whom and where and how. Accounts of persons who have returned to life after being legally declared dead report moving though a long dark tunnel into the great illumination on the other side—so that I now wait with interest for the great illumination and the poignancy of saying good-bye to friends who will be the last page of my growing old.

Nancy Grace

8

Communicating With Health Care Practitioners

Effective communication with doctors and other health care practitioners improves health. Understanding how to communicate effectively and how to go about it are not so simple. As the old expression goes, "The devil is in the details."

Communicating effectively with an individual health care practitioner becomes more difficult when several practitioners are involved. In fact, the more people providing care, the greater the potential for miscommunication. For example, a person may incorrectly assume he has already mentioned an important detail to a particular practitioner, when in fact he mentioned it to someone else. Or differences of opinion among the various practitioners may become overwhelming and confusing.

Miscommunication can be minimized by establishing a consistent relationship with a primary care practitioner. Most often a primary care practitioner is a doctor, although a nurse practitioner or physician's assistant sometimes fills this role. In many ways, a primary care doctor is the health care version of an air traffic controller, keeping track of the actions of each of the practitioners involved and of the comings and goings of medical information.

Having a primary care doctor has many advantages and usually leads to better care. A primary care doctor is most familiar with the person's overall medical history and also learns about the person's values and how they affect health care decisions. Anxiety may diminish knowing that a primary care doctor is coordinating care. Also, the primary care doctor can explain the types of care needed, why such care is necessary, and how often visits should be scheduled. In general, preventive visits are needed more frequently by older people than by younger people.

SELECTING A PRIMARY CARE DOCTOR

Virtually any kind of doctor can function as a primary care doctor. Those from the fields of family medicine (family doctors), internal medicine (internists), and general practice (general practitioners) do so most often. Some doctors have additional training and expertise in geriatric medicine (geriatricians)—a field devoted to the health care of older people.

When selecting a primary care doctor, a person may wish to consider what three or four qualities or characteristics are most important to him in a doctor (for example, friendliness and patience). Asking family members, friends, and other health care practitioners for recommendations is a good idea. Especially helpful is information from other older people about how well their doctor communicates with them.

Information about the credentials of most doctors is available by calling the American Board of Medical Specialties (866-275-2267 toll-free), by visiting their web site (www.abms.org), or by reviewing their book, which is available in many public libraries. The American Medical Association has similar information on their web site (www.ama-assn.org). Some state medical licensing boards and medical societies offer additional information.

Some practical issues to consider include whether the doctor participates in the person's health insurance plan and whether new patients are being accepted.

COMMUNICATING WITH A NEW PRIMARY CARE DOCTOR

The first meeting with a new doctor is the best time to begin establishing effective communication and ways in which to take an active role.

Before a Visit

Advance preparations can improve communication and help a first visit go more smoothly. Information about past hospitalizations, use of home health services, or care from any specialists or other health care practitioners (including any complementary or alternative medicine practitioners) should be given to the primary care doctor. If copies of written records have already been obtained, then a copy should be given to the new primary care doctor. Listing the names, addresses, and telephone numbers of practitioners and institutions where health care has been received assists the new doctor in acquiring important health information and records.

Bringing along the containers of any drugs currently being taken, including prescription and nonprescription drugs, is very important. Containers of vitamins, other nutritional supplements, and medicinal herbs should also be included. Bringing notes on any side effects experienced while taking drugs is a good idea and saves time. Also helpful is a list of the names and telephone numbers of pharmacies where the prescriptions were filled.

A medical history form may need to be completed in the waiting room, although sometimes the doctor's office mails this form before a visit. All medical forms should be completed as accurately as possible. Ideally, the person visiting the doctor answers the questions. However, if the person is unable to complete a medical history form alone, whoever provides assistance should strive to involve the person as much as possible.

Before the visit, it can be worthwhile to think about and possibly write down brief notes about exercise, sleep, diet, and use of caffeine, tobacco, and alcohol.

During a Visit

Difficulties with vision, hearing, or speech may make communication less effective. Glasses, hearing aids, or dentures, if normally used at home, should be worn during the visit. Informing the doctor and the office staff about a loss of vision, hearing, or speech at the outset of a visit creates an opportunity to improve communication. The doctor may be able to change the lighting of the examination room or provide an amplification device. Sometimes a person who has a loss of vision or hearing is tempted to find out if the doctor notices and, if the doctor notices, how long it takes. Some people simply do not want to admit to any vision, hearing, or speech loss. However, communication between the person and the doctor is more effective if honesty and pragmatism are the order of the day. If the person needs a translator, it is important that someone who can

IS THIS DOCTOR RIGHT FOR ME?

The process of choosing a primary care doctor can be aided by asking friends and family members the following questions concerning their doctor:

• What are the doctor's normal office hours and days?

• Is the doctor's office easy to get in and out of?

• Is the doctor prompt with appointment times?

• Who takes care of the doctor's patients outside of normal business hours or when the doctor is away?

• Who else is routinely involved in taking care of the doctor's patients (for example, nurses, physician's assistants)?

• Does the doctor take time to listen to your concerns?

• Does the doctor adequately explain a diagnosis?

• Do you trust the doctor's opinion?

• Does the doctor routinely blame old age as the cause of your problems?

• Does the doctor prescribe drugs without discussing their benefits and risks?

• Does the doctor prescribe drugs without discussing other alternatives?

• Does the doctor ask you about your wishes for end-of-life care and is he in accepting of your stated wishes?

• Does the doctor respond to your phone calls or electronic mail (e-mail)? If so, how quickly?

translate accompany the person or that the doctor be forewarned so that a translator is available.

A person should expect questions about his health habits. Questions may address sensitive topics, such as sexual practices or mistreatment by a caregiver. Other sensitive topics include problems with memory, bladder control, and balance. Clear and honest answers to all questions make the communication more effective.

A person's personal, religious, and cultural beliefs and values affect health care decisions and should be discussed with the primary care doctor. During this discussion, the doctor's attitudes and policies concerning the use of a living will or a durable power of attorney for health care should be asked about.[1] Mental preparation for such a discussion can help save time and improve future communication with the doctor.

Whether to bring a family member along to the office and whether to have this person in the examination room for part or

1. see pages 954 and 955

all of the visit are important considerations. A family member can help the person recall an important piece of information or provide perspective on aspects of illness. Some types of information, such as information on diet, are best received by several family members so that all of the information is retained. However, having a family member in the room can interfere with communication. A person may be reluctant to share certain kinds of information with the doctor when a family member is present, such as mental health symptoms, alcohol use, or sexual practices.

COMMUNICATING DURING SUBSEQUENT VISITS

Once a person has settled into a routine with a primary care doctor, communication is easy to take for granted. The person may assume that responsibility for effective communication falls on the doctor's shoulders. However, with a little planning, a person can form habits that will make him an equal partner in sharing information and thus enhance communication during future visits.

Before a Visit

Preparing a brief list of concerns or problems can prove very helpful. If more than a few items make their way onto the list, some priorities must be set. Keeping in mind the brevity of a typical visit, important items should be brought up first. Writing down questions for the doctor is also useful. Insurance information and payment for the office visit should be brought as well.

Letting the doctor know what has happened since the last visit is helpful. The person should bring information about any health care that has taken place elsewhere, including where it took place, who was involved, and a telephone number or address where additional details can be obtained. Records of measurements taken at home, such as blood pressure or blood sugar levels, should be brought as well. The doctor should also be told of any changes in drugs or of any major life changes, such as retirement, a move into a different home, or the death of a loved one.

QUESTIONS THAT GENERATE MORE QUESTIONS DURING A VISIT

General Question	Specific Questions	Comment
Is more information needed?	Is a test needed? How does one prepare for the test? Does the test have risks or side effects? What might be learned from the test? How will the test results be reported?	Having adequate information about a test helps increase the chances that a person will be well prepared. Good preparation improves the likelihood that the test will provide useful results.
What is the problem (diagnosis)?	What might have caused the problem? Does having the problem put anyone else at risk of developing the problem?	Information about the cause(s) of a problem helps give a sense of control to some people, because they may then be able to use this information to prevent future problems or to explain their problem to family members.
What is the outlook (prognosis)?	How long will this problem last? Is it permanent? Life threatening? What are the possible short-term effects of the problem? What are the possible long-term effects of the problem?	This type of information helps reduce fear of not knowing what to expect and allows people to plan.
What are the plans for taking care of what is wrong?		
• Drugs	For each drug, what are the common side effects? What	Information about using drugs helps reduce the chances of misusing a

General Question	Specific Questions	Comment
	should be done if too much of the drug is taken or if a dose is missed? Does this drug interact with foods or other drugs to cause side effects?	drug or of incurring a preventable side effect. It also increases the likelihood that a person will adhere to the doctor's recommendations.
• Surgery	For a planned operation, what is the goal of surgery? What is the likelihood of achieving that goal?	Information about surgery increases the chances that a person will have the assistance he needs when he returns home.
• Advice to change behavior	For a recommended change in behavior, what are the specific goals to be achieved, and what resources are available to help a person achieve those goals?	Behavior change often takes time and multiple trial-and-error attempts.
Who else will be involved?	Is a second opinion from a doctor who specializes in this type of problem needed?	Knowing the reason(s) why a particular specialist is recommended improves the chances that the person will follow through with the visit and with the specialist's recommendations.
What other resources are available?	Is useful and trustworthy information about the problem available in books or on the Internet?	Discussing ways to become better informed reduces the likelihood that a person will use unreliable information.

During a Visit

Being honest is a basic guiding principle of effective communication with a doctor. Unless a person is honest, the doctor cannot give the best care possible. For example, a person who under-reports or over-reports the pain he is experiencing greatly hinders the doctor's ability to help. A smoker who denies smoking or inaccurately describes his smoking habit undermines the doctor's efforts to assist. A person who has not been taking drugs as prescribed needs to tell the doctor and provide an explanation (for example, "I seem to get stomach cramps from the medicine" or "I can't afford the medicine").

Besides being forthcoming about symptoms and health habits, a person needs to express when he is unhappy with something the doctor has said or done. The doctor can acknowledge the person's feelings and take steps to resolve differences, but only if the person's viewpoint is known.

Usually, more is said or more takes place than is likely to be recalled after the visit. A person who brings a specific concern or problem to a visit may be told what tests are needed to gather additional information. The person may be given an explanation and a diagnosis for his concern or problem and the typical outlook for people with that particular problem. The doctor is also likely to describe detailed plans for treating the problem. Ways to prevent health problems may be discussed during some visits. The person should request an explanation of anything that is not understood.

A person may have to rely on more than memory to retain information. The doctor may offer to write down important information or provide handouts or other materials. However, the person may also wish to take notes or ask the doctor's permission to use a recording device during a visit. Such strategies help reduce the need for continually repeating questions and answers.

Toward the End of a Visit

The last portion of a visit is critical in determining the effectiveness of communication with the doctor. This is not the best time to bring up something completely new, because the doctor usually will not be able to take more time to address a last-minute item. Most doctors dread hearing the words, "Doctor, there is one more thing I would like to speak with you about today."

Rather, the end of a visit is an opportunity to have the most important information reviewed and summarized. A person can briefly repeat instructions and directions while the doctor listens, so that the doctor can verify that key points have been heard and understood. If certain issues were not addressed because of limited time, arrangements can be made to discuss those issues at the next visit. A longer visit can be scheduled for the next appointment, if necessary.

9

Continuity of Care

The days are long gone when one doctor, with the help of a nurse, provided all the health care a person needed. Now, older people are likely to see several health care practitioners. They may receive care from doctors, nurses, nurse practitioners, physician assistants, pharmacists, dietitians, physical or occupational therapists, social workers, and nurses' aides. They may have several doctors, each specializing in one organ system or problem.

Older people are also likely to move from one place of care to another. They may receive care in a doctor's office, in a hospital, in a rehabilitation facility, in a board-and-care facility, in an assisted living facility, in a nursing home, or at home. At the end of life, they may receive hospice care.

Ideally, all people involved in a person's health care, including the person receiving care, communicate and work with each other to coordinate health care. Also, all should agree on and understand the goals for health care. Then, changes in practitioners and places of care would occur smoothly, without disrupting care. This ideal is called continuity of care.

As worthwhile as continuity of care sounds, it is not always easy to accomplish because the health care system in the United States is complicated and fragmented. Once people enter the health care system, care seems to happen automatically, according to rules they do not understand and cannot change. So many health care practitioners are involved that if people have questions, they do not know which practitioner to ask. As a result, people may feel like a stone rolling downhill, with no control over what is happening or where they will end up.

People can help improve the continuity of their care. For example, they can learn more about what can interfere with continuity, how the health care system works, and what the system is doing to improve continuity of care. This information can help them take a more active part in their care.[1]

What Can Interfere With Continuity?

Having so many practitioners at so many places may disrupt the continuity of a person's health care. For example, one health care practitioner may not have up-to-date, accurate information about the care provided or recommended by other practitioners. That practitioner may not know who the other practitioners involved are or may not think to contact them. Information about care may be miscommunicated or misunderstood. The person receiving care may mention an important detail to one practitioner and forget to mention it to the others. If the practitioners involved do not have complete, up-to-date, and accurate information, inappropriate drugs or other treatments may be prescribed. Diagnostic tests may be needlessly repeated. Preventive measures may not be taken because each practitioner assumes someone else has provided them.

Different practitioners may have different opinions about a person's health care. For example, practitioners in a hospital may disagree with a person's primary care doctor about whether the person should go to a nursing home after being discharged. The person receiving care and family members may be overwhelmed and confused by differences of opinion among the various practitioners.

The health care system has many rules that affect continuity of care. The rules may be made by the government, insurance companies, or professional organizations for health care practitioners. For example, some insurance companies limit which

1. see page 112

DOCTORS BY ANY OTHER NAME

In the United States, most doctors are medical doctors (MDs), sometimes called allopaths. They are trained in conventional Western medicine. Some doctors, called doctors of osteopathic medicine (DOs) or osteopaths, also train in osteopathy. Osteopaths are taught that the whole person (body, mind, and spirit) and lifestyle should be considered and that the body has the ability to heal itself. Both types of doctors often obtain special training (specialize) in one area of medicine. Consequently, doctors go by many different names, indicating their specialty.

Allergists diagnose and treat allergies and certain sinus disorders.

Anesthesiologists provide care (particularly pain relief) just before, during, and just after surgery. They choose and administer the anesthetic. During surgery, they monitor the person so that they can adjust the amounts of anesthetic, other drugs, and fluids as needed.

Cardiologists are internists who diagnose and treat disorders of the heart.

Dermatologists diagnose and treat disorders of the skin, nails, and hair.

Endocrinologists are internists who diagnose and treat disorders of glands and hormones.

Family practice doctors study the needs of people from birth through old age. Thus, these doctors can provide continuous, comprehensive care for a person. They diagnose and treat a wide variety of disorders, referring people to other doctors as needed.

Gastroenterologists are internists who diagnose and treat disorders of the digestive tract.

Gynecologists provide health care for women. They perform preventive screening tests (such as yearly breast and pelvic examinations and Papanicolaou tests). They diagnose and treat disorders of the female reproductive system and perform surgery (such as hysterectomies).

Hematologists are internists who diagnose and treat disorders of blood and the organs that produce blood (such as the bone marrow).

Internists who provide comprehensive health care for adults are called general internists. They diagnose and treat a wide variety of common and complex disorders—an area called internal medicine. Some internists specialize in one area of medicine.

Nephrologists are internists who diagnose and treat kidney disorders. They also perform dialysis.

Neurologists diagnose and treat disorders of the brain, spinal cord, nerves, and muscles (which may be affected when nerves malfunction).

Oncologists are internists who diagnose and treat cancer. They may further specialize in cancers of one body system (such as the female reproductive system) or in a particular treatment of cancer (such as radiation or surgery).

Ophthalmologists diagnose and treat vision problems and eye disorders. They perform eye examinations, prescribe glasses and contact lenses, prescribe drugs to treat eye disorders, perform surgery, and manage eye problems due to other disorders.

Orthopedists, also called orthopedic surgeons, diagnose and treat disorders of the muscles and skeleton (including bones, ligaments, and tendons). They may further specialize in one part of the body (such as the foot) or in one area of care (such as trauma).

Otolaryngologists (otorhinolaryngologists) are surgeons who diagnose and treat ear, nose, and throat (ENT) disorders.

Physiatrists specialize in rehabilitation. They focus on helping people who have been disabled recover lost functions.

Psychiatrists diagnose and treat mental disorders (such as schizophrenia and bipolar disorder) and substance abuse. Some psychiatrists focus on counseling (psychotherapy), but most use a variety of treatments, including drugs. Geropsychiatrists specialize in mental health care for older people.

Pulmonologists are internists who diagnose and treat lung disorders.

Radiologists read x-rays and other images of internal structures taken to make a diagnosis. Radiologists also supervise imaging tests used for guidance during biopsies.

Rheumatologists diagnose and treat arthritis and other disorders that affect joints, muscles, bones, skin, and other tissues.

Surgeons perform operations for various disorders. They may further specialize in a specific part of the body, such as the heart and chest (as a cardiothoracic surgeon), or type of problem, such as malformed, missing, or lost tissues (as a plastic surgeon).

Urologists are surgeons who diagnose and treat disorders of the kidneys and urinary tract and male reproductive system.

hospital a person can go to. The person's doctor, if not on staff at that hospital, may be unable to provide care there.

Continuity of care may be disrupted when people do not have access to health care. Some older people do not have transportation to a doctor's office. Some do not have insurance and cannot afford to pay for health care themselves, so they may not see a doctor or specialist.

Who Provides Care?

For the best health care, a person may need to see several types of health care practitioners. Sometimes a group of health care practitioners work together to provide care for a person. This type of care is called interdisciplinary care.[1]

Doctors: Older people may see many different kinds of doctors: family practice doctors, general internists, specialists in

1. see page 112

WHO ARE GERIATRICIANS?

Geriatricians are internists or family practice doctors trained specifically to care for older people. This care often involves managing many disorders and problems at once. Geriatricians have studied how the body changes as it ages, so that they can better distinguish when a symptom is due to a disorder rather than to aging itself. They evaluate older people in terms of social and emotional as well as physical needs, then they can help older people live as independently as possible.

People who are most likely to benefit from seeing a geriatrician include those who are very frail, those who have many disorders, those who need to see several different types of health care practitioners, and those who take many drugs and are thus likely to experience side effects.

---

such areas as heart disorders (cardiologists) or cancer (oncologists), and surgeons.

Some doctors, called geriatricians, are trained specifically to care for older people. A geriatrician may be the person's primary care doctor or may be called in for a short time for consultation.

Nurses: Nurses check vital signs (blood pressure, pulse, and temperature), take samples of blood, give treatments, and teach people how to care for themselves. Nurses may ask about the person's health (for the medical history) and home situation. They may help coordinate care by communicating information to the different practitioners involved, the person, and family members.

Registered nurses (RNs) often provide most of a person's health care. Registered nurses supervise care provided by licensed practical nurses (LPNs) and nurses' aides. Registered nurses are taught to do a physical examination and check for changes that need to be evaluated by a doctor. They also can administer drugs to the person, as prescribed by a doctor. Licensed practical nurses may perform many functions but always under the supervision of a registered nurse.

Some nurses, called nurse practitioners, receive additional training in diagnosis and treatment. Thus, these nurses have more responsibilities than registered nurses. Some nurse practitioners, those called geriatric nurse practitioners, are specially trained to care for older people.

ADDING TO THE CONFUSION: OTHER SPECIALISTS

Some health care practitioners receive specialized training in one area of medicine but are neither medical doctors, doctors of osteopathy, nor nurses. Usually, they are licensed and certified in their specialty.

Audiologists evaluate the type and degree of hearing loss using a wide variety of tests. They prescribe and fit hearing aids. They also evaluate dizziness and provide balance training. They have a master's degree or doctorate in audiology and have completed a clinical internship.

Gerontologists have a master's degree or doctorate in gerontology—the study of the aging process, including physical, mental, and social changes. Gerontologists analyze information about older people to develop strategies and programs for improving their lives. They may work directly with older people or do research about them. Some gerontologists also have a medical degree and are geriatricians.

Orthotists fit braces and other supportive devices. They may be involved in rehabilitation.

Opticians translate an ophthalmologist's or optometrist's prescription into glasses or contact lenses that are suitable for a person's lifestyle and visual needs. They may grind the lenses of glasses and fit the lenses into the frame. To fit contact lenses, they measure the curve of the eye.

Optometrists are doctors of optometry—the evaluation of vision and use of lenses to correct vision. They perform the same functions as ophthalmologists except they do not prescribe drugs or perform surgery. However, they may care for people just before and just after surgery.

Podiatrists are doctors of podiatry. They diagnose and treat disorders of the foot and ankle and perform surgery on the foot.

Prosthetists fit replacements for body parts. They may be involved in rehabilitation.

Psychologists are doctors of psychology. They use talk therapies (counseling) to help people with phobias, depression, or emotional or family problems. In most states, they, unlike psychiatrists, cannot prescribe drugs.

Physician assistants: Physician assistants (PAs) perform some of the same functions as doctors and nurse practitioners but always with a doctor's supervision. Physician assistants ask about the person's health (for the medical history), perform physical examinations, order diagnostic tests, help doctors develop treatment plans, and assist in surgery. They do routine procedures, such as giving shots and stitching up wounds. Physician assistants also provide people with information about following their treatment plan and taking care of themselves (such as information about a healthy diet and exercise).

Physician assistants work in most places of care, including long-term care facilities. They may provide health care in a person's home. Some physician assistants specialize in treating older people.

Pharmacists: In addition to dispensing drugs, pharmacists evaluate prescriptions to make sure that appropriate drugs are being used. Pharmacists can check to make sure that older people are not taking drugs that pose special risks for them.[1] Pharmacists also make sure that instructions are clear and include information about how much and how often a drug is to be used. They keep track of a person's prescriptions and refills. In this way, they can check for interactions between drugs.

Some pharmacists specialize in the care of older people. They are sometimes called consultant (senior care) pharmacists. They often work in nursing homes. They provide other practitioners with information about how to use drugs appropriately.

Dietitians: Dietitians assess how well nutritional needs are being met. When needs are not being met, they provide specific recommendations about which foods to choose and how to prepare foods.

Therapists: Different types of therapists may be needed, depending on the disorders and problems a person has. Physical therapists evaluate and treat people who have difficulty moving—for example, difficulty walking, changing positions (standing up, sitting down, or lying down), transferring from bed to chair, lifting, or bending.[2] They work with people who have had problems such as a stroke, amputation of a limb, or hip surgery. Treatments may include exercise, heat, and ultrasound. Occupational therapists evaluate and treat people who have difficulty caring for themselves (for example, dressing or bathing), working, and doing other daily activities.[3] Speech therapists help people who have difficulty using and understanding language.[4]

Social workers: Social workers help coordinate discharges from hospitals and transfers between institutions. They may help people fill out insurance and other forms. They help people

1. see table on pages 52 to 57
2. see page 171
3. see page 177
4. see page 179

identify services that can be provided in the home and community and often help arrange for these services. They also evaluate how people are responding to the care and services obtained.

Social workers may bring family members together for discussions about important health care issues. Many social workers counsel people with anxiety, depression, or difficulty coping with a disorder or disability.

Most social workers are familiar with the special needs of older people. But some are specially trained to counsel older people and to determine whether they need supervision or additional help.

Nurses' aides: Nurses' aides care for people in hospitals, rehabilitation facilities, nursing homes, assisted living communities, or other medical facilities under the direction of nurses, doctors, and other medical staff members. They are sometimes trained to do some simple assessments of health. For example, an aide may measure temperature, pulse, and blood pressure. Nurses' aides may respond to signal lights or bells indicating that someone needs help. They bathe, dress, and undress people. They serve and collect food trays and feed people who need help eating.

Home health aides: Employed by home health care agencies, home health aides do many of the same tasks that nurses' aides do, but in the home. They help with daily activities, especially with dressing and grooming. These aides may prepare meals, help the person out of a wheelchair, or take the person for a walk. They sometimes help with light housework. They may also do some simple health assessments under the supervision of a registered nurse.

Medical ethicists: Medical ethicists help resolve conflicts over moral issues that come up during health care. For example, health care practitioners and family members may disagree about whether a treatment that appears to be ineffective should be stopped. Medical ethicists may be doctors, other health care practitioners, lawyers, or other people who have been specially trained in medical ethics. Some hospitals have a medical ethicist or a team of medical ethicists on staff.

Where Is Care Provided?

Health care practitioners may work in a variety of places.

Doctor's office: Most older people receive medical care as outpatients. That is, they see their doctor in an office, then they go home. A doctor's office is a suite of rooms where a doctor can take a person's medical history and perform a physical examination. The office may be in a medical office building, a clinic, a hospital, or elsewhere. Diagnostic tests, such as blood tests or x-rays, are often done in a doctor's office. If not, they may be done at a nearby clinic. Some doctors' offices offer certain treatments, such as physical therapy.

Hospitals: Hospitals provide the most comprehensive medical care, usually to people who are very sick. Older people may enter the hospital through the emergency department, or they may be scheduled for admission by a doctor.[1]

A doctor (who may be the person's primary care doctor, a specialist, or a staff doctor at the hospital) is in charge of the person's care in the hospital. Sometimes several other doctors are involved. Nurses, who are available 24 hours a day, provide much of the care. A nurse is always available, but doctors may come and go at more irregular times.

Many other people may help provide care in a hospital. They include pharmacists, dietitians, physical and occupational therapists, social workers, medical technicians, nurses' aides, and volunteers.

How long a person stays in the hospital depends partly on how sick the person is, what the diagnosis is, and, if needed, what arrangements for continuing care can be made after discharge. The health care practitioners involved determine whether and what type of continuing care is needed. This care may be provided in a rehabilitation facility, in a long-term care facility, or in the person's home by a visiting nurse.

Rehabilitation facilities: After discharge from the hospital, people with a severe disability may need to continue their recovery in a rehabilitation facility.[2] A facility may be located in a hospital or a nursing home. These facilities provide skilled nursing care and physical, occupational, and speech therapy. When people are discharged to a rehabilitation facility, doc-

1. see page 143
2. see page 167

tors predetermine how long their stay will be. For older people, the stay ranges from several weeks to a few months. Goals for progress are set, and progress is evaluated every day. Thus, the types and amount of therapy can be adjusted as needed. Some older people need to come to a rehabilitation facility periodically for therapy. Appointments can be scheduled for them.

Long-term care facilities: When older people need more help than can be provided at home and need it for an indefinite time, a long-term care facility may be appropriate. Older people or family members can choose among several living arrangements that provide different services and levels of health care.[1]

Board-and-care facilities provide a room, meals, and some help with daily activities. Some facilities provide certain basic health care. Assisted living communities are similar. But they provide more health care, and most provide 24-hour supervision of the resident if needed. Some of these facilities have a registered nurse on site.

Nursing homes provide nursing care, including giving residents their drugs, in addition to help with daily activities. Nursing homes have at least one registered nurse on site at all times. They also employ licensed practical nurses and nurses' aides. Some homes provide physical and occupational therapy.

Life-care communities provide different levels of services and care, depending on need. Life-care communities guarantee that people, regardless of their health, are cared for within the community for the rest of their life.

Home health care: After discharge from the hospital, many older people who are well enough to go home need some health care services. Often, home health care agencies also provide some help with daily activities. These agencies employ registered nurses, therapists, home health aides, and social workers.

Some people need home health care for a short time after they leave the hospital. For example, a nurse may be needed to change wound dressings. Other people, especially those with a chronic disorder, need home health care for a longer time. People with a heart or lung disorder may need a nurse to visit regularly and check whether they are worsening or improving. The nurse can also adjust a drug dose if needed. Or a nurse may regularly visit people with diabetes to make sure they are following

1. see page 190

their treatment plan, to monitor drug use, and to adjust doses as needed. A physical therapist may be needed to help people regain strength and balance or recover from a stroke. A home health aide may be needed to help with shopping, preparing meals, going out in a wheelchair, taking a walk, or bathing. A social worker can assess whether people are receiving the services they need and recommend additional services if needed. A social worker may help arrange for rides to and from medical appointments.

Community services: In the United States, one source of support services and health care in the community is senior centers. In addition to social, recreational, and educational activities, some senior centers serve meals—an important service for people who cannot prepare their own. Often, senior centers are a place where family members who care for a person full-time can take the person and get a break from care (a service called respite care).

Many senior centers also provide some health care. For example, some senior centers have a nurse on duty at least a few days a week. The nurse can check blood pressure, make sure people are taking their drugs as instructed, and teach people about their disorders. The nurse also helps people with health problems determine whether they need to see a doctor. Sometimes the nurse contacts a person's doctor or family members. Some senior centers provide day care for people with mild to moderate dementia, and some provide physical and occupational therapy.

Other services available in the community include meal programs (such as Meals on Wheels), transportation services, help with daily activities, support groups, and respite care. Some religious communities provide many of these services. These services are usually inexpensive, and some are free.

Information about community services, including senior centers, can be obtained from the hospital (discharge planning or case management department), home health care agencies, local health departments, and religious communities. Senior centers can also be found by looking in a local telephone book or on the Internet.

Day hospitals: Day hospitals provide hospital care only during the day. They are usually located in a hospital. They enable people to have complex tests and treatments without having to check into an overnight (inpatient) hospital. Day hospitals are particularly useful for people who need rehabilitation over a period of time—for example, for people who have had a stroke or amputation of a leg. These hospitals also provide meals and transportation to and from medical appointments and therapy sessions.

The primary care doctor or a hospital may send a person to a day hospital. Day hospitals are usually used for a limited period of time (6 weeks to 6 months).

Hospice care: For people who have a progressive, incurable disorder, hospice care provides the treatments and services needed to control symptoms, ease pain, and help people and their family members prepare for the death.[1] Hospice care may be provided in a person's home, in a nursing home, or in a hospice facility.

Hospice care usually involves a doctor, nurse, and social worker trained to care for dying people. Pharmacists, counselors, physical therapists, ethicists, and volunteers may also be involved. These practitioners are needed to make sure that all of the person's physical and psychologic needs are met as well as possible. Most people who receive hospice care do not have to transfer to a hospital before they die. Thus, they can die in a more comfortable, intimate environment, often with loved ones around them. Hospice care also involves helping family members prepare for the death and understand what to do when a person dies.

How to Improve Continuity

Improving continuity of care requires efforts by the health care system, by the people receiving care, and by their family members.

Health care system: Managed care organizations[2] and some government health care plans coordinate all health care and thus contribute to continuity of care. Also, the health care system has developed several strategies to improve continuity of care. Examples are interdisciplinary care and geriatric case managers.

Interdisciplinary care is coordinated care provided by many

1. see page 223
2. see page 968

types of practitioners, including doctors, nurses, pharmacists, dietitians, physical and occupational therapists, and social workers. These practitioners make a conscious, organized effort to communicate, cooperate, and agree with each other about a person's care. Interdisciplinary care aims to ensure that people move safely and easily from one place of care to another and from one health care practitioner to another. It also aims to ensure that the most qualified health care practitioner provides care for each problem and that care is not duplicated. Interdisciplinary care is not available everywhere.

Interdisciplinary care is important when treatment is complex or when it involves movement from one place of care to another. People who are most likely to benefit include those who are very frail, those who have many disorders, those who need to see several different types of health care practitioners, and those who experience side effects from drugs.

The practitioners who care for a particular person are called the interdisciplinary team. One practitioner, often the person's primary care doctor, coordinates care.

Sometimes the interdisciplinary team consists of health care practitioners who do not work together on a regular basis (an ad hoc team). In other situations, the team has the same team members—a group of practitioners who usually work together and who care for many people (an established team). Some nursing homes, hospitals, and hospice organizations have established teams.

Team members discuss plans for treatment and inform each other about changes in the person's health, changes in treatment, and results of examinations and tests. They make sure that the person's records are up-to-date and that the records accompany the person through the health care system. Such efforts help make changes in places of care or in health care practitioners smoother and less traumatic. Also, tests are less likely to be repeated unnecessarily, and mistakes or omissions in treatment are less likely.

The interdisciplinary team also includes the older person being cared for and family members or other caregivers. For effective interdisciplinary care, these people must actively participate in care and must communicate with the health care practitioners on the team.

Geriatric care managers are specialists who make sure that an older person receives all the help and care needed. Most geriatric care managers are social workers or nurses. They may be members of an interdisciplinary team. Geriatric care managers can make arrangements for the services needed and supervise these arrangements. For example, care managers may arrange for a home nurse to visit several times a day or for an aide to help with housecleaning and preparation of meals. They may locate a pharmacy that delivers drugs or arrange for transportation to and from the doctor's office. Geriatric care managers are relatively uncommon.

People receiving care: Actively participating in health care is crucial to improving continuity of care. Active participation begins with communication—giving and getting information.[1] When older people have special health care needs, they or their family members should tell their health care practitioners. For example, some older people need help determining which health care costs are covered by Medicare, Medicaid, and other health care insurance.

When an interdisciplinary team or geriatric care manager is unavailable, people who are receiving care or their family members may need to become proactive in care. For example, they may need to ask one health care practitioner to call and talk with another to make sure treatment is appropriate. They need to establish a good relationship with at least one health care practitioner, usually the primary care doctor, to minimize the problems created by having several health care practitioners.

Active participation includes seeing a health care practitioner (usually the primary care doctor) regularly and following the instructions of health care practitioners. It means asking questions about a disorder, treatment, or other aspect of care. It includes learning how to prevent disorders and taking the appropriate steps to do so.

For people who have a disorder, active participation may involve self-monitoring. For example, people with high blood pressure can regularly monitor their blood pressure. People with diabetes can regularly check the level of sugar in their blood.

Keeping a copy of their medical record can help people participate in their health care. They can often obtain a copy from

1. see page 93

their doctor. Keeping a copy of the medical record is useful as a reference for information about disorders present, drugs being taken, treatments and tests done, and payments made. This information can also help people explain a problem to a health care practitioner. File boxes, binders, computer software, and Internet programs have been designed for this purpose.

When people go to a hospital or to a new health care practitioner, they should check with someone at the new location to make sure that their medical record has been received.

Buying all drugs (prescription and nonprescription) at one pharmacy or through one mail order service and getting to know a pharmacist there are also important.[1] Older people can ask their pharmacist questions about the drugs they are taking. They can also ask for containers that are easy to open and labels that are easy to read.

10

Understanding Medical Tests

Much of health care revolves around the use of tests. Medical tests—some of which may also be referred to as procedures or studies—allow health care practitioners to gather information about a person's health and ability to function. Few medical tests are designed specifically for older people. But older people tend to undergo more medical tests in large part because they are at higher risk of developing many diseases. Moreover, older people, compared with younger people, often face very different challenges while preparing for and undergoing many medical tests. In addition, as people age, their test results and the way in which those results are interpreted often change.

1. see pages 59 and 107

Types of Medical Tests

Medical tests generally fall into one of six categories:

- Analysis of body fluids and contents
- Imaging tests
- Endoscopy
- Measurement of body functions
- Biopsy
- Analysis of genetic material in cells.

In many instances, two or more types of tests are combined in a single procedure, and the lines that separate the categories become blurred. For example, endoscopy of the stomach enables the examiner to view the inside of the stomach and obtain tissue samples for examination in a laboratory.

Analysis of body fluids and contents most often consists of tests of blood, urine, and the fluid that surrounds the spinal cord and brain (cerebrospinal fluid). Less often, fluids such as sweat and saliva and the contents of the digestive tract (for example, gastric juices and stool samples) are analyzed. In some instances, fluids being analyzed are present only in the case of disease. For example, in many liver diseases, fluid accumulates in the abdomen (ascites). In some lung diseases, fluid accumulates in the space between the membranes that surround the lungs (pleural effusion).

Imaging tests provide a picture of the inside of the body. Ordinary x-rays are the most common imaging tests. Others include mammograms, ultrasound scans, radioisotope (nuclear) scans, computed tomography (CT) scans, magnetic resonance imaging (MRI) scans, and positron emission tomography (PET) scans.

Endoscopy is the use of a tube to directly view the inside of body organs or spaces (cavities). Most endoscopes are flexible, although a limited number are rigid. The tip of the endoscope is usually equipped with a light and a camera so that the images can be seen simultaneously on a television monitor. Tools passed through a channel in the endoscope can be used to cut and remove tissue samples, destroy abnormal tissue, and close off bleeding blood vessels.

The endoscope is usually passed through an existing body opening. For example, esophagogastroduodenoscopy (EGD)

VIEWING THE DIGESTIVE TRACT WITH AN ENDOSCOPE

A flexible tube called an endoscope is used to view different parts of the digestive tract. The tube contains several channels along its length. One channel is used to transmit light to the area being examined. Another channel has a camera at its end. The camera lens can be used for viewing. Fluids or air can be pumped in or out through another channel. Biopsy or surgical instruments can be passed through yet another channel. When an endoscope is passed through the mouth, it can be used to examine the esophagus, the stomach, and some of the small intestine. When passed through the anus, an endoscope can be used to examine the rectum and the entire large intestine. The instrument used in the different procedures varies only in length and size of the tube.

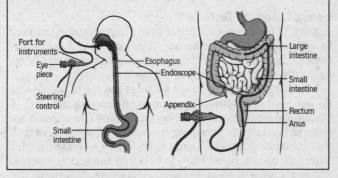

involves passing an endoscope through the mouth. Colonoscopy involves passing an endoscope through the anus. However, sometimes a small cut (incision) is made in the skin so that an endoscope can be passed into a body cavity. For example, arthroscopy involves passing an endoscope through an incision to view a joint, such as the knee.

Measurement of body functions often involves recording and analyzing the electrical activity of an organ. For example, electrical activity of the heart is measured with electrocardiography (ECG); and electrical activity of the brain is measured with electroencephalography (EEG). Other body functions that can be measured include how much and how fast air moves in and out of the lungs, the amount of blood pumped by the heart over a certain amount of time, and the ability of the kidneys to excrete waste products and excess water.

Biopsy involves examining tissue samples, usually with a microscope. This examination usually is used to determine the presence of abnormal cells that might provide evidence of inflammation or a cancer. Tissues commonly examined include skin, breast, lung, liver, kidney, and bone marrow.

Analysis of genetic material usually involves testing cells from skin, blood, or bone marrow. Older adults do not commonly undergo genetic testing for the purpose of determining whether they themselves have or are at increased risk of developing a disease. More often, they may undergo genetic testing to help determine the likelihood that their children or grandchildren will develop certain diseases.

Uses of Medical Tests

Medical tests have a variety of uses. Frequently, they are used to screen for or diagnose disease. Tests may also be used to determine the severity or extent of disease and to monitor how well a disease is responding to treatment.

Screening tests are designed to detect disease in people who do not have symptoms. For example, measuring the level of cholesterol may identify an abnormality that can increase the risk of a heart attack. Screening is usually performed when finding and treating a disease early is preferable to doing so later. Screening tests are most likely to be useful and widely accepted if they are accurate, pose few health risks, cause little or no discomfort, and are relatively inexpensive.

Diagnostic tests, on the other hand, are designed to confirm the presence of a disease when there is already suspicion or evidence that a person has the disease. For example, a doctor who suspects coronary artery disease in a person who gets chest pain during an exercise stress test might recommend cardiac angiography.

Cardiac angiography is not a good choice for screening because it can produce serious side effects, can be uncomfortable, and is expensive. These drawbacks are outweighed by the need for cardiac angiography, however, when the presence or absence of coronary artery disease must be confirmed.

Medical tests are also used to classify diseases into categories for the purpose of planning specific and effective treatment. For example, after a diagnosis of breast cancer is confirmed,

THE MEDICAL HISTORY AND PHYSICAL EXAMINATION

Doctors have long been taught that much can be learned about a person's health simply by taking a medical history and performing a thorough physical examination. Sometimes this is all that the doctor needs to do to screen for, diagnose, or monitor a disease. However, in many cases, the history and examination may not provide enough information.

Doctors may ask questions in a specific way. For example, they may inquire about sadness by inquiring of every person, "Have you felt sad nearly every day for at least 2 weeks?" They may also consistently check for physical findings in a specific way. For example, they may check strength in the arms by asking every person to hold a fist up to the shoulder joint and keep it there while trying to pull it away.

Some doctors go one step further by using a standardized questionnaire or a standardized performance test. Standardized means that the exact same questions are asked in the same way, or the exact same tasks are performed. Standardized questionnaires may be used, for example, to screen for depression, confusion, excessive use of alcohol, and limitations in the ability to function.

additional tests are performed to determine if the cancer cells have special sites, called receptors, where estrogen attaches. The results influence decisions about which drugs to use to treat breast cancer.

Tests are sometimes used to monitor how well a person is responding to treatment. For example, blood tests are performed periodically in people with hypothyroidism to determine if the dosage of thyroid hormone replacement needs adjustment.

Certain tests lend themselves to both gathering information and treating disease. A colonoscopy, for example, may be done to detect abnormal growths, such as polyps, and then, if growths are found, to remove them immediately.

Making Decisions About Tests

Medical tests may give rise to a variety of questions. The best decisions about medical tests are reached when the doctor's experience and knowledge are combined with the person's knowledge, wishes, and values.

Most doctors rely heavily on their experience when recommending and ordering tests. Doctors learn more about tests by reading medical books and journals, consulting with colleagues, attending educational conferences, and referring to other resources, such as the Internet. They may also review recommendations (practice guidelines) published by groups of experts. In addition, doctors evaluate the results of research studies and consider how the findings might be applied.

People rely most heavily on their doctors for information on medical tests. Many people also turn to an ever-growing number of resources in print and on the Internet, but determining whether these resources are based on scientifically sound information can be challenging.

When deciding whether to recommend a screening test for a disease, the doctor estimates how likely it is that a person has the disease. The doctor considers whether the person has risk factors. The doctor may also consider how common the disease is in a population of people who have many of the same characteristics as the person (prevalence) and how many new cases of the disease occur during a specific period of time in that population (incidence). With this information, the doctor can then begin to select the best test with which to confirm or exclude the presence of the disease.

When deciding whether to perform a test, a doctor must consider what the range of possible results may mean. Unfortunately, medical tests are not perfect. Sometimes tests produce normal results in people who in fact have the disease (false-negative results). On the other hand, tests sometimes produce abnormal results in people who do not have the disease (false-positive results). Therefore, the doctor considers the test's sensitivity and specificity. Sensitivity is the likelihood that the test will produce abnormal results in people who do have the disease. Specificity is the likelihood that the test will produce normal results in people who do not have the disease.

A test must also be reliable. A reliable test gives the same result or nearly so when a person undergoes the test more than once under the same circumstances. In contrast, results from an unreliable test may change each time the test is done, making interpretation difficult or impossible.

A doctor must also consider how the results will be used. A test may not be warranted if the results will not change the recommended treatment plan. For example, if a test is being considered to determine the advisability of starting a particular treatment but the person and his doctor have already decided not to undergo that treatment, then the test need not be performed. Before performing a test, a doctor weighs the potential harm against the potential benefit.

Challenges Faced by Older People

Older people face a variety of challenges in preparing for and undergoing medical tests. Most tests, even many considered simple and safe, pose potential problems for older people. The higher risk of a problem occurring may be due in part to aging and to a higher likelihood of having one or more chronic diseases. The potential problems also depend on the specific test being considered. Few, if any, tests are problem free.

Following test instructions or understanding explanations may be difficult for some older people and may impede test taking. Such difficulty may arise because of vision or hearing loss. Written instructions may benefit some people. Large-print versions of written instructions may help, as may a simple voice amplifier. Memory or the ability to understand and follow instructions (cognition) may be impaired. People with severe cognitive impairment may become frightened or upset because they are not able to understand instructions or explanations. A family member or caregiver may need to remain with the person during testing to provide reassurance. Soft, soothing music played during the test may have a calming effect.

Problems with balance and moving around (mobility) may also affect testing. Older people are more likely to have diseases that interfere with balance and mobility. Decreased mobility and balance can make it difficult, for example, to get to the testing facility or to climb onto the tables used in magnetic resonance imaging (MRI) and computed tomography (CT) scanners. Testing may be made easier and safer if railings, assistive devices (such as walkers), and small portable steps or stools are available. Surroundings that are well lit also improve safety.

Chronic pain may make it difficult to lie motionless or to change positions during certain tests. Cushions or pillows may be used to reduce pain and pressure on a specific area of the body.

The fragile, thin skin of older people may be easily torn or cut in the process of moving on or off equipment. A bit of extra time and caution may be needed to avoid damaging the skin.

Questions to Ask the Doctor

An older person as well as family members and friends can become better informed about an upcoming medical test by asking the doctor the following questions:

- Why is the test being done?
- How is the test done?
- How do I prepare for the test?
- What can I expect to happen during and after the test?
- What are some potential problems that the test may cause?
- What are considered to be normal results?

The person may also want to know how long the test takes, what factors may affect test results, when test results will be available, and what may need to be done after the test results are known.

SPECIFIC TESTS

Hundreds of different medical tests exist. Some tests are performed so often that it almost seems odd to find an older person who has not undergone such a test at least once. Other tests are done so infrequently that most people will never have them done. But many tests, because they fall somewhere in between, are likely to generate questions. Several such tests are discussed below.

Bone Densitometry

Other names: Dual-energy x-ray absorptiometry (DEXA).

Related tests: Closely related bone densitometry tests include single- or dual-energy photon absorptiometry and single-energy x-ray absorptiometry.

Why the test is done: Bone densitometry measures bone density to determine whether a person has or is at high risk of developing osteoporosis. In osteoporosis, porous (less dense) bones are weak and more likely to break. Certain bones, including those of the hip, spine, and wrist, are especially likely to become porous and warrant particular attention.

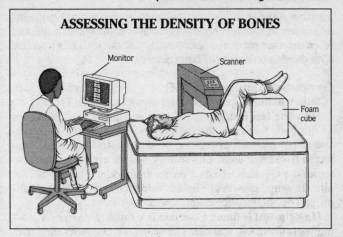

ASSESSING THE DENSITY OF BONES

Monitor

Scanner

Foam cube

How the test is done: A bone densitometry scanner analyzes changes in x-ray beams as they pass through the body. These changes are then analyzed to calculate bone density.

Preparing for the test: Minimal preparation is needed. The person is usually instructed to wear comfortable, loose-fitting clothes that are free of buttons, snaps, zippers, and wire supports. Medications are not affected by the test and need not be changed.

What to expect during the test: The person is helped onto a special table and is instructed to lie flat. A scanner is then positioned overhead. The technician remains in the room while the test is underway. The person can hear soft buzzing and can watch the scanner as it changes positions to obtain views of specific bones. The test usually lasts about 10 to 20 minutes.

Most people find the test to be simple and painless. People who find it difficult to lie flat, such as those with arthritis or chronic obstructive pulmonary disease (COPD), may experience discomfort.

What to expect after the test: Usual activities can be resumed immediately after the test is finished.

Potential problems: Bone densitometry is very safe. The small amount of radiation the person is exposed to is less than that from a simple chest x-ray.

Results in older people: Test results may be more difficult to interpret. Osteoarthritis, accumulation of calcium in ligaments, or a history of broken bones (especially in the spine, a site that often receives particular attention during the test) can interfere with the determination of bone density.

Computed Tomography (CT)

Other names: Computed axial tomography (CAT).

Why the test is done: A CT scan is done to provide images of the body's interior for the purpose of detecting structural abnormalities, such as tumors, dead tissue (infarctions), or infected tissue that cannot be seen on simple x-rays. In some instances, a CT scan assists a doctor in guiding a hollow needle into abnormal growths or tissue inside the body so that a sample can be obtained for examination.

How the test is done: Continuous x-rays are taken by a moving part of the CT scanner. The scanner's computer then uses information on how the x-rays penetrated specific tissues to generate pictures. The detailed pictures show the body in "slices" (cross-sectional views) from head to toe (as if looking down through the head or up through the feet). Some newer scanners can create 3-dimensional images of the body. In contrast, simple x-rays view the body from front to back, back to front, or side to side. In CT scanning, sometimes a dye is injected into a vein to highlight certain structures, such as blood vessels and specific organs. Alternatively, people undergoing CT scanning of the digestive tract may be asked to swallow dye mixed in a drink.

Preparing for the test: The person is asked to wear comfortable, loose-fitting clothing free of buttons, snaps, zippers, and wire supports. When use of a dye is planned, the person is asked about allergies to the dye. If a dye is to be injected or swallowed, the person is asked to refrain from eating for several hours and from drinking for at least 1 hour before the test. Most medications are not affected by the test and need not be changed. Metformin, a drug for diabetes, can be harmful if dye is used.

What to expect during the test: The person is asked to remove any jewelry that might interfere with the quality of the pictures. The person lies flat on a motorized scanner table. If dye is to be injected, an intravenous line is inserted. If dye is to be swallowed, a drink containing the dye is provided. Once the person is properly positioned, the table moves into a large tube that contains the x-ray device. The tube then rotates around the person, taking multiple pictures. With older scanners, the test may take 10 to 20 minutes, depending on how much of the body is being scanned. With newer scanners (helical, or spiral, scanners; high-speed multi-slice scanners), the table moves quickly and steadily through the tube. A complete scan of the entire body may take less than a minute.

Most people find the test to be simple and painless. However, a few experience discomfort, especially those who find it difficult to lie flat. Occasionally, people who fear being in a confined space (claustrophobia) may be uncomfortable during a CT scan of the head or upper body. When the test involves injection of a dye, the person may experience a brief sensation of warmth and a metallic taste.

What to expect after the test: Usual activities can be resumed immediately after the test. If dye has been used, usually the person is advised to drink extra fluids for the rest of the day.

Potential problems: The amount of radiation to which the person is exposed, although more than that from a simple chest x-ray, is still considered to be safe. Uncommonly, a person has an allergic reaction to the dye.

Magnetic Resonance Imaging (MRI)

Other names: Magnetic resonance scanning.

Why the test is done: An MRI scan is done to provide images of the body's interior for the purpose of detecting abnormalities, such as tumors and dead or infected tissue, that cannot be seen on simple x-rays.

How the test is done: An MRI scanner, which is a large magnet, produces a magnetic field. The magnetic field causes certain molecules within the person's body to undergo a very brief change. Radio waves are then passed through the body. A computer creates detailed pictures using information about how the radio waves were affected by different tissues and structures. The pictures show the body in "slices" (cross-sectional views) from head to toe (as if looking down through the head or up through the feet), from side to side, and from front to back. A dye is sometimes injected into a vein to highlight certain structures, such as blood vessels and specific organs.

The strength of the magnetic field makes undergoing an MRI unsafe for people with certain electronic or metallic materials in their body, such as pacemakers, cochlear implants, and clips used to repair blood vessels. People who have had recent surgery should not undergo an MRI scan.

Preparing for the test: The person is asked to wear comfortable, loose-fitting clothing that is free of buttons, snaps, zippers, and wire supports. Items with magnetic strips (such as credit cards) and most kinds of metal cannot be worn or otherwise taken into the scanner room because of the effects of the strong magnet even when the machine is not scanning. Medications are not affected by the test and need not be changed.

What to expect during the test: The person lies flat on a scanner table and is told to remain as still as possible. If dye is to be injected, an intravenous line is inserted. If a closed scanner is being used, the table moves the person into a large tube that contains the magnet. In open scanners, the table is open on all four sides. The magnet is contained within an overhead arm. The scanner produces a thumping or knocking sound that can be heard while pictures are being produced. The sound from closed scanners is louder than that from open scanners. The test usually takes about 20 to 30 minutes, although some complex scans may take 45 to 60 minutes.

Most people find the test to be simple and painless. A few experience discomfort, especially those who find it difficult to lie flat. People who find the thumping or knocking sound disturbing or worrisome are usually offered ear protectors to help dampen the noise. Recordings of music or soothing sounds may also help the person relax. People who fear being in a confined space (claustrophobia) may be uncomfortable in a closed scanner. An open scanner may be an alternative, or a drug may be given to help reduce or control anxiety.

What to expect after the test: Usual activities can be resumed immediately after the test.

Potential problems: MRI scanning is very safe. Rarely, a person has an allergic reaction to the dye.

Positron Emission Tomography (PET)
Other names: None.
Why the test is done: Most often, a PET scan of the entire

body is done to detect cancer, to determine if cancer has spread, or to monitor how well cancer is responding to treatment. Sometimes a PET scan is done to determine how well a part of the body, such as the brain or heart, is functioning. The test can also measure blood flow. These results help detect tissue that has been damaged by a disease or an injury.

How the test is done: A substance that is known to be used by specific cells or tissues in the body, such as glucose, is attached to radioactive material. A small amount of this combination is then injected into the blood. The radioactive material gives off particles, called positrons, which can be measured with a special detecting instrument. Abnormal areas are then displayed. Some devices combine PET scanning and CT scanning to produce cross-sectional (slices as if looking down through the head or up through the feet) or 3-dimensional views.

Preparing for the test: The person is asked to wear comfortable, loose-fitting clothing. For about 24 hours before undergoing a PET scan of the brain, the person is told to avoid alcohol, caffeine, and any tobacco products or drugs that might alter mental function (such as sedatives). For several hours before undergoing a PET scan that includes the abdomen, the person is asked to refrain from eating or drinking. Most medications are not affected by the test. However, the scheduling of certain drugs, for example, those used to treat diabetes, may need to be adjusted.

What to expect during the test: Before the test is started, an intravenous line is inserted so that the radioactive material can be injected. Throughout much of the test, the person lies flat. At times the person may be asked to perform certain activities, depending on the part of the body being studied. For example, if the test is measuring brain function, the person may be asked to perform mental tasks that stimulate certain parts of the brain. The test takes about 1 to 2 hours. Most people find the test to be simple and painless. A few experience discomfort, especially those who find it difficult to lie flat.

What to expect after the test: Usual activities can be resumed immediately after the test.

Potential problems: A PET scan is safe.

Nuclear Scan

Other names: Radionuclide scan.

Why the test is done: A nuclear scan may be done for a variety of reasons, depending on the type of scan. A thyroid scan is done to determine whether nodules are producing thyroid hormone. A cardiac scan is done to assess damage after a heart attack or to determine how well the heart is able to pump blood. A lung scan may be done to determine if a clot is present (pulmonary embolus) and to assess the resulting damage. A gallbladder scan is used to identify inflammation and to determine if bile is draining appropriately from the gallbladder. A renal (kidney) scan is done to identify kidney problems and disorders, including abnormal blood flow, tumors, and infections. A gallium scan (named for gallium, which is the radioactive material used in the test) is done to locate areas of infection or tumor. A bone scan is done to find cancer or infection in bones.

How the test is done: A small amount of a radioactive material is injected into the blood. The radioactivity can be measured with a special detecting scanner to determine where the radioactive material is accumulating and how long it is taking to do so. Areas of activity are used to construct images of the body.

Preparing for the test: Preparation depends on the type of scan. Many types, such as bone scans, heart scans, and gallium scans, may not require any preparation. However, before undergoing a gallbladder scan, the person is asked to refrain from eating or drinking for several hours. Generally, medications are not affected by the test. However, the scheduling of certain drugs, for example, those used to treat diabetes, may need to be adjusted.

What to expect during the test: Because radioactive material is to be injected, an intravenous line is inserted. The person lies flat on a scanner table, under the scanner and camera, and is told to remain as still as possible while a set of pictures is taken.

Some types of nuclear scans involve taking several sets of pictures over several hours to measure the accumulation of radioactive material. Picture taking is separated by periods when the person can rest or get up and move about. Each set of pictures may be completed in 20 to 30 minutes, but repeated sets can take up to 3 days to complete.

Most people find nuclear scans to be simple and painless. However, some experience discomfort, for example, because of the need to lie flat.

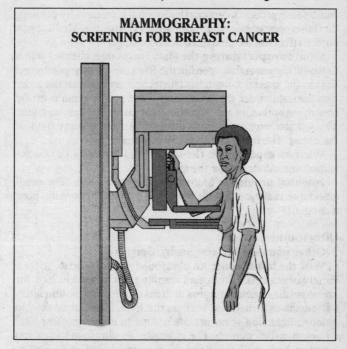

**MAMMOGRAPHY:
SCREENING FOR BREAST CANCER**

What to expect after the test: Usual activities can be resumed immediately after the test.

Potential problems: Nuclear scanning is safe in almost all people.

Mammography

Other names: None.

Why the test is done: A screening mammogram is done to look for evidence of breast cancer in women who do not have symptoms of breast cancer. A mammogram may also be done to further evaluate a previously identified lump.

How the test is done: Simple x-rays are taken from at least two views of each breast to generate pictures of the internal structures of the breasts.

Preparing for the test: The woman is asked not to use underarm deodorants or powders on the morning of the test, because these products can interfere with the pictures by creating the false appearance of abnormalities (artifacts). Medications do not affect the test and need not be changed.

What to expect during the test: The woman changes into a loose-fitting gown that opens in the front. She is then positioned next to the special x-ray unit. The technician places a flat x-ray film cassette under the breast and a flat plastic plate over the breast, compressing the breast so that an image can be taken. The woman may experience discomfort from compression of the breast. The test takes about 30 minutes.

What to expect after the test: Usual activities can be resumed immediately after the test.

Potential problems: Mammography is very safe. The small amount of radiation that the woman is exposed to does not pose a danger.

Ultrasound

Other names: Ultrasonography, Doppler.

Why the test is done: An ultrasound scan may be done for a variety of reasons. Ultrasound scanning can be used to look for abnormalities, such as tumors or areas of infection, within internal organs or structures, such as the liver, kidneys, or thyroid gland. Ultrasound scans are often done to determine how well an organ is functioning. For example, an ultrasound scan can measure how well the heart is pumping blood (echocardiogram). A special type, called a Doppler ultrasound scan, measures blood flow and can be used to determine if blood vessels are blocked.

Ultrasound scanning can be done to determine if a mass is solid, liquid, or a combination of the two. Occasionally, an ultrasound scan is done to determine if an excessive amount of urine remains in the bladder after urination. In some instances, ultrasound scanning assists a doctor in guiding a hollow needle into a growth or tissue inside the body so that a sample can be obtained for examination.

How the test is done: A hand-held device called a transducer produces high-frequency sound waves. Most often, the transducer is used to pass waves through skin and muscle. When waves strike organs and abnormal growths inside the body, echoes bounce back. The echoes are captured by the transducer, and an image is produced.

The examiner applies gel to the skin over the approximate location of any organ or growth that is being examined. The gel improves the passage of sound waves through the skin. The examiner glides the transducer on the skin, over the area where the gel has been applied.

In some instances, the transducer can be passed inside the body. For example, a smaller type of transducer may be passed through the anus into the rectum for images of the prostate gland or into the vagina for images of the uterus and ovaries. Also with the use of an endoscope, a transducer can be passed through the mouth and into the bottom portion of the esophagus for images of the heart. When ultrasound involves passing the transducer through the esophagus, preparation for the test and what happens during and after the test are similar to the experience of undergoing esophagogastroduodenoscopy.[1]

Ultrasound images can be produced continuously, usually for several minutes, so that movement can be shown, such as blood flowing through vessels or muscles contracting and relaxing. In some instances, a graph is produced to show the speed and strength of movement. Sometimes ultrasound compares the tendency of sound waves to bounce off of versus to pass through a structure. Bone density, for example, is sometimes measured in this way.

Preparing for the test: Preparation is often unnecessary. When the test involves looking at structures or growths within the abdomen, the person is told to refrain from eating or drinking for about 6 hours before the test. If the test involves the urinary tract or the lowest part of the abdomen (pelvis) the person is asked to drink a large amount of water about 1 to 2 hours before the test. Most medications are not affected by the test and need not be changed. However, the scheduling of certain drugs, for example, those used to treat diabetes, may need to be adjusted.

What to expect during the test: The person usually changes into a loose-fitting gown. Then, depending on the area of the body being tested, the person may be asked to sit or lie down on a stretcher or examination table. Most people find an ultrasound in which the transducer is on the outside of the body to be simple and painless. They may experience slight pressure as the ex-

1. see page 136

aminer moves the transducer about and presses downward occasionally to adjust the images that are being produced. Some people experience discomfort if they must lie down for the ultrasound, especially people who find it difficult to lie flat.

If the ultrasound involves passing a transducer inside the body, additional steps are taken, as in esophagogastroduodenoscopy[1] and prostatic biopsy.[2] The person may experience some discomfort.

What to expect after the test: Most often, usual activities can be resumed immediately after the test.

Potential problems: Ultrasound on the outside of the body is very safe. Rarely, when ultrasound involves passing the transducer inside the body, for example, the rectum, vagina, or esophagus, an injury occurs. Bleeding and infection may occur with such an injury.

Coronary Angiography

Other names: Coronary arteriography, cardiac catheterization, cardiac cath, heart cath.

Related tests: Angiography is done to evaluate arteries in many areas of the body. Kidney or renal angiography is done to look for blockages of arteries that supply the kidneys. Cerebral angiography is done to look for blockages of the arteries that supply the brain or to evaluate blood flow to tumors. Peripheral or extremity angiography is most often done to look for blockages of arteries that supply the legs.

Why the test is done: Coronary angiography is done to look for blockages in the arteries that supply the heart with blood (coronary arteries). Most often, the test is performed in people with symptoms. It may be done in people who have already had a heart attack to assess blood flow to the undamaged parts of the heart. If the test is done for reasons other than evaluating arteries, the term "catheterization" may be used. For example, it may be done to look for abnormal bulges in the wall of the heart (aneurysms) or damaged heart valves. Tissue samples may be obtained if infection or inflammation is suspected. The test may also be used to assess how well a transplanted heart is functioning.

1. see page 136
2. see page 140

How the test is done: A catheter is inserted into a blood vessel, usually an artery in the leg or arm. The catheter is threaded through larger and larger arteries until it reaches the aorta (the largest artery, which carries blood from the heart) and the heart. Dye is injected through the catheter, usually several times during the course of the test, to highlight the coronary arteries and the chambers of the heart. In some cases, the tip of the catheter has a camera that can transmit pictures of the inside of the arteries and heart to a video monitor. If tissue samples are needed, an instrument can be inserted through the catheter to obtain samples.

Preparing for the test: Because driving is not allowed until the day after the test, the person is told to arrange for a ride home. The person is also told to refrain from eating or drinking for 12 hours before the test. Adjustments to the scheduling and dosages of medications may be needed.

What to expect during the test: The person changes into a loose-fitting gown. The person lies on a table and is asked to remain as still as possible throughout the test. If the catheter is to be inserted into a blood vessel in the groin, hair is shaved from the area. A numbing drug (anesthetic) is injected at the site where the catheter is to be inserted. A small cut is made so that the catheter can be inserted safely into the vessel. After the catheter is inserted, a sedative may be given, which results in drowsiness but not sleep. The test itself usually requires about 1 hour.

Coronary angiography may be uncomfortable for some people, especially for those who find it difficult to lie still for a prolonged period. Each time dye is injected through the catheter, a brief sensation of warmth and a metallic taste may be experienced.

What to expect after the test: Pressure is usually applied after the catheter is removed. A bandage is placed over the incision site. Pressure is then continued, often by placing a small bag filled with sand on the bandage. The person is monitored in a recovery area for several hours, with blood pressure, heart rate, and breathing rate measured regularly. After about 4 hours, the person is allowed to sit and then stand and walk a bit. Usually the person is able to return home after about 6 hours but is advised to rest at home for the remainder of the day. The person is asked to call if bleeding or swelling occurs at the site where the catheter was inserted.

Potential problems: Uncommonly, a person has an allergic reaction to the dye. A blood clot may develop in the vessel where the catheter was inserted (thrombus), or bleeding (hematoma) may develop at the insertion site. Occasionally, the blood vessel may be damaged where the catheter was inserted, and a bulge (aneurysm) can develop. Rarely, other complications can occur, such as a heart attack, abnormal heart rhythm, stroke, or even death.

Colonoscopy

Other names: Lower endoscopy.

Why the test is done: Often, a colonoscopy is done to screen the lower digestive tract for evidence of cancer in people who have no symptoms. Also, it may be performed to look for noncancerous (benign) tumors or cancer in people who have been found previously to have noncancerous tumors. Colonoscopy may be used to look for recurring cancer in people who have had colorectal cancer. The test is also done to identify the source of bleeding from the digestive tract. Less often, the test is performed to look for a cause of persistent diarrhea or constipation.

Colonoscopy sometimes has a role in treatment, because it allows a doctor to remove polyps (noncancerous growths that can become cancerous), stop bleeding, or open up the large intestine or rectum in people who have a narrowing or partial blockage.

How the test is done: A type of flexible endoscope called a colonoscope is inserted through the anus and then passed along the length of the large intestine. A doctor can view the inside of the large intestine by looking through the colonoscope or at a television monitor.

Preparing for the test: Many medications are not affected by the test. However, the scheduling and dosage of some medications may need to be adjusted on the day before and the day of the test.

The person is told to refrain from taking aspirin and other nonsteroidal anti-inflammatory drugs (NSAIDs) during the week before the test. These drugs increase the risk of bleeding.

Almost always, warfarin, an anticoagulant (a drug that prevents clots), must be temporarily stopped before the test. Often, when warfarin is stopped, another anticoagulant is given by injection or intravenously until just before the test and briefly afterward, until warfarin can be safely restarted. People with artificial heart valves or certain types of prostheses are given antibiotics before and just after colonoscopy to prevent infection.

The person is told to refrain from eating and to drink only clear liquids on the day before the test. To clean out the intestine of all stool, the person consumes a special laxative. The laxative is mixed with or taken with a large amount of water.

Because driving is unsafe for several hours after the test, the person is told to arrange for a ride home.

What to expect during the test: The person changes into a loose-fitting open-backed gown and lies on a stretcher or examination table. An intravenous line is inserted so that a sedative can be given. The sedative causes the person to become very drowsy or to fall asleep. If the person wishes to remain alert enough to watch the television monitor along with the doctor, a smaller dose of sedative may be given. A small device is clipped onto the person's finger so that the level of oxygen in the blood can be monitored. The person is then positioned on his side with one knee bent, and the colonoscope is inserted. Air is sometimes blown into the large intestine to widen (dilate) it and water is sometimes used to flush out any remaining stool.

The test is usually completed in as little as 30 minutes. It may take up to 90 minutes, especially if the large intestine has not been completely emptied or if polyps are removed or other tissue samples are taken. Colonoscopy may be uncomfortable for some older people, especially for those who find it difficult to lie still for a prolonged period.

What to expect after the test: The person remains in a recovery area for about 1 to 2 hours while blood pressure, heart rate, and breathing rate are monitored. The person is then instructed to rest or to greatly reduce usual activities for the remainder of the day. Large amounts of gas may be passed for many hours, and normal bowel function may take a few days to return. The person is told to refrain from taking aspirin and other NSAIDs for several days after the test.

Potential problems: Older people may find taking the laxative before the test to be a bit stressful. They can become dehydrated from the laxative and from the restrictions on drinking and eating that are necessary for test preparation.

Rarely, a heart valve or a prosthesis becomes infected. In rare cases, the large intestine or rectum is torn or the wall is penetrated (perforated) by the colonoscope. Older people, especially those who have multiple bulges (diverticula) in the wall of the large intestine, are more likely to have their intestine perforated than are younger people. Perforation usually results in bleeding and infection and often requires surgery.

Esophagogastroduodenoscopy (EGD)

Other names: Upper gastrointestinal endoscopy.

Why the test is done: An EGD is done to check the inside lining of the esophagus, stomach, and upper part of the small intestine (duodenum) for problems such as inflammation, ulcers, tears, blockages, and noncancerous (benign) or cancerous (malignant) tumors. Usually the test is done when a person has difficulty swallowing, persistent nausea and vomiting, vomiting of blood, or pain that is not relieved by drugs.

How the test is done: An endoscope is inserted through the mouth and throat and passed into the esophagus, stomach, and duodenum. The doctor can view the inside of these organs by looking through the endoscope or at a television monitor.

Preparing for the test: Most often, medications are not affected by the test and need not be changed. However, the scheduling and dosage of some medications may need to be adjusted.

The person is told to refrain from taking any aspirin or other nonsteroidal anti-inflammatory drugs (NSAIDs) during the week before the test. These drugs increase the risk of bleeding during the test. Almost always, warfarin, an anticoagulant (a drug that prevents clots), must also be temporarily discontinued a week before the test. Often, when warfarin is discontinued, another anticoagulant is given by injection or intravenously until just before the test and briefly afterward, until warfarin can be safely restarted. People with artificial heart valves or certain types of prostheses are given antibiotics prior to and just after EGD to prevent infection.

Because driving is unsafe for several hours after the test, the person is told to arrange for a ride home. Eating and drinking are prohibited for 8 hours before the test.

What to expect during the test: The person removes all clothing above the waist and changes into a loose-fitting open-backed gown. The person lies partly reclined on a stretcher or examination table. The back of the throat is sprayed with a numbing drug (topical anesthetic) to prevent gagging. A mouth-piece is inserted to prevent biting on the endoscope. An intra-venous line is inserted so that a sedative can be given.

As the endoscope is inserted, the person is asked to swallow so that the endoscope can be passed easily into the esophagus. The sedative may then be increased slightly if the person prefers to sleep through the procedure. Tissue samples are sometimes taken for a biopsy. EGD is sometimes completed in as little as 10 minutes but often lasts 20 to 30 minutes, especially if tissue samples are taken. The test may be uncomfortable, especially for people who find it difficult to lie still for a prolonged period.

What to expect after the test: The person remains in a recovery area for about 1 to 2 hours while blood pressure, heart rate, and breathing rate are monitored. Afterward, the person is instructed to rest or to greatly reduce usual activities for the remainder of the day. The person is told to refrain from eating or drinking for a few more hours. Gas may be passed for many hours. The person is told that aspirin or other NSAIDs should not be taken for several days after the test.

Potential problems: Rarely, the esophagus, stomach, or duodenum is injured by the endoscope. Such an injury, which is a bit more likely for older people than for younger people, may result in bleeding and infection. The risk of aspiration, in which gastric juices travel up the esophagus and down into the lungs, is higher for older people as well. Aspiration may result in a fever and pneumonia. Rarely, an artificial heart valve or prosthesis becomes infected.

Polysomnography

Other names: Sleep study.

Why the test is done: Polysomnography is done to diagnose disorders that can cause insomnia or excessive daytime sleepiness. Such disorders include sleep apnea; rapid-eye-movement

(REM) sleep behavior disorders; limb movement disorders, such as restless legs syndrome; and narcolepsy.

How the test is done: Polysomnography is performed in a sleep laboratory, almost always within a hospital. Sensors are attached to the person, allowing for various body functions to be continuously recorded during sleep, and the person is video-taped. The body functions recorded may include electrical activity of the brain; oxygen levels in the blood; the rate of air flow in and out of the lungs; heart rate; blood pressure; and movement of muscles in the eyes, jaw, and legs. The results are analyzed to determine how long it takes a person to fall asleep, how long the person sleeps, and how frequently the person awakens. Information is also available on the time spent in different stages of sleep and whether the person has periods during which breathing stops briefly (apnea) or becomes very shallow (hypopnea).

Preparing for the test: The person is told to maintain regular sleep habits up to and including the night before the test. The person is asked to bring comfortable clothing suitable for sleep. Most medications are not affected by the test and need not be changed. However, the person is told to avoid taking any drugs that affect sleep, such as sleep aids, stimulants, and alcohol.

What to expect during the test: Sensors are attached to the scalp, face, chest, and legs. After the sensors are attached, the person has several minutes to relax and become accustomed to wearing all the sensors and wires.

The test usually involves recordings of body functions for an entire night of sleep (a full study). Alternatively, the test may involve recordings for about half a night of sleep followed by a period when recordings are performed while various treatments are tried (a split study). The second half of the study is performed to measure the response to treatment if a problem is identified during the first half of the night. Occasionally, the test is continued the following day to measure naps and daytime sleepiness (multiple sleep latency test).

Many people worry at first that they will be unable to sleep while attached to the sensors and wires. However, once the study gets underway, most people are able to get comfortable and fall asleep.

What to expect after the test: Usual activities can be resumed immediately after the test.

Potential problems: Polysomnography is safe. Problems are very infrequent.

Electromyography (EMG) and Nerve Conduction Velocity (NCV)

Other names: None.

Why the test is done: EMG and NCV testing provide information about how well the muscles and nerves are functioning. The pattern of any abnormalities detected often suggests possible causes, such as pressure on or entrapment of a nerve. Results can also help distinguish between and diagnose diseases of muscles and diseases of nerves.

How the test is done: When muscles contract, measurable electrical signals are generated. Electrical signals traveling along nerves can also be recorded. An EMG requires that very thin needles (similar to pins) be inserted through the skin so that they are situated in or very near muscles at specific points of the arms or legs. The needles are electrodes that transmit the electrical activity of the muscles to a monitoring device. An NCV test requires that a nerve stimulator be placed on the skin, together with a recording electrode located farther along the nerve. Information on the velocity and the strength of the electrical activity is sent to a monitoring device.

Preparing for the test: Most medications are not affected by the test and need not be changed. However, the person may be told to refrain from taking any aspirin or other nonsteroidal anti-inflammatory drugs (NSAIDs) during the week before the test, because these drugs can increase the risk of bleeding during the test. Similarly, the scheduling and dosage of warfarin (a drug that prevents clots) may need to be adjusted. On the day of the test, the person is asked to refrain from using hand cream or lotion that might interfere with adherence of electrodes to the skin and to wear comfortable, loose-fitting clothes.

What to expect during the test: Depending on the area being tested, the person may be asked to change into a gown. The person then sits or lies on a table. Sometimes only one test is done, but often EMG and NCV tests are done together. Both can usually be done in about 30 to 60 minutes.

For an EMG, skin in the area where each needle is to be placed is cleaned with alcohol. A brief but painful prick is felt as each needle is inserted. Usually only a few needles are used. For an NCV, the placement of electrodes is on the surface of the skin.

What to expect after the test: Aching in the areas that were tested may persist for several hours. Most often, usual activities can be resumed immediately after the test.

Potential problems: Very rarely, a person develops an infection or bleeding at the site where a needle was inserted.

Prostatic Biopsy

Other names: Biopsy of the prostate.

Why the test is done: A prostatic biopsy is done to examine the prostate gland for evidence of cancer. The test is performed in men suspected of having cancer on the basis of the physical examination, blood tests, and ultrasound scanning.

How the test is done: A doctor inserts into the rectum a device that combines an ultrasound probe with a thin, hollow needle guide. Once the device is positioned appropriately, a thin needle is repeatedly passed through the guide, penetrating through the wall of the rectum and into the prostate, until several tissue samples have been obtained. The tissue is then examined under a microscope in a laboratory.

Preparing for the test: Most medications are not affected by the test. However, the person is told to refrain from taking aspirin or other nonsteroidal anti-inflammatory drugs (NSAIDs) during the week before the test. These drugs increase the risk of bleeding during the test. Warfarin, an anticoagulant (a drug that prevents clots), must also be temporarily discontinued during the week before the test. Often, when warfarin is discontinued, another anticoagulant is given by injection or intravenously until just before the test and briefly afterward, until warfarin can be safely restarted. An antibiotic is taken, usually the day before, the day of, and the day after the test. The man is usually told to take an enema the morning of the test and to eat a light breakfast.

What to expect during the test: The man changes into a loose-fitting open-backed gown. He then lies on a table and must remain as still as possible. A numbing drug (anesthetic) and a sedative are given. The man feels pressure when the doctor inserts the ultrasound probe–needle guide combination into the rectum. This may be followed by a pricking sensation as the needle is passed through the needle guide repeatedly to obtain several tissue samples. The test takes about 20 to 30 minutes.

What to expect after the test: Usual activities can be resumed immediately. However, for a few days after the test, the rectum may feel sore, and a small amount of blood may be visible in urine or in ejaculate. The man is asked to call his doctor if blood remains visible for more than a few days or if he experiences a fever or bleeding from the rectum.

Potential problems: There is a small risk that the needle used to obtain tissue samples will cause bleeding. Infections, although uncommon, may occur.

Skin Biopsy

Other names: Biopsy of the skin.

Why the test is done: A skin biopsy is done to examine skin growths or other abnormal areas of skin tissue for evidence of cancer or inflammation.

How the test is done: A doctor performing a skin biopsy can choose from several options. With a growth that is raised above the level of the surrounding skin, a shave biopsy can be performed. In a shave biopsy, a sharp blade (scalpel) is used to shave off the growth. If the growth extends deeper into the skin, a scalpel is used to perform an excisional biopsy. In an excisional biopsy, some or all of the growth is removed. In some cases, especially when inflammation is suspected, a punch biopsy is performed. In a punch biopsy, a sharp circular punch is used to push through the skin. When the hollow punch is pulled back, it contains a core of tissue from the full thickness of the skin. The biopsy is examined under a microscope in a laboratory.

Preparing for the test: Often, preparation is not needed. However, if the doctor expects to obtain tissue from deeper layers of the skin, the person may be asked to refrain from taking aspirin and other nonsteroidal anti-inflammatory drugs (NSAIDs) the week before the test. These drugs can increase the risk of bleeding. Warfarin, an anticoagulant (a drug that prevents clots), may also be temporarily discontinued a week before the test. Often, when warfarin is discontinued, another anticoagulant is given by injection or intravenously until just before the test and briefly afterward, until warfarin can be safely restarted.

What to expect during the test: The person can remain dressed if the test involves an easily accessible area, such as the lower arm. Otherwise, the person changes into a loose-fitting open-backed gown. The person may sit or lie on a table and must remain as still as possible. The skin surrounding the area where the tissue is to be removed is cleaned and injected with a numbing drug (anesthetic). The person may feel pressure from the scalpel or punch used to remove the tissue. The test usually takes about 5 to 15 minutes. A solution that stops bleeding may be applied, or 1 or a few stitches (sutures) may be used to close the small wound.

What to expect after the test: Usual activities can often be resumed immediately if the wound is very small. However, if stitches are needed, the person may be advised to keep the area of the wound dry and to avoid heavy lifting or vigorous exercise until the stitches are removed.

Some steps must be followed to care for the wound. If stitches are not needed, the site is covered with a dressing or bandage. The person is given directions to care for the wound until it heals in a few days or several weeks, depending on the type of biopsy. Directions usually involve changing the dressing at least once a day after cleansing the site and applying antibiotic ointment. The person may be advised to check the site each day and to report any bleeding or increasing redness or pain.

Potential problems: A scar may form. The size of the scar depends on the type of biopsy performed. Rarely, the site becomes infected or bleeds excessively.

11

Hospital Care

More than one third of people admitted to the hospital are older people. And at any time, almost half of people in the hospital are 65 or older.

Older people may go to a hospital when they have a serious or life-threatening problem (such as a heart attack) or when a disorder (such as heart failure) suddenly worsens. They may go to the hospital when a less serious problem (such as a sprained ankle) requires immediate attention. Or they may be scheduled for admission to a hospital by a doctor because they need certain tests, intensive treatment, or surgery.

A hospital can be a frightening and intimidating place. Often, the need for care occurs quickly and without explanation. Knowing what to expect can help people cope and actively participate in their care during their stay.

Hospital care is needed only when appropriate treatment cannot be provided in another place. The main goal is to restore or improve health so that people can return home. Thus, hospital stays are intended to be relatively short. Leaving the hospital as soon as it is safe is usually best for older people.

If further care is needed temporarily or permanently after a hospital stay, people are sent to another facility. They may go to a rehabilitation facility or a nursing home (skilled nursing facility).[1] Sometimes care can be continued at home.[2]

1. see pages 109 and 110
2. see page 110

GOING TO THE EMERGENCY DEPARTMENT

Most older people need emergency medical care at some time. The most common reasons include heart attacks, heart failure, strokes, and injuries. Almost half of older people seen in an emergency department are admitted to the hospital. Older people may be taken to the emergency department by a family member or friend or in an ambulance. They may leave from their home or from a long-term care facility.

Knowing when to go to an emergency department can be difficult. When emergency care is not needed, going to an emergency department can be more harmful than helpful. In the United States, emergency departments are often crowded and uncomfortable, with little privacy and loud noises. Staff members sometimes have little time to ease people's anxieties. People sometimes wait several hours before seeing a doctor.

People should know what problems their health insurance plan considers an emergency. Some plans require people to call their insurance company or primary care doctor before they go to the emergency department, except for serious injuries (such as a hip fracture) or life-threatening situations (such as chest pain or a stroke).

Before going to an emergency department, older people should call their primary care doctor regardless of whether their health insurance plan requires such a call. The doctor can often determine whether such a visit is needed. The doctor may meet the person in the emergency department or call there to advise staff members about the person. If the primary care doctor is not available, calling the emergency department before going can help. Staff members there ask about symptoms and can help determine whether coming in is necessary. They can explain what to bring and what to do after arrival.

People should ask a family member or friend to accompany them to the emergency department. Having another person who can help fill out the forms and provide support makes the experience less overwhelming.

When people go to the emergency department, they should bring any medical information they have at home. This information may include a list of drugs they are taking, a copy of the most recent medical summary, or records of hospital stays. Otherwise, the information must be obtained from the primary care doctor or, for residents of a long-term care facility, from that facility. Family members can help by asking whether the emergency department has received the information.

In the emergency department, a staff member asks the person, if able, to describe the problem. The person is asked to fill out registration and health insurance forms and to sign a form consenting to treatment. If the person cannot fill out the forms, staff members try to locate someone, such as a close family member, to help.[1] Then a nurse evaluates the seriousness of the problem. The more serious the problem, the more quickly a person is seen by a doctor.

BEING ADMITTED TO THE HOSPITAL

A doctor—the primary care doctor, a specialist, or an emergency department doctor—determines whether a person has a medical problem serious enough to warrant admission to the hospital.

The first step in admission is registration. Sometimes registration can be done before arriving at the hospital. A person fills out forms requiring basic information (such as name and address) and health insurance information. Telephone numbers of family members or friends to contact in case of an emergency are listed. The person also signs forms consenting to being treated, releasing information to insurance companies, and agreeing to pay the charges. The person is given an ID bracelet to be worn on the wrist.

A person should bring a list of the drugs and doses being taken and any written instructions from the doctor. Hospitals also recommend that a person bring advance directives[2] to the hospital. All of this information should be given to the nurse responsible for getting the person settled into a hospital room. A person should bring toiletries, a robe, sleepwear, slippers, and, if needed, eyeglasses, hearing aids, and dentures. All personal items should be marked or labeled. Prescription drugs and any valuables (such as a wedding ring or other jewelry, credit cards, or large sums of money) should be left at home.

1. see page 956
2. see page 953

SPECIAL CARE UNITS

Some people need different types of care in the hospital. They are put in special care units.

Intensive care units (ICUs) are for people who are seriously ill. People may have had a sudden, general malfunction (failure) of an organ, such as the liver, lungs (requiring assistance with breathing), or kidneys (requiring dialysis). People who are in shock, have a severe infection, or who have had major surgery are likely to be placed in an ICU.

Coronary care units (CCUs) are for people who are having or have had a heart attack. People who are likely to have a heart attack (such as people with angina or an abnormal heart rhythm) and people with heart failure may be admitted to a coronary care unit or, if it is unavailable, to an ICU.

In intensive care and coronary care units, people are monitored constantly with electronic equipment. Various lines or wires may connect people with a machine to monitor heart rate (electrocardiography, or ECG), blood pressure, and breathing rate. Thus, staff members can continuously evaluate vital body functions. Staff members usually also insert a flexible catheter into a vein (an intravenous line). Through it, people may be given drugs, fluids, and sometimes nutrients. These units have ventilators to help people with breathing and defibrillators to restore heart rhythm to normal. Visiting hours and rules are more restrictive in these units.

Isolation is used to prevent a person from infecting others. Isolation may be complete (when a disorder can be transmitted through the air). Or it may be incomplete (when a disorder is transmitted only by contact with the skin, blood, or stool). Incomplete isolation requires fewer precautions.

Reverse isolation is used to prevent a person from being infected by others. Reverse isolation is needed when a person's immune system is not functioning well—for example, after a bone marrow transplantation.

For isolation, the person is placed in a single room. Anyone who goes into the room must wear a mask, gown, cap, and gloves, which are sterilized or burned after use. All items that come in contact with the person are also sterilized. The air in the room may be filtered. Visitors are usually limited to the immediate family.

After admission, the person may be taken to a laboratory to be tested or to a hospital room. Hospital rooms may be private (one bed) or shared (more than one bed).

Various tests, such as blood or urine tests, may be done to evaluate the person for other problems. Staff members may ask questions to determine whether the person is likely to develop problems in the hospital or to need extra help after discharge from the hospital. They may ask about eating habits, mood, vaccinations, drugs taken, problems with walking, the amount of help needed with daily activities, and living arrangements. The person may be asked a standard series of questions to evaluate mental function.[1]

During the hospital stay, a doctor examines the person at least once a day. Nurses and other staff members usually come in several times a day and provide most of the care. Physical therapists may come in regularly to help the person exercise.[2] Some older people need special care, such as help with eating. Family members and volunteers at the hospital may provide this care. Family members can also talk with a social worker at the hospital about making arrangements for extra help. Sometimes an attendant can be hired to help the person eat and walk.

How aggressively a disorder is treated in a hospital does not depend on age. However, less aggressive treatments are sometimes appropriate for older people, depending on their wishes and outlook—that is, how the disorder is expected to progress and how long the person is expected to live. Family members and older people can talk with a doctor or another health care practitioner about options for treatment to make sure those offered are based on the severity of the disorder, not on age.

PROBLEMS DUE TO HOSPITALIZATION

Hospitals are a place where people go expecting to get better, at least eventually. However, when many older people leave the hospital, they are in worse shape than before they became ill. Many older people cannot care for themselves when they are ready to be discharged from the hospital. Some of these people leave the hospital only to go to a nursing home. Part of the reason for the decline in function is that older people tend to have serious and debilitating disorders when they enter the hospital. However, part of the reason is just being in a hospital.

In the hospital, older people who already have problems caring for themselves tend to decline even more, as do those whose mental function is impaired, who are depressed, or who are undernourished. Many older people have difficulty bouncing back psychologically and physically from the experience of being in

1. see table on page 345
2. see page 171

a hospital as well as from the disorder they have had. Sometimes mistakes are made in hospitals. For example, the wrong drug may be given. Also, many hospitals do not adequately deal with the needs of older people.

Problems Due to Bed Rest

Staying in bed for a long time, as is sometimes necessary in a hospital, can cause many problems. Examples are weak muscles, stiff joints, blood clots, dizziness, weak bones, pressure sores, constipation, kidney stones, incontinence, infections, and depression.

When muscles are not used, they become weak. This effect may be greater in older people because muscles may already be weak. Older people tend to lose muscle tissue (a condition called sarcopenia) if they do not stay active. Staying in bed can make muscles and the tissues around them (ligaments and tendons) stiff. Stiffness can result in joints that are permanently bent (a contracture). A vicious circle may result: Staying in bed because of a disorder or surgery makes moving difficult, resulting in weak muscles and stiff joints, which make movement (including standing and walking) even more difficult.

When the legs are not being used, blood moves more slowly from the leg veins to the heart. Blood clots are more likely to form in slow-moving blood.[1] Blood clots sometimes travel from the leg veins to the lungs and cause blockage of an artery in a lung (pulmonary embolism). Pulmonary embolism can be life threatening. Also, if blood moves slowly from the leg veins, the heart may not be able to pump enough blood to the brain when a person stands up. Then, standing up may make the person feel dizzy or light-headed—a disorder called orthostatic hypotension.[2]

When bones do not bear weight regularly (that is, when a person does not spend enough time standing or walking), bones become weak and more prone to fractures.[3]

When people stay in one position in bed for too long, pressure is put on the areas of skin that touch the bed. The pressure cuts off the blood supply to those areas. If the blood supply is

1. see page 649
2. see page 273
3. see page 311

cut off too long, tissue breaks down and a sore (bedsore or pressure sore[1]) forms. Pressure sores can begin to form in as few as 2 hours. Pressure sores are more likely to develop in people who are undernourished or incontinent. Being undernourished makes the skin thin, dry, inelastic, and more likely to tear or break. Being incontinent exposes the skin to urine, which irritates it. Pressure sores usually occur on the lower back, tailbone, heels, elbows, and hips. Pressure sores can be serious and can result in discharge to a nursing home rather than home.

When people stay in bed or are less active, stool (feces) moves more slowly through the intestine and rectum and out of the body. Thus, constipation is more likely to occur.

When people are restricted to bed rest or are too weak or ill to get out of bed by themselves, urinating and having bowel movements become complicated. Such people need a bedpan or urinal or someone's help getting to a toilet. Often, the needed help is delayed. Thus, these functions take more time than they usually do and require planning. A delay getting to the toilet may result in leakage of urine (a type of urinary incontinence called functional incontinence) or of stool (fecal incontinence).[2]

When getting to the bathroom is delayed, the bladder may become overstretched because urine accumulates and stretches it. When the bladder is overstretched, a catheter is often inserted into the bladder to drain urine. Bacteria are more likely to enter the bladder when a catheter is inserted, making urinary tract infections more likely.

People who stay in bed do not use their lungs as much, and the muscles that control breathing may weaken. Then, taking a deep breath or coughing forcefully may become difficult. If mucus accumulates in the airways, coughing may not be forceful enough to clear the mucus out. Thus, people are more likely to become short of breath and to develop pneumonia and lung infections.

Depression is common among people who stay in bed for a long time. One reason is that bed rest results in so many other problems. Also, staying in bed may make people feel helpless and useless. They have less contact with other people, which may contribute to depression.

1. see page 503
2. see page 153

Steps to prevent problems related to bed rest may seem bothersome or too demanding, but they are necessary for a good recovery. Moving as soon and as much as possible can help prevent most problems. People are encouraged to get out of bed as soon as they can. If they cannot get out of bed, they should sit up, move, or do exercises in bed. Flexing and relaxing muscles in bed can help keep muscles from weakening. For people who cannot exercise on their own, a physical therapist or another staff member moves their limbs for them. Furnishings, such as handrails, grab bars in the bathroom, raised toilet seats, low beds, and carpeting, can make movement easier.

If a person has difficulty moving, staff members periodically change the person's position in bed. This measure helps prevent pressure sores from forming and mucus from accumulating in airways. The person's skin is inspected for any sign of pressure sores. Pads may be placed over parts of the body that are in contact with the bed, such as the heels, to protect them.

Deep breathing and coughing exercises can help keep breathing muscles from weakening.

Undernutrition

Generally, older people are more susceptible to undernutrition for many reasons.[1] For example, they may have a disorder or take a drug that interferes with the way the body uses some nutrients or may cause the appetite to decrease. Food may taste unfamiliar and unappetizing. Some people are put on a restricted diet, such as a low-fat or low-salt diet. Meals are served and removed at set times. People may be served foods they do not like or cannot eat for philosophical or religious reasons (for example, because the foods are not kosher). Also, eating in a hospital bed with a tray may be difficult.

Some people need help or more time while eating. Often, by the time someone arrives to help with eating, the food has cooled and is even less appetizing. If dentures are left at home, are misplaced, or do not fit right, chewing can be difficult.

Water may be difficult to reach from a hospital bed. Even if water can be reached, older people may not drink enough because they tend to feel thirsty less quickly or less intensely than younger people. As a result, older people may become dehy-

1. see page 231

drated in the hospital. If dehydration becomes severe, they can become confused, making them less likely to eat and drink.

Undernutrition is a serious problem. People who are undernourished cannot fight off infections. Sores and wounds heal more slowly, and recovery is less likely. Vitamin D deficiency is particularly common among people who are hospitalized.[1] This deficiency increases the risk of fractures.

Hospital staff members can make sure that restrictive diets are changed as soon as possible and can check how much a person eats each day. Letting the staff members know what foods are preferred or not eaten can also help prevent undernutrition. Hospital diets can be modified to some degree. Family members may bring in the person's favorite foods. Having family members present at meals helps, because people tend to eat more when they eat with others. A pitcher of fresh water should be placed within easy reach from the bed unless fluids must be limited because of a disorder. Family and staff members can also regularly offer the person something to drink.

For people who cannot take food by mouth, a fluid containing nutrients can be given through a tube inserted into the stomach or a vein (intravenously).[2] Such feedings may be necessary for a short time or indefinitely. If a person cannot take food by mouth (even if only temporarily), family members should check with staff members to make sure adequate nutrition is provided.

Loss of Independence

In hospitals, staff members do many of the tasks people normally do by themselves, largely because doing so is easier. People are brought food and are bathed. When people have to go to another location for a test or treatment, they are often taken by wheelchair. However, if older people do not continue to care for themselves, they tend to lose the ability to do so.

Family and staff members should encourage older people to do as much as possible for themselves. The more people do for themselves, the more likely they are to return home.

1. see box on page 298
2. see page 239

Confusion and Decline in Mental Function

Being ill or taking drugs for pain can make anyone somewhat confused. But in older people, an illness or a drug may cause sudden, noticeable confusion (delirium).[1] Delirium is more likely because of changes that occur as people age.

The hospital environment can also contribute to confusion. Without their personal effects and clothing, people may feel as if they are losing their identity. They are in a strange place without familiar landmarks and usual routines. In their residence, these landmarks and routines help them compensate for various problems, such as impaired vision or memory loss.

Often, hospitals provide little stimulation (such as sights, sounds, and interaction with other people). A person may be alone or with an uncommunicative roommate in a room that has blank white walls and bland, institutionalized furnishings. For most of the time, there may be no one to talk with. The only sound available may be that from a television.

Hospital procedures and schedules can be disorienting. For example, people may be awakened frequently during the night. They may be unable to get their bearings in an unfamiliar, dimly lit room. The many tests and the complicated equipment may be overwhelming. Forgetting to bring eyeglasses or hearing aids can add to a person's confusion and disorientation.

Intensive care units (ICUs) can be even more confusing. People in ICUs are alone, often with no windows or clocks to help them orient themselves. The constant beeping of electronic monitors, constant bright light, and frequent interruptions to take blood, change intravenous (IV) tubes, or give drugs may interfere with sleeping. People who are tired are more easily confused and disoriented. Sometimes confusion is so severe that people develop a type of delirium called ICU psychosis.[2]

If family members notice that an older person becomes unusually confused while staying in a hospital, they should tell staff members. Delirium can usually be cured if its cause (a disorder, drug, or stressful situation) is corrected.

Staff and family members can help keep the person oriented. If the person wears glasses or a hearing aid, they can make sure the person has these items. They may also need to help the per--

1. see page 346
2. see page 348

son use these items. For example, they may need to clean the lenses of the glasses or change the battery in a hearing aid. Adequate lighting in the room can help orient a person. Staff and family members can encourage the person to get out of bed, walk regularly, and do as many usual daily activities as possible. Talking with the person about what is going on outside the hospital helps keep the person's mind active. Explaining tests and treatments helps the person understand what is happening and why. Making sure the person eats, drinks, and sleeps enough also helps.

Incontinence

In the hospital, many people 65 and older lose control of their bladder or bowels (urinary or fecal incontinence). In these cases, incontinence often results from the environment rather than from the person's physical condition. For example, older people may have trouble getting out of bed because the bed is too high. A disorder or surgery may make walking difficult. Equipment such as IV or oxygen lines, heart monitors, and catheters may be in the way. Thus, getting to a toilet may take more time. The alternative—bedpans—may be hard to use or uncomfortable. Help may be needed. People who have dementia or who have had a stroke may be unable to use a call bell to request help. After the call bell is pushed, help may be delayed in coming. Such delays may result in incontinence. Also, some drugs and disorders can make incontinence more likely to develop.[1]

Staff members can set up regular times to help a person go to the toilet. Placing a toilet chair (commode) by the bed is sometimes useful. Having access to a urinal is helpful for men.

Falls

Conditions in a hospital can increase the risk of falling, particularly for older people. Bed rest can make muscles weak. It can cause people to feel dizzy or light-headed when they stand. They may be given drugs that make them feel dizzy, drowsy, or confused. A bed may be too high or have rails, making getting out of bed more difficult. Lighting may be dim, so people may not see obstacles. People who are confused or disoriented are more likely to fall.

1. see page 860

If people who are hospitalized or their family members realize what can cause falls in a hospital, they can take steps to prevent falls.[1] For example, to counter weak muscles, people can get out of bed as soon as possible and exercise. Family or staff members can accompany people while they walk down hospital corridors until muscle strength is regained. Bed rails are usually unnecessary.

Most falls occur when people get out of bed. So family or staff members should make sure people can get out of bed safely. People may need to be shown how high the hospital bed is. They also need to be careful and move slowly when getting out of bed. Wearing slippers or shoes with nonskid soles helps prevent falls. Knowing where the toilet is and how to get there can prevent missteps and bumping into furniture. People should be shown how to call for help.

Often, staff members try to identify and provide extra help to people who are likely to fall. Staff members may check on them at regular intervals or put them in rooms near the nursing station. Family members can ask a doctor to check the drugs being taken to identify any that can increase the risk of falling. If such a drug is being used, family members can ask the doctor about possibly changing the drug or reducing the dose.

Side Effects of Drugs

Generally, but particularly in the hospital, older people experience more side effects from drugs than younger people.[2] The main reason is that older people tend to take more drugs. During one stay in a hospital, older people may take 6 to 12 different drugs. Drugs may be given to help with sleep. But these drugs may make older people more likely to fall or become confused. In the hospital, new drugs may be started, and old ones discontinued. When older people are discharged, half of the drugs they are taking may be new to them.

Older people who are entering the hospital or their family members can talk with staff members about reviewing the drugs being taken. Making sure older people take drugs as instructed is also important. Before discharge, older people or family members should make sure they completely understand the instructions for taking the prescribed drugs.

1. see page 291
2. see page 50

IMPLEMENTING PREVENTIVE STRATEGIES

Some hospitals have developed strategies to prevent problems that can result when older people are hospitalized. These strategies are designed to help older people continue to function as well as they did before they became ill. One such strategy is an interdisciplinary team of health care practitioners who work together to care for an older person.[1] Team members evaluate the person's needs and coordinate the person's hospital care. Team members look for possible problems and correct or prevent them.

Another strategy is a team that focuses on preventing and managing one specific problem, such as undernutrition or pressure sores. Such teams are often led by a nurse, who checks the person for the problem and develops a care plan.

Some hospitals have geriatricians, who are trained specifically to care for older people. These doctors can help prevent problems common among older people. For example, they avoid prescribing drugs that are particularly likely to cause problems.[2] Hospitals may also follow guidelines for care (protocols) developed specifically for older people.

Sometimes a person is assigned to a nurse who has primary responsibility for and monitors that person's care. This nurse makes sure that other staff members understand the treatment plan for the person.

A few hospitals have nursing units that are designed for older people and staffed with people trained in caring for older people. In these units, older people are encouraged to get out of bed as soon and as much as possible. They are encouraged to dress each morning, to follow their usual daily routine as much as possible, and to eat in a group dining room. If older people are going to be in the hospital a long time, they are encouraged to personalize their room with photographs, pillows, and other familiar items. Staff members encourage family members and friends to participate in care.

Even when these strategies are unavailable, hospitals can take general measures to help prevent problems. For example, restraints are used only when absolutely necessary. Bed rails may

1. see page 112
2. see table on pages 52 to 57

be used to enable people who are too weak to sit up. Drugs are given in the lowest dose and for the shortest time possible.

Family members can alert doctors and other hospital staff members if the older person has problems that may become worse in the hospital. Family members can also talk with staff members about potential problems related to hospital care.

If family members know that the person may have a problem communicating, they should tell hospital staff members. Communication may be difficult if English is not the person's first language or if hearing is impaired. Staff members can take measures to help. For example, if the person has difficulty communicating in English, they can arrange for someone to translate.

BEING DISCHARGED FROM THE HOSPITAL

When people have recovered sufficiently or can be appropriately treated elsewhere, they are discharged from the hospital. Most older people leave the hospital before they have fully regained their strength and their ability to function. So making plans to help people function safely after discharge is important. For example, an older person may need a short stay in a rehabilitation facility. They may need special equipment (such as oxygen tanks), transportation, health care at home, or help with daily activities (such as preparing meals, doing housework, dressing, or bathing). Or a long-term care facility may have to be chosen. A discharge planner or a social worker at the hospital can anticipate which problems are likely, then make suggestions about and arrange needed services. However, the person and family members should be involved in the plans to make sure they are appropriate.

Before leaving the hospital, older people or their family members should make sure that they have detailed instructions for follow-up care. Getting a written schedule for using the prescribed drugs and for follow-up appointments can help. If older people are being discharged to another facility, a written summary of their treatment plan should be sent with them and another copy faxed to the facility.

Rowing can prolong the health of both body and mind. At least it seems to have done so for the two of us who have been rowing together for the 62 years of our married life.

Our preference for rowing stems from the happy coincidence that both of us have been enthusiastic sailors since our youth when the normal way of getting to a sailboat was by rowing, not by outboard motors.

Most of our rowing together has been in a 12-foot Jarvis Newman dory. Our usual routine is to row about 1½ miles out of our harbor and to a mid-channel buoy. Our usual starting time is 6:30 a.m., just after sunrise.

We each have two oars and the boat goes best when our strokes are in perfect sync. It is the responsibility of the person in the stern of the craft to set the rhythm, and the responsibility of the person in the bow is to follow precisely.

Assuming that in a married couple the husband is both larger and stronger than the wife, the necessity for synchronized rowing makes it advisable to position the wife in the stern of the boat where she can set both the timing and length of the stroke. It is the husband's responsibility to follow her lead. This configuration of a married couple has many psychological advantages when practiced over a long span of years together. It can also subordinate, and soon eradicate, any minor differences that may be bothering them before the trip begins.

During the 9 months of the year when the weather is suitable in our home in Down East Maine, we row nearly every morning before breakfast. Only rain or high winds interfere with this routine.

Our boat is tied to a float within an easy walk of our house, just long enough to get some of the kinks out of our joints before climbing aboard. Rowing has become as natural to us as walking, so that we can enjoy the beauty and interesting sights that await us: eagles, osprey, cormorants, seals, and an occasional lobsterman heading out to his traps.

Donald and Beth Straus

12

Undergoing Surgery

In the mid-1900s, surgeons often hesitated to perform even simple operations on people over age 50. Times have changed! Now, more than one third of all operations in the United States are performed on people 65 or over.

Despite an increased willingness to perform surgery on older people, aging does increase the risk of complications during and after surgery. For example, older people are much more likely than younger people to develop delirium after surgery. They are also more likely to experience complications from bed rest that might occur after surgery. The risk of death during or after surgery also increases with aging. More than three quarters of deaths in the period immediately after surgery occur in older people. Further, when emergency surgery is performed or when surgery involves the chest or abdomen, the risk of death goes up in all age groups, but much more so for older people.

Although age itself is a risk factor, overall health and the presence of certain disorders increase surgical risk far more than age. Having had a heart attack within 6 months is a particularly high risk factor, as is poorly controlled heart failure. Coronary artery disease, certain abnormal heart rhythms, and poorly controlled high blood pressure increase the risk of surgery in older people. Lung problems, such as chronic obstructive pulmonary disease, are of some concern when determining the risks of surgery, particularly in smokers. Impaired kidney function and problems with mental function, such as dementia, may also increase the risk.

Certain surgical procedures pose more risk than others. For example, surgery involving the abdomen or chest ranks high on the list of risky procedures. Many procedures that older people commonly undergo, such as cataract surgery and joint replacement surgery, pose lower risk. If an older person is generally well, most operations, including ones considered to be higher risk, can be performed safely.

When the risks of surgery are high, they still may be outweighed by the potential benefits. For example, surgery that involves some risk of death, such as repair of a large aortic aneurysm, should be considered if the person is expected to live for another 8 to 10 years, because such aneurysms increase the risk of death if they are not repaired. However, such surgery should probably be avoided if other illnesses limit life expectancy to only 1 to 2 years. When the risks of surgery are low, the low risk may be outweighed by a lack of benefit. For example, some people believe that the risk of tooth-extraction surgery, which usually is very low, is still much too great to justify putting a person with advanced dementia through such an operation.

BEFORE AN OPERATION

Before surgery, the surgeon explains the operation and its possible complications. The person is then asked to sign an informed consent agreement. If the person is mentally incapacitated and cannot understand the benefits and risks of the proposed operation, any advance directives (for example, a living will or durable power of attorney for health care agreement[1]) are reviewed. If there is no advance directive or if available advance directives do not address the person's wishes regarding surgery, the surgeon must involve an appropriate alternative person (a surrogate) in the decision making.[2]

The doctor obtains a thorough medical history before surgery. During this process, other disorders and past problems are reviewed. A careful accounting of drug use, including prescription and nonprescription drugs, and use of nutritional supplements and vitamins are part of the history as well. The doctor also performs a physical examination to determine whether the person is physically ready to undergo surgery.

Laboratory tests and imaging tests such as x-rays are some-

1. see page 953
2. see page 956

times necessary. More specialized tests, such as a measurement of breathing (for example, pulmonary function testing) or heart function (for example, an echocardiogram), may be needed if the person has known diseases that might affect lung or heart function.

Assessment of surgical risk may involve consultation with other health care practitioners. Sometimes these consultations are coordinated by doctors who specialize in addressing the health needs of older people (geriatricians). Surgery may be postponed until any potential problems revealed in the assessment are addressed.

Assessment before surgery can help identify needs that an older person might have after surgery. Often a social worker or discharge coordinator helps with this assessment. These needs also exist among people who are undergoing operations that do not involve a hospital stay (ambulatory, or same-day, surgery). Plans for aftercare must be made before the operation. For example, if a person is expected to have difficulty walking after surgery, planning may involve arranging for someone to assist the person, making an appointment with a physical therapist, and obtaining an assistive device, such as a cane or walker.

AT THE TIME OF AN OPERATION

Many older people undergoing surgery have multiple health problems, and some may be very frail. These people often need special assistance during surgery. Special equipment (for example, step stools or grab bars) or extra personnel can help people with limited mobility move safely from the bed to a stretcher or from the stretcher to an operating table. People who feel pain during movement (for example, those with a hip fracture) can be given a drug to relieve pain (analgesic) before they are moved. A pillow or cushion can be placed under the person's knees to relieve stress on back muscles while on the operating table. Foam padding can be placed in a way that relieves or reduces pressure on vulnerable points of the body, such as bony prominences of the hips or the spine. Arms and legs can be positioned to avoid injury. In addition, the skin, which is much more fragile in older people, needs to be protected. Restraining devices, monitoring devices, and tape can tear or rub the skin, causing sores.

Monitoring

During surgery, the monitoring of blood pressure, heart rate and rhythm, breathing, the balance of body fluids, and urine output is similar in people of all ages. But monitoring of older people must often be more vigilant, in part because of their greater likelihood of having chronic diseases that can increase risks during surgery. Death rates among older people undergoing surgery have dropped steadily in recent years, due in part to improved tools for monitoring vital body functions during surgery. Additional monitoring of older people may include measurements of body temperature and the amount of oxygen in the blood.

Temperature in central parts of the body (core body temperature) is monitored—usually with a special probe in the esophagus or rectum—during long operations. In many older people, core body temperature is lower and more difficult to maintain than in younger people. For older people, the body's normal mechanisms to increase body temperature (for example, shivering) demand more oxygen and energy. Therefore, specific steps are taken to maintain a reasonable body temperature. These measures include using special warming systems, using warmed fluids that are given intravenously, maintaining adequate operating room temperature, and minimizing the amount of time that body organs are exposed to room temperature. Despite these measures, older people may lose significant body heat during surgery. If this occurs, doctors make every effort to rewarm the body as soon as possible.

The amount of oxygen in the blood is generally monitored with a device called an oximeter, which typically is placed on a finger or earlobe.

Anesthesia

Anesthesia is prevention of pain through the use of drugs (anesthetics) that cause a temporary loss of sensation or deep relaxation. With increasing age, the body undergoes changes that affect the type and amount of anesthetics that can be used. The use of anesthetics creates more risks for older people compared with younger people, in part because older people take longer to recover from the effects of the drugs. Also, the likelihood of developing side effects from anesthetics and the severity of side effects tend to increase.

Anesthesia is provided in several ways, some of which are safer than others. Local anesthesia blocks sensation in a very limited area. An anesthetic is injected as close as possible to the area to be operated on. Local anesthesia is commonly used for cataract surgery, placement of a heart pacemaker, and repair of certain types of hernias. When surgery involves the skin, an anesthetic is sometimes sprayed on the skin surface. With local anesthesia, mild sedatives may be added if needed, an approach called monitored anesthesia. Local anesthesia is generally the safest form of anesthesia. Occasionally, however, someone is allergic to the drug used or develops some other unexpected reaction.

Regional anesthesia blocks sensation in a specific region; thus, regional anesthesia involves a larger area than local anesthesia. For example, in an operation to repair or replace a joint, such as the hip or knee, anesthetic drugs may be injected very close to the spinal cord to numb the nerves going to the leg. By injecting anesthetics into nerves near the arm pit, a surgeon may be able to operate on an arm. Regional anesthesia poses more risk than local anesthesia but far less than general anesthesia.

General anesthesia produces temporary loss of consciousness, loss of memory of the events immediately before loss of consciousness, pain relief, and muscle relaxation. General anesthesia is the riskiest type of anesthesia but is often essential for surgery. A general anesthetic generally is given as a gas. If surgery is brief, an anesthesiologist may administer the gas through a mask. For longer operations, a tube is inserted into the trachea, and the person is connected to a ventilator (a machine that does all or some of the breathing for a person). Sometimes, a general anesthetic is administered by injection. This technique, however, is usually reserved for very brief procedures.

Anesthesiologists have many drugs to choose from. They try to select the safest drug for a particular person and his disorder. Whenever possible, they avoid using drugs with so-called anticholinergic effects. Drugs with anticholinergic effects block the action of acetylcholine, which is a substance that helps carry messages between nerves or from a muscle to a gland.[1]

1. see box on page 58

Anticholinergic effects are particularly vexing in older people, causing confusion, blurred vision, constipation, dry mouth, lightheadedness, and an inability to start or continue urinating.

AFTER AN OPERATION

After a low-risk operation, such as knee-replacement surgery, the person may be monitored for only a few hours in a recovery unit or intensive care unit before being moved to a standard hospital room. However, if the low-risk operation is performed on a person with several other disorders, more intensive monitoring is needed. After a high-risk operation, such as one involving the heart or lungs, the person is monitored for several hours in a recovery unit. Recovery units are staffed by nurses and other health care practitioners specifically trained to care for people just out of surgery. In many cases, the person is then moved to an intensive care unit. Intensive care units are staffed by doctors, nurses, and other health care practitioners who are trained to prevent or recognize and quickly treat complications of surgery—even if the operation is uneventful and completed without complications. If no new problems arise after a few days in an intensive care unit, the person is usually moved to a standard hospital room.

After a brief initial recovery period, older people are encouraged to take certain preventive measures, even when convalescence seems to be uncomplicated. Getting out of bed and sitting in a chair is often the first goal. Older people also benefit from getting up to walk as soon as is permitted after surgery. Not doing so may result in many complications of bed rest,[1] such as a rapid loss of muscle strength and an increased risk of pressure sores, blood clots in the legs, and pneumonia. Getting up and about also helps improve digestion and speeds return of normal bowel movements. Older people may need more help, because they are at risk of getting dizzy or of fainting when they attempt to stand. Dizziness or fainting may occur because the body's normal means of regulating blood pressure when changing position adapts more slowly with increasing age.

1. see page 148

Complications

Pain: Pain is to be expected after any type of surgery. Older people may be particularly stoic and may not report pain after surgery. If a person is temporarily unable to talk because of the need for an oxygen mask or hoarseness after anesthesia, health care practitioners and family members must be particularly vigilant for indications that the person is experiencing pain. Some hospitals ask people who are unable to talk to view illustrated facial expressions and to point to the one that best depicts the amount of pain they are experiencing.[1] Generally, effective pain control after surgery helps get people back on their feet sooner. It allows for deeper and more effective breathing and improves the ability to function, hastening the person's return to everyday activities. However, doctors must be careful about the type and dosage of drugs used to control pain, because older people are at high risk of side effects from some drugs used to control pain, particularly opioid analgesics. Side effects of opioid analgesics include confusion, drowsiness, nausea, constipation, urinary retention (causing excessive urine to remain in the bladder after urinating), and impaired breathing (slower and shallower than normal).

Confusion: Some degree of sudden confusion (delirium) occurs in many older people in the first week after surgery.[2] Delirium seems to increase the risk of other complications, and it can prolong a hospital stay. For example, people with delirium may remove devices such as tubes draining the bladder, intravenous tubing, or wound drains. Or, they may fall and injure themselves when getting out of bed.

Several factors increase the risk of developing delirium. One is the use of certain drugs, such as opioid analgesics and drugs with anticholinergic effects, just before, during, and after surgery. A sudden imbalance of fluids and dissolved salts (electrolytes) in the body, lack of or disruption of sleep, and lack of reminders and cues about time and where one is also contribute to delirium. People with dementia who undergo surgery are particularly susceptible to delirium.

If delirium does develop, possible causes are remedied as quickly as possible. At the same time, steps to ensure the per-

1. see art on page 333
2. see page 346

SOME POTENTIAL COMPLICATIONS OF SURGERY*

Complication	Cause	Symptoms
Low levels of oxygen in the blood (hypoxemia)	Drugs that cause slow or shallow breathing	Confusion (initially). If severe, may cause an awareness of heartbeats (palpitations), irregular heartbeat, coma, or death
Low blood pressure (hypo-tension)	Blood loss; movement of fluids into body cavities that normally do not contain fluid (such as the abdominal cavity); use of certain drugs; heart failure and infection, which are complications of some types of surgery	Light-headedness; confusion; weakness. If severe, may lead to coma, abnormal heart rhythm, or death
Airway problems	Removal of the breathing tube (used to protect the airway during surgery) while there are lingering effects of the anesthetics. Lying flat can further compromise the airway	Coughing resulting from mucus, food, or drugs entering the lungs
Urinary retention	Removal of a catheter before the body has regained control over muscle contractions. Alternatively, if left in place too long, a catheter can trigger spasms that interfere with normal bladder muscle contraction once the catheter has been removed. Certain drugs also interfere with bladder muscle contraction	Feelings of being unable to start or complete urination, pressure or fullness in the lower part of the abdomen due to enlargement of the bladder. A sudden urge to urinate, sometimes with so little warning that leakage (incontinence) occurs

Table continues on the following page.

Complication	Cause	Symptoms
Imbalance of fluids and dissolved salts (electrolytes)	Heart failure, breathing problems (too much fluid); decreased blood pressure, reduced kidney function (too little fluid)	Light-headedness, weakness, tiredness, confusion

*Although these complications can occur at any age, they are more likely to occur or to be more severe in older people.

son's safety are undertaken. Having someone in constant attendance (for example, a family member or special aide) is always preferable to using physical or chemical restraints. If sedatives are used, low doses of short-acting drugs are best.

Confusion persists in some older people after surgery. This type of problem is most likely with coronary artery bypass surgery and other long, complicated operations.

Undernutrition: Special nutritional support is needed for people who were malnourished before surgery and for people who cannot resume normal eating immediately after surgery.[1] Supplements are sometimes needed and are given by mouth whenever possible. If swallowing is impaired, doctors may place a temporary feeding tube through the esophagus and into the stomach or small intestine. If digestion or absorption of nutrients is impaired, doctors can give nutrition intravenously.

1. see page 237

13

Rehabilitation

Rehabilitation helps people recover lost function. Many people think of rehabilitation in terms of recovering a physical ability (physical rehabilitation). But it can include any therapy or service that helps people function better and more independently. Rehabilitation may include doing physical exercises, using devices that make doing activities easier, modifying the person's living environment, and teaching family members how to help the person.

Most people who have been disabled can benefit from rehabilitation. A disability is any reduction in the ability to function requiring a change in normal daily activities. Conditions that can disable people include a stroke, hip surgery, replacement of a knee, amputation of a limb, a severe injury, an infection, cancer, or a chronic progressive disorder (such as arthritis). Even a few days of bed rest (for example, after surgery) can cause muscles to become weak and stiff and result in disability.

After an illness, an injury, or surgery, rehabilitation is particularly important for older people. Rehabilitation helps them remain independent—able to live on their own and take care of themselves.

Services and Settings

Which therapies and services are used in rehabilitation depends on the person's needs. Physical therapy, occupational therapy, recreational therapy, and speech therapy are commonly used. Some people need social services, such as help finding appropriate services or home care after discharge from the hospital. Rehabilitation can also involve techniques to relieve pain and inflammation, which can interfere with the movements required by therapy.

Because rehabilitation can include so many services, it is usually provided by a team of health care practitioners. The rehabilitation team may include doctors, nurses, therapists, psychologists, and social workers, as well as the person and family members. Sometimes specialists who fit braces and supportive devices (orthotists) or who fit replacements for body parts (prosthetists) are also included.

The severity of the person's disability determines the type of rehabilitation program. Programs may be informal. In such cases, the person's primary care doctor may provide an exercise program directly to the person or family members. Or programs may be formal, requiring a referral (similar to a prescription) from the person's doctor. The referral may be to a doctor who specializes in rehabilitation (physiatrist), an occupational or a physical therapist, or a rehabilitation center.

If the disability is severe, rehabilitation in a hospital or rehabilitation center is needed. If the disability is milder, rehabilitation can be started in other places, such as a nursing home, a clinic, a doctor's office, or the person's home.

For people who have been hospitalized, rehabilitation is usually started in the hospital. It may be continued at a rehabilitation center, where the person stays for a relatively short time, usually several days to several weeks. When possible, it is then continued elsewhere. Sometimes people can continue the exercise programs set up during rehabilitation at fitness centers.

Rehabilitation can occur at home if a person understands instructions and can transfer from a bed to a chair without help or with help from one person. Rehabilitation at home is desirable for several reasons. The person can learn how to function at home under normal living conditions. The person may be more comfortable at home. Also, the home can be assessed in terms of the person's limitations and, if needed, modified. Family members or a caregiver can be trained to help with rehabilitation. Sometimes a visiting physical therapist, occupational therapist, or home health aide can help. However, rehabilitation at home can be physically and emotionally taxing for all involved. Family members may become exhausted, funds for outside help may be limited, or therapists may be unable to come as often as needed.

Goals of Rehabilitation

The immediate goals of rehabilitation are to help people become independent and to prevent them from losing the ability to function.

The long-term overall goal of rehabilitation is usually to enable people to function as well as they did before the problem that prompted rehabilitation. This goal may mean something different for older people than it does for younger people. For example, older people may have a chronic disorder, such as heart failure, that already limits their ability to function. If they have a stroke or a hip fracture, functioning as well as before may simply mean being able to take care of basic needs: eating, dressing, bathing, moving (transferring) between a bed and a chair, and using the toilet without help from others. (Such activities are called basic activities of daily living.)

Before rehabilitation is started, the therapist or another rehabilitation team member reviews what the long-term overall goals are and how long rehabilitation is expected to take. Then the person can better understand what to expect from rehabilitation. Specific short-term goals and a time frame for accomplishing each goal are also discussed. For example, goals may be to enable the person to move a shoulder more freely, to walk better, to eat without assistance, and to open a jar. Team members encourage the person to achieve each short-term goal, and they track the person's progress. The goals of rehabilitation may be changed if the person progresses more rapidly or slowly than expected or if rehabilitation has to be cut short because the person is unwilling or unable (financially or otherwise) to continue.

Outcome and Support

Regardless of the severity of the disability or the skill of the rehabilitation team, the person's motivation greatly influences the final outcome. Many older people have doubts about their ability to recover. Family members and friends may need to help with motivation.

Rehabilitation for people who have depression may take longer. Sadness or lack of interest blunts the motivation to improve. For people with dementia, rehabilitation may be particularly difficult because they cannot understand what they need to do or why. However, people with dementia can often benefit from rehabilitation if it is tailored to their needs.

Rehabilitation programs designed specifically for older people can be helpful. Then older people will not be tempted to compare their progress with that of younger people. Doing so can be discouraging. Programs that are designed for a particular situation (such as recovery after hip surgery) can also be helpful. Then people with similar problems can empathize with, encourage, and help each other.

Family members and friends are taught to enable the person to be as independent as possible. If they help or protect the person too much, the person may lose improvements in function gained through rehabilitation. The person may become more dependent on others than is necessary—a quality called learned helplessness. On the other hand, if family members and friends do not help when help is needed, the person may be injured, give up trying to function independently, or become depressed.

TREATMENT OF PAIN AND INFLAMMATION

A disorder or injury that produces pain and inflammation can interfere with rehabilitation therapy. So physical therapists and other members of the rehabilitation team treat pain and inflammation before and during therapy. Techniques used include heat therapy, cold therapy, electrical stimulation, traction, massage, and acupuncture.

Heat therapy helps make joints less stiff and easier to move. It reduces pain and muscle spasms. Heat therapy is used for such problems as sprains, strains, muscle spasms, and various forms of arthritis. Heat may be applied to the surface of the body with hot packs, an infrared heat lamp, whirlpools (hydrotherapy), or heated wax. A limb may be immersed in heated wax (paraffin baths), or heated wax may be applied to part of the body. For diathermy, heat may be applied to deeper tissues through sensors (electrodes). For ultrasonography, a high-frequency sound (ultrasound) device placed on the skin is used to apply heat. Heat is applied carefully to avoid burns.

Cold therapy (cryotherapy) may help relieve pain and muscle spasms. It may reduce swelling after an injury occurs. Cold may be applied to the surface of the body with an ice bag, a cold pack, or fluids that evaporate quickly (and thus cool). Therapists apply cold carefully to avoid damaging tissues and lowering the body temperature too much (resulting in a disorder called hypothermia), particularly in older people.[1]

Traction is occasionally used to reduce pain and muscle spasms as well as to keep bones aligned while fractures heal.[2] Traction involves applying a gentle, steady pulling action. Traction may be applied to different parts of the body. For traction of the neck (cervical traction), a sling is fitted under the chin and wrapped around behind the head. This type of traction may relieve chronic neck pain.

Massage may relieve pain and reduce swelling. It may help make tight muscles, ligaments, and tendons easier to move. Massage may help people who have low back pain, arthritis, bursitis, neuritis, fibrositis, multiple sclerosis, cerebral palsy, or various degrees of paralysis.

Acupuncture may be used in rehabilitation to relieve pain. The application of a low electrical current through hair-thin needles inserted at specific body sites may stimulate nerve activity.[3] Chiropractic may be used to relieve low back pain.[4]

Most people feel some pain during the first few days of rehabilitation. Pain relievers (analgesics) can be taken. If pain seems excessive, people should tell a health care practitioner.

PHYSICAL THERAPY

Physical therapy helps people move better. It includes several types of exercise, transfer training, walking (gait) training, and techniques that make movement safer or easier. It aims to increase endurance, make joints less stiff, strengthen muscles, reduce pain, and improve coordination and balance. Techniques to treat pain and inflammation are also used. Physical therapists work closely with occupational therapists.

Aerobic exercise: Aerobic exercise strengthens the heart and lungs and helps increase endurance.[5] As endurance increases, any physical activity becomes less tiring. Walking, bicycling,

1. see page 258
2. see page 317
3. see page 87
4. see page 86
5. see page 905

and swimming are aerobic exercises. Consulting with a doctor before starting an aerobic exercise program may be important, especially for people who have had a heart or lung disorder or who have been very inactive.[1]

Range-of-motion exercises: Moving joints through their range of motion helps make muscles and joints less stiff. Inactivity for several days (for example, after a stroke or surgery) makes the muscles around joints stiff. So joints may become less flexible. That is, their range of motion may become limited. Limited range of motion can cause pain, and the person cannot function as well. Range-of-motion exercises can help the person do daily activities.

Before range-of-motion exercises are started, physical therapists evaluate the person's range of motion with an instrument that measures angles of joint motion (goniometer). If flexibility or range of motion is extremely limited, surgery or special casts are sometimes needed before range of motion can be improved.

Range-of-motion exercises may be passive (in which a therapist moves the joint), active-assistive (in which the person needs some help moving the joint), or active (in which the person moves the joint without any help). During passive or active-assistive range-of-motion exercises, therapists move the joint gently to avoid injury, although some discomfort may be unavoidable. For improvement to occur, a joint with limited range of motion must be moved far enough to cause some discomfort. A person may begin with passive or active-assistive exercise and, as strength increases, move to active exercise.

Muscle-strengthening exercises: To make a muscle stronger, a person must exercise against resistance that is gradually increased. When a muscle is very weak, no extra resistance is needed. The force of gravity provides enough. As a muscle becomes stronger, resistance is gradually increased with elastic bands or weights. This type of exercise also increases muscle size (mass) and endurance.

The two main types of muscle-strengthening exercises are isotonic and isometric.[2] Isotonic exercises involve contracting a muscle to move a joint. Isometric exercises involve contracting

1. see page 907
2. see also page 905

a muscle without moving a joint. Isometric exercises can be done in bed, for example after hip or knee surgery.

Coordination exercises: Exercises to improve coordination involve repeating a movement that works more than one joint and muscle. Examples are picking up an object or touching a body part. Such exercises are often used for people who have had a stroke.

Balance exercises: Exercises can improve the ability to maintain balance while standing, sitting, and moving. Standing on one leg is an example. Tai chi may be used to improve balance. Exercises that improve strength and coordination may also help with balance.

Transfer training: Some people need to learn a safe way to move (transfer) from one place to another—for example, from a bed to a chair (or wheelchair) or from a chair to a toilet. The need may be temporary (until the ability to walk is recovered) or permanent.

Different techniques are used in transfer training depending on whether the person can bear weight on one or both legs, has good balance, or is paralyzed on one side of the body. Special devices, such as a chair with a raised seat, can sometimes help. Some people cannot transfer by themselves. They can learn how to help another person help them transfer. They may need to wear a special cloth strap around the waist called a gait belt. A therapist or a caregiver trained to use the belt can grasp it securely and thus help people transfer safely. A transfer board can be used as a bridge to slide across from wheelchair to bed, toilet, or bathtub seat. These boards are light-weight planks of smooth wood or plastic. Mechanical lifts may be used by a caregiver to help with transferring. Therapists teach caregivers how to help with transferring.

Gait training: This training improves the ability to walk, with or without help. Before starting gait training, some people need to do exercises that improve strength, range of motion, balance, and coordination. Gait training may be needed after bed rest, a stroke, or the amputation of a leg. A gait belt may also be used during gait training to help prevent falls.

After walking safely on a level surface, the person may be taught to step over curbs or climb stairs. For going up stairs, the stronger or uninjured leg goes first. For going down stairs, the

CHOOSING AND USING A CANE

People who need a cane have several options. Most canes have one tip (called a single-point cane) or four tips (called a quad cane). The more tips, the more stability provided, but the heavier the cane. People can choose a pistol-grip handle or a curved handle. The pistol grip is easier to grasp.

Regardless of the cane's style, getting a cane that is the right height is important. A cane that is too long or too short can cause low back pain and poor posture. It can also make walking unsteady. The handle should come to the crease in the wrist when the arm hangs down by the side. A cane should be held in the hand opposite the weak or painful leg.

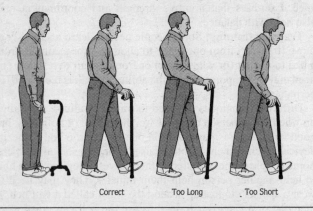

Correct   Too Long   Too Short

weaker or injured leg goes first. The phrase "good is up, bad is down" can help people remember. If possible, the person should go up and down the stairs with the railing on the uninjured side.

Some people require an assistive device for walking. If a joint does not support weight and buckles readily, a leg or an ankle brace is needed. If the legs are weak or balance is a problem, a cane or walker can be used.

Crutches are seldom recommended for older people because their arms may not be strong enough to use crutches safely. Even when used correctly, crutches can make arthritis in the shoulders worse.

If people cannot walk with a cane or walker, a wheelchair or scooter can help them stay active. A wheelchair or scooter may be needed all the time or only for long distances. Wheelchairs come in many varieties. Choosing the most suitable one, getting

CHOOSING AND USING A WALKER

Walkers come in many varieties. They may or may not have wheels, and the number of wheels may vary. Walkers without wheels are seldom recommended for older people because they are hard to use correctly.

Walkers with two wheels and two rubber tips are the most common. They are the easiest to use and provide the most support. Walkers with three wheels are small and maneuverable. They may be recommended for people who live in a small home (such as a trailer) with narrow doors. Walkers with four wheels may be recommended for people with Parkinson's disease. They may have difficulty lifting walkers with two or no wheels. Sometimes four-wheel walkers with a seat and hand brakes are recommended for people with a heart or lung disorder. Such people may tire more easily. The seat enables them to rest when needed. They should always apply the hand brakes before they sit down.

Walkers cannot be used on stairs. As people walk, they should keep the walker close to their body. They should not use a walker to help them get up or sit down because it may tip over.

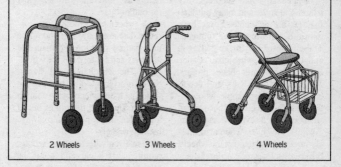

2 Wheels   3 Wheels   4 Wheels

one that fits properly, and learning how to use it correctly are important for safety and comfort.

Tilt table: Some older people need therapy for dizziness due to an excessive fall in blood pressure that occurs when they stand (orthostatic hypotension[1]). A tilt table is commonly used for this purpose. For the procedure, a person lies face up on a padded table with a footboard and is held in place with safety belts. The table is tilted very slowly until the person is nearly upright. How long the position is held and how often the procedure is repeated depend on the person's response.

1. see page 279

Electrical stimulation: Sometimes muscles do not function normally because nerves are damaged. Such muscles can be stimulated electrically to help prevent them from wasting away (atrophying). An electrical current is transmitted through electrodes placed on the skin. The current stimulates the muscle to contract automatically. Electrical stimulation may help prevent muscle wasting in people who are paralyzed (for example, after a stroke or an accident).

Another type of electrical stimulation, called transcutaneous electrical nerve stimulation (TENS), is used to treat certain kinds of pain. TENS uses a gentle oscillating current. TENS produces a tingling sensation without increasing muscle tension. TENS may be applied through electrodes attached to the

WHEELCHAIRS AND SCOOTERS

Wheelchairs and scooters vary in size and style, and many optional features are available. Some have removable armrests and footrests. These features may make getting in and out of the wheelchair easier. Some wheelchairs have motors. Motorized wheelchairs and scooters are useful for people who cannot push a wheelchair because of weak arms or a severe heart or lung disorder. However, when arm muscles are not used to push the wheels, these muscles may progressively weaken (become deconditioned).

People who are likely to develop pressure sores may need a special cushion, designed to redistribute weight and relieve pressure. These people include those who cannot shift their weight, those who are incontinent, and those who have had a pressure sore.

People who have had a stroke may need a wheelchair that is shorter than standard. Then, they can use their good foot to help propel the wheelchair. Some wheelchairs are designed primarily for indoor use, and others are designed for outdoor use.

A wheelchair should fit correctly. The arms and feet should be in a natural position when on the armrests and footrests of the wheelchair. The wheelchair seat should be comfortably wide but not so wide that it does not provide enough support. Before getting in or out of a wheelchair, people should always lock the wheels.

Usually, a wheelchair or scooter requires that a car and home be modified somewhat. Usually, a special lift that is attached to the back of the car is needed to transport the motorized wheelchair or scooter. The car must have heavy-duty shocks installed to support the lift. Even then, some cars cannot support a wheelchair lift. For the home, ramps may need to be placed over steps, and doors may need to be widened.

Payment for motorized wheelchairs and scooters by Medicare or other health insurance can be a problem, even with a doctor's prescription.

skin or through a hand-held device. It may be applied several times a day for 20 minutes to several hours each time. The timing and length of stimulation vary because each person responds differently. Often, people are taught to use the TENS device at home, so that they can use it as needed.

OCCUPATIONAL THERAPY

Occupational therapy helps people do their normal daily activities, including caring for themselves, working, and participating in leisure activities. Occupational therapists work closely with physical therapists.

Many types of problems can make doing even simple activities difficult. Joints may be stiff and have a limited range of

---

DEVICES THAT HELP PEOPLE FUNCTION

• Grab bars on the side and back of the bathtub or toilet for people with balance problems or weak legs

• Shower chairs for people who cannot stand for a long time because of weakness or dizziness

• Bathtub benches for people who have balance problems or who have difficulty getting in and out of the bathtub because of pain or weakness in the legs

• Raised toilet seats and chair leg extenders (which make the chair's seat higher) for people who have trouble standing up

• Eating utensils, shoehorns, and other tools with large, built-up handles for people with a weak grip

• Weighted eating utensils, cups with lids, and swivel spoons for people with tremors

• Plates with rims and rubber grips (to prevent slipping) for people who have coordination problems

• "Grabbers" that can pick items off the floor or from a shelf

for people whose reach or movement is limited

• Tools with spring-loaded or electronic controls for people with hand problems

• Devices that turn electrical appliances (such as lamps, radios, and fans) on or off at the sound of the voice for people whose movement or coordination is limited

• Computer-assisted devices for people whose arms and legs are paralyzed or who have other disorders that greatly limit function

• Larger dials on telephones for people with impaired vision

• Telephones and doorbells that display a flashing light when they ring for people with hearing loss

• Automatic dialing on a telephone, devices that remind a person about when to take a drug, and pocket devices that record and play back messages (reminders, instructions, and lists) at the appropriate time for people who have trouble remembering

motion. Muscles may be weak, and endurance may be short. Balance, dexterity, or coordination may be lacking. Shaking (tremor) may make carrying objects difficult. There may be problems with thinking (cognitive problems). These difficulties may make a person feel incompetent, frustrated, and unable to cope with relearning old skills or learning new ways to do old activities.

Occupational therapists try to identify such problems. They watch the person do a specific activity. They may also ask family members or other caregivers about the disability. Sometimes specific tests, such as a test to assess balance, are done.

Occupational therapists also try to identify other problems that can make an activity difficult. For example, the attitudes of family members can affect the person's ability to do an activity. Or the physical environment can make doing an activity difficult. For example, lighting may be inadequate, or electrical cords across walkways can make walking hazardous.

Occupational therapy includes many of the techniques and activities used by physical therapists. However, occupational therapy focuses on the person's living environment and equipment, devices, and physical abilities needed to do specific activities, especially those done with the arms and hands.

The occupational therapist and person choose the techniques and activities that seem appropriate and set goals for each. For example, if a person has problems using eating utensils, therapy may consist of repeating an activity that requires similar movements, such as inserting pegs on a peg board. A memory game may be used to improve recognition and recall. A person with a paralyzed arm is taught adaptive techniques, such as how to dress, tie shoes, and fasten buttons with one arm. Adaptive techniques help a person use strengths to compensate for disabilities. A person who has trouble concentrating and planning may be taught to limit activities and put them into routines.

Occupational therapists also suggest tips for simplifying activities. For example, a person who has trouble with dressing may be advised to wear pullovers, which are easier to put on than cardigans. Therapists may also suggest devices that can help a person function more independently (assistive devices).

SPEECH THERAPY

Speech therapy varies depending on the type of speech problem.[1] Speech exercises can help retrain people to use the muscles involved in speech. Exercises can help train the brain to understand words, numbers, or gestures and to learn new ways to concentrate, remember, and process information. Therapists may help people who cannot speak find alternative ways to communicate.

Some of the same muscles used in speaking are used in breathing, swallowing, and eating. So speech therapy can also help people who have problems with these functions. Exercises may improve control of mouth and throat muscles. Therapists may suggest techniques to help with eating. For example, holding the head in a certain position may make chewing and swallowing easier. A special diet may be recommended because some kinds of foods are easier to swallow than others. Examples are soft foods, foods with a consistent texture, and thick liquids. Therapists may recommend using gelatin to thicken liquids.

REHABILITATION FOR SPECIFIC PROBLEMS

Rehabilitation can be tailored for many specific problems. Examples are heart disorders, stroke, hip surgery, replacement of a knee, amputation of a leg, speech disorders, blindness, and hearing loss.

Heart Disorders

Rehabilitation for people with a heart disorder is called cardiac rehabilitation. It may help after a heart attack[2] or heart surgery. It may also help when heart failure develops or worsens.[3] The goals are to enable people to care for themselves—at the least, to do the basic activities of daily living—and to live as independently as possible.

Cardiac rehabilitation is started as soon as possible, usually while the person is still in the hospital. Before rehabilitation can

1. see page 186
2. see page 676
3. see page 686

begin, some people, such as those who have had a heart attack, must be stabilized. For example, they may need to be treated to stop sudden changes in blood pressure.

Typically, cardiac rehabilitation begins with a relatively undemanding activity, such as transferring to and sitting in a chair. All activities are supervised by a trained attendant. When these activities can be done comfortably, usually by the second or third day, the person tries somewhat more demanding activities, such as dressing, grooming, and walking short distances. More demanding activities are tried as the person progresses. Before a person is discharged from the hospital, doctors measure the person's heart and breathing rates while the person does certain activities. Then doctors and other members of the rehabilitation team can tell the person which activities are safe and which are not. The person is also given a detailed description of exercises to be done at home.

The number and intensity of activities are slowly increased. The goal is full resumption of normal activities after about 6 weeks. Most people benefit from a cardiac rehabilitation program. Typically, there are 3 sessions a week for about 8 to 12 weeks after discharge from the hospital.

Cardiac rehabilitation programs provide help handling the psychologic effects of having had a heart attack or heart surgery. People are also taught about changes in lifestyle that can help prevent or slow the progression of a heart disorder or reduce the risk of another heart attack. Examples are quitting smoking, losing weight, controlling blood pressure, reducing cholesterol levels (by changing the diet and taking drugs), and doing aerobic exercises at least 3 times a week.

These programs improve endurance (making physical activity less tiring), improve quality of life, and decrease the risk of dying after a heart attack or bypass surgery. The benefits of cardiac rehabilitation are at least as great for older people as for younger people.

Stroke

Rehabilitation can help people recover some or all of the abilities they have lost as a result of a stroke. However, the extent of recovery depends heavily on how well the damaged areas in the brain heal on their own. How much and how quickly the brain will heal cannot be predicted. How successful rehabilitation is depends partly on the person's general condition, including flexibility of joints, muscle strength, motivation, and the ability to understand and learn.

Rehabilitation is begun as soon as the person can tolerate being moved and exercising. Starting rehabilitation soon helps prevent problems, such as weakening of muscles, stiffening of joints, undernutrition, pneumonia, development of blood clots, pressure sores, and depression.[1]

Rehabilitation usually begins with a therapist moving the person's affected limbs through their range of motion (as passive range-of-motion exercises). When able, the person is encouraged to help move (as active-assistive range-of-motion exercises) or to move the affected limbs alone (as active range-of-motion exercises). The unaffected limbs should also be exercised to prevent them from weakening. As soon as the person is able (often within 1 week), coordination exercises are started.

The person is expected to practice other activities, such as moving in bed, turning, changing position, and sitting up. When able, the person is taught to transfer from the bed to a chair or wheelchair safely and independently. Being able to get out of bed as soon as possible helps physically—in terms of exercising—and mentally—in terms of feeling independent and making progress in recovery.

Some of the problems caused by a stroke require specific therapies. Exercises to improve strength, balance, and coordination and gait training may be needed. People may need help learning how to compensate for problems with vision, hearing, speech, swallowing, or thinking (cognitive problems).

If one leg is greatly weakened, walking (gait) training focuses on teaching people to walk safely, not necessarily to walk as they did before. Such training can help prevent falls.[2] A cane with four tips is useful because it provides more support than a cane with one tip. A leg or an ankle brace can enable people with one paralyzed leg or with tight, stiff (spastic) muscles to walk. If one arm is paralyzed, therapists teach people how to dress with one arm.

After a stroke, many people cannot do activities that require

1. see page 147
2. see page 291

fine coordination. That is, they cannot move their hands precisely or coordinate the movement of their hands and eyes. Occupational therapy may help. People may learn new ways to do activities, such as fastening clothing, opening and closing containers, and getting objects that are too far to reach. Devices, such as Velcro closures for clothing and dinner plates with rims and rubber grips (to prevent slipping), may be recommended.

After a stroke, some people are partially or completely blind in one or both eyes. People who are blind in one eye are taught ways to avoid bumping into door frames or other obstacles. Turning the head toward the affected side can help. Specific therapies are used for people who are blind in both eyes.[1]

Rehabilitation for cognitive problems is a very slow process. It requires a one-on-one approach. Also, it must be tailored to the person's situation. A stroke can cause different types of cognitive problems, depending on which area of the brain was damaged.[2] Therapy includes specially designed exercises to retrain the brain and ways to compensate for problems.

Speech therapists can retrain people to use the muscles involved in speaking and breathing (which is necessary for speaking.[3] If necessary, people are taught other ways to communicate effectively. Speech therapists also help people with swallowing problems learn to eat more safely.

Hip Surgery

Hip surgery may be done to repair or replace bones in the hip joint that are damaged by arthritis or broken. After surgery, rehabilitation is begun as soon as possible. Depending on the type of surgery, rehabilitation may begin on the same day as surgery. The initial goals of rehabilitation are to help the person become mobile and to prevent loss of muscle tone and other problems that result from bed rest, such as blood clots and pressure sores. The ultimate goal is to enable people to walk as well as they could before the problem occurred.

After surgery, hospital staff members encourage the person to resume activities as soon as possible. To a person who is tired and in pain after surgery, this prodding may seem bothersome,

1. see page 187
2. see page 381
3. see page 179

too demanding, or even cruel. However, resuming activities is necessary for a good recovery. The person is encouraged to sit in a chair as soon as possible, sometimes within hours of surgery. Sitting in a chair helps counter the effects of too much bed rest. Sitting also makes the transition to standing easier. The person is taught range-of-motion exercises and exercises to strengthen the trunk, leg, and arm muscles. These muscles may have to be used more because the lower body is injured. Exercises should be done daily.

Usually within a day of surgery, the person is encouraged to stand on the unaffected leg (the one not operated on) with the help of a chair, a bed rail, or another person. The surgeon and therapist decide when and how much weight can be put on the affected leg. Sometimes the affected leg can bear full weight on the second day after surgery.

Walking (gait) training is started as soon as the affected leg can safely bear some or all of the person's weight without discomfort and the person can balance well enough—often just a few days after surgery. Stair-climbing exercises are started soon afterward.

An assistive device, such as a walker or cane, is often needed. People learn how to sit, stand, and walk in ways that will not reinjure the hip. They learn how to prevent falls.[1] Therapists teach them exercises to strengthen the hip and maintain its range of motion. Doing them regularly aids recovery.

Therapists may recommend special equipment for the bathroom, such as a raised toilet seat or a bathtub bench, to make using the bathroom easier and to protect the hip.

Replacement of a Knee

One or both knees may need to be replaced because of arthritis. Rehabilitation for people who have had a knee replaced is similar to that for people who have had hip surgery. That is, rehabilitation emphasizes range-of-motion and strengthening exercises and walking (gait) training. However, the specific exercises vary.

1. see page 291

Amputation of a Leg

Older people who have diabetes or peripheral arterial disease (usually due to atherosclerosis) may have to have one or both legs surgically removed (amputated). A leg may be amputated below the knee, above the knee, or at the hip. Sometimes only a toe or part of the foot is amputated.

Rehabilitation after amputation is extensive. Doctors usually recommend an artificial leg (prosthesis). An artificial leg consists of a foot, knee unit (if the leg is amputated above the knee), and socket. (The socket enables the artificial leg to be attached.)

After surgery, the remaining part of the leg (stump) must heal before an artificial leg can be worn. The stump is also swollen. A permanent artificial leg cannot be fitted until the swelling goes down, but a temporary one can be used. Therapists teach the person or a family member how to apply an elastic sock (called a stump shrinker), which helps the stump shrink. Exercise, including walking with a temporary artificial leg as soon as possible, also helps the stump shrink. Taking care of the stump is important. It should be kept clean and dry. The skin of the stump should be checked daily for irritation, breaks, and redness. Any problems should be reported to a doctor.

After surgery, physical therapy is started as soon as the person is able. Therapy varies somewhat depending on whether one or both legs were amputated and whether the amputation was above or below the knee. Exercises to stretch the hip and knee are started as soon as possible. These exercises help prevent muscles from stiffening. Exercises to strengthen arm and leg muscles are also started. Endurance exercises may be needed. At first, exercises are done in bed, then in a chair. The person is encouraged to do standing and balancing exercises with parallel bars as soon as possible.

People who have decided to use an artificial leg are taught how to walk with the leg on. Walking begins with assistance from one or more therapists and progresses to walking between parallel bars to using a walker, then a cane. Therapists teach people to use stairs, walk up and down hills, and walk on other uneven surfaces.

After amputation of one leg below the knee, most older people who are fitted with an artificial leg can learn to walk without a cane. However, people who have had a leg amputated above the knee may not. Controlling an artificial leg with a knee joint requires more skill, strength, endurance, and energy than controlling one without a knee joint. Some artificial legs for amputations above the knee are controlled by a microcomputer, enabling a person to control movements more precisely. Walking with an artificial leg of either type is more tiring than walking with a natural leg.

Gaining weight should be avoided because added weight makes walking with an artificial leg more difficult and may affect the fit of the leg.

When both legs have been amputated—regardless of where—walking may be limited, and a wheelchair is sometimes needed.

The person's home usually needs some modification. For example, grab bars in the shower or a hoist over the tub may be needed. Sometimes a new living arrangement is needed. Driving is often possible, but a car may need to be modified.

Problems after amputation: Rehabilitation can help with problems that may occur. The most common problem is stump pain. Pain may be felt when the stump is touched or when the artificial leg is worn. The pain may have a visible source (such as a sore) or an internal source in the bone or nerves (such as an irregular projection of bone called a bone spur). Pain may also be caused by a poorly fitted artificial leg, swelling, or weight gain. When such problems occur, the therapist works closely with the prosthetist.

After amputation, many people have a feeling that the amputated leg is still there (called phantom limb sensation). Sometimes people feel a mild tingling where the leg was. The sensation is so real that they can sometimes describe the position of the foot. Sometimes, usually at night when waking up to use the bathroom, people try to stand up as if they had both legs, and they fall down. Phantom limb sensation may last several months or years but usually disappears without treatment. Frequently massaging the stump often helps.

Some people feel extreme pain in the amputated leg (called phantom limb pain). It may be more likely to occur when pain was present before amputation or was not controlled well during or after amputation. Exercising both legs and using an artificial leg help relieve the pain. Often, massaging the stump or using a vibrator or an ultrasound device also helps. Certain antidepressants (such as nortriptyline or desipramine) or anticonvulsants (such as gabapentin or carbamazepine) are sometimes helpful.

Many people feel loss and grief when they lose a body part. Getting support from family members and talking with a counselor may help with these feelings and with the lifestyle changes required after amputation.

Speech Disorders

Different types of speech therapy are used depending on the speech disorder.

Aphasia: Some people have difficulty using or understanding spoken or written language. Others completely lose the ability to do either. These people have aphasia. Aphasia often results from a stroke that damages the part of the brain that controls language.

The goal of therapy is to find the most effective way to communicate. For mild cases of aphasia, a speech therapist points to an object or picture, the person says what the object is, and the therapist nods to reinforce the person's efforts to communicate. For more severe cases, words are repeatedly spoken to the person. Also, objects are named and presented to the person. Being able to touch and see an object as well as to hear the name of an object can help the person relearn words.

Family members and caregivers of a person with aphasia need to be patient and appreciate the person's frustration. For example, they should not interrupt when the person is speaking slowly. They should encourage the person to speak (for example, by nodding). A person with aphasia may think normally. So using baby talk is inappropriate and can increase the person's frustration. Instead, family members and caregivers should speak in simple sentences and, if necessary, use gestures or point to objects. Asking questions that can be answered with "yes" or "no" can make communicating easier.

Dysarthria: Some people have difficulty physically forming words. They have dysarthria. People who have dysarthria produce sounds that approximate what they mean and that are in the correct order. Dysarthria is caused by damage to the nervous system (for example, by a stroke or by multiple sclerosis). The damage affects control of the muscles involved in speaking, including those of the lips, tongue, palate, and vocal cords and those used in breathing (which help with speaking).

Depending on the cause of dysarthria, the goal of therapy may be to restore and preserve speech or to maintain the ability to speak for as long as possible.

Speech therapists can retrain people to use the muscles involved in speaking and breathing. For mild cases of dysarthria, therapy may involve making different sounds or repeating sounds, words, or sentences. These exercises may help the person relearn how to use facial muscles and the tongue. The person may be taught to speak more slowly and to use shorter phrases. For severe cases, the person may need to communicate using a board with letters, words, or pictures (sometimes homemade) or a specially designed electronic communication device.

Verbal apraxia: Some people cannot initiate, coordinate, or sequence the muscle movements needed to talk. They have verbal apraxia. They randomly mispronounce words and seem to have forgotten how to make the sounds of language. Verbal apraxia is caused by damage to the nervous system (for example, by a stroke, a head injury, or brain surgery).

A speech therapist may ask the person to say sound patterns over and over again. Or a therapist may teach the person to use natural melodic patterns for common phrases. Usually, each phrase has a melody (the voice goes high and low in a pattern) and a rhythm. The speech therapist encourages the person to speak using an exaggerated melodic pattern and rhythm. As speech improves, the person can gradually speak with less exaggeration.

Blindness

For people whose vision is impaired or who become blind, rehabilitation includes learning new ways to do daily activities. For example, food is always arranged on the plate in the same places. Clothing, furniture, and other objects should be kept in the same place. People may learn how to use a cane to get from one place to another. A cane can also be used to check for objects in the way.

Sometimes people who are blind need guidance when walking. So family members and other caregivers are taught how to guide them. For example, caregivers are taught to have the blind person hold onto their arm and to lead the person, rather than hold onto the blind person's arm and try to push him one way or another.

Blind people may learn how to get around with a seeing eye dog and may learn Braille. Until they learn Braille, audio books can be used. Household items, such as stoves, microwaves, and cooking ingredients, can be labeled with tags written in Braille. Items specially designed for the blind, such as talking watches, may be useful.

Hearing Loss

Rehabilitation for people with hearing loss (partial or complete) includes learning to read lips and to use a hearing aid. People with hearing loss learn how to modulate their speaking volume because they tend to speak loudly. Audiologists can help people choose a hearing aid that suits their needs.[1] They can recommend devices that are specially designed for the deaf, such as doorbells, telephones, and alarms that display a flashing light when they ring. Some people benefit from having a dog trained to respond to certain sounds and then alert them.

I was born on May 9, 1925. From the start, life was a struggle. I suffered with rickets, and doctors told me that I might not be able to walk. With the help of my lovely wife, a good diet, and plenty of exercise, I overcame that prognosis. My wife believes the syrup and bread that I have been eating for years has kept me going.

In 1935, I moved to Virginia. I attended school and worked as a field hand. This is where I found my love for horses, I even bought a horse.

During 1943, I enlisted in the Army. I was a private in the 10th Calvary (known as the Buffalo Soldiers) in Fort Bliss, TX. When I was patrolling, my horse became frightened by a snake and threw me. I was stranded there for 3 days and 3 nights. In the dry desert terrain, temperatures were 110° in the daytime and 30° to 40° at night, and I suffered from hypothermia, dehydration, and early starvation. All that was in my possession was a compass and flashlight. My other gear was lost, because my horse had run off. To keep the coyotes away I started fires from desert weeds and matches I had attached to my belt.

After completing rehabilitation, I enrolled at Tuskegee Institute. There I met my wife, Sylvia, to whom I have been married for 56 years. We had 7 boys and 1 girl. I have been active in my community. As far as aging goes, I have worked hard, lived hard, and loved hard, and I never believed in the word "can't." I have lost my driving privileges, but I still get around with help from my family and friends, public transportation (the senior pass is great), and even my motor scooter. I never give up, so I always try to show my support for my family, friends, church, and the community. I may get weak and weary, or wake up with arthritis and need to lay back down with liniment, but I still keep on going like a Buffalo Soldier should.

Henry Washington

14

Long-Term Care

The prospect of long-term care concerns many older people. The likelihood of needing long-term care increases greatly as people age. Older people are more likely to develop chronic disorders and to have problems functioning. Learning about the many types of long-term care can help people choose the right time and place for this care. How long care is needed varies from weeks to years to indefinitely.

Long-term care focuses on helping people function. It helps them do the activities necessary to care for themselves and to live as independently as possible. These activities include basic daily activities (such as eating, dressing, bathing, grooming, and walking) and other activities (such as shopping, balancing a checkbook, doing laundry, and cleaning). Long-term care usually includes help with health care. Most long-term care facilities also provide social and recreational activities.

Many people have their first experience with long-term care after a hospital stay. During a hospital stay, many older people lose some or all of the ability to care for themselves.[1] Thus, they may need to go to a long-term care facility for rehabilitation and recovery. This move can be physically and psychologically demanding. People have to adjust to many new faces and to new routines for sleeping, bathing, dressing, eating, and other daily activities. The move happens quickly, with little time to adjust.

Most people associate long-term care with a change in residence: to a retirement community, an assisted living community, a board-and-care facility, a life-care community, or a nursing home. However, only one third of older people who receive long-term care live in an institutional setting. The others receive care in their own home or the home of a family member. This care is usually provided by family members or friends. If needed, health care practitioners may visit the home to provide additional care.[1] People who receive care in institutions usually have more physical and thinking (cognitive) problems and less social support from family members and friends.

What type of arrangement is possible depends partly on the person's needs (medical, functional, social, and emotional). However, it also depends on the person's preference, finances, and social support (for example, the family's willingness and ability to help). One person may be able to live at home with the help of a spouse. Another person with similar problems but without family support may need to go to a nursing home.

After the type of arrangement needed is determined, a particular facility must be carefully chosen. Within each type, facilities differ considerably in environment, services (including health care), activities, living arrangements, and rules. Sometimes the difference is simply a matter of what a person can afford, but even within a price range, quality varies.

Retirement Communities

Retirement communities are designed for people who can live independently but who need or want some help, mainly with caring for a home. Some older people choose to move to a retirement community before they need additional help. They may move because they do not want the responsibility of maintaining a large house and yard or because they have become lonely or isolated.

Retirement communities consist of a group of apartments, townhouses, or detached homes. These communities provide some services, such as transportation, entertainment facilities, some on-site nursing services, community meals, laundry services, and house cleaning and maintenance. Such services enable older people who are reasonably well to live independently. Retirement communities may arrange group activities, such as trips, game nights, or lectures by guest speakers. Some have recreational facilities, such as swimming pools and golf courses. The homes are usually designed for older people. For example, they may have only one floor. Retirement communi-

DELAYING THE NEED FOR A LONG-TERM CARE FACILITY

The idea of going to a long-term care facility, particularly a nursing home, does not appeal to most people. The following problems are common reasons for entering a long-term care facility. However, sometimes problems can be solved, and the need for a long-term care facility can be delayed or avoided.

Urinary incontinence: People with urinary incontinence may be hard to care for at home. However, urinary incontinence may be caused by a disorder that can be treated. Treating the disorder may cure the incontinence. People with urinary incontinence, their family members, or their caregivers should talk with a doctor about incontinence to find out whether treatment is possible.

Problems with doing daily activities: Certain devices can help people function better. A physical or occupational therapist or a home health nurse can observe people in their home and can sometimes help

them choose appropriate devices that will enable them to continue to function safely at home.

Dementia: Taking care of people with dementia is difficult and frustrating. However, family members can learn ways of dealing with the behavior. For example, to deal with wandering, family members can place an identification bracelet on the person or purchase or rent monitoring devices. Learning more about how to care for people with dementia may delay the need for a long-term care facility.

Caregiver burnout: Strongly motivated family members can usually provide elaborate and detailed care. However, providing such care can wear them out physically and emotionally. Talking with health care practitioners can help. They can provide information about caregiving support groups and about groups that provide temporary (respite) care.

ties enable some people to postpone a move to a facility that provides more intensive long-term care.

Some retirement communities are part of a life-care community. Life-care communities provide as much care as people need for the rest of their life.

Because retirement communities vary so much, people should ask questions to make sure the community they are considering is suitable for them.

• Is there an entrance fee in addition to the monthly fee? Which services, activities, and amenities are included in the monthly fee?

• What services, activities, and amenities are available? Is

TYPES OF LONG-TERM CARE

Type	Typical Services	Typical Living Arrangement	Funding
Assisted living communities	Meals (in a common dining room or in the person's room)	Apartments or occasionally just a bedroom with a private bath	Mostly private funds or long-term care insurance
	Social and recreational activities		Help from Medicaid in some states
	Help with daily activities		
	In some facilities, monitors for emergencies (such as intercoms and personal emergency response systems), services of nurses and physical therapists, and 24-hour supervision if needed		
Board-and-care facilities	Meals (in a common dining room or in the person's room)	Rooms on a common hallway	Mostly private funds
	Transportation to medical appointments or shops		
	Social activities		
	Help with personal care and sometimes		

Table continues on the following page.

Type	Typical Living Services	Arrangement	Funding
	some help with taking drugs (for example, reminding people to take their drugs)		
Life-care communities	Meals (usually in a common dining room, except for residents who need more care and who have meals in their room) Transportation Social and recreational activities As much help with daily activities and health care as needed	Varied arrangement according to need	Mostly private funds Help from Medicare and Medicaid for skilled nursing care when it is needed
Nursing homes	Meals Help with daily activities 24-hour skilled nursing care, rehabilitation (physical, occupational, respiratory, and speech therapy) Hospice care Oversight by a doctor	Rooms on a common hallway	Private funds Medicaid Medicare for skilled care for a short time in certified nursing homes if care is needed daily after a hospital stay lasting 3 days or more

there a bank, beauty salon, post office, or general store? Is transportation readily available for trips to local shopping areas, doctors' offices, and other health care facilities? What social and physical activities are available?

- What is the minimum age to live in the community?
- Are the facilities well maintained? Are the living units and their setting pleasant? Is there enough parking?
- Are there service people to help?
- Are meals provided?

Assisted Living Communities

Assisted living communities are designed for people who can care for themselves if they have some help with daily activities. These communities can help older people who have problems with memory, who get confused, or who have physical problems. Some communities have special units for people with dementia where residents can be closely monitored.

Assisted living communities vary from small and homey to large and elaborate. Residents usually have their own apartment or a bedroom with a bathroom. These communities provide meals, help with daily activities (including personal care), and offer some social and recreational activities. Residents can choose which activities and services they want. Most assisted living communities provide some health care, including 24-hour supervision if needed. Doctors and nurses may visit regularly, and physical therapists may be available. Services and activities offered vary greatly from community to community. Also, regulations for these communities differ from state to state.

When people need intensive treatment, they may have to move to another facility, such as a hospital or rehabilitation center. They may move back to the assisted living community if they are able. But to hold their living space while they are gone, they must continue to pay for it.

People who move to assisted living communities usually need help with daily activities because they have some limiting health problems. Assisted living communities prefer people who do not need help moving (transferring), for example, from bed to chair. But even when people become relatively impaired, they may be able to stay in these communities because of the help provided. How much help is provided varies considerably from community to community. Generally, an assisted living community is not an alternative to a nursing home. More often, it is a transitional living arrangement, followed eventually by a move to a nursing home. Assisted living communities are usually less expensive than nursing homes because they provide less care. However, they can still be expensive. Usually, Medicare and Medicaid do not pay for assisted living communities.

Board-and-Care Facilities

Typically, board-and-care facilities, also called rest homes, are similar to assisted living communities. They are for people who need some help, particularly with personal care. Board-and-care facilities provide a room, meals, help with daily activities, and occasionally some health care. In board-and-care facilities, people usually live in rooms, as in a college dormitory, rather than in apartments. Some facilities have a very homelike atmosphere.

Board-and-care facilities are not as closely regulated as nursing homes or even some assisted living communities. Many provide good care, but some do not. Some facilities attempt to care for people with very different needs. For example, younger people, many of whom have an untreated or a poorly treated mental disorder, live side by side with older people who do not have a mental disorder. In such an arrangement, the older people may feel uncomfortable or awkward.

Older people and their family members must carefully evaluate a board-and-care facility. They should ask what the facility does and does not provide and make sure that the staff members can meet the needs of the residents and treat them well.

Life-Care Communities

Life-care communities (also called continuing care retirement communities) are for older people who want to move only once, to a place that will provide as much care as they need for the rest of their life. These communities guarantee that residents are cared for within the community regardless of their health.

A person may begin by living in a house or apartment. But later, if health deteriorates, the person can move to an assisted living community and finally to a nursing home, all on the same property. Life-care communities offer the security of continued care in one location, without having to move very far. However, many life-care communities are expensive. Some require a large deposit as well as monthly payments and fees for additional services. Sometimes there is an upper limit (cap) for monthly payments and fees. But in many communities, costs increase when the level of services needed increases.

Medicare and Medicaid usually do not pay for residence in a life-care community but may help pay for skilled nursing care when it is needed.

Nursing Homes

Nursing homes are for people who need help with health care for chronic conditions but do not need to be hospitalized. The decision to move to a nursing home may be triggered by a change in circumstances. A disorder may suddenly worsen, or an injury may occur. Function may deteriorate suddenly or slowly but steadily. Family circumstances may change, making care at home difficult.

"Nursing home" is sometimes used as a general term for any long-term care facility. But it specifically refers to skilled nursing facilities. "Skilled" indicates that some of the care included can be provided only by trained health care practitioners. "Nursing" indicates that nurses provide most of the care in the facility. Nurses give residents their drugs, monitor disorders, supervise treatments, consult with doctors about care, and organize most of the activities in the nursing home. The nursing staff includes registered nurses (the most highly trained), licensed practical nurses, nursing assistants, and a director of nursing, who oversees nursing care in the home.

Each nursing home also has a medical director, a doctor who oversees the medical care. In some nursing homes, the medical director is the only doctor who provides medical care. But in most nursing homes, several doctors provide care. Sometimes a doctor who has been taking care of the person before the move continues to provide care. Otherwise, the person chooses or is assigned to a doctor. According to regulations, a doctor must see every nursing home resident at least once every other month. Many residents see a doctor more often because they tend to develop additional disorders, such as infections or confusion. Also, nurses may call a doctor to discuss problems and changes in treatments.

Many nursing homes provide other health care services, such as oxygen treatments and drugs or fluids given by vein (intravenous therapies). Almost all nursing homes provide rehabilitation, including physical, occupational, respiratory, and speech therapy. Many people are admitted to nursing homes specifically for rehabilitation, then are discharged after several weeks.

Dentists and medical specialists, such as ophthalmologists, neurologists, or psychiatrists, may examine and treat residents on site. But most often, people with a specific problem have to be transported to a different site for treatment. Some nursing homes have special units for people with dementia. These units are staffed by specially trained nurses. Many nursing homes provide hospice care for people who are dying.[1]

Almost all nursing homes have a social worker on staff. Social workers help residents adjust to the home. They identify residents who are lonely and withdrawn and help residents, staff members, and family members communicate with each other. They may also help residents and family members make financial arrangements. For example, they may show family members how to apply for Medicare and Medicaid coverage.

Social workers often help coordinate the care provided by the different health care practitioners in a nursing home. These practitioners work together to enable each resident to function as well as possible and to have the best possible quality of life.

Some nursing homes provide the minimum of services in an institutional, impersonal environment. They may resemble hospitals more than homes. However, many nursing homes are trying to change from a more institutional environment with rules and regulations to a more homelike environment that gives residents more control over their care. Some nursing homes permit pets, encourage residents to maintain existing hobbies or develop new ones, and provide many opportunities for contact between residents and people of all ages who live in the community around the nursing home. Providing this kind of environment is complicated because the residents of nursing homes are usually sick and frail. Many nursing homes have din-

---

1. see pages 112 and 223

CHOOSING A NURSING HOME

Environment

• Is the nursing home attractive, friendly, homelike, and relaxed?

• Are there any unpleasant odors? Is the nursing home clean and well maintained?

• Are the dining room and other common areas bright, cheery, and pleasant?

• How is the noise level in common areas monitored to prevent it from disturbing residents whose rooms are nearby?

• Are there safe, accessible walking paths on the grounds?

• Is there a garden or patio?

• Does the nursing home have appropriate safety devices, such as fire alarms and sprinklers? What are the plans for emergencies, such as fires?

Residents

• Do the residents seem reasonably happy and active, or are they wandering aimlessly or sitting and doing nothing?

• Are the residents clean and properly dressed?

• Are any of the residents restrained?

Staff Members

• Do the staff members treat the residents with respect, patience, and friendliness?

• Are staff members experienced and qualified?

• Is there a high turnover in staff members?

• Do staff members respond to requests for help in a reasonable amount of time?

• What is the staff member to resident ratio?

Rooms

• Is there enough storage or closet space?

• Are the residents' rooms bright and cheery?

• Are private rooms available?

• How are roommates selected?

• How are private items stored or secured?

• Can residents have their own telephone and television?

• Is water available and within reach for residents?

• Can residents decorate their rooms with personal items?

• Are there safety features, such as grab bars and pull cords (to call for help)?

• Can residents keep food in their rooms?

Meals

• What time are meals served?

• Are meals served hot?

• Are snacks available between meals?

• Can residents get from their room to the dining area easily?

• Can meals be provided in a resident's room if needed?

• Are the meals tasty and nutritious?

• How are special dining or menu requests handled? Are choices available at meals?

• Can the nursing home provide special diets when needed? Is there an additional cost?

• Are staff members available to help with feeding during meals?

Health Care

• Can residents keep their own doctor rather than use the nursing home's doctor?

• Does the nursing home have an arrangement with a nearby hospital?

• If residents have to be hospitalized, will a bed be available afterward?

• Are other health care practitioners (such as dentists, podiatrists, physical therapists, optometrists, counselors, and social workers) available?

• Are therapy programs (such as physical, occupational, or speech therapy) provided?

• Does the nursing home have special programs for people who have such disorders as Alzheimer's disease or HIV infection?

• What services does the nursing home provide for residents with a terminal disorder?

• How are prescription drugs ordered and given to residents? How is the use of drugs monitored?

• What is the policy on residents keeping nonprescription drugs?

• Are residents and family members encouraged to participate in developing a plan for care?

Services

• Is help with daily dental care provided?

• How is personal laundry done?

• Is reading material available?

Visiting

• Is the nursing home conveniently located for frequent visits by family members and friends?

• Can family members visit any time?

Activities

• What activities are offered?

• Are residents encouraged to participate? How are the residents informed of the activities?

• Is there an activity director?

• Does participation in activities cost extra?

• Are there rooms for other activities, such as a TV or game room?

• Are religious services held on the premises?

Costs

• Are all the services that residents need covered in the basic charge?

• What services (such as beauty salons or laundry) cost extra and what is the cost?

Residents' Rights and Privacy

• Are residents allowed to go in and out as they please?

• Are restraints used? When and why?

• Is there a lock on the door to private rooms? Do staff members knock before entering?

• Can married couples live together? Are they given privacy?

• Are the sexual needs of residents respected?

• How often are residents bathed? Can residents have a bath or shower whenever they want? Are bath and shower areas kept warm enough? How much privacy is provided in these areas?

• Are pets allowed? Can visitors bring pets?

• Can residents keep food or alcohol in their rooms?

• What is the nursing home's policy on lost or missing valuables?

• Who contacts family members in case of an emergency?

• If residents wish to leave, what are the policies on giving notice or refunds?

ing rooms, recreation rooms, beauty salons, patios, and gardens. All nursing homes provide recreational and social activities.

Nursing homes are highly regulated by the government. State health departments conduct surveys and inspections to monitor and evaluate quality in nursing homes. A copy of this evaluation is kept at the nursing home and can be reviewed by residents and their family members. Many homes also use other programs that monitor and help improve the quality of care. For example, nursing homes that are part of a network or chain usually have their own monitoring programs in addition to those of the government.

Even though nursing homes are monitored and regulated by government, they vary considerably in quality, personality, and cost. So people or family members who are interested in a nursing home should try to get as much information as possible. They can ask the administrator of the nursing home to see the state's evaluation of the home. Similar information is available on the Internet. One evaluation called the Quality Indicator Report looks at how well a nursing home handles specific problems. These problems commonly develop or worsen in residents of nursing homes but can be prevented with attentive care. They include a decline in the ability to do daily activities, undernutrition, weight loss, pressure sores, incontinence, constipation, infections, depression, and use of too many drugs. Whether these evaluations are valid is debated. Nonetheless, they provide information that can help people better compare nursing homes.

Other important questions to ask the administrator include whether the nursing home is certified to provide Medicare and Medicaid coverage, how often care of residents is reviewed, and whether residents and family members are included in the review of care. For some questions, the administrator may direct people to the nursing home's medical or nursing director.

Talking to other people who are familiar with the home is helpful. Such people include long-term care ombudsmen (who visit nursing homes and investigate complaints), doctors, clergy, family members of residents, residents, and employees of the nursing home. Some homes have resident organizations, consisting of family members and friends of residents who meet to discuss issues that come up in the nursing home. These organizations can provide family members of prospective residents with helpful information. However, visiting a home for several hours is usually the best way to determine whether the quality of services is good and whether the home will be a good place for a loved one.

In the United States, Medicaid and private funds pay for most nursing home care. Medicare pays for skilled care for a short time in certified nursing homes if care is needed daily after a hospital stay lasting 3 days or more.

15

Caregiving

Most people cherish their independence. But many older people eventually need and depend on help with performing either minor or essential tasks. The people who provide this help are usually referred to as caregivers.

Of the nearly 36 million people aged 65 or older in the United States, about 7 million need a caregiver's help on a daily basis. This need develops primarily because of the effects of diseases that become more common with aging. The types of needs vary greatly. Some older people need help with everyday activities, such as eating, dressing, and bathing. Others need help with household chores, such as cooking, cleaning, shopping, paying bills, and mowing the lawn. Even people who are largely independent benefit from occasional help—such as receiving a ride to a friend's house or assistance with transporting a heavy item—and from the interest and involvement of family members and neighbors.

The costs of caregiving are enormous. The United States spends more than $130 billion a year on the care of older people with a disability or chronic disease. About two thirds of this cost is paid for by the federal and state governments, and the remaining one third is paid for by the older person or family members. This estimate does not include indirect costs, such as those incurred when caregivers miss work to care for a loved one. Nor does it include the additional amounts that would be needed if family and friends did not provide care free of charge. This family care is estimated to be worth about $200 billion.

Who Are Caregivers?

The number of caregivers continues to grow. More than 22 million caregivers in the United States provide ongoing care for older people for periods of time ranging from a few hours a week to around-the-clock.

Most caregivers are the spouses or children of the people they care for, and most are women. About two thirds of caregivers work full- or part-time in addition to filling their caregiving role. Many come to the role having never imagined they would have to take responsibility for their partner or parent and having no special caregiving skills. They learn these skills on the job.

Other relatives, friends, neighbors, and members of religious or other groups may assist family caregivers or take over the role altogether. Occasionally, families hire health care practitioners, such as licensed practical nurses (LPNs) or nurse's aides, to help care for a parent or spouse.

Rewards of Caregiving

Caregiving can be very rewarding, even when it is hard work and causes stress. Many people choose to care for a spouse, partner, or parent out of love and respect. They find new meaning in their own life by making a difference in another person's life, even if their efforts are not always appreciated. Some caregivers report great satisfaction in giving back to someone who has given so much to them. Others report that caring for a parent provides a good role model for their own children. Caregivers who provide care out of love and a desire to help another person report greater personal benefits from caregiving than those who provide care merely out of a sense of duty.

Challenges in Caregiving

No one can ever be fully prepared for the challenges of caregiving. The tasks and responsibilities involved can be demanding, even more so when caregivers themselves are frail, have been thrust into their role unexpectedly or reluctantly, or must care for someone who is uncooperative or combative.

Physical challenges: Caregiving presents physical challenges to the person who provides care. The caregiver may need to assist with or even assume complete responsibility for physically demanding tasks, such as doing laundry or housekeeping. Or the caregiver may need to help with more basic needs, such as bathing or dressing the person. The caregiver must be sure of her physical capability to provide care. For example, a man who has had a stroke may need his wife's support while rising from

---

DOES THIS PERSON NEED CARE?

Family and friends concerned with an older person's ability to care for himself can ask themselves the following questions to determine whether the help of a caregiver is needed:

• **Eating:** Are clothing items frequently stained by food? Is the person losing weight without an obvious explanation?

• **Getting in and out of a chair or bed:** Does the person rock back and forth several times before actually getting up? Are nearby furniture items or objects used for support? Does sitting seem to involve falling backward into a chair?

• **Toileting:** Are clothing items soiled or wet?

• **Bathing:** Are the person's skin and hair dirty?

• **Grooming:** Does the person have a rumpled or disheveled appearance?

• **Walking:** Does the person seem unsteady? Have falls occurred?

• **Taking medicine:** Do prescriptions last longer than they should? Are prescriptions used up faster than they should be?

• **Using the telephone:** Does the person seem to understand phone conversations? Is the phone consistently answered when the person is known to be home?

• **Managing money** (paying bills, balancing a checking account): Do bills go unpaid, leading to overdue notices? Has the person repeatedly been notified of overdrafts on accounts?

• **Preparing food:** Are food items kept past expiration dates? Do pots and pans seem to become scalded repeatedly? Has the stove been found left on?

• **Doing laundry:** Are clothes clean?

• **Housekeeping:** Is the home increasingly unkempt? Can the person find things readily when they are needed?

• **Using transportation:** Has the person repeatedly become lost while traveling in ways or on routes that are familiar?

• **Shopping:** Is the kitchen or pantry stocked with a reasonable amount and variety of food items?

a bed, chair, or toilet or while walking. But his wife may be unable to lift him if he falls and could be at risk of injuring herself if he falls while leaning on her for support.

Mental challenges: People who are confused because of dementia often are unable to carry out everyday activities that require cognitive skills, such as the ability to remember, organize, and plan. The caregiver may need to assist with or assume responsibility for the person's medications, including understanding what they are for and how they are to be taken. Or the caregiver may have to manage the person's money. The caregiver also needs to plan activities and modify the home in ways that provide a safe environment that is stimulating yet not overwhelming for the person with dementia. Doing so requires attentiveness to details and some creativity.

Financial challenges: Many older people subsist on limited funds available from savings, pensions, and Social Security payments. The medical disorders that make older people dependent often pose enormous financial burdens that overwhelm their assets.

Caregivers must be aware of any financial responsibilities that they face when they begin to care for people. For example, children may need to assume some financial responsibility for their dependent parents and, without financial help, may spend their life's savings in the process. A caregiver may face additional household expenses for food, utilities, and transportation. If remodeling must be done, additional expenses may be incurred. A caregiver who is employed may need to reduce work hours or quit altogether to provide care. The resulting loss of income can in turn create more financial challenges.

Emotional challenges: Family caregivers commonly experience conflicting feelings of affection, frustration, a wish to help, anger, sadness, satisfaction, guilt, and a sense of loss for the deteriorating health or abilities of their partner, spouse, parent, or friend. These varying emotions can occur unpredictably and simultaneously and can be made worse by the expectations of the person who needs care. For instance, some older people come to expect more from their caregivers than is necessary, because relying on others may be easier and more emotionally rewarding. Other truly needy older people may refuse all outside help, instead insisting that family members attend to their own needs. This puts a responsible caregiver in the position of mak-

LONG-DISTANCE CAREGIVING

In a modern, mobile society, family members sometimes live hundreds or even thousands of miles apart. Such distances can complicate efforts to ensure that aging loved ones receive the care that they need. Indeed, long-distance caregivers—usually adult children—are presented with unique challenges. First and foremost, good communication is often difficult to maintain. Family members may feel that they never get a complete or accurate impression of how their distant loved one is managing or what his needs are. Just as important, even when needs are understood, family members may feel there is little they can do for their loved one unless they themselves are there to do what is needed.

Several steps can be taken to assist with the challenges of helping from a distance. Scheduling a regular time for phone calls, for example, is a simple step that can be reassuring for everyone involved. Newer technologic options for communicating include phones that can send and receive pictures or video and computers, wireless hand-held devices, and devices that hook directly into a telephone line that transmit electronic mail. Family members can sometimes identify a person who can visit their loved one regularly and who agrees to call them immediately if questions or concerns arise. If family members have concerns about how well their distant loved one is coping with shopping, meal preparation, and eating, they may be able to arrange for participation in some type of meal program to help ensure that the older person is eating properly. If concerns about security arise, a home security system may be useful. If the family is concerned that a loved one might fall and be unable to call for help, a personal emergency response system (medical alert device) might be an option. And family members should have copies of any advance directives, such as a living will or durable power of attorney for health care, if their involvement is required should their loved one need emergency treatment.

With the many challenges of helping from a distance, getting assistance from someone familiar with resources in the community where the loved one resides can be valuable. The primary care doctor for the loved one's medical care may be helpful in arranging for local help. A geriatric care manager can oversee the caregiving and health care of older people in the absence of a primary caregiver. If none of these measures is sufficient, sometimes the family members believe they have no other choice than to go to their loved one and help directly. The Family Medical Leave Act permits a person to keep a job while taking up to 12 weeks of unpaid leave to attend to a dependent family member. This protection extends only to larger employers, however, and has other restrictions.

ing major personal sacrifices for an unrealistic parent or partner or arranging needed care over the person's fierce objections. Either solution brings mixed feelings with it. In addition, many caregivers, especially women, believe that society expects them to give up their own lives to care for others.

Caregiving often involves sacrifices, restrictions, and competing responsibilities. Younger caregivers have less time to spend in activities they enjoy and may get caught between caring for an older parent or friend and caring for their own spouse or partner or for their dependent children. They are sometimes referred to, therefore, as the sandwich generation.

Siblings may argue over dividing caregiving responsibilities, the burden of which almost always falls disproportionately on one. The patience of family members may be sorely tested when a person needing care lives under the same roof. And caregivers who are themselves old, such as the spouse of a person needing care, may have their own complex health and financial concerns that require almost as much attention as those of the person they care for.

The many conflicts and responsibilities that come with caring for an older person can isolate a caregiver, compromise relationships, threaten job opportunities, and lead to mounting anger, frustration, guilt, anxiety, stress, depression, and a sense of helplessness and exhaustion that is sometimes called caregiver burnout. Burnout can affect anyone at any time but is more likely when the person being cared for cannot be left alone or is disruptive overnight. In the worst cases, when caregivers are unaware of or are unable to obtain help, burnout can lead to abandonment and even abuse of their older charges.[1]

Getting Help

A caregiver must find a balance between the rewards and challenges of caregiving. Although there is no easy fix for the challenges, there are strategies for coping with the conflicts and mechanisms for occasionally relieving the burdens. Determining what kind of help an older person needs and how to get that help often involves working with many different practitioners, including doctors, nurses, physical and occupational therapists, social workers, and case managers.[2]

1. see page 945
2. see pages 104 to 108

Physical help: Often, caregivers can help people with physical disabilities gain greater independence by making or arranging for minor home modifications.[1] For example, installing grab bars over the bed or grip bars in the bathroom by the toilet and tub can help a person rise from the bed, toilet, or tub without assistance. Other equipment, such as a shower chair or bathtub bench, can help a person shower or bathe safely. Placing a night light in the bathroom or a commode by the bed can help prevent overnight problems, such as falls and episodes of incontinence. A chair- or bed-bound person can use mechanical pincers to grab distant objects or objects on the floor without getting up or bending down.

Nurses and occupational therapists often can evaluate a home and recommend these and other measures to improve an older person's safety and reduce his physical dependence. Physical therapists can teach special techniques that can reduce the risk of injury and exercises that can improve strength and balance. Health care practitioners can also teach caregivers techniques to improve their ability to provide care. For example, they can teach a caregiver how to use a gait belt (a canvas strap wrapped around the older person's middle section) to help the person walk more safely.

Mental help: Paper and pen organizers or computer software can help caregivers list, organize, and track information about appointments, medications, and finances related to the person for whom they are caring.

Financial help: Meeting the additional expenses that may arise with caregiving begins with understanding and taking advantage of the financial resources of the person for whom care is being provided. Long-term care expenses of dependent older people may require several forms of insurance.[2] Inexpensive forms of Medigap and other private supplemental insurance cover only the deductibles and co-payments that a person with basic Medicare coverage incurs, whereas more costly forms cover many more expenses, such as prescription drugs.

When finances are limited, older people can pay for expenses with a reverse mortgage on a home; by using a life insurance policy as collateral for a bank loan; by borrowing money di-

1. see box on page 293
2. see page 957

rectly from the policy (viatical loan); or by selling the policy to a third party for a portion of its cash value (viatical settlement).

Caregivers have other ways to control their expenses or increase their financial resources. Some caregivers can benefit from the medical-expense deductions and other tax credits that come from claiming an older person as a dependent. They may also be able to take medical-expense deductions for home modifications that provide a clear medical or safety benefit. Employed caregivers may have access to flexible-spending accounts, which allow allocation of pre-tax dollars toward meeting predictable expenses incurred through providing care. Free or low-cost programs may be available through state or local programs, churches, or other community organizations that assist with expenses relating to transportation, home modifications, or in-home help from a nurse's aid.

Emotional help: Many strategies are available for relieving the emotional burdens of caregiving, the most important of which is taking personal time out. Relaxing or engaging in enjoyable activities allows caregivers to recharge their batteries. Support groups for caregivers, in which the challenges of caregiving are discussed, can be helpful.

Help from the community: Caregivers can do only so much as individuals, and the help they may receive from other family members or friends may not be enough. Additional help may come from the community. Programs in the community that provide assistance with and relief from the various demands of constant caregiving are sometimes referred to as respite-care programs.

One option may be to locate and use a program that offers supervision and activities for the older person for a few hours. The caregiver can then run errands, get a haircut, or perhaps just take a nap. Adult day care centers have filled this need in many parts of the country. An older person can be taken to an adult day care center for an occasional visit or scheduled for several days a week. Most adult day care centers provide transportation, and all provide supervised activities, hot lunches, snacks, and drug monitoring. Some adult day care centers also provide check-ups with health care practitioners, such as nurse practitioners, dentists, doctors, and podiatrists, and assistance with bathing.

Alternatively, home health care agencies can provide a home health care worker with the necessary skills to assume caregiving responsibilities for a period of time during the day. Cooperatives are sometimes formed by families who provide assistance to each other, thus allowing for an inexpensive form of care. However, because of the difficulties of transporting people with multiple disabilities, cooperatives are not used too often.

Nursing homes, personal care homes, and assisted living communities that already have 24-hour staffing can sometimes provide overnight care, often for several days or longer, and include some nursing care. These options are particularly helpful when a caregiver wants to take several days of vacation and the older person needs 24-hour assistance. However, these facilities are typically more expensive than adult day care centers.

STRATEGIES FOR AVOIDING CAREGIVER BURNOUT

• Learn about the cause, symptoms, and course of the person's condition. Anticipate changes.

• Let the older person make his own decisions and solve problems if he is able. Set limits to the amount of assistance offered if necessary.

• Avoid taking an older person's anger, frustration, or difficult behaviors personally. These behaviors may be symptoms of a disorder such as dementia.

• Avoid arguments.

• Delegate responsibilities and ask other family members and friends to help whenever possible.

• Ask for help from trustworthy family members, friends, or neighbors. Be explicit but reasonable about expectations. Avoid criticism as long as the person helping is responsible.

• Discuss feelings and experiences with others, either informally or through a support group.

• Eat and exercise regularly, and schedule regular time for relaxing, enjoyable activities.

• Obtain information about the older person's financial resources; avoid depleting personal finances.

• Contact organizations that can provide information and referrals for caregivers.

• Consider day care or respite care before the burden of isolation or of caregiving grows too great.

• Remember that assisted living facilities and nursing homes may be the best option.

16

Palliative and End-of-Life Care

Most people envision living "the good life" in their later years and devote decades to preparing for it. But few people devote much thought to how they might live with a serious or life-threatening disease or to how they will die. Thus, most people do not discuss their feelings or make adequate plans to ensure that their wishes will be followed.[1]

Until a few generations ago, there was very little to think about concerning death and dying. Many people died very quickly after becoming infected or injured. Others died quickly after developing a disease such as coronary artery disease or cancer, because no effective treatments existed.

Much has changed in the last few generations, however. Some people still die of infections or injuries, although far fewer than ever before. And some people still die instantly or very quickly of diseases that strike with little or no warning. For example, a person without any prior evidence of coronary artery disease may die abruptly of a massive heart attack. A person who has had very few symptoms may die very soon after being diagnosed with an aggressive cancer that has already spread widely. However, most Americans now develop one or more serious chronic diseases with which they will live for many years before they die.

More than three fourths of deaths in the United States are due to chronic diseases, such as heart disease (including coronary artery disease and heart failure), cancer, stroke, chronic obstructive pulmonary disease (COPD), and dementia. People are now living much longer after they learn of having a chronic disease. After receiving such a diagnosis, a person's health and

SIGNS OF APPROACHING DEATH

Most people with a life-threatening chronic disease want to know how much time they have left to live. Family members often want to be present at the time of death and may need to make arrangements to ensure their availability. Predicting the timing of death is imperfect. For a variety of reasons, doctors almost always overestimate the amount of time that their patients have to live. More experienced doctors seem somewhat better at making this prediction, although the longer a doctor has known a patient, the less objective and accurate the prediction seems to be.

Despite the difficulties involved in predicting when death will occur, some signs indicate that death is approaching or imminent.

• **Change in level of alertness:** When near death, people typically spend increasingly more time sleeping. When awake, they may be less alert or interactive. Confusion or disorientation is common.

• **Decreased interest in eating or drinking:** People near death typically refuse most food, although they may still request or accept sips of fluid.

• **Absence of urination:** Once a person stops urinating, death typically follows within a few days to a few weeks.

• **Changes in the skin:** The hands and feet often become cool and bluish or develop a lacy pattern. These changes are expected and are markers that death is likely in hours to days.

• **Changes in breathing:** The breathing pattern changes as death approaches. Breathing may become rapid and shallow or may alternate between periods of slow and rapid breathing. The person may stop breathing for increasingly prolonged periods, only to resume breathing again. A rattling noise may be heard when the person breathes (the death rattle). This noise is caused by accumulation of secretions, such as saliva, that the dying person cannot swallow or spit out and by relaxation of muscles in the throat. The dying person is usually unaware of this noise, but family members may be very distressed by it, fearing that their loved one is choking.

---

ability to function tend to decline gradually, but death is still very often sudden. It becomes difficult to know when a person goes from living with one of these diseases to dying of the disease.

The medical care received by people with life-threatening chronic diseases is, on the whole, successful at helping them live longer. But the health care system has not been nearly as successful at providing support and comfort. The system also falls short of addressing why many treatment decisions are at odds with a person's previously stated wishes or why there is so little advance care planning.

When asked, people with life-threatening chronic diseases often have simple goals. These goals may include the following:

• Relief from pain and other troubling symptoms
• Involvement whenever possible in decisions about their care
• Assurance that their previously stated wishes will be honored and respected when they are no longer able to be involved in decision making
• A sense of completion and relief of any burdens on family and friends

Family, friends, and health care practitioners of a person with a life-threatening chronic disease can often approximate the person's goals of care. However, in most cases, the person must state his own goals, discuss these goals, and revise them periodically when appropriate. Continued, open communication with family, friends, and health care practitioners about these goals of care can make the difference between a peaceful death and one characterized by unnecessary suffering.

REDUCING SUFFERING

Pain

Pain is a common symptom for people living with a life-threatening chronic disease. It is particularly common for those very near the end of life. The disease itself can cause pain, such as when cancer spreads to the bones or the spinal cord. Certain treatments for disease can cause pain, such as when anticancer drugs or radiation alter nerve activity (neuropathic pain). In addition, certain conditions that accompany dying can cause pain, such as when immobility leads to stiff joints, constipation, or pressure sores.

Some types of pain are better tolerated than others, but pain of any type generally diminishes the quality of a person's life—and death. Pain is affected by a person's other symptoms, mood, quality of sleep, emotional and social support systems, and spirituality or religious beliefs.

A doctor carefully assesses the pain to determine the best treatment approach. People with pain and those who care for them need to know that pain can be controlled satisfactorily without serious side effects.

Because a person with a life-threatening chronic disease often has several types of pain, treatment that involves several approaches is often most effective. Pain relievers (analgesics) are a mainstay of treatment.[1] However, the effectiveness of drug treatment is often improved when combined with other kinds of treatment, such as massage and the use of heat. Once treatment is started, health care practitioners continue to assess the effectiveness of pain control. It is important that people with severe pain alert their health care practitioners when pain is poorly controlled or when side effects of treatment develop.

People with severe pain often need opioid analgesics as part of their treatment plan. Opioid analgesics are extremely effective in relieving pain. Side effects include constipation, sleepiness, confusion, nausea, and itching. All of these side effects can be controlled so that opioid analgesics can be used without fear. Opioid analgesics may also slow breathing, but this side effect is extremely rare when dosages are adjusted properly.

People should discuss their preferences for drug and nondrug treatments. These discussions should also clarify specific goals of treatment, such as whether to treat pain aggressively, even when doing so may increase sedation at the end of life. There is no evidence that properly administered analgesics hasten death. On the contrary, evidence suggests that people live longer when their pain is under better control. And, dying people need not worry about becoming dependent on analgesics. Finally, knowing possible indications of pain, such as grimacing and fast breathing, gives family and friends a way to monitor pain when a dying person can no longer speak for himself.

Information about what to expect can help a dying person tolerate new or worsening symptoms. Companionship, emotional encouragement, and spiritual counseling all may lessen the anxiety, anger, depression, fear, insomnia, and loneliness that make pain worse.

1. see page 335

Shortness of Breath and Coughing

Shortness of breath and coughing are experienced by many people with life-threatening chronic diseases, especially near the end of life. Shortness of breath is any unpleasant feeling of uncomfortable breathing. It can be frightening for the person suffering it as well as for family members.

Many complications can cause shortness of breath and coughing: infection, spread of cancer, fluid accumulation in or around the lungs, fluid collection around the heart (pericardial effusion) or in the abdomen (ascites), blood clots in the lung (pulmonary embolus), or compression of large veins in the chest due to cancer. Some medical treatments may also contribute to shortness of breath at the end of life. For example, fluids given to maintain hydration or provide nutrition may interfere with breathing if they unintentionally accumulate in the lungs, the space that surrounds the lungs (pleural space), and the space that surrounds organs within the abdomen (abdominal cavity). The extra fluid may prevent the person from breathing normally.

Often there is no clear cause of shortness of breath. A low red blood cell count (anemia), a high level of carbon dioxide in the blood, weakness, poor positioning in bed, a feeling that there is not enough air in the room, and anxiety all contribute to the sensation. Fear and stress expressed by family members as well as restless activity in a dying person's room can also worsen breathing.

Treatment of shortness of breath and coughing involves treating the underlying causes. Therefore, any treatment that is contributing to the problem, such as intravenous fluids, may need to be discontinued. When the underlying cause cannot be easily treated, a person may feel best while sitting up and breathing cool air in a room free of crowding and unnecessary commotion. A fan sometimes provides a sense of relief, as do physical touch, massage, and other calming distractions. Oxygen therapy is sometimes helpful. Some people may breathe more restfully when moisture is added to the air. Moisture can be added either by humidifying the entire room or by adding mist to oxygen received through a face mask or through a device that fits into both nostrils (nasal prongs).

When these remedies do not sufficiently relieve symptoms, opioid analgesics, such as morphine, can relax a person's breathing and can actually have helpful effects on the heart, lungs, and blood vessels. Antianxiety drugs (such as benzodiazepines) are also useful. Bronchodilators may help, as may drugs that decrease mucus secretions, such as scopolamine and hyoscine. Coughing can also be treated with codeine and other cough suppressants; corticosteroids may also help.

Digestive Problems

Digestive problems, including nausea and vomiting, loss of appetite (anorexia), mouth problems, constipation, and diarrhea, are common in people with life-threatening chronic diseases, especially near the end of life.

Nausea and vomiting can, like pain and shortness of breath, prevent a person from thinking of anything else. Nausea and vomiting have dozens of causes, including opioid and anticancer drugs; constipation; infection; sores (ulcers) in the mouth, esophagus, or stomach; blockage of the stomach and intestines; liver and kidney failure; and altered calcium and sodium levels in the blood.

The underlying causes are treated if possible. A nauseated person who cannot eat may still enjoy ice chips. Antinausea drugs are almost always helpful. Some of these drugs can be used anytime. Others are used in specific situations, such as when an anticancer drug, constipation, or intestinal blockage causes nausea. Acupuncture and acupressure (which involve stimulating certain parts of the body with needles or with pressure) appear to be effective against nausea due to anticancer drugs, cancer itself, and other causes.

Loss of appetite can result from difficulty chewing due to dry mouth, mouth sores, or mouth infections or from difficulty swallowing due to a tumor. Severe pain, nausea, constipation, or changes in taste due to illness or treatment can also affect appetite. More commonly, however, loss of appetite occurs because of a serious disease or condition, such as cancer or an infection. The disease can cause protein and fat to break down in the body. These changes often cause significant weight loss (cachexia) in a dying person.

In the uncommon event that a person appears to be distressed by loss of appetite, family members and friends can try offering small portions of soft foods (such as eggs; gelatin, or sherbet) or of the person's favorite foods on a flexible schedule. Some drugs can be used to increase appetite, including cortico-steroids, hormonelike drugs (progestins and androgens), drugs that speed up digestion (metoclopramide), and a drug related to marijuana (dronabinol). These drugs can take weeks to take effect. In rare circumstances, the person fares better with food given by feeding tubes or intravenously.

Family members and friends often do not understand that loss of appetite near death is nearly universal, and dying people are rarely hungry. Near the end of life, loss of appetite does not distress the dying person, although it may greatly concern loved ones. Coaxed or forced nutrition rarely increases a dying person's weight and may cause the person greater distress. Artificial feeding and hydration through tubes or intravenously usually does not prolong life and often worsens symptoms such as shortness of breath. Thirst is much more successfully managed by allowing sips of liquids or by keeping the dying person's mouth moist with liquids or sprays intended for this purpose or even with a moistened cloth.

Mouth problems come from ulcers due to anticancer drugs, fungal infection, dryness due to radiation treatment and dehydration, and poor hygiene. Treatment includes taking frequent sips of water or other liquids, brushing the teeth twice a day, and rinsing the mouth with an anesthetic solution. Antifungal drugs such as nystatin, used as a mouth rinse or dissolving lozenge, or fluconazole, taken as a pill, are effective against fungal infection.

Constipation may seem trivial compared with other symptoms, but it can greatly compromise comfort. Constipation occurs because a seriously ill person nearing the end of life is typically inactive or immobile, is dehydrated, eats little dietary fiber, and takes constipating drugs, especially opioid analgesics. Other contributing factors are an inability to get out of bed to reach a toilet, confusion, depression, and such disorders as spinal cord compression, intestinal blockage, and high calcium levels in the blood.

Constipation can sometimes be managed by remedying the underlying cause, which may include taking periodic walks, sucking on ice chips, and using a bedside commode. Laxatives taken by mouth or as suppositories are useful, as are enemas. Increased fiber intake, which is usually helpful in treating constipation in healthy, active people, should be avoided in people who are nearing the end of life, because their reduced fluid intake can cause the fiber to be useless or even harmful.

Diarrhea is much less common than constipation. Diarrhea is often caused by drugs, including anticancer drugs, antibiotics, and laxatives; by diseases such as some cancers; and by surgery on the stomach or intestine that speeds up the movement of materials in the digestive tract and decreases their absorption. Diarrhea can also be a sign of constipation when hard stool stimulates the large intestine to push liquid stool around it. Treatment is usually with antidiarrhea drugs, such as loperamide and diphenoxylate.

Inflammation of the Anus

The anus sometimes becomes irritated and inflamed because of constipation, diarrhea, changes in the skin and the lining of the anus that may occur if weight is lost, and increased pressure on the skin during long periods without moving around. Zinc oxide and corticosteroid creams may relieve irritation and inflammation around the anus.

Pressure Sores

Pressure sores (bedsores)[1] occur because dying people usually lie in one position for long periods without moving. Pressure sores are easier to prevent than to treat. Prevention involves changing positions frequently and cushioning areas prone to pressure sores, such as the heels, ankles, hips, and lower back. Treatment involves reducing pressure, changing positions frequently, applying dressings, removing dead tissue, and maintaining proper nutrition.

Itching

Itching affects some people with life-threatening chronic diseases because of incontinence, sweating, poor hygiene, dehydration, dry skin, dermatitis and other skin conditions, and liver and kidney failure. Often the cause is unknown. Treatment involves correcting the underlying cause combined with applying moisturizing and corticosteroid creams and taking drugs that decrease itching (such as antihistamines) as needed.

1. see page 503

Fatigue

Fatigue is extremely common and often is due to many factors, including pain, sleep disturbance, low red blood cell count (anemia) or low blood oxygen level, organ failure, drugs, infection, and depression.

Often it is best to simply let a person rest as much as he needs to. Sometimes, other treatment seems appropriate and may involve treating the underlying cause with analgesics, sedatives, antibiotics, antidepressants, oxygen, or a blood transfusion or erythropoietin (a drug used to increase the red blood cell count). Occasionally, psychostimulants such as methylphenidate or dextroamphetamine are useful.

Anxiety

Anxiety is common in people with life-threatening chronic diseases. It may be a normal response to physical symptoms or to the prospect of death. Pain and shortness of breath are common triggers, as is the appearance of a new or unfamiliar symptom. Some drugs can cause anxiety. Anxiety is also caused by conflicts with family members, recognition of one's own mortality and limitations, fear of abandonment, regret over past actions, and financial concerns. Anxiety is a problem when it causes sleeplessness or other disturbing symptoms and when it overwhelms people's thoughts or limits their ability to do the things they would like to do.

Anxiety can be relieved by emotional support and reassurance from family members and by health care practitioners, who can patiently explain symptoms, treatments, and choices. Music, prayer, or other relaxing activities may also help. Antianxiety drugs, including benzodiazepines and antidepressants, are effective when other measures fail.

Depression

Depression affects many people with life-threatening chronic diseases and needs to be distinguished from the sadness a person might normally feel. Although depression near the end of life may be common, it is never considered normal. Depression near the end of life is just as burdensome as at any other time of life and can rob the dying person of a sense of purpose and the energy and interest needed to communicate with and enjoy the company of family members and friends. Depression should be identified and treated at the end of life as at any other time.[1]

Depression may be worse for those with uncontrolled pain or nausea, little family or social support, and financial or other stresses. A primary symptom of depression is sleeplessness, which in turn may worsen pain, nausea, and fatigue. Depression also affects appetite.

Alleviating pain and nausea often relieves depression, as does allowing people as much control as possible over treatment decisions and over their surroundings. Spiritual counseling or other empathic support may also help. Sometimes, antidepressant drugs are needed and can be highly effective in treating depression in people who are nearing the end of life. For those for whom death is anticipated sooner than the time required for traditional antidepressants to take effect, a more rapid elevation in mood can be achieved with psychostimulants, such as methylphenidate or dextroamphetamine.

Confusion

Sudden confusion (delirium) is especially common at the end of life. Drugs used to treat pain, shortness of breath, anxiety, and depression contribute to confusion, as do fever, dehydration, and sleep disturbance. For many people, however, confusion reflects changes in the brain and body that are a natural part of dying. Confusion is often more a problem for family members than for the dying person.

Treatment involves keeping the person safe, usually by having someone with him as often as possible. Drugs that cause confusion should be stopped or the dose decreased whenever possible. Treating fever and dehydration and creating a calm, quiet environment with few distractions may help. Antipsychotic drugs, such as haloperidol, often help reduce fear or hallucinations in people nearing the end of life. If the person is agitated and restless, sedatives such as benzodiazepines may also be helpful.

1. see page 442

RETAINING CONTROL OVER DECISIONS

People can retain control over the decisions that they confront near the end of life, even as they become less able to care for and speak for themselves.

Advance Directives

A living will allows a person to explicitly state his wishes regarding health care in the event that he can no longer speak for himself.[1] A durable power of attorney for health care (called a health care agent or health care proxy in some states) authorizes a specific person, often a spouse or adult child, to make health care decisions for a person who can no longer speak for himself.[2]

In many cases, when a living will or a durable power of attorney for health care does not exist, several family members participate in making decisions. However, problems may arise when family members disagree over the best course of action for a sick relative. The family's wishes may contradict those communicated by the dying person, or the dying person's wishes may be unknown to the family. To avoid such problems, family members should try to follow the dying person's preferences and interests regarding treatment rather than their own. In addition, family members should do their utmost to resolve their differences before becoming involved in treatment decisions. It is also often helpful to have a family meeting to communicate those decisions, ask questions, and receive information from health care practitioners. However, a single family spokesperson should be appointed to improve the efficiency and clarity of communication between meetings.

Assisted Suicide

In assisted suicide, a dying person asks a doctor to help him end his life, usually by prescribing a lethal dose of drugs to be taken at the time of his choosing. Assisted suicide is currently legal in only one state in the United States (Oregon). Euthanasia, in which a doctor personally administers a treatment with the intended purpose of bringing about death, is illegal in the

1. see page 954
2. see page 955

United States but is legal in the Netherlands. A small number of dying people ask their doctor to assist them in ending their life, even in places where it is illegal.

Depression and hopelessness are among the main reasons for these requests. Other reasons include a sense of being a burden to others; loss of independence; loss of control of bodily functions; inability to participate in enjoyable activities; a wish to control the circumstances of death; and physical suffering. A request for assistance in dying should be considered a sign of extreme distress and should never be ignored. Exploring the reasons for the request, asking about fears and worries, and listening to the person making the request are important.

AT THE BEDSIDE OF A DYING PERSON

Just as the beginning of life begins with what doctors refer to as "active labor," so the ending of life begins with "active dying," during which signs of approaching death develop. Once active dying has begun, the focus of care often shifts from treating medical problems to providing immediate comfort. Family members may begin to gather to visit, care for, and say goodbye to the dying person. Nonetheless, many people are unsure of what to do when at the bedside of a dying person.

The actively dying person is often minimally responsive or even unresponsive (comatose). Nonetheless, people at the bedside should assume that the dying person can hear and is aware of those around him. This assumption is based on the experiences of people who have been sedated or in a coma but who could describe events that occurred in their presence. Loved ones can take the opportunity to express thoughts that they have been meaning to share (for example, "I love you" or "You were a wonderful mother") and to say goodbye.

Loved ones frequently take comfort and pride in the personal care they are able to provide to an actively dying person. Keeping the dying person clean, changing his position occasionally to enhance comfort or to help with clearing secretions, and keeping his mouth clean provide comfort to the caregiver as well. Loved ones may also provide comforting touches or massage or apply skin moisturizers.

Helping to create a peaceful and soothing atmosphere is an important aspect of care. Whether a person is dying at home or in an institution (for example, a nursing home or hospital), filling the room with the comforting, familiar sounds of loved ones' voices or favorite music should be encouraged. Family disagreements or discussions that might distress the dying person should be avoided. Pastoral visits from clergy members may be very important and can provide tremendous support for many families.

PALLIATIVE CARE AND HOSPICE CARE

Palliative care focuses on relieving burdensome symptoms and improving the quality of life for people and families living with a life-threatening chronic disease. Ideally, palliative care would be offered early in the course of a chronic disease, when treatment intended to lengthen life begins. Early palliative care helps to ensure that concerns about quality of life are addressed. Early palliative care also helps to ease the transition into the period when the disease is more advanced and when treatment intended to lengthen life is no longer seen as being desirable or useful. In reality, palliative care often begins more abruptly, at the point at which everyone agrees that the goal is more to improve comfort and less to extend the length of the person's life.

Physical suffering is not inevitable or unavoidable after a person is diagnosed with a life-threatening chronic disease. People have a right to expect adequate control of symptoms and tolerable side effects from treatment. However, people who experience symptoms that do not respond well to treatment sometimes have to choose between relief of those symptoms and side effects that might occur if treatments are intensified or more treatments are added. For example, a person with pain that is relieved by potentially sedating analgesics might face a choice of increasing the drug dosage to gain further relief at the expense of becoming sedated. Such choices, however, are the exception and not the rule.

If symptoms are poorly controlled, consultation with a specialist in palliative medicine may be worthwhile. Palliative medicine specialists work with people and their primary health care practitioners to relieve suffering and maximize quality of life. Referral to a palliative medicine specialist or to a palliative care team is appropriate at any time during the course of a chronic, potentially life-threatening disease when symptoms do not respond to treatment or when side effects of treatment interfere with the person's comfort.

Unlike palliative care, hospice care, as defined by the hospice benefit provided for by Medicare, is reserved exclusively for people expected to die within 6 months. Medicare-certified hospice programs aim to provide comprehensive services that help dying people and their families maximize the quality of life in the very late stages of a disease and to prepare for death. Doctors, nurses, nurse's aides, and social workers form the core of a hospice team. The team may also include nutritionists, psychologists, pharmacists, therapists, chaplains, ethicists, and volunteers.

Together the hospice team offers a broad range of services, from medical care to personal care (such as bathing, dressing, and grooming). In addition, the hospice team helps family members become more comfortable caring for their dying loved one and provides psychologic and spiritual counseling to help the dying person and family members prepare for death. Perhaps most importantly, the hospice team coordinates care, which is typically a great relief to families who have experienced the frequently fragmented care that characterizes much of modern medicine.

Hospice care can be provided in any setting, including a person's home (where more than 95% of hospice care in the United States is provided), a nursing home, or a hospital. People in hospice can choose to die in a variety of settings, depending on where they are most comfortable.

The cost of hospice is covered by most health care insurances, including Medicare, under two conditions. First, a doctor must certify that a person is expected to live less than 6 months. Because the time a person has left may be difficult to predict with some diseases, such as heart failure and lung disease, not everyone who might benefit from hospice care is deemed eligible. Second, a dying person must agree that relief of distress rather than cure is the goal of treatment.

Treatments that are intended to eliminate or reverse certain short-term symptoms or complications of a disease are allowed under the many insurance plans that cover hospice expenses as long as they are intended to relieve symptoms and not cure the underlying disease. For example, a person who has trouble breathing and a low number of red blood cells (anemia) might receive blood transfusions if the hospice team believes that increasing the number of red blood cells is an effective way to help relieve the person's shortness of breath. Hospices do try to avoid providing burdensome or minimally effective treatments. For most people this leads to more appropriate care and an improved quality of life for the entire family. People in hospice who decide they want to discontinue hospice care are free to leave.

PEACE AND RESOLUTION

For the dying person, the prospect of death provokes essential questions, such as "What have I accomplished in my life?" "Has my life been meaningful?" and "What happens to me after death?" Some people find answers to these questions in spiritual and religious traditions. Others look to their work or to their family for a sense of meaning. Still others find no comfort from these sources and instead face a spiritual, religious, or personal crisis. They may ask questions such as "Why has God done this to me?" "Why now?" and "What could I have done differently that would have prevented this?" People with these questions need spiritual, religious, or mental health counseling as much as they need medical care so that they can live meaningfully and die peacefully with a sense of completion. Many hospitals and hospice programs can provide such counseling through clergy, prayer groups, and mental health services.

Peace and resolution at the end of life are important not only for dying people but for their families as well. Yet family members who are grieving may find it impossible to find peace and resolution. Although grieving is a normal process, it is always painful. It involves feelings of shock, denial, regret, anger, sorrow, uncertainty, and painful longing. A peaceful death, characterized by caring, love, a chance to say goodbye, and resolution of conflicts and unvoiced feelings, helps minimize these reactions but cannot prevent grieving. Indeed, a long-expected death can still seem unanticipated and unbelievable when a loved one finally dies.

For some people, death of a loved one brings tremendous anxiety in the months after. A loved one may develop symptoms such as headaches or vague chest, abdominal, or other pain. Some people have vivid dreams of the deceased person, sense the deceased person's presence in familiar places, or hear the deceased person's voice. These reactions are generally normal.

Tremendous variation exists among individuals and cultures as to what constitutes normal grief. For many, grief may be so intense that the ability to function is impaired. However intense grief becomes, it diminishes in most people over a period of 6 to 12 months. People who experience more prolonged periods of disabling grief may face expectations "to get over it." At the same time, they may have less support from family and friends. When the bereaved become stuck in their grief and show no sign of resuming previous life activities, counseling is appropriate.

Every person and every culture has a different timetable for working through grief. Family members should be aware that older men are especially likely to become depressed and to contemplate suicide after the death of their wives. Family gatherings and anniversaries of important events are common triggers for memories and grief. Even long after the time of death, thoughts of the deceased person never completely go away. Effective grieving is marked by the bereaved's ability to move beyond the point where loss and sadness dominate thoughts to a time when painful memories about the deceased give way to fond ones.

After retirement, time remains for rest plus interesting and enjoyable projects: time with friends, hobbies, repayment for years of hard labor.

I spent a great deal of time with my friend Robert Bates, watching him as he built ship models. He talked me into building ship models. I built my first model in his shop. It was a whaling ship, the *Charles Morgan*. The ship has been restored and is at the dock at Mystic, Connecticut.

A friend of Bates' from Annapolis visited, saw the model, and made an appointment with the famous Howard I. Chapelle at the Smithsonian Institution. Chapelle became a close friend. He kept me very busy and happy building several models that are on display at the Smithsonian. It is a pleasure to create models, and working on them is not a big task for an old man.

The greatest thrill of my model career was the *Half Moon*, which I built for the Statue of Liberty. This ship was used when Henry Hudson discovered the Hudson River. The model is mounted on a wall in an exhibit located in the base of the Statue. When I see the Statue on TV, I am so excited and proud knowing my work is on display.

I built models for my friends and relatives, and they proudly display them. I know the gifts are appreciated. This helps me as I spend time reliving the wonderful times of my past. Life is worth remembering. I pray a lot, thanking the good Lord for longevity and the happy days I continue to love. I love life, and I try to help others feel the same. In my 92 years, I try to remember the formula for happiness: comfort, remembrance, hope, and friendship.

Herbert Kendrick

SECTION 3

MEDICAL CONDITIONS

Everyone hopes that their experience with aging will be healthy and trouble-free. However, many medical disorders and conditions can make doing daily activities more difficult and limit independence. Some can worsen quality of life and even shorten life. Understanding these conditions can help people live as healthy a life as possible. Reading about them is a good start.

This section contains in-depth discussions of a wide range of topics: from abdominal aortic aneurysms to Zenker's diverticulum—and with coronary artery disease, dementia, diabetes, falls, hypertension, incontinence, osteoarthritis, and many, many others in between. The focus is on conditions that are particularly common among older people or that affect older people differently.

17

Nutritional Disorders

As people age, their nutritional needs change.[1] Consequently, older people may develop a nutritional disorder, even when they follow standard nutritional recommendations.

Nutritional disorders may result from eating too little or too much food. Or they may result from eating too little or too much of a particular nutrient, such as a vitamin or mineral.[2] Nutritional disorders may also develop when the body cannot use the nutrients it gets, regardless of whether a person eats appropriate amounts of a variety of foods.

UNDERNUTRITION

Undernutrition is what happens when the body does not get the nutrients it needs for good health or cannot use the nutrients it gets.

Many people think undernutrition is not a problem in the United States. But about 1 out of 6 older people are undernourished. Undernutrition is a problem for many older people who live alone or who live in a nursing home.

Undernutrition and weight loss do not always go together. People can be undernourished without losing weight. They can be overweight and undernourished. And people can lose weight, particularly if they are trying to do so, without becoming undernourished.

Most people who do not consume enough food also do not consume enough vitamins and minerals, sometimes resulting in

1. see page 41
2. see page 240

a vitamin or mineral deficiency.[1] Many do not drink enough fluids, sometimes resulting in dehydration.[2]

Causes

Undernutrition may result from eating too little food (that is, too few calories). But it may result even when enough food is eaten if the foods chosen do not contain enough of the needed nutrients, particularly protein, vitamins, and minerals. People may choose foods that are low in nutrients but high in calories (called empty-calorie foods). People may eat only a few foods rather than the variety needed to provide enough nutrients. Undernutrition may also result when the body cannot absorb nutrients from foods.

Older people are more susceptible to undernutrition for several reasons.

• **Changes due to aging:** In some older people, changes due to aging itself cause the appetite to decrease. So less food may be eaten.

• **Disorders and drugs:** Many older people have disorders or take drugs that change the body's nutritional needs or make the body less able to meet those needs. For example, a disorder can cause the body to burn more calories, so more food is needed. Or a disorder (such as depression) or drug can decrease the appetite. Some disorders (such as a stroke or dental problems) can make eating difficult.

• **Living situation:** Many older people live and eat alone and thus are less motivated to prepare and eat meals. Older people may also eat less because funds are limited or because shopping for or preparing food is difficult. Caregivers providing meals for older people may be unaware of which foods are nutritious. In nursing homes, older people may not be served foods they like. Or they may not receive the help or time they need to eat. Older people who are hospitalized may have some of the same problems.[3]

1. see page 240
2. see page 249
3. see page 150

EATING IN A NURSING HOME

Living in a nursing home can make undernutrition more likely. Residents of nursing homes usually do not get to choose the foods they are served. If they do not like the food, they may not eat enough. Some residents are placed on restricted diets that are unappealing, such as a low-fat or low-salt diet.

Residents cannot get food when they want it. Meals may be served and taken away at specific times without any consideration of whether a person is hungry. Occasionally, residents are neglected. They may not be given the help or time they need to eat. The food may become cold while they are waiting for someone to help them eat. Or the food may be cold when it arrives. Consequently, they may not eat enough.

Family members can help by talking with staff members about ways to make sure the resident's nutritional needs are being met. They can talk about the resident's food preferences with staff members. This information is especially important if the resident will not eat certain foods.

Family members may offer to bring some of the resident's favorite foods to the nursing home. They can visit during mealtimes. Having family members present may make the resident more interested in eating. They can talk with staff members about making sure that the resident is given enough time to eat and, if needed, help with eating and snacks between meals.

Sometimes undernutrition has one cause. But more often, several conditions work together to cause undernutrition.

ADDITIONAL DETAIL

As people age, the body changes in several ways that may cause older people to eat less. The aging body produces more hormones that decrease appetite and fewer chemical messengers (neurotransmitters) that stimulate appetite. Thus, older people tend to feel satisfied with less food. The ability to taste or smell gradually diminishes, so food becomes less appetizing.[1] Some older people produce less saliva, making the mouth feel dry. As a result, chewing and swallowing food may be difficult. When older people become less physically active, they may eat less. Physical activity stimulates the appetite.

Disorders can increase the risk of undernutrition by changing the body's nutritional needs or by changing the body's ability to

1. see page 13

meet those needs. For example, an overactive thyroid gland (hyperthyroidism) increases the amount of nutrients needed because it changes the way the body uses nutrients.

Some disorders cause symptoms that interfere with the body's ability to meet nutritional needs. For example, nausea makes a person eat less. Vomiting or diarrhea prevents the body from absorbing as many nutrients. Liver or kidney failure can cause these symptoms. Some disorders, sometimes called malabsorption disorders, interfere with the absorption of nutrients in the digestive tract. Examples are liver failure, lactose intolerance, and disorders of the pancreas. A stroke can make swallowing difficult.

Dental problems, such as tooth decay, gum disease, missing or loose teeth, and poorly fitting bridges or dentures, can make eating and drinking awkward or painful. Thus, eating may become more of a necessity than a pleasure, even for relatively healthy older people.

Some disorders, such as Parkinson's disease, can make shopping for, preparing, and eating food more difficult. Being frail, apart from any disorder, can also make these tasks difficult.

Depression or anxiety disorders can decrease appetite. Depression is more likely to lead to undernutrition in older people than in younger people.

Some disorders change the body's nutritional needs and the ability to meet those needs. For example, some disorders increase the body's requirements for energy and decrease appetite. That is, even though the disorder causes the body to use more calories, people with one of these disorders tend to eat less. Examples are cancer, infections, chronic obstructive pulmonary disease (COPD), and rheumatoid arthritis. Such disorders typically cause weight to be lost slowly over time. COPD also may make people breathless while eating, so that they eat less.

Diabetes changes the body's nutritional needs by changing the way the body handles sugar. Consequently, people with diabetes should substitute complex carbohydrates (found, for example, in beans, many other vegetables, and whole-grain foods) for simple sugars (found, for example, in ice cream, candy, syrups, jellies, and sodas). Also, diabetes can interfere with the body's ability to meet nutritional needs by changing how quickly food moves through the digestive tract. Nausea and abdominal pain may result, causing a person to eat less.

Drugs can increase the risk of undernutrition by changing the body's nutritional needs. Some drugs (such as thyroxine and theophylline) increase the body's requirements for energy. Other drugs can change the way the body uses nutrients.

Drugs can also change the body's ability to meet nutritional needs. Many drugs can decrease appetite. Examples are some drugs used to treat depression (such as fluoxetine and sertraline), high blood pressure (such as diuretics), heart failure (such as digoxin), and chemotherapy drugs (such as cisplatin). If older people notice a decrease in their appetite after they start taking a new drug, they should tell their doctor.

Some drugs can have side effects that interfere with meeting nutritional needs. These side effects include nausea, upset stomach, diarrhea, and constipation (which can greatly decrease appetite). Other drugs alter taste or smell. As a result, many foods may no longer taste good, so less food is eaten. Some drugs (such as cholestyramine) interfere with the absorption of nutrients, as does taking too many laxatives. Certain drugs (such as some antidepressants and antipsychotics) increase appetite. When people stop taking these drugs, they may eat less and thus lose weight.

Drinking too much alcohol can lead to undernutrition. Alcohol has little nutritional value. It also decreases appetite. Alcohol can interfere with the absorption and use of nutrients partly because it damages the liver.

Smoking dulls taste and smell, so smokers may eat less. Smoking increases the metabolic rate, causing the body to burn more calories. Smoking also causes many types of cancer, which can lead to weight loss and sometimes undernutrition.

Many older people live alone. For them, preparing meals just for themselves may seem like too much trouble. Or they may not enjoy eating alone. They may make the same meals for themselves day after day. As a result, they may not consume enough of some nutrients. Or they may snack throughout the day without eating a well-balanced meal. Older people who live alone may not have transportation to a grocery store. Or they may be afraid of going out alone or be physically unable to do so. They may need help preparing meals. Loneliness, especially after losing a partner, may make people feel less like eating.

Older people who have a caregiver may develop undernutrition. Caregivers may not know what the nutritional needs of older people are. They may not realize how little the person is eating. Or they may not think about nutrition at all.

Symptoms

The appearance of people who are undernourished may not change. If only a specific nutrient (such as protein) is lacking, their weight may be normal or higher. However, many undernourished people are obviously underweight and have little or no body fat. They may notice that their clothes fit more loosely or that they have lost muscle.

As undernutrition becomes more severe, the temples may look hollow and bones may protrude. The skin may become thin, dry, inelastic, pale, and cold. The hair may become dry and sparse. It may fall out easily. Undernourished people often lose muscle. They may feel tired, sleepy, weak, and dizzy. As a result, they are more likely to fall.[1] Infections may develop more often. Sores or wounds may be slow to heal.

In older people, undernutrition is often part of a general decline. People may gradually become less able to think clearly and to take care of themselves. They may become depressed and withdraw from friends and family. This decline is called failure to thrive.

Many older people do not notice any changes or symptoms as they become undernourished. Family members and caregivers may notice the changes first. However, caregivers may think that weight loss in older people is normal. Also, older people may not think losing weight is a problem. They may not connect symptoms they are having with what they are eating or not eating.

Diagnosis

Undernutrition can sometimes be identified based on appearance. Maintaining a weight that is too low or losing weight without trying, even for people who are overweight, may indicate undernutrition.

To determine whether people are undernourished, health care

1. see page 287

practitioners measure weight and height. From these measurements, they can calculate body mass index (BMI).[1] Practitioners may ask whether weight has recently been lost and, if so, how much and over what period of time. They also ask people what and how much they eat and drink each day. However, for most people, this information is difficult to recall. Practitioners may ask whether people consider themselves well-nourished and generally healthy. Whether people recognize the problem affects their willingness to participate in a treatment plan.

Practitioners may measure around the arm or waist to estimate the percentage of fat and muscle (body composition). Blood tests may be done to measure the levels of cholesterol and albumin (the main protein in the blood). Cholesterol levels become low when not enough calories are consumed. The albumin level may decrease when not enough protein is consumed.

Health care practitioners ask about problems that may be contributing to undernutrition: disorders, drugs, alcohol consumption, mood, living situation, and the need for help (with paying for, shopping for, preparing, or eating meals).

Prevention and Treatment

Preventing undernutrition is better than treating it. Restoring people to their previous level of health and functioning takes a lot longer than undernutrition takes to develop. Many of the same measures help prevent and treat undernutrition.

Generally, to prevent undernutrition, older people should eat a varied diet. It should include lots of fruits and vegetables, protein-rich foods (such as fish and poultry), and high-fiber breads and cereals.[2] Drinking plenty of fluids is also important. Water, fruit or vegetable juices, and caffeine-free coffee and tea are good choices. For most healthy, active older people who eat a varied diet, eating large amounts of a particular food or using dietary supplements is not necessary.

For people with a small appetite, making meals more appetizing may help. For example, foods with different flavors, textures, colors, and temperatures can be included in a meal. Tastes and smells can be enhanced by using spices. However, people with high blood pressure or heart failure should use salt moder-

1. see table on page 47
2. see page 41

ately. Too much salt can make these disorders worse. Eating with other people can make meals more appealing. Physical activity such as walking before meals helps stimulate appetite.

If preparing food is difficult, prepared foods (such as frozen dinners) can be purchased. Periodically, family members or friends can help cook foods in quantity. Then the foods can be packaged in appropriate portions to freeze and be eaten later. A microwave or toaster oven may make food preparation easier. Some gadgets (such as electric can openers) are also helpful.

If shopping is difficult, family members or friends may be able to help. Churches, synagogues, mosques, and community organizations sometimes provide shopping services. Some senior centers offer meals, and some organizations, such as Meals on Wheels, bring meals to the home. These meals are inexpensive or free.

Help with buying appropriate foods and preparing healthy meals may be all that is needed to prevent or treat undernutrition. The companionship and stimulation that come with this kind of help may also boost a person's interest in eating.

If funds are limited, organizations and programs (such as food stamps) can help. They are often listed in the telephone book. People can ask a health care practitioner for help with getting this information.

Dental problems should be treated. Having a tooth extracted or getting dentures that fit properly can make eating easier. If eating remains difficult, foods that are hard to chew can be chopped finely, mashed, or blended. Peanut butter, eggs, cheese, yogurt, or beans can be substituted for meat as sources of protein.

Treating disorders that contribute to undernutrition can help. If depression or an anxiety disorder is interfering with eating, antidepressants or antianxiety drugs may lessen these feelings. However, some of these drugs can decrease appetite.

People who are undernourished should limit their consumption of alcohol to one drink a day.

A dietitian can teach a family member or caregiver which foods help an undernourished person and which foods do not.

Nutritional supplements that are rich in carbohydrates, protein, and fat are often useful for people who are not eating enough. Supplements are available as powders or thick liquids with or without a prescription. There are many nutritional supplements. All are equally effective.

When other measures are ineffective, undernourished people may be given drugs to stimulate appetite and promote weight gain. Corticosteroids, growth hormone, other hormones, and dronabinol may be used but are often ineffective. Also, whether these drugs can be safely taken for a long time is unclear.

Some people cannot take nutritional supplements by mouth. For example, some people who have had a stroke cannot swallow. In such cases, supplements can be given through a tube inserted through the nose and throat into the stomach. If feeding through a tube is needed for a long time, the tube may be inserted directly into the stomach or small intestine through a small incision in the abdomen.

Tube feeding can cause problems. Among older people, the most common problem is the movement of food backward into the esophagus and throat (reflux). Food in the throat can be breathed into the lungs (aspirated). Aspirating food can result in pneumonia. Food is less likely to be aspirated when the head of the bed is raised. Tube feeding can also cause diarrhea and abdominal discomfort.

The tube, whether inserted through the nose and down the throat or through an incision in the abdomen, can irritate tissues, causing inflammation and infection.

For people whose digestive tract cannot absorb enough nutrients, a solution containing nutrients can be given through a tube inserted in a vein (intravenously). Food given intravenously is called parenteral nutrition. When all of a person's food is given this way, it is called total parenteral nutrition.

In older people, intravenous feeding is usually used only for a short time. When used for a long time, it can cause problems. Infections are more likely because bacteria can enter the body through the incision for the tube. Also, when there is no food in the intestine, bacteria can pass through the wall of the intestine into the bloodstream. Intravenous feeding may lead to vitamin and mineral deficiencies. Electrolyte levels can become dangerously high or low if people are fed too fast, too much, or too little or if they have been undernourished for a long time.[1]

1. see page 253

VITAMIN AND MINERAL DEFICIENCIES

Getting enough vitamins and minerals from foods is prefer-able to getting them from supplements, but it can be difficult. Most older people do not eat a healthy diet every day. So taking a multivitamin that contains the recommended daily allowances for vitamins and minerals is a good idea—in addition to, not as a substitute for, trying to eat a healthy diet.

Taking a multivitamin is particularly useful for people who have a vitamin or mineral deficiency or who are at risk of a de-ficiency. People at risk of a deficiency include those who are not eating enough food and those who have a disorder or take drugs that can cause undernutrition.[1] Older people who live in a nurs-ing home and those who have been in the hospital for a long time are also at high risk.[2] Older people who must be fed in-travenously for a long time may develop vitamin and mineral deficiencies.

Some people believe that taking high doses of specific vita-mins (such as vitamin C or E) or minerals (such as zinc) can help prevent disease. However, there is little evidence that con-suming high doses of vitamin or mineral supplements or foods that contain large amounts of these nutrients provides more benefits than consuming the recommended amounts.

Deficiencies that older people may develop include deficien-cies of folic acid (folate), vitamin B_{12}, vitamin C, vitamin D, calcium, magnesium, phosphorus, potassium, sodium, and zinc. Usually, nutritional deficiencies are diagnosed based on symptoms and the results of blood tests that measure the levels of nutrients. Treatment varies depending on the deficiency but often involves taking a supplement.

Disorders may develop when minerals that are dissolved in fluids of the body are out of balance.[3] Some of these minerals are called electrolytes. Examples are sodium, chloride, and potassium.

1. see page 232
2. see page 150 and box on page 233
3. see page 253

SOME VITAMIN AND MINERAL DEFICIENCIES

Deficiency	Causes	Symptoms	Treatment
Folic acid (folate)	Not consuming enough folic acid in the diet Drinking too much alcohol Not being able to absorb folic acid from food in the digestive tract (malabsorption) Taking drugs such as methotrexate, trimethoprim, phenytoin, or triamterene	A low number of red blood cells (anemia) Fatigue An increased risk of heart and blood vessel disorders and possibly cancer	Eating foods rich in folic acid (such as fortified breads, pastas, and cereals; raw leafy green vegetables; and citrus fruits) Taking supplements of folic acid
Vitamin B_{12}	Not being able to absorb vitamin B_{12} from food in the digestive tract because of decreased levels of stomach acid (hypochlorhydria) Having stomach infections due to *Helicobacter pylori* Following a strict vegetarian diet Having surgery on the stomach or a disorder affecting the small intestine	Anemia Tingling or numbness in the feet and hands Loss of balance Weakness Personality changes If the deficiency is severe, mental confusion or even dementia	Being given vitamin B_{12} monthly by injection into a muscle or taking vitamin B_{12} supplements
Vitamin C	Not consuming enough	Easy bruising Bleeding and	Eating foods rich in vitamin C

Table continues on the following page.

Deficiency	Causes	Symptoms	Treatment
	vitamin C in the diet Smoking (which increases the body's requirement for vitamin C) Undergoing hemodialysis	swollen gums Slow healing of sores and wounds	Taking vitamin C supplements
Vitamin D	Not spending enough time in sunlight Not consuming enough vitamin D in the diet Having a liver or kidney disorder Taking drugs such as anticonvulsants	Increased risk of fractures because bones become less dense and weaker	Drinking milk (which is fortified with vitamin D) Taking vitamin D supplements Spending time in sunlight
Calcium	Not consuming enough calcium in the diet Having a deficiency of vitamin D (which helps the body absorb calcium) Having a kidney disorder, a parathyroid disorder, or pancreatitis	Increased risk of fractures because bones become less dense and weaker Muscle spasms Confusion	Eating foods rich in calcium (such as milk and other dairy products) Taking calcium supplements
Magnesium	Not consuming enough magnesium in the diet Having a kidney disorder, diabetes, or a digestive	Loss of appetite Nausea and vomiting Drowsiness Muscle weakness and spasms Tremors	Eating foods rich in magnesium (such as leafy vegetables, nuts, cereal grains, and seafood) Taking

Deficiency	Causes	Symptoms	Treatment
	disorder that interferes with absorption Having diarrhea Taking a diuretic Drinking too much alcohol		magnesium supplements If the deficiency is severe, being given magnesium intravenously or by injection into a muscle
Phosphorus	Not consuming enough phosphorus in the diet Having a kidney disorder or a digestive disorder that interferes with absorption	Usually, no symptoms If severe, loss of appetite and muscle weakness If very severe, coma and death	Drinking large quantities of milk Taking phosphate supplements If the deficiency is severe, being given phosphate intravenously
Potassium	Taking a diuretic Having diarrhea or vomiting for a long time	Fatigue Confusion Muscle weakness and cramps If the deficiency is severe, paralysis and abnormal heart rhythms (arrhythmias)	Eating foods rich in potassium (such as milk, whole-grain cereals, green leafy vegetables, most beans, prunes, and many fruits such as bananas and oranges) Taking potassium supplements
Sodium	Drinking a lot of water or nutritional supplements that are low in sodium without consuming enough salt	Confusion Drowsiness Abnormal breathing Loss of muscle tone Seizures	Being given sodium and water intravenously Eating salty foods

Table continues on the following page.

Deficiency	Causes	Symptoms	Treatment
	Being given large amounts of fluids intravenously without enough sodium Taking a diuretic Vomiting or having diarrhea for a long time Having heart failure, cirrhosis, or a kidney disorder		
Zinc	Not consuming enough zinc in the diet Having diabetes or cirrhosis Taking diuretics Drinking too much alcohol Not being able to absorb zinc from food in the digestive tract	Decreased appetite Decreased sense of taste Slow healing of sores and wounds Increased susceptibility to infections	Taking zinc supplements (which may upset the stomach and cause other problems)

OBESITY

Obesity refers specifically to having too much body fat. It usually also means being very overweight. People may be overweight without being obese.

Some people think that being overweight or obese is the opposite of undernutrition, that overweight or obese people are overnourished. However, overweight or obese people may not consume enough of the nutrients needed for good health and may therefore be undernourished. For example, they may not consume enough fiber, vitamins, or minerals.

In the United States, the percentage of older people who are obese has been increasing during the last few years. People may be obese throughout most of their life, or they may become obese late in life.

Some extra body fat is not necessarily bad for older people. Fat is the way the body stores energy. Some disorders, such as cancer or infections, can increase the body's need for energy. Some extra body fat may come in handy if one of these disorders develops. Fat around the hips and buttocks helps protect bones from being broken during a fall. And people who weigh more are less likely to develop osteoporosis.

But too much body fat is unhealthy for older people as well as for younger people. The risk of health problems increases as body fat (and weight) increases. For example, heart disorders, high blood pressure, stroke, diabetes, some cancers, osteoarthritis, gallbladder disorders, and obstructive sleep apnea are more common among obese people.

Causes

In one sense, the cause of being overweight or obese is simple. The cause is consuming more calories than the body needs over a period of time. But why people consume more than the body needs and what determines how many calories the body needs are more complex questions.

Most people gain body fat and weight as they age. These changes may occur if older people become less physically active but do not eat any less. Physical inactivity is considered one of the main causes of obesity.

Also as people age, levels of hormones, such as growth hormone and testosterone, decrease. When growth hormone and testosterone levels decrease, the amount of muscle decreases and the amount of body fat increases. Muscle burns more calories than fat, so this change may contribute to weight gain as well as to increased body fat.

People may eat too much for many reasons. Some people eat more when they are bored, lonely, or under stress.

Eating foods that are high in calories, even when the amounts are relatively small, can result in weight gain. Many convenience foods and foods eaten in a restaurant are high in fat and in calories.

Many drugs used to treat common disorders promote weight gain. Examples are some antidepressants, insulin, and corticosteroids. Taking corticosteroids causes an unusual type of obesity. Fat accumulates only in the trunk. The arms and legs may become thinner because muscle is lost.

Rarely, hormonal disorders cause obesity. A disorder of overactive adrenal glands (Cushing's disease) causes the same type of obesity as corticosteroids. A low level of thyroid hormone (hypothyroidism) slows the rate at which calories are used (metabolic rate). Thus, this disorder may result in weight gain.

The nicotine in tobacco decreases appetite and increases the metabolic rate. Stopping smoking usually results in weight gain because the metabolic rate slows and the body thus burns fewer calories. People who smoke may remain thin, but fat tends to accumulate around their waist and abdomen. This accumulation increases their risk of health problems, even if they remain within a normal weight range.

Symptoms

Obesity may cause no specific symptoms other than a change in appearance and in the way clothes fit.

Osteoarthritis of the hips and knees is more common among obese people because excess weight puts more stress on the joints. Low back pain is also common. Obese people may tire easily and become short of breath after slight exertion.

Some obese people have difficulty sleeping because of obstructive sleep apnea.[1] This disorder interferes with breathing during sleep. When the muscles of the throat relax during sleep, tissue in the wall of the throat may partially block the airway. As a result, people snore loudly, sleep restlessly, and may suddenly wake up gasping and choking. They may feel sleepy during the day.

Obese women may feel pain in their pelvis or pressure on the bladder, rectum, or uterus. The pressure of excess weight can weaken the muscles and other tissues that support pelvic organs (bladder, rectum, and uterus). This pressure may cause or worsen a pelvic support disorder.[2]

1. see page 437
2. see page 879

Diagnosis

Usually, obesity can be identified based on appearance. However, health care practitioners usually measure weight and height and use these measurements to calculate body mass index (BMI).[1] The BMI indicates whether people are overweight or obese and how severe the obesity is.

Treatment

Treatment of weight gain and obesity involves exercising and decreasing the number of calories consumed. Any exercise, such as regularly walking in a mall or around the neighborhood or lifting light weights, can lead to gradual weight loss as long as the number of calories consumed is not increased. To lose weight, a person must consume fewer calories than the body burns. So decreasing the number of calories consumed is usually also recommended. Avoiding between-meal snacks may be all that is needed.

Learning to identify activities and feelings that trigger overeating may help people stop overeating. For example, snacking while watching television can be replaced with other activities, such as exercise or crafts. An absorbing, purposeful activity or hobby, such as painting or gardening, may take the mind off anxieties, which can trigger overeating.

Older people who are trying to eat less should drink plenty of fluids. They may need to take a multivitamin with minerals. Obese older people who are losing weight should be evaluated periodically to check for serious disorders that may be causing the weight loss.

Most drugs that help reduce body weight are not recommended for older people because of their side effects. But orlistat may be useful for obese older people who cannot exercise or change their diet. Orlistat blocks fat absorption from the digestive tract. However, deficiencies of some vitamins and minerals can develop. People taking orlistat are monitored closely by their doctor.

1. see table on page 47

18

Water and Electrolyte Balance

Water is the main component of blood and cells. It fills most of the spaces around cells. To function normally, the body must keep the amount of water in these areas in balance and relatively constant. Too little water (dehydration) or too much water (overhydration) in the body can cause problems.

The water in the body contains dissolved minerals called electrolytes. They include sodium, potassium, and calcium. The body must also keep levels of electrolytes in balance and relatively constant. The balance of electrolytes is closely tied to the balance of water in the body: If one changes, the other usually also changes.

To maintain water and electrolyte balance, the body must replace water and electrolytes that are lost as the body performs its necessary functions. The body loses water and electrolytes primarily in urine, produced by the kidneys. Water and electrolytes are also lost in sweat, feces, and air that is breathed out. The body obtains water and electrolytes primarily from beverages and foods consumed. A healthy body can adjust the amount of water and electrolytes lost and consumed. Thirst, hunger, and the kidneys help with these adjustments. For example, a person who feels thirsty usually drinks more fluids. When a person becomes dehydrated, the brain releases a hormone called antidiuretic hormone. This hormone signals the kidneys to retain more water by making and excreting less urine.

As the body ages, it changes in ways that make older people more likely to have problems with water and electrolyte balance. The older body contains less water. Water accounts for 60% of body weight in healthy young people but for only 45% in healthy older people. In older people, the kidneys are less able to regulate the excretion of water and to concentrate urine as needed. Therefore, more water may be lost in urine. Also, older people often do not drink enough water, especially on hot days, partly because they tend to be less thirsty. If older people have problems with walking, they may not be able to get themselves enough water to drink. Older people who have urinary incontinence may drink less because they are worried about getting to a bathroom in time.

Many disorders, especially those that cause fever, vomiting, or diarrhea, can result in problems with water and electrolyte balance. These disorders may be short-lived (for example, pneumonia) or chronic (for example, kidney failure). Many drugs, especially diuretics, can also cause problems.

DEHYDRATION

Dehydration is not having enough water in the body.

Sometimes people dismiss dehydration as a minor nuisance. However, without treatment, dehydration can have serious effects, including confusion (delirium), dizziness, falls, and death.

When a person is dehydrated, blood pressure falls, the body's organs do not receive enough blood and nutrients, and the body cannot cool itself adequately. Also, the levels of many electrolytes tend to become abnormal. The body tries to keep blood pressure from falling by moving water from cells and the spaces around the cells into the blood vessels. Then, the tissues dry out. The kidneys try to conserve water by concentrating urine more or by not making any urine.

Dehydration can occur at any age. But older people are prone to dehydration because of changes that occur as the body ages—for example, older people sense thirst less quickly and intensely, and the kidneys function less well. Other conditions that make dehydration more likely include the following:

- Hot weather, because sweating is increased
- Fever, because sweating is increased and breathing becomes more rapid (causing more water to be lost in the air that is breathed out)
- Diarrhea, because water is lost in the stool

- Vomiting, because water is lost in the vomit
- Diabetes that is poorly controlled, because the body produces more urine
- Kidney disorders, because the kidneys are less able to concentrate urine as needed
- Problems with walking, because getting water is difficult
- Dementia, because the sense of thirst is reduced and the ability to get water when needed is impaired
- Use of diuretics, because these drugs increase the amount of water (and salt) excreted by the kidneys

Symptoms and Diagnosis

When dehydration is mild, the skin and the membranes of the nose and eyes become dry. A dehydrated person may feel confused and sluggish. After standing up, the person may feel lightheaded and may faint. As dehydration becomes more severe, the body makes less urine, and the urine becomes dark. Severe dehydration can lead to a fall in blood pressure that can be life threatening.

Blood and urine tests help doctors diagnose dehydration and determine how severe it is. Doctors measure levels of certain electrolytes and other substances that indicate how well the kidneys are functioning.

Treatment

Treatment involves replacing lost fluids. How rapidly they are replaced depends on how severe dehydration is. People who have mild dehydration are usually given about 2 to 3 liters of water to drink over a period of a few hours. People who have moderate dehydration are usually given a fluid that contains some salt (sodium) and other electrolytes. Dilute broths and rehydration formulas (available in pharmacies without a prescription) are a good choice.

Some people must be given fluids through a tube inserted in a vein (intravenously). Such people include those who are severely dehydrated, those who cannot swallow, and those who are in a coma. If electrolytes must also be replaced, they are given intravenously with the fluids.

OVERHYDRATION

Overhydration is having too much water in the body.

When more fluid is consumed than can be excreted, overhydration occurs. The blood vessels overfill, and fluid moves from the blood vessels into the spaces around cells, causing swelling (edema).

Overhydration has many causes. The most common is heart failure, which occurs when the heart cannot pump blood adequately.[1] Kidney disorders can cause overhydration if the kidneys cannot excrete enough water. Overhydration can also occur when the body produces too much antidiuretic hormone (which signals the kidneys to retain more water). Overproduction of antidiuretic hormone may be caused by disorders such as pneumonia and stroke and by drugs such as carbamazepine (an anticonvulsant) and sertraline (an antidepressant). Some drugs, especially nonsteroidal anti-inflammatory drugs (NSAIDs), and foods that are high in sodium cause fluids to be retained and may lead to mild overhydration. People who are hospitalized can become overhydrated if they are given intravenous fluids or blood transfusions too rapidly.

Symptoms and Diagnosis

Overhydration often causes swelling in the legs or, if people are confined to bed, in the lower back. However, swelling in the legs is not always caused by overhydration. Often, it is caused or worsened by poor circulation due to a blood vessel disorder[2] (such as chronic venous insufficiency), particularly in people who sit a lot.

Overhydration can cause shortness of breath because fluid backs up in the lungs. Often, shortness of breath is worse when a person lies down, because fluid moves from the feet and legs into the abdomen and chest. The person may wake up shortly after lying down, gasping for air.

If overhydration is suspected, a doctor looks for swelling and enlargement of organs, such as the heart and liver. The veins in the neck are examined to see whether they are overfilled. With a

1. see page 680
2. see page 649

stethoscope, the doctor listens to the heart and lungs for any signs of heart failure.

Other tests may be done to determine whether symptoms are due to overhydration or to poor circulation in the legs. Blood tests may be done to measure levels of electrolytes or other substances that indicate how well the kidneys are functioning. A chest x-ray can show the backup of fluid in the lungs. Tests may be needed to determine whether heart failure is present.[1]

Treatment

For people who are overhydrated, treatment involves helping the body excrete the excess water. Diuretics are drugs that help the kidneys do just that. There are several types of diuretics. Thiazide diuretics are often used first, because they are mild and tend to have few side effects. However, more potent diuret-

℞ TYPES OF DIURETICS

Type	Examples	Comments
Loop diuretics	Bumetanide Ethacrynic acid Furosemide	These diuretics help the kidneys excrete water and salt (sodium). Thus, they reduce the amount of fluid in blood vessels.
Thiazide and thiazide-like diuretics	Chlorthalidone Hydrochlorothiazide Indapamide Metolazone	The effects of these diuretics are usually milder than those of loop diuretics. Combinations of the two types of diuretics are particularly potent.
Potassium-sparing diuretics	Amiloride Spironolactone Triamterene	These diuretics reduce the amount of potassium excreted in urine. Usually, a potassium-sparing diuretic is not used by itself because it is weaker than other types of diuretics. Thus, it may be given in addition to thiazide or loop diuretics. Some drug products contain both a potassium-sparing diuretic and another type of diuretic.

1. see page 686

ics, such as furosemide, are often needed. Diuretics can be taken by mouth or given intravenously.

Most diuretics cause the kidneys to excrete more potassium as well as more water. Therefore, most people who take diuretics have to take potassium supplements or eat foods rich in potassium.[1] Some people are also given another type of diuretic, which reduces the amount of potassium excreted (potassium-sparing diuretic).

Taking a diuretic can cause or worsen urinary incontinence. Taking a diuretic can also worsen the need to urinate during the night (nocturia). However, a dose of a diuretic can usually be timed so that the diuretic's maximum effect does not occur when a bathroom is unavailable or when a person is sleeping.

If edema due to overhydration is bothersome, support stockings can help reduce the amount of fluid that accumulates in the legs. Consuming less salt also helps. If edema is due to poor circulation rather than overhydration, increasing physical activity can help. Usually, the blood vessel disorder that is causing poor circulation is treated.

If possible, the cause of overhydration is corrected. If the cause was giving intravenous fluids too rapidly, doctors give them more slowly. Heart failure[2] and kidney disorders can be treated. If the cause is a drug, the drug may be discontinued. However, some older people need to take NSAIDs for arthritis or pain. Such people may have to tolerate a small amount of edema or take a diuretic. If the cause of overhydration is over-production of antidiuretic hormone, the amount of fluids consumed each day may have to be limited.

PROBLEMS WITH ELECTROLYTE BALANCE

The level of any electrolyte in the blood can become too high or too low. The main electrolytes in the blood are sodium, potassium, calcium, magnesium, chloride, phosphate, and carbonate. Most commonly, problems occur when the level of sodium, potassium, or calcium is abnormal. Often, electrolyte levels change when water levels in the body change.

Doctors refer to a low electrolyte level with the prefix "hypo-"

1. see table on page 243
2. see page 686

and to a high level with the prefix "hyper-." The prefix is combined with the scientific name of the electrolyte. For example, a low level of potassium is called hypokalemia, and a high level of sodium is called hypernatremia.

Older people are more likely to develop abnormalities in electrolyte levels for the same reasons that they are more likely to become dehydrated or overhydrated. The main reason is that as the body ages, the kidneys function less well. The use of certain drugs, including diuretics and some laxatives, can increase the risk of developing electrolyte abnormalities. Problems with walking can increase the risk of developing electrolyte abnormalities because getting fluids and food may be difficult. Many chronic disorders (such as Paget's disease) and any disorder that causes fever, vomiting, or diarrhea can result in electrolyte abnormalities.

Electrolyte abnormalities can be diagnosed by measuring electrolyte levels in a sample of blood or urine. Other tests may be needed to determine the cause of the abnormalities.

To treat a low level of some electrolytes, such as sodium or potassium, doctors usually advise eating foods rich in the electrolyte or taking supplements. If the level is very low, the electrolyte may be given through a tube inserted in a vein (intravenously). If the level is high, treatment consists of consuming more fluids. Sometimes fluids must be given intravenously. Sometimes treatment is more complex because the disorder causing the electrolyte abnormality must be treated.

Sodium

Hyponatremia: A low sodium level (hyponatremia) may result from not consuming enough sodium in the diet, excreting too much (in sweat or urine), or being overhydrated. The sodium level may decrease when a person drinks a lot of water without consuming enough salt (sodium chloride), typically during hot weather when a person also sweats more. The sodium level may decrease when large amounts of fluids that do not contain enough sodium are given intravenously. Diuretics help the kidneys excrete excess sodium and excess water. However, diuretics may cause the kidneys to excrete more sodium than water, resulting in a low sodium level.

A low sodium level (and overhydration) can result when the

body produces too much antidiuretic hormone, which signals the kidneys to retain water. Overproduction of this hormone can be caused by disorders such as pneumonia and stroke and by drugs, including anticonvulsants (such as carbamazepine) and a type of antidepressant called selective serotonin reuptake inhibitors (SSRIs—such as sertraline). Other disorders that can cause a low sodium level include poorly controlled diabetes, heart failure, liver failure, and kidney disorders.

Having a low sodium level can cause confusion, drowsiness, muscle weakness, and seizures. A rapid fall in the sodium level often causes more severe symptoms than a slow fall. A low sodium level is restored to a normal level by gradually and steadily giving sodium and water intravenously.

Hypernatremia: A high sodium level (hypernatremia) is usually caused by dehydration or use of diuretics. (Diuretics may also cause the kidneys to excrete more water than sodium.) Typically, thirst is the first symptom. A person with a high sodium level may become weak and feel sluggish. A very high sodium level can cause confusion, paralysis, coma, and seizures.

If the sodium level is slightly high, it can be lowered by drinking fluids. If the sodium level is very high, fluids are given intravenously. Once the body's fluids are replaced, the high level of sodium returns to a normal level.

Potassium

Hypokalemia: A low potassium level (hypokalemia) is often caused by use of a diuretic. Many diuretics cause the kidneys to excrete more potassium (as well as more water) in urine. A low potassium level can also result from having diarrhea or vomiting for a long time.

A slight decrease in the potassium level rarely produces symptoms. If the potassium level remains low for a long time, the body tends to produce less insulin. As a result, the level of sugar in the blood may increase. If the potassium level becomes very low, fatigue, confusion, and muscle weakness and cramps typically occur. A very low potassium level can cause paralysis and abnormal heart rhythms (arrhythmias). For people who take digoxin (used to treat heart failure), abnormal heart rhythms tend to develop when the potassium level is even moderately low.

Treatment involves taking potassium supplements by mouth as a tablet or liquid or eating foods rich in potassium. People who are taking a diuretic that causes potassium to be excreted are sometimes also given another type of diuretic, which reduces the amount of potassium excreted (potassium-sparing diuretic).

Hyperkalemia: A high potassium level (hyperkalemia) is much more dangerous than a low potassium level. Most commonly, the cause is kidney failure or use of drugs that reduce the amount of potassium excreted by the kidneys. These drugs include the diuretic spironolactone and angiotensin-converting enzyme (ACE) inhibitors (used to lower blood pressure).[1] When a person who takes one of these drugs also eats potassium-rich foods or takes a potassium supplement, the kidneys cannot always excrete the potassium. In such cases, the potassium level in the blood can increase rapidly.

The first symptom of a high potassium level may be an abnormal heart rhythm. When doctors suspect a high potassium level, electrocardiography (ECG)[2] may help with the diagnosis. This procedure can detect changes in the heart's rhythm that occur when the potassium level is high.

People with a high potassium level must stop eating potassium-rich foods and stop taking potassium supplements. They may be given drugs that cause the body to excrete excess potassium, such as diuretics. If the potassium level is very high or is increasing, treatment must be started immediately. If the heart rhythm is abnormal, calcium is given intravenously. This treatment helps protect the heart. Then diuretics or drugs that prevent potassium from being absorbed are given to reduce the amount of potassium in the body. These drugs may be given intravenously, taken by mouth, or given as enemas.

Calcium

Hypocalcemia: A low calcium level (hypocalcemia) can result when a disorder such as a widespread infection in blood and other tissues (sepsis) develops suddenly. A low calcium level can also result when the body produces less parathyroid hormone, as may occur if the parathyroid glands are removed or

1. see table on pages 618 and 619
2. see page 661

damaged during neck surgery. A low level can also result from a deficiency of vitamin D. Vitamin D helps the body absorb calcium from foods. People may develop a vitamin D deficiency when they do not eat enough foods that contain vitamin D or when they do not spend much time outside. (Vitamin D is formed when the skin is exposed to direct sunlight.) Certain drugs, such as the anticonvulsants phenytoin and phenobarbital, can interfere with the processing of vitamin D, resulting in a deficiency of vitamin D. Several disorders, such as an underactive thyroid gland (hypothyroidism) and pancreatitis, can result in a low calcium level.

A low calcium level makes a person weak and causes numbness in the hands or feet. It can cause confusion or seizures. Treatment involves taking calcium supplements by mouth. If a disorder is the cause, it should be treated.

Hypercalcemia: A high calcium level (hypercalcemia) can result when bone is broken down and releases calcium into the bloodstream. Calcium may be released when cancer spreads to the bone or when Paget's disease (a bone disorder) becomes so severe that it makes a person unable to move around. Normally, parathyroid hormone helps the body control the level of calcium in blood. An abnormally high level of parathyroid hormone can result in a high calcium level. Usually, the cause is production of an excessive amount of hormone by a tumor in the parathyroid gland. But some cancers, including certain lung cancers, can also produce parathyroid hormone. A high calcium level can also result when the level of thyroid hormone is abnormally high.[1]

A slight increase in the calcium level may not cause any symptoms. A very high level can result in dehydration because it causes the kidneys to excrete more water. A very high level can also cause loss of appetite, nausea, vomiting, and confusion. A person may even go into a coma and die.

If the calcium level is very high, rapid treatment is needed. Giving fluids intravenously helps. Often, drugs such as calcitonin and bisphosphonates must be given intravenously for short periods of time. These drugs decrease the amount of bone being broken down and thus the amount of calcium released into the bloodstream. Other treatments may be needed, depend-

1. see page 468

ing on the cause of the high calcium level. When the cause is cancer or Paget's disease, bisphosphonates are often taken by mouth indefinitely. When the cause is a tumor in the parathyroid gland, surgery to remove the tumor or part of the parathyroid gland may be done.

19

Hypothermia and Hyperthermia

When it comes to temperature control, the body runs a tight ship. The body carries out its business best at about 98.6° Fahrenheit (F), so the healthy body prevents its temperature from varying more than $1\frac{1}{2}°$ F from this desirable level. When the body's temperature gets much hotter or colder than 98.6° F, people generally feel terrible, functioning becomes impaired, and the results can be deadly.

Aging decreases the body's ability to control its temperature. In addition, older people are more likely than younger people to have diseases and to take drugs that decrease the body's ability to control its temperature. It should come as no surprise, then, that older people, compared with young and middle-aged adults, are much more susceptible to disorders in which body temperature falls dangerously low (hypothermia) or climbs dangerously high (hyperthermia).

HYPOTHERMIA

Hypothermia is a decrease in body temperature to 94° F or lower. At low temperatures, the body's organs become sluggish and less effective.

When the body temperature is low, messages travel more slowly through the brain and the rest of the nervous system. Abnormal heart rhythms (arrhythmias) may occur. The heart also slows down, and blood pressure falls. The kidneys make less urine, and digestion slows because muscles in the digestive tract contract less. If body temperature falls below about 86° F, organs are likely to stop working altogether, and death is likely.

Causes

An older person's body temperature may begin to fall whenever the body is exposed to temperatures cooler than it. The fall in body temperature is not likely to make a difference when the surrounding temperature is above 80° F, but it can become a problem when the surrounding temperature starts dipping below 70° F. Heat loss is also increased by wind, by sitting or lying on a cold surface, and by being immersed in cold water.

ADDITIONAL DETAIL

The body is equipped with ways of generating additional heat when the surroundings are cooler than the body's temperature. For example, muscles contract and produce additional heat by shivering. The body is also equipped with ways of keeping what heat it has. For example, small blood vessels just below the surface of the skin narrow (constrict) so that more blood goes to the heart and brain. However, aging itself takes its toll on the body's ability to adapt to the cold. With aging, the body becomes less efficient at shivering or at diverting blood away from the surface of the body. Also, the layer of fat just under the skin thins, so there is less insulation to prevent heat loss.

The body's ability to produce heat is decreased by diseases that commonly affect older people, such as hypothyroidism. The body's ability to retain heat is decreased by diseases such as diabetes. A person who is less able to move around because of an injury or a disease such as a stroke or arthritis is also at a greater risk of dangerous cooling, because the decreased movement generates less heat-producing muscle activity. Alcohol and certain drugs, such as antidepressants, increase the risk as well.

Symptoms

Initial symptoms of hypothermia come on slowly and without fanfare; thus hypothermia may sneak up on a person. When body temperature falls to between 95° and 97° F, the person may report feeling cold and, more than likely, will begin to shiver. However, by the time body temperature has fallen to 94° F or lower, reports of feeling cold and shivering usually stop. Instead, the skin may feel cold to the touch, even in such areas as the back and abdomen, which tend to be better insulated from the cold.

Movements become slow and clumsy, and the person becomes stiff or even rigid. Speech is thick and slow, and balance worsens. The person may stumble or fall. Some people appear to be intoxicated or to be experiencing a stroke. Thinking becomes less clear, and judgment is usually impaired. Rather than seeking a source of heat, some people actually remove their clothing.

Other changes may become apparent. The heartbeat slows down and may become irregular. Breathing also slows down.

If the body temperature falls below about 86° F, an older person usually becomes sleepier and sleepier, slips into a coma, and, in all likelihood, dies a short time later.

Diagnosis

The diagnosis of hypothermia is made when the body temperature is measured at or below 94° F. Most ordinary thermometers do not record temperatures below 96° F. A doctor may use a special thermometer that reads very low temperatures.

Once a doctor has determined that a person has hypothermia, an electrocardiogram may be performed to determine how much the cold temperature has affected the heart, and routine blood tests indicate whether other organs have been affected.

Prevention

Hypothermia is almost always preventable. Older people are advised to take the following precautions to prevent hypothermia:

• **Maintain a warm environment:** Older people sometimes keep their homes at a lower-than-desirable temperature as a means of saving money, but the thermostat should be set at 68° F or higher. It is especially important that the bedroom be kept warm. Fuel assistance programs and home winterization programs may help defray costs.

• **Wear several layers of clothing:** Clothing made of wool or synthetic materials such as polypropylene are especially useful, because these materials insulate even when they become wet. Because the body loses a large amount of heat from the head, wearing a hat is important. Fingers and toes must also be protected.

• **Eat warm foods and drink warm fluids:** Food provides the body with fuel to be burned, and warm fluids provide heat and prevent dehydration.

• **Avoid alcoholic beverages:** Alcohol dilates blood vessels in the skin, which makes the body temporarily feel warm but actually causes greater heat loss.

• **Exercise regularly:** Exercise can increase the body's production of heat.

Outlook and Treatment

Hypothermia requires emergency medical treatment. Chances of recovery depend on how long the person has been cold, how low the body temperature has fallen, and the person's general health before hypothermia developed. The longer the amount of time, the lower the temperature, and the worse the person's general health, the lower the chances are of recovery.

The first goal when hypothermia is suspected or diagnosed is to keep the person warm and dry so that body temperature does not fall further. The person must be handled gently, because sudden movements may cause a dangerous abnormal heart rhythm. The person is also kept still, because exertion pumps very cold blood from the extremities back to the heart.

If the person appears to be in a coma or even to have died, the heart may still be beating, although very slowly and weakly. Cardiopulmonary resuscitation (CPR) should not be started unless it is certain that there is no pulse, because chest compressions could stop the heart.

Emergency treatment focuses on warming the person, but

problems already caused by the cold body temperature, such as abnormal heart rhythms and dehydration, must also be corrected. The person is placed in a warm room and covered with special blankets or insulating materials to retain whatever heat the body is still producing. These measures may be all that is needed to warm the body in cases of mild hypothermia. Doctors want the warming to be slow and steady, increasing the body temperature by about 1° to 2° F per hour. It might seem as though warming should be done as fast as possible. However, rapid warming can sometimes increase the risk of very low blood pressure (shock) or life-threatening abnormal heart rhythms. Therefore, rapid warming is done only if the person is extremely ill and the body temperature is below 90° F.

Rapid warming is carried out by having the person breathe heated oxygen through a face mask or by passing heated fluids into the blood through a vein (intravenously) or into the abdominal or chest cavity through a plastic tube. Special heating blankets may also be used. In addition, the blood may be warmed by pumping it out of the body, warming it, and returning it to the body.

Some people with hypothermia who have arrived at the hospital with no signs of life recover. Efforts to restart the heart while a person is hypothermic often fail. Therefore, a decision to discontinue these efforts is not made until after the person's body temperature has been raised above 94° F.

HYPERTHERMIA

"Hyperthermia" is an increase in body temperature above 99° F, but most often the term is used to refer to a dangerously high body temperature.

"Fever" is a more general term that describes any increase above 99° F. It is usually reserved for situations in which body temperature is elevated for reasons other than a warm environment, such as a response to infection.

When an older person's surroundings are hotter than his body temperature, heat cramps, heat exhaustion, or heatstroke can occur. Heat cramps and heat exhaustion usually involve an increase in body temperature, although some people with these disorders have a normal body temperature. Heatstroke always involves a dangerously high body temperature.

High body temperature is never the sole cause of the symptoms of heat cramps, heat exhaustion, and heatstroke. Symptoms also stem from the loss of body fluids and dissolved salts (electrolytes), especially sodium and potassium, in the blood.[1]

Causes

An older person's body temperature may rise whenever the body produces too much heat or when it is unable to get rid of excess heat. The body gains excess heat when the air is warmer than 98.6° F. When high humidity accompanies high air temperature, the body has difficulty getting rid of excess heat, because humid air makes evaporation of sweating less effective. Heat is also produced during physical activity by muscles. Thus, most cases of hyperthermia occur on hot days, especially humid ones, and in people who are exerting themselves.

The chance of developing hyperthermia increases when a person is exposed to high heat suddenly. Such a situation might occur when an older person stays inside during a heat wave with windows closed and with no air-conditioning because of poverty or loss of electrical power. As a person is exposed to longer periods of high heat and humidity, the body gradually adjusts (acclimates) and is better able to maintain usual body temperature. Older people, however, are not as able as younger people to acclimate to higher temperatures and humidity. In addition, they more commonly have underlying diseases or take drugs that interfere with their ability to eliminate heat.

ADDITIONAL DETAIL

The body has different ways of ridding itself of excess heat. When the body is warmer than its surroundings, heat flows from warmer to cooler areas of the body, which promotes cooling. The body also produces moisture that cools the skin as it evaporates (sweating). Wearing tight or heavy clothing makes sweating less effective by preventing evaporation from the skin surface. Humidity (the presence of moisture in the air) also

1. see page 253

slows evaporation, making sweating less effective. For example, an air temperature of 90° F might be tolerable for many people if humidity is only 40%. But 90° F or even 80° F would be dangerous for many of those same people if the humidity were to rise to 80%. The body also gets rid of some heat through the evaporation that occurs during breathing, but this too is decreased by humidity. Getting rid of excess heat is therefore more difficult in hot, humid weather.

Older people in particular tend to have difficulty increasing the flow of blood to all skin surfaces. Certain drugs, such as antipsychotics and antidepressants, and some diseases that affect the skin, such as scleroderma and psoriasis, can also interfere with sweating. Other disorders, such as heart failure and obesity, can interfere with the body's ability to cool itself as well. Aging itself also affects thirst; older people do not get thirsty as readily as younger people. Thus, older people tend to get dehydrated, which in turn means they are less able to sweat in warm surroundings.

Symptoms and Diagnosis

Hyperthermia produces symptoms proportional to its severity.

Heat cramps, the mildest form, can develop with modest losses of fluids and electrolytes. Heat cramps are felt as waves of painful contractions in muscles of the hands, shoulders, feet, calves, or thighs. The muscles become hard and tense.

Heat exhaustion often results in dizziness that is typically described as light-headedness. Fainting may occur, especially upon standing after a period of sitting or lying down. Drenching sweats are common. Mild confusion, headache, blurred vision, weakness, fatigue, muscle aches, nausea, or vomiting may develop.

Heatstroke, the most severe form, sometimes develops without any warning symptoms. The first sign of trouble may be severe confusion, bizarre behavior, or a coma. In some cases, however, light-headedness, mild confusion, headache, blurred vision, weakness, fatigue, muscle aches, nausea, or vomiting may develop early on. Seizures may occur. Some people with heatstroke, especially people who have been physically exerting themselves, are still sweating. More commonly, however, the skin becomes hot, flushed, and dry. Sweating often stops despite the heat, and the person urinates very little or not at all.

A doctor makes the diagnosis of heat exhaustion and heatstroke on the basis of symptoms. A physical examination often shows the heart rate and breathing rate to be increased. Blood pressure may be low in heat exhaustion and is often extremely low in heatstroke. In heat exhaustion, body temperature can be normal or high, but not higher than 104° F. In heatstroke, body temperature usually exceeds 105° F and may be so high that it can no longer be read on a typical thermometer. Blood tests are done to determine if the levels of sodium and potassium are low.

Prevention

Common sense is the best tool for preventing hyperthermia. During hot, humid weather, older people are advised to take the following precautions:

• **Avoid strenuous exertion:** When exertion in a hot environment cannot be avoided, drinking plenty of liquids and frequently cooling the skin by misting or wetting it with cool water can help keep body temperature near normal.

• **Wear light, loose-fitting clothing** made of cloth that allows air and moisture to pass through easily, such as cotton.

• **Replace fluids and salts lost through sweating** by consuming lightly salted foods and beverages, such as salted tomato juice or cool bouillon. Many commercially available drinks contain extra salt. To adequately replace fluids, drinking must continue even after thirst is quenched.

• **Use air-conditioning or fans:** It is especially important that the bedroom be air-conditioned. People who live in homes without air-conditioning or fans should open windows at night and create cross-ventilation by opening windows on two sides of the building. Windows should be covered with curtains, shades, or blinds during daylight hours to reduce the heat from the sun. When transportation is available, older people who live in homes that are not air-conditioned can go to public places that are air-conditioned, such as shopping malls, movie theaters, or libraries.

Outlook and Treatment

Mild heat cramps can often be treated by moving to a cooler environment and drinking beverages that contain salt. Severe heat cramps are treated with fluids and salts given intravenously. Drugs to treat fever, such as acetaminophen and aspirin, are ineffective and should not be used.

If body temperature continues to rise, untreated heat cramps or heat exhaustion can progress to heatstroke. Fortunately, most older people with heat cramps or heat exhaustion recover fully when appropriately treated.

Many older people do not survive heatstroke. Because of the danger and the need for specialized treatment and monitoring, people with heatstroke are usually best treated in an emergency department and then admitted to an intensive care unit of a hospital.

An older person with heatstroke must be cooled immediately. After calling for medical assistance, the caller should remove the person's clothing, splash water on his skin, and then fan him. Ice packs should not be used to cool the person, because shivering produces heat. At the hospital, body cooling is usually accomplished by spraying the body with tepid water. To speed evaporation and body cooling, a fan is used to blow air on the body. Ice packs are also placed over large blood vessels in the neck, genital region, and armpits. Body temperature is measured continuously. Cooled fluids may be given intravenously. To avoid overcooling, efforts to cool the body are halted when the temperature is reduced to about 102° F.

After recovery, body temperature may remain abnormal and fluctuate for weeks. The brain may not fully recover, and an older person who has had heatstroke may be left with personality changes, clumsiness, or poor coordination.

20

Dizziness and Fainting

Dizziness and fainting are symptoms. They may indicate that a disorder is present. Both dizziness and fainting are common. They sometimes occur together and may have similar causes. But most people who have dizziness do not faint, and many people who faint do not have dizziness.

Dizziness makes daily activities difficult and can worsen a person's quality of life. But dizziness rarely indicates a life-threatening disorder. Fainting is less common than dizziness and tends to interfere less with daily activities. But it can result in injuries and may indicate a serious or even life-threatening disorder.

DIZZINESS

Dizziness is an uncomfortable, troubling sensation that can feel like spinning, unsteadiness, or light-headedness.

While standing still, some people feel as if the world is spinning around them, making them feel nauseated. While walking, some people feel their knees go wobbly, and they feel unsteady and shaky. Just after standing up, some people sway, feel as if their head is swimming, and sometimes drop right back down in the chair. After standing for a while, some people feel light-headed. All of these people may say they feel dizzy.

Because so many different feelings can be described as dizziness, doctors often try to put dizziness into categories. These categories help people understand each other when they talk about dizziness. Four categories are usually used.

Vertigo is a sensation of motion when there is no motion. It is often described as spinning. Vertigo is what some people have just after they ride on a carousel. They briefly feel as though they are still moving, even after they have both feet planted firmly on the ground. People with vertigo may feel that they are moving or that the surroundings are moving while they remain still. Vertigo usually occurs when a person is standing. But it sometimes occurs while a person is sitting, lying down, or changing position. People with vertigo may also have nausea, sometimes with vomiting, and abnormal jerky eye movements (nystagmus).

Dysequilibrium is a sense of unsteadiness or loss of balance that involves the legs or trunk. Dysequilibrium may occur while a person is standing or walking.

Light-headedness is a feeling that fainting may occur in the next few moments. Light-headedness usually occurs when a person gets up quickly after sitting or lying down for a while.

Mixed dizziness is a miscellaneous category. It refers to dizziness that does not fit neatly into one of the other three categories.

The categories seem to work fairly well for dizziness that lasts less than a month (temporary or acute dizziness). But for dizziness that lasts more than a month (persistent or chronic dizziness), the categories start to blur together. For example, dizziness may seem like light-headedness and vertigo at the same time. Or dizziness may seem to change from one category to another over time. Older people usually have chronic dizziness, so the categories are less helpful.

Causes

Dizziness may occur when the brain gets wrong or conflicting information about the body's position in relation to the surroundings and to the body's movements. Several parts of the body provide this information. They include the eyes, a structure in the inner ear (called the vestibular labyrinth), and the nerves that carry information from large joints (in the neck, hips, knees, and ankles) to the brain. The brain constantly uses information from these body parts to direct the activities of muscles and joints so that balance and stability are maintained. When the body cannot maintain balance and stability, dizziness sometimes occurs.

PROBLEMS THAT CAN CONTRIBUTE TO DIZZINESS

Problem	Possible Causes	Possible Solutions
Impairment of vision	Cataracts	Have surgery to remove cataracts
	Macular degeneration	For wet macular degeneration, have laser treatment. Install bright lighting, and use a magnifying lens
	Glaucoma	Take drugs that reduce eye pressure or have laser treatment
	Difficulty judging the distance of objects while wearing glasses	Do not wear bifocals or trifocals if possible
Impairment of hearing	Accumulation of wax in the ear	Use small amounts of mineral or baby oil or other nonprescription preparations to thin the ear wax so that it can drain out. Have a doctor remove the wax
	Changes in nerves (such as that due to presbycusis)	Wear a hearing aid. Attend a hearing rehabilitation program to learn lip reading and other strategies for coping with hearing loss
	Changes in bone (such as that due to otosclerosis)	Wear a hearing aid. For otosclerosis, have surgery
Malfunction of inner ear	Side effects of certain drugs (such as certain antibiotics, aspirin in high doses, or the diuretics ethacrynic acid or furosemide)	Talk to the doctor about using a different drug
	Infections	Have the infection treated. Attend a rehabilitation program

Table continues on the following page.

Problem	Possible Causes	Possible Solutions
		to learn exercises that help prevent dizziness
	Strokes	Attend a rehabilitation program to learn exercises that help prevent dizziness
	Benign positional vertigo	Be treated with the Epley maneuver
	Meniere's disease	Limit consumption of salt and caffeine. Talk with the doctor about possible treatments
Malfunction of the nerves that carry information between the brain and other parts of the body	An unidentified cause (most commonly)	Wear appropriate footwear (flat heels and firm soles) Attend training to improve balance and walking
	Diabetes	Take insulin or other drugs for diabetes Wear appropriate footwear. Attend training to improve balance and walking
	Vitamin B_{12} deficiency	Take vitamin B_{12} supplements by mouth or by injection
	Hypothyroidism	Take thyroid hormone
Pressure on nerves in the neck	Arthritis	Attend a rehabilitation program to learn exercises that help prevent dizziness
	Degeneration of the disks and vertebrae in the neck (cervical spondylosis)	Attend a rehabilitation program to learn exercises that help prevent dizziness. Rarely, surgery is needed
Reduced blood flow due to blockages in the arteries	Atherosclerosis	Take drugs to help prevent blockages from worsening or new ones from

Problem	Possible Causes	Possible Solutions
that carry blood to the brain		forming, such as aspirin and drugs that lower fat (lipid) levels in the blood. Have surgery to remove material blocking an artery
Low blood pressure after eating (postprandial hypotension)	Malfunction of the mechanisms that control blood pressure and blood flow	Eat small meals that are low in carbo-hydrates. Near meal-times, do not take drugs that may lower blood pressure. Drink caffeinated beverages with the morning meal
Low blood pressure when standing up after sitting or lying down (orthostatic hypotension)	Side effects of drugs	Talk to the doctor about discontinuing the drug that may be contributing to dizziness, substituting another drug, or reducing the dose
	Dehydration	Drink enough fluids to replace those that were lost. Increase the amount of salt consumed
	Loss of muscle tone and strength	Flex the feet repeatedly before getting up. Stand up slowly after sitting or lying down. Wear waist-high support stockings
	Diabetes	Take insulin or other drugs for diabetes. Follow the suggested solutions for loss of muscle tone and strength. Do exercises to strengthen the legs.
	Parkinson's disease	Take drugs such as fludrocortisone and

Table continues on the following page.

Problem	Possible Causes	Possible Solutions
		midodrine, which help prevent blood pressure from falling excessively. Follow the suggested solutions for loss of muscle tone and strength
Impairment of the heart's ability to pump blood	Heart failure	Take drugs used to treat heart failure
	Abnormal thickening of the heart muscle (hypertrophic cardiomyopathy)	Take drugs used to treat thickening of the heart muscle, such as drugs that lower blood pressure (antihypertensives)
	Heart valve disorders	Take drugs used to treat heart valve disorders or have a heart valve repaired or replaced
	Abnormal heart rhythms (arrhythmias)	Take drugs used to treat abnormal heart rhythms (antiarrhythmic drugs) or have a pacemaker implanted
Reduction in the oxygen level in the blood	Any chronic lung disorder, especially chronic obstructive pulmonary disease (COPD)	Use oxygen therapy (for example, from tanks) at home
Reduction in the sugar level in the blood	A low blood sugar level (hypoglycemia) in people who are treated for diabetes	Ask the doctor about changing the dose or schedule of insulin or other drugs used to treat diabetes
Side effects of drugs	Antidepressants, antipsychotics, antihistamines, benzodiazepines (used mainly to treat anxiety), beta-blockers, diuretics, and nitrates (used to treat angina)	Talk to the doctor about discontinuing the drug that can contribute to dizziness, substituting another drug, or reducing the dose. Talk to the doctor about taking the lowest reffective dose of all drugs needed

Aging itself can cause some of the body parts involved in balance to function less well. But the effect is not enough to cause dizziness unless a person also has a disorder or takes a drug that adds to the effect. Having problems with several of the body parts involved in balance is a common cause of dizziness in older people. For example, a person may have vision problems, inner ear (vestibular) problems, and nerve damage or arthritis (which can interfere with information sent from the joints to the brain). In such cases, the brain does not get enough information to maintain balance and stability.

Many disorders can cause dizziness. Among older people common causes include two disorders of the inner ear: benign positional vertigo and Meniere's disease.

• **Benign positional vertigo:** Vertigo occurs when the head is moved—for example, when a person lies down, gets up, turns over in bed, or looks up. Benign positional vertigo develops when particles that are normally distributed evenly in the fluid-filled canals of the inner ear clump together.

• **Meniere's disease:** Vertigo is usually accompanied by hearing loss and a low roaring or ringing in the ears (tinnitus). Meniere's disease is caused by excess fluid in the inner ear.

Some disorders cause light-headedness only during or after certain activities. For example, an excessive fall in blood pressure after standing up quickly (orthostatic hypotension) or after eating a meal (postprandial hypotension) can make people feel light-headed after those activities. In both cases, the brain does not get enough blood because blood pressure is too low.

Some disorders tend to cause temporary dizziness. For example, a person who has a heart attack may suddenly feel dizzy (usually light-headed) and continue to feel that way for a few days to a few weeks. As the heart heals, the feeling goes away. With other disorders, how long dizziness will last is uncertain. For example, if a person with diabetes develops dysequilibrium, it may go away in a month, or it may last for a lifetime (although its severity may vary). Depression sometimes causes dizziness. People who are depressed may lose confidence in their ability to interact with their surroundings. They may then feel unsteady or light-headed.

A low number of red blood cells (anemia), a low or high level of sugar (glucose), or a low level of vitamin B_{12} may contribute to dizziness. An underactive thyroid gland (hypothyroidism) can cause dizziness.

Dizziness can also be a temporary side effect of certain drugs, including many taken for high blood pressure. This type of dizziness often goes away after a person takes the drug for a week or two. Antihistamines and sleep aids, including nonprescription ones, can contribute to dizziness.

Certain situations can cause temporary dizziness in healthy people. For example, turning around or standing up very quickly can cause a brief period of dizziness. Wearing bifocals may cause dizziness when a person goes down stairs or looks down.

Diagnosis

People who experience dizziness should report it to their doctor. A doctor tries to identify what is causing the dizziness and whether the dizziness fits into a specific category, such as vertigo. To do so, the doctor asks the person to describe the dizziness. For example, the doctor asks whether the dizziness is accompanied by other symptoms, such as nausea. The doctor also asks how long the dizziness has been present. If dizziness has been present for less than a month, the doctor may ask whether the person started taking any new prescription or nonprescription drugs and whether the dosages of any drugs have changed recently. If the dizziness has lasted more than a month, the doctor checks for certain disorders that may be causing the dizziness.

The doctor performs a physical examination. Hearing is tested to help determine if an ear is malfunctioning. If one ear hears better than the other, the person may have an inner ear disorder, which may be contributing to dizziness. Vision is tested, and the eyes are checked for specific problems that can limit vision, such as cataracts.

The doctor sometimes observes the eyes for abnormal jerking movements (nystagmus), which may indicate an inner ear disorder. The doctor may perform a simple maneuver, called the Hallpike maneuver. For this maneuver, the person sits on a table. The doctor rapidly lays the person down with the person's head hanging over the edge of the table. In the same movement, the doctor turns the person's head to the right or left. If the dizziness is caused by an inner ear disorder, the Hallpike maneuver may quickly produce nystagmus and dizziness.

The doctor uses a stethoscope to check the rate, rhythm, and sound of the heartbeat. Blood pressure is measured after the person has been lying down for about 5 minutes and immediately after the person stands up. Sometimes it is measured again after 3 minutes. These measurements help determine whether the cause of the dizziness is orthostatic hypotension.

The doctor checks some aspects of brain and nerve function, particularly the senses of position and balance. For example, a person may be asked to stand still with the eyes open, then with the eyes closed. If the person sways more than expected, the dizziness may be caused by an inner ear disorder, a brain disorder, or a problem with the body's ability to send information from the large joints to the brain.

Blood tests may be done. Typically, the number of red blood cells and levels of sugar, vitamin B_{12}, and thyroid hormones are measured.

If evidence suggests a heart disorder, especially an abnormal heart rhythm, electrocardiography (ECG) may be done to record the electrical activity of the heart.[1] The person may be asked to wear a small, battery-powered ECG device (Holter monitor)[2] for 1 or 2 days. If evidence suggests a brain disorder, computed tomography (CT) or magnetic resonance imaging (MRI) may be done to obtain images of the brain.

Treatment and Prevention

The goals of treatment are correcting or controlling possible causes of dizziness and enabling people to prevent or control dizziness so that they can do daily activities safely.

Sometimes dizziness can be cured. For example, if a drug is causing it, the drug can be stopped and changed to something else. If the cause is benign positional vertigo, the Epley maneuver may provide a cure. The Epley maneuver resembles the Hallpike maneuver, which is used for diagnosis. If persistent light-headedness is related to episodes of low blood

1. see page 661
2. see art on page 698

pressure that occur when a person stands up or after a person eats, wearing support stockings (compression stockings) may help. Drugs such as fludrocortisone and midodrine may be used.

People who have experienced dizziness should not take non-prescription drugs that may contribute to dizziness, such as antihistamines or sleep aids. Antihistamines can worsen dizziness in older people, even though low doses of these drugs help a few younger adults who have persistent vertigo.

If dizziness persists despite treatment, people can learn how to avoid movements that tend to trigger dizziness. Examples are looking up, reaching up, or bending down. One way to avoid these movements is to store household items between waist and eye level. Getting up slowly after sitting or lying down for a while can help. Clenching the hands and flexing the feet sometimes helps, especially if the dizziness feels like light-headedness.

Outlook

For some people, dizziness goes away or lessens without treatment. For others, dizziness goes away or lessens only after the cause is corrected. For still others, dizziness, even when treated, lasts for months or years. However, most of these people can cope and continue everyday activities, especially when treatment controls the dizziness to some degree.

FAINTING

Fainting (syncope) is a sudden and temporary loss of consciousness. A person who has fainted cannot be aroused for several seconds to several minutes.

Fainting can be frightening. People who have fainted open their eyes and find themselves slumped in a chair or sprawled on the floor, just moments after they had been going about their business. They may find themselves surrounded by a throng of concerned people.

THE EPLEY MANEUVER:
A POSSIBLE CURE FOR VERTIGO?

Some people experience vertigo when they change the position of their head rapidly. This type of vertigo is usually benign positional vertigo. It develops when particles that are normally distributed evenly in the fluid-filled canals of the inner ear clump together. Often, the disorder can be cured by the Epley maneuver. This maneuver may redistribute the clumps of particles in the inner ear.

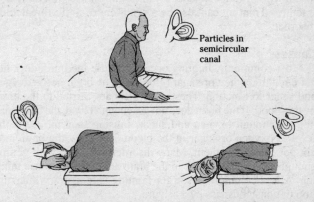

Particles in semicircular canal

The head may be rapidly turned even further (so that the person nearly faces the floor). The person is returned to a seated position and should remain at least semiupright for the next 24 hours.

The doctor rapidly lays the person down with the person's head hanging over the table edge. The head is turned to the same side as the affected ear.

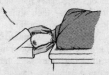 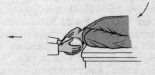

The head is rapidly turned further (so that the ear is parallel to the floor).

The head is rapidly turned to the other side.

Some people faint only once. Others faint over and over again. Anyone can faint, but older people are much more likely to do so. Sometimes symptoms related to the cause of fainting occur before, during, or after fainting. People who have fainted may limit their daily activities because their doctor has advised them to so or because they are afraid of fainting again. Fainting often results in a fall, which increases the risk of injuries and disability.[1] In older people, a fall is more likely to result in a fracture.[2] Fainting can also be a symptom of a life-threatening disorder.

Causes

Most commonly, fainting occurs because the brain does not get enough oxygen or sugar (glucose). The brain needs oxygen and sugar to function. These vital fuels are carried to the brain by the blood. If the brain does not get enough blood, the brain may not get enough oxygen and sugar, causing fainting. Or if the level of oxygen or sugar in the blood decreases, the brain may not get enough of them. Many disorders interfere with getting enough oxygen and sugar to the brain and thus can cause fainting. A less common reason for fainting is temporary interruption of consciousness by a seizure.

BEFORE, DURING, AND AFTER FAINTING

Sometimes before fainting occurs, people experience sensations warning that they may faint. For example, when fainting is caused by orthostatic hypotension, people may feel light-headed before they faint. When fainting is caused by an abnormal heart rhythm, people may feel the heartbeat skip or race—sensations called palpitations. Such people usually recover quickly and can function normally soon after they regain consciousness.

When fainting is caused by a seizure, people may lose control of the bladder or bowel while they are unconscious. They may need a long time to clear their thoughts after they regain consciousness.

When fainting is caused by straining while having a bowel movement or urinating, injuries are more likely, because bathrooms tend to be small and full of hard surfaces. For example, people may bump their heads on the edge of a sink.

---

1. see page 287
2. see page 311

As the body ages, blood flow to the brain and the amount of oxygen available to the brain decrease. These changes alone are not enough to cause fainting. But because of them, other problems—certain disorders, certain drugs, and sudden stressful events—are more likely to cause fainting. For most older people, fainting results from several problems, not just one.

Certain disorders and situations can cause blood pressure to fall. As a result, the brain may not get enough blood, and fainting may occur. Blood pressure may fall after standing up quickly (orthostatic hypotension) or after eating a meal (postprandial hypotension). Coughing strenuously, straining while having a bowel movement, or urinating under certain circumstances (for example, when straining) can cause a fall in blood pressure. Blood pressure may fall when a person becomes dehydrated.

Fainting can result from overstimulation of the vagus nerve, which helps control heart rate and blood pressure. Stimulating the vagus nerve causes the heart rate to slow and blood pressure to fall. This type of fainting is sometimes called a vasovagal attack or vasovagal (neurocardiogenic) syncope. It can result when a person is having trouble swallowing something, is startled, is in a stressful situation, suddenly has severe pain, or becomes nauseated.

Some disorders keep the brain from getting enough blood. For example, a heart attack, an abnormal heart rhythm (arrhythmia), or a heart valve disorder can interfere with the heart's ability to pump blood. In a stroke, an artery that carries blood to the brain may be blocked.

The two large arteries in the front of the neck (carotid arteries)—one on each side—have a specialized area that helps control blood pressure. This area, called the carotid sinus, can become overly sensitive to pressure caused by movements of the neck or by a tight collar. This disorder is called carotid sinus syndrome. In people with this disorder, pressure on the carotid sinus can cause the heart rate to slow dramatically or blood pressure to fall. Fainting can result.

Blood flow through the arteries that carry blood to the back of the brain may be decreased because atherosclerosis has narrowed the arteries or because bony outgrowths due to osteoarthritis press on them. People with either disorder may faint when they tilt the head backward or turn it sharply to the side. This disorder is called vertebrobasilar insufficiency.

A low number of red blood cells (anemia) increases the risk of fainting. Red blood cells carry oxygen. Thus, anemia reduces the amount of oxygen the blood carries to the brain. Fainting sometimes results from a fall in the level of sugar in the blood, which may happen in people with diabetes.

Many prescription drugs may contribute to fainting, particularly when a drug is first started. They include drugs used to treat heart disorders and high blood pressure, such as beta-blockers (which slow the heart), diuretics (which cause the kidneys to excrete more water and salt), and angiotensin-converting enzyme (ACE) inhibitors (which lower blood pressure by widening arteries). Other drugs that can cause fainting include some antidepressants and alpha-blockers (often used to treat an enlarged prostate gland).

Diagnosis

Fainting is easy to recognize. A doctor focuses on identifying the cause, particularly whether the cause could be life threatening, such as an abnormal heart rhythm or a heart valve disorder. The doctor begins by asking questions and by performing a physical examination. Often, these steps are enough to identify possible causes of fainting.

The doctor asks what the person was doing before fainting. For example, if the person had eaten a large meal within an hour before fainting, the cause may be postprandial hypotension. The doctor also asks what the person felt like before fainting and what the person remembers immediately after regaining consciousness. The symptoms that occurred before, during, or after may suggest a possible cause. The doctor asks whether the person has started taking any new prescription or nonprescription drugs and whether the dosage of any drug has been changed.

The physical examination includes measuring blood pressure after the person has been lying down for about 5 minutes and immediately after the person stands up. Sometimes it is measured again after 3 minutes. If blood pressure falls excessively when the person stands, orthostatic hypotension may have contributed to fainting.

If blood pressure falls occasionally, a person may be asked to measure blood pressure at home with an automatic device. The person measures and records blood pressure at specific times when fainting has previously occurred. The doctor can then review the blood pressure record to determine how often and when it falls too low.

The doctor listens to the heart with a stethoscope. If the sound of turbulent blood flow (a heart murmur) is heard, a heart valve disorder may have caused the fainting. The doctor checks the functioning of the brain and nerves. This check (called a neurologic examination) can determine whether sensation or muscle control was lost. Such a loss may indicate that a stroke caused the fainting.

Blood tests are usually done. The number of red blood cells is determined to check for anemia. The sodium and urea nitrogen levels in the blood are measured to check for dehydration. The sugar level in the blood is measured to check for diabetes.

More complex procedures are done only if evidence suggests a specific cause that needs to be confirmed.

Electrocardiography (ECG), which records the electrical activity of the heart, is done to check for a heart disorder.[1] Sometimes the person is asked to wear a small, portable ECG device (Holter monitor) for 1 or 2 days.[2] If the monitor detects an abnormal heart rhythm just before or at the same time as a fainting episode, the abnormal heart rhythm is likely to have caused or contributed to the fainting. Another type of monitor is used when the person must be monitored longer. This monitor is similar to the Holter monitor except it records the heart's rhythm only when the person or someone assisting the person pushes a button. The button is pushed when the person feels he is about to faint or immediately after regaining consciousness after fainting.

Echocardiography, which uses sound waves to produce a picture of the heart, can show whether the heart has an abnormality that may decrease blood pressure or blood flow to the brain.

If seizures may be the cause, electroencephalography (EEG) may be done. In this procedure, small adhesive sensors (electrodes) are placed on the person's scalp. The electrodes are con-

1. see page 661
2. see art on page 698

nected by wires to a machine that records the electrical activity of the brain.

To confirm a suspected cause, the doctor may try to re-create a fainting episode under safe conditions. For example, while monitoring the heartbeat with electrocardiography, a doctor may gently press on the person's neck over the carotid sinus. This pressure temporarily increases blood pressure inside the carotid sinus. Thus, the body is tricked into thinking that blood pressure has increased throughout the body. A signal is then sent to the brain to reduce blood pressure. If the brain's response is exaggerated, blood pressure may fall excessively, and the person may feel faint or even faint.

Another procedure, called tilt table testing, involves tilting a person who is lying flat to an almost standing position. Tilt table testing is used to confirm a diagnosis of vasovagal syncope. For the procedure, the person is strapped to a padded motorized table. The table is then tilted until the person is nearly upright. The person is kept in position for up to 45 minutes. Blood pressure and heart rate are continuously monitored. If blood pressure does not decrease, the person is given a drug that stimulates the heart, and the procedure is repeated. Use of this drug makes the procedure more likely to detect a problem. During the procedure, the person should report any feelings of faintness or light-headedness to the doctor or nurse.

Prevention

Learning about and then avoiding conditions that can cause fainting can help prevent fainting. For example, older men who have felt faint or have fainted while urinating can sit down when they urinate. Avoiding straining during a bowel movement can help prevent fainting. If needed, a stool softener can be used, or the fiber content of the diet can be increased.

For people who must continue taking a drug that increases the risk of fainting, lying down after taking the drug—for example, taking the drug before going to bed—can help.

If fainting sometimes occurs after eating a large meal, eating smaller, more frequent meals that are low in carbohydrates and lying down after eating can help. Antihypertensive drugs, if being used, should not be taken immediately before a meal. For people whose blood pressure falls when they stand up, drinking plenty of fluids and increasing the amount of salt consumed helps. These measures increase the amount of fluid in the bloodstream and thus help keep blood pressure from falling. However, consuming too much salt may be dangerous for people who have heart failure. People should consult a dietitian or doctor about how much salt to consume.

Sitting up and flexing the feet before getting out of bed can also help. This maneuver improves blood flow to the heart and thus helps maintain blood pressure. In general, older people should sit or stand up slowly, particularly when getting out of bed in the middle of the night.

To prevent dehydration and thus reduce the risk of fainting, older people should drink plenty of fluids, particularly during hot weather or an illness. People who take diuretics (used to treat high blood pressure or heart failure) should ask their doctor about discontinuing the drug temporarily during very hot weather or an illness. These drugs cause the kidneys to excrete more water. The increased loss of body fluids lowers blood pressure. Thus, diuretics may increase the risk of fainting. People who have fainting episodes should not drink alcohol because it tends to make them lose body fluids and lowers blood pressure.

Exercising the legs to keep the muscles toned can help prevent fainting. Strong leg muscles are needed to help move blood from the legs back to the heart.

People who have fainted can take steps to prevent serious injury and accidents if they faint again. For example, people can learn to recognize the warning symptoms of fainting and to lie down immediately when these symptoms occur. If the cause of the fainting cannot be identified and corrected, they should not drive for at least 6 months after the last fainting episode.

Treatment

Treatment focuses on several areas. Any injuries due to fainting are treated. If a potentially life-threatening disorder, such as an abnormal heart rhythm, a heart attack, or rapid bleeding is suspected, hospitalization and immediate treatment are needed. However, for most people, hospitalization is not needed and diagnosis can be done more slowly.

Measures are taken to correct or control other possible conditions that may contribute to or cause fainting. If the cause of fainting appears to be orthostatic hypotension, increasing the amount of salt consumed, wearing waist-high support stockings (compression stockings), and raising the head of the bed may help. If orthostatic hypotension occurs after a long period of bed rest, the person may be instructed to sit on the side of the bed a few times to get used to being upright again before trying to stand. Occasionally, a tilt table is used.[1] It helps reprogram the body to adjust blood pressure in response to changes in position. If orthostatic hypotension persists despite these measures, drugs such as fludrocortisone or midodrine may help.

If a potentially life-threatening disorder is the cause, surgery is sometimes necessary. The type of surgery depends on the disorder. For example, a pacemaker may be implanted to correct an abnormal heart rhythm.[2] After a heart attack, coronary angioplasty or coronary artery bypass surgery can improve blood flow to the heart.[3] After a stroke, surgery to improve blood flow through arteries in the neck (carotid endarterectomy) may be needed. A heart valve may need to be repaired or replaced.[4]

If the cause is carotid sinus syndrome, a pacemaker may be implanted or a drug such as midodrine may be used.

If anemia is detected, vitamins, iron supplements, drugs that stimulate the production of red blood cells, or transfusions may be given.

Drugs that may increase the risk of fainting are discontinued whenever possible or replaced with another drug less likely to cause fainting. When a potentially harmful drug cannot be discontinued or replaced, the dose is reduced to the lowest effective dose.

People who have fainted several times can get a personal emergency response system (a medical alert device). Most of these systems include an alert button worn on a necklace. Pressing the button calls for help.

Outlook

Most people who faint recover completely within minutes to hours. However, fainting can cause injuries when a person suddenly falls to the floor. Older people may bump their head or

1. see page 282
2. see art on page 703
3. see pages 671 to 673
4. see art on page 719

break a bone. Sometimes the fracture is a serious one, such as a hip fracture.[1]

When fainting is due to a life-threatening heart disorder, the person's outlook depends on whether the heart disorder can be treated effectively.

In 1899, Merck published a small book of all the maladies known to the medical world, along with a comprehensive listing of all the medicines available to treat these diseases. Just one year before that book became available, a baby was born on a farm in southeast Georgia. I am that baby 105 years later.

When I was born there were no baby foods and no prepared formulas; if a mother did not nurse or chew for her baby, it stood a poor chance of surviving. Surgery in 1898 was almost nil; except for smallpox vaccinations, there were no immunizations; anesthetics were primitive; and x-rays had been discovered only 3 years earlier. Then, early in the 20th century, immunization was being developed; with better anesthetics, surgery became more sophisticated; antibiotics were also being developed, as were dramatic diagnostic procedures. These things have taken place during the lifetime of the child of 1898, that is, during *my* lifetime. As a practicing pediatrician for more than 70 years, retiring in 2001, I watched these marvels unfold, and what blessings they have proved to be in saving, prolonging, and enhancing life!

In modern times, we have little excuse for a baby's losing his life. We have immunizations, baby food, surgeons who can put in a new heart or liver, and neonatal care that saves the lives of scores of babies who, 100 years ago, would not have survived.

However, with all that we have to keep a baby alive, we have more sick children today per capita than we had 100 years ago. When I started in practice, there were no day cares, mothers' mornings-out, or church nurseries. Children were cared for by their parents. Today, tremendous numbers of children never get parental guidance. What we really need today—and I speak after nearly 100 years of observation—is better parental guidance so that these wonderful medical advances can be used to give every child a chance.

Leila D. Denmark, MD

21

Falls

Many older people fear falling. And with good reason. Falls are common among older people. About one third of older people who live at home fall at least once a year. Those who are hospitalized or live in a nursing home fall more often.

Falls often cause injuries. Some of the injuries, such as a broken hip, can be serious.[1] Older people are more likely to break bones in falls because many older people have porous, fragile bones (osteoporosis).[2]

Fear of falling can lead to problems. People may worry about doing their usual activities and thus lose their self-confidence and even their independence. As Gabriel García Márquez said in *Love in the Time of Cholera*, "Old age begins with the first fall and ends with the second."

Older people can do many things to help overcome their fears and to reduce their risk of falling. Knowing what causes falls can help.

Causes

Falls can be caused by a person's physical condition, hazards in the environment, or potentially hazardous situations. Most falls occur when several causes interact. For example, a person with Parkinson's disease and impaired vision (the person's physical condition) may trip on an extension cord (an environmental hazard) while rushing to answer the telephone (a potentially hazardous situation).

A person's physical condition is affected by changes due to aging itself, physical fitness, disorders present, and drugs used.

1. see page 320
2. see page 295

A person's physical condition probably has a greater effect on the risk of falling than do environmental hazards and hazardous situations. Not only does the person's physical condition increase the risk of falls, but it also affects how the person responds to hazards and hazardous situations.

Hazards in the environment are involved in many falls. Falls may occur when a person does not notice a hazard or does not respond quickly enough after a hazard is noticed. Environmental hazards include:

- Inadequate lighting
- Throw rugs and slippery floors
- Electrical or extension cords or objects that are in the way of walking
- Uneven sidewalks and broken curbs

Most falls occur indoors. Some happen while a person is standing still. They sometimes result from fainting.[1] But most occur while a person is moving—getting in and out of bed or a chair, getting on or off a toilet seat, walking, or going up or down stairs. While moving, a person may stumble or trip, or balance may be lost. Any movement can be hazardous. But if a person is rushing or if a person's attention is divided, movement becomes even more hazardous. For example, rushing to the bathroom or to answer the telephone or talking on a cordless phone can make walking more hazardous.

ADDITIONAL DETAIL

Some changes due to aging can increase the risk of falling. As the body ages, sensation in the feet may decrease. So when older people step on or bump into an obstacle, they may not notice it right away and may fall. Also, the body responds to changes in position less well. For example, when a person stands, the body may be unable to make the necessary changes in blood flow and blood pressure. Blood pressure may decrease excessively, making the person feel light-headed. This disorder, called orthostatic hypotension, can increase the risk of falling. Abnormal heart rhythms (arrhythmias) and heart failure can

1. see page 276

also cause low blood pressure with light-headedness and thus increase the risk of falling.

The eyes and specialized structures in the inner ear help the body maintain balance. The eyes and ears also help people notice and avoid hazards. The nervous system helps the body know what its position is (for example, standing up straight or bending over). The muscles and bones help the body maintain and change position. Disorders that affect any of these body parts can increase the risk of falling. Disorders that interfere with walking (such as Parkinson's disease) or that weaken muscles (such as an underactive thyroid gland, or hypothyroidism) are common causes of falls.

Drugs that cause drowsiness can increase the risk of falling. These drugs include sleep aids and opioid pain relievers (analgesics). Drugs that lower blood pressure (such as antihypertensives and certain antidepressants) can also increase the risk of falling. A drug is most likely to cause a fall when a person first starts taking the drug or when the dose is changed.

Symptoms

Often before falling, a person has no symptoms. When an environmental hazard or a hazardous situation results in a fall, there is little or no warning. However, if a fall is partly or completely due to a person's physical condition, symptoms may be noticed before falling. Symptoms may include dizziness, light-headedness, or irregular or rapid, pounding heartbeats (palpitations). Before falling the first time, a person may have had a close call, almost falling but being able to prevent it.

After a fall, pain is common because injuries are common. More than half of all falls result in at least a slight injury, such as a bruise, sprained ligament, or strained muscle. More serious injuries include broken bones, torn ligaments, deep cuts, and damage to organs such as a kidney or the liver. About 2% of falls result in a broken hip. Other bones (in the upper arm, wrist, back, and pelvis) are broken in about 5% of falls. Some falls result in loss of consciousness or a head injury.

Falls can cause even more pain if a person cannot get up right away or summon help. Such a situation may be frightening and may make a person feel helpless. Remaining on the floor, even for a few hours, can also lead to problems such as dehydration and skin sores due to pressure (pressure sores).

The effects of a fall may last a long time. About half of people who could walk before they fell and broke a hip cannot walk as well afterward, even after treatment and rehabilitation. People who have fallen may develop a fear of falling that robs them of their self-confidence. As a result, they may stay at home and give up activities, such as shopping, visiting friends, and cleaning. When people become less active, joints can become stiff and muscles can become weak. Stiff joints and weak muscles can further increase the risk of falling and make remaining active and independent more difficult. For all these reasons, falls can greatly reduce a person's quality of life. Falls seem to be an important consideration in the decision of many people to move to a nursing home or another assisted living facility.

Rarely, falls result in death. Death may occur immediately—for example, when the head hits a hard surface and causes uncontrolled bleeding in the head. Much more commonly, death occurs later, resulting from complications of serious injuries caused by the fall.

Diagnosis

People who have fallen may be reluctant to discuss the problem with anyone, including a doctor, especially if they have not been injured. But even people who have been seriously injured during a fall and have been treated in an emergency department may be reluctant to admit they have fallen. People may be reluctant because they think falling is just part of getting older. And they do not want others to think they are helpless and now must move from their home into a more supervised environment such as a nursing home. Because of this reluctance, many doctors routinely ask all of their older patients if they have fallen in the recent past.

If a person has fallen, doctors try to identify the cause of the fall. To do so, they ask about the circumstances of the fall, including any symptoms experienced just before the fall and any activities that may have contributed to the fall. Doctors also ask about the use of drugs—prescription and nonprescription—that may have contributed to the fall. Doctors may ask people who witnessed the fall what they noticed.

Doctors perform a physical examination first to check for injuries and to obtain information about possible causes of the fall. Blood pressure is measured. If it decreases when a person stands up, the fall may be caused by orthostatic hypotension. With a stethoscope, doctors listen to the heart for evidence of abnormal rhythms and heart failure. They assess muscle strength and the ability to fully move various parts of the body (range of motion). Vision and some aspects of the nervous system, including the senses of position and balance, are also assessed. Doctors sometimes ask the person to do some usual activities, such as sitting in a chair and then standing up or stepping up on a step. Observing these activities may help doctors identify conditions that contributed to the fall.

If the fall resulted from an environmental hazard and no major injury occurred, no tests may be done. However, if the person's physical condition could have contributed to the fall, tests may be needed. For example, if the physical examination detected evidence of a heart problem, heart rate and rhythm may be recorded using electrocardiography (ECG).[1] This test may last a few seconds and be done in the doctor's office. Or the person may be asked to wear a portable ECG device (Holter monitor) for 1 or 2 days. If a person has been experiencing dizziness or light-headedness, blood tests, such as a complete blood count and measurements of electrolyte levels, may be helpful. If the nervous system appears to be malfunctioning, computed tomography (CT) or magnetic resonance imaging (MRI) of the head may be helpful.

Prevention

Older people can do many simple, practical things to help reduce the risk of falling.

• **Exercising regularly:** Weight training or resistance training may help strengthen a weak limb and thus may improve steadiness during walking. Tai Chi and balancing exercises such as standing on one leg can help improve balance.

• **Wearing appropriate shoes:** Shoes that have firm, nonslip soles and low heels are best.

• **Standing up slowly** after sitting or lying down and taking a moment before starting to move. This strategy can help prevent

1. see page 661

dizziness because it gives the body time to adjust to the change in position.

• For some older people who feel dizzy when they move, **learning a simple head maneuver,** called the Epley maneuver.[1] It involves turning the head in specific ways. Doctors usually perform the maneuver the first time, but people can learn how to do it themselves if it needs to be repeated.

• For older people who feel dizzy when they stand (because blood pressure decreases), wearing support stockings.

• **Asking a doctor** or another health care practitioner to review all prescription and nonprescription drugs being taken to see if any of the drugs could increase the risk of falling. If such drugs are being used, the doctor may be able to lower the dose or discontinue the drug.

• **Having vision checked regularly:** Getting the correct glasses and wearing them can help prevent falls. Treatment of glaucoma or cataracts, which limit vision, can also help.

• **Consulting with a physical therapist** about ways to reduce the risk of falling. Some older people need a physical therapist to train them to walk, particularly if they need to use a walker or cane.

Falls cannot always be prevented. So, people who are likely to fracture a hip—such as those who have osteoporosis and fall frequently—may consider wearing a hip protector to prevent hip fractures. The most effective type is a thigh-length undergarment with plastic and foam padding inserted along its sides.

Hazards in the environment can sometimes be removed or corrected. For example, lighting can be improved by increasing the number of lights or changing the types of lights. Light switches can be positioned so that they are easily reached. Or lights that turn on when they are touched or when they detect nearby motion can be used. Adequate lighting for steps (inside and outside) and for outdoor areas used at night is particularly important. Steps should have sturdy, secure handrails. Electrical or extension cords that are in the way of walking can be eliminated by adding more electrical outlets, or the cords may be tacked over doorways. Other items that clutter floors and stairways can be stored out of the way of walking.

1. see art on page 277

PREVENTING FALLS IN THE HOME

All rooms:	Reachable light switch
	No electrical or extension cords in the way of walking
	No throw rugs
	Cordless phone
Kitchen:	Reachable cabinets (so that bending and stretching are unnecessary)
	Nonslip mats
Bedroom:	Reachable bedside light
	Night-light
	Wall-to-wall carpet
Bathroom	Raised toilet seat
	Grab bars
	Nonslip mats
	Night-light
Living room:	Tacked down or wall-to-wall carpet
Steps: (inside and outside)	Good lighting
	Sturdy railing
	Nonslip treads

Grab bars can be installed next to toilets, tubs, and other places for people who need something to hold onto when they stand up. Grab bars must be installed properly, so that they do not pull out of the wall. Raised toilet seats can also help. Loose throw rugs can be removed or taped or tacked down. Nonslip mats should be used in the bathroom and kitchen. Frequently used household items can be stored in cabinets, cupboards, or other spaces between waist and eye level, so that they can be reached without stretching or bending.

Learning how to safely handle potentially hazardous situations may be more important than removing an environmental hazard. Sometimes people need only to think about ways to accomplish daily tasks more carefully. For example, they can install an intercom so that they do not have to rush to answer the door. They can place cordless phones around the home so that they do not have to rush to answer phone calls.

Knowing what to do if a fall occurs can help older people be less afraid of falling. If they fall and cannot get up, they can turn onto their stomach, crawl to a piece of furniture (or other structure that can support their weight), and pull themselves up.

Older people should also have a good way to call for help. People who have fallen several times may keep a telephone in a place that can be reached from the floor. Another option is installing a personal emergency response system (a medical alert device) that signals someone to check in on them. Most of these systems include an alert button worn on a necklace. Pressing the button calls for help.

Treatment

When a person falls, the first priority is treatment of injuries, such as fractures, sprained ligaments, and strained muscles. The next priority is to prevent subsequent falls and injury due to falls.

Disorders that may have contributed to the fall are treated. For example, if a person who has fallen has a very slow heart rate accompanied by light-headedness, a pacemaker for the heart may be implanted. If possible, potentially harmful drugs are discontinued, the dose is reduced, or another drug is substituted.

Physical and occupational therapists can help improve a person's self-confidence after a fall.[1] They can provide tips on how to avoid falling. Therapists can also encourage the person to remain active. Physical therapy and supervised weight training and stretching can help improve muscle strength and balance.

1. see page 167

22

Osteoporosis

"Osteoporosis" means porous bones. In people with osteoporosis, bones become less dense or more porous.

Because bones are less dense, they are very weak and more likely to break. However, not all people with osteoporosis break a bone, and not every older person who breaks a bone has osteoporosis.

Osteoporosis is common. In the United States, about 8 million women and 2 million men over 50 have osteoporosis. In millions of other women and men over 50, bone density (mass) is low but not low enough to be considered osteoporosis. These people have osteopenia (which means deficient bone). They are at risk of developing osteoporosis as they grow older.

Bones do not become porous overnight. Bones slowly begin to become less dense long before people reach old age. And the process continues as people age. Consequently, osteoporosis used to be considered an unavoidable part of aging. It was associated with becoming stooped over, breaking bones, and not being able to live independently. But now osteoporosis is recognized as a disorder that can be detected early, treated effectively, and often prevented.

To keep bones dense, the body needs an adequate supply of minerals (mainly calcium and phosphorus) and vitamin D. Minerals are incorporated into bones, making them dense and strong. This process is called mineralization. Vitamin D helps the body absorb calcium from food and incorporate it into bones. Calcium, phosphorus, and vitamin D can be consumed in foods. The body needs sunlight because vitamin D is formed when the skin is exposed to sunlight. To keep bones dense, the body also needs to produce appropriate amounts of several hor-

POROUS BONE: A DECREASE IN BONE DENSITY

Bone looks something like a sponge. When bone becomes more porous, or less dense, the holes in the sponge become larger. Porous bone is weaker and more easily broken. Bone becomes more porous because in the normal process of breaking down and re-forming bone, more bone is broken down than is re-formed.

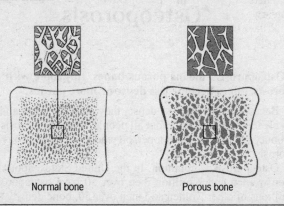

Normal bone   Porous bone

mones. They include estrogen, testosterone, parathyroid hormone, and growth hormone. Calcitonin, another hormone, may play a role.

Bone is a constantly changing tissue. In response to the changing demands placed on bones, small areas of bone are continuously broken down and re-formed. For example, when physical stress is placed on bones, the body responds by forming more bone. The process of breaking down and re-forming bone is called remodeling. It occurs continuously in healthy bone.

Until about age 30 to 35, more bone is re-formed than is broken down, and bones progressively increase in density. Around this age, bones are at their densest and strongest. At some point after this age, bones begin to decrease in density slowly and progressively because more bone is broken down than is re-formed. Thus, as people age, bones become less dense, more fragile, and more likely to break.

Fractures due to osteoporosis are more likely to occur in some bones than in others. They include the thighbone (femur) at the hip, the arm bones (radius and ulna) at the wrist, and the bones of the spine (vertebrae), usually in the middle to lower back.

Causes

There are two main types of osteoporosis: primary and secondary.

Primary osteoporosis, by far the most common type, has no specific cause but usually occurs in people over 50. Primary osteoporosis is more likely to develop in some people than in others. The following characteristics or conditions (called risk factors) make a person more likely to develop primary osteoporosis:

- Being middle-aged or older
- Being female
- Being white, Asian, or Hispanic
- Being thin
- Having close relatives with (a family history of) osteoporosis
- Consuming an inadequate amount of calcium
- Consuming an inadequate amount of vitamin D

WHAT IS OSTEOMALACIA?

"Osteomalacia" means soft bones. Like osteoporosis, osteomalacia weakens the bones and makes bones more likely to break. However, the process is different from that in osteoporosis. In osteoporosis, bone is broken down faster than it is re-formed. In osteomalacia, the two activities are balanced, but the bone that is formed does not become dense and hard (mineralized). Among older people, osteomalacia is much less common than osteoporosis.

Osteomalacia is usually caused by vitamin D deficiency or by a digestive tract or kidney disorder. These disorders can interfere with the body's use of vitamin D. Rarely, osteomalacia is caused by a low phosphate level.

Osteomalacia causes fatigue and pain in the back, ribs, and hips. Muscles in the upper arms and thighs become weak. People with osteomalacia may have trouble getting up from a chair or climbing steps. They may waddle when they walk. Like osteoporosis, osteomalacia leads to bone fractures.

Doctors diagnose osteomalacia with blood tests, x-rays, and sometimes a biopsy. Osteomalacia is treated with vitamin D or phosphate supplements depending on the cause.

- Spending an inadequate amount of time in sunlight
- Being physically inactive
- Smoking cigarettes

Drinking large amounts of alcohol may increase the risk of developing osteoporosis. However, consuming 1 to 6 drinks of alcohol a week does not seem to harm bones. If osteoporosis is already present, drinking large amounts of alcohol and smoking can make it worse.

Whether consuming a lot of caffeine increases the risk of osteoporosis is unclear. Consuming a lot may increase the amount of calcium excreted in urine. However, consuming a moderate amount of caffeine has only a small effect on bone density as long as enough calcium is also consumed.

Secondary osteoporosis is caused by a specific disorder or a drug. Disorders include inflammatory bowel disease, liver disorders, chronic kidney failure, rheumatoid arthritis, lupus (systemic lupus erythematosus), and hormonal disorders (especially hyperparathyroidism, Cushing's disease, hyperthyroidism, and diabetes mellitus). Drugs that can cause osteoporosis include corticosteroids (such as prednisone), thyroid hormones, phenytoin and phenobarbital (anticonvulsants), and cyclosporine

---

VITAMIN D: KEEPING BONES STRONG

Vitamin D helps the body absorb calcium and phosphorus from the intestine. Calcium and phosphorus are two of the main components of bone. Thus, vitamin D is necessary for the formation of normal bones. Good sources of vitamin D are milk (which is fortified with vitamin D), green vegetables, egg yolks, fish, and fortified cereals. Also, vitamin D is formed when the skin is exposed to sunlight.

Vitamin D deficiency may develop because not enough vitamin D is consumed in foods. For example, many older people do not drink a lot of milk. Vitamin D deficiency may also develop because the skin is not exposed to enough sunlight. For example, older people tend to spend less time outdoors. Some older people are confined to their bed and do not go outside. Also, in older people, less vitamin D is formed when the skin is exposed to sunlight. Disorders or drugs that interfere with the body's use of vitamin D can cause a deficiency. Examples are digestive tract, liver, and kidney disorders and the anticonvulsants phenytoin and phenobarbital.

Treatment of vitamin D deficiency depends on the cause. But it almost always includes vitamin D supplements.

(an immunosuppressant, taken to prevent rejection of transplanted organs). If primary osteoporosis is already present, these disorders and drugs can make it worse.

ADDITIONAL DETAIL

Primary osteoporosis: The longer a person lives, the higher the risk of osteoporosis. Bone density decreases partly because levels of hormones (such as estrogen and testosterone) decrease as people age. Estrogen, the main female hormone, helps prevent bone from being broken down and therefore helps keep it dense and strong. Testosterone, the main male hormone, stimulates bone formation.

Older women are affected by the decrease in hormone levels more dramatically than older men. Until menopause, bone density in women may decrease a little. But at menopause, the decrease in bone density speeds up dramatically because estrogen levels decrease rapidly. During the first few years after menopause, bone density may decrease by as much as 3 to 5% each year. After that, it decreases by about 1 to 2% each year. Thus, women are more likely than men to develop osteoporosis. Also, on average, women usually have lower bone density to begin with than men.

Women who have produced less estrogen before menopause are at even higher risk of developing osteoporosis. Such women include those who started menstruating late, reached menopause early, or had their ovaries surgically removed (a procedure called oophorectomy) before menopause.

As men age, testosterone levels usually decrease slowly. Testosterone levels may decrease abruptly if prostate cancer is treated by surgically removing the testicles or using drugs that prevent the testicles from producing testosterone. Men produce small amounts of estrogen. As men age, estrogen levels also slowly decrease. Men with low testosterone or low estrogen levels are more likely to develop osteoporosis.

Of racial groups, white people are most prone to osteoporosis. Asians are next, then Hispanics. Black people are less prone to osteoporosis, possibly because black people tend to have denser, stronger bones during young adulthood. Thus, they can better tolerate the decrease in bone density that occurs with aging and at menopause.

Thin people tend to have less dense bones than heavier people. Part of the reason is that body weight puts stress on bone, stimulating it to form more bone. Also, thin women may have lower estrogen levels than heavier women, because thin women usually have less body fat. Fat tissue produces some estrogen.

People who have close relatives with osteoporosis are more likely to develop it. The risk of developing osteoporosis is even higher when a relative has had a fracture related to osteoporosis.

People who do not consume enough calcium or who have vitamin D deficiency are also more likely to develop osteoporosis.

Physical activity affects the risk of developing osteoporosis. Bone is formed in response to weight-bearing activity (such as walking). Bone is broken down in response to inactivity. People who are less physically active throughout life are more likely to develop osteoporosis.

Smoking cigarettes increases risk because it interferes with the re-formation of bone.

Secondary osteoporosis: Disorders and drugs can cause osteoporosis by interfering with the body's absorption or use of calcium or vitamin D, by directly affecting the process of breaking down and re-forming bone (remodeling), or by doing both. For example, in hyperparathyroidism, the parathyroid glands produce too much parathyroid hormone. Normally, this hormone helps keep bone remodeling in balance. If too much parathyroid hormone is produced, more bone is broken down than re-formed, and calcium is removed from bone.

In Cushing's disease, the adrenal glands produce too much cortisol. Cortisol inhibits the cells that form bone. Thus, overproduction of parathyroid hormone or cortisol results in loss of bone density. Taking corticosteroids (such as prednisone), which act like cortisol, has the same effect. These drugs also decrease the amount of calcium that is absorbed from food and increase the amount of calcium lost in the urine.

An overactive thyroid gland (hyperthyroidism) produces too much thyroid hormone. Overproduction of this hormone speeds up the bone remodeling process, eventually resulting in loss of bone density. Thyroid hormones, taken to treat an underactive thyroid gland (hypothyroidism), can have the same effect.

In diabetes, more calcium is lost in urine. In inflammatory bowel disease, less calcium is absorbed from food. Rheumatoid arthritis and lupus (systemic lupus erythematosus) interfere with bone remodeling.

Anticonvulsants, such as phenytoin and phenobarbital, may interfere with the activity of vitamin D.

Symptoms

Usually, osteoporosis does not cause any symptoms at first. The most common symptoms are pain and broken bones. People may not know they have osteoporosis until they break a bone, often after a slight jarring or a fall. Occasionally, a bone breaks for no apparent reason.

Some people lose height and become stooped with a bent back, called a dowager's hump (kyphosis). These changes may occur because the bones of the spine (vertebrae) gradually collapse within themselves and become squashed (compressed). This type of fracture is called a compression or crush fracture.[1] Compression fractures may be painless or painful. Pain may develop gradually and be aching, or it may begin suddenly and be sharp. The shape of the chest and abdomen may change. As a result, clothes may be looser around the shoulders and chest and tighter around the waist. The changes in shape may put pressure on the lungs, heart, or intestine, and these organs may function less well.

People with osteoporosis may break other bones, particularly the hip and wrist. Hip and wrist fractures often occur after a fall.[2] A broken hip is especially serious.[3] It can lead to loss of independence and function and to serious, even life-threatening problems. However, all broken bones in people with osteoporosis are serious, because bones that are less dense tend to heal slowly and sometimes incompletely. Also, if people with osteoporosis break one bone, they tend to break other bones.

1. see page 325
2. see page 287
3. see page 320

HOW OSTEOPOROSIS CAUSES STOOPING

When the bones of the spine (vertebrae) become less dense, they may gradually collapse within themselves and become squashed. This type of fracture is called a compression or crush fracture. The normally drum-shaped part of a vertebra becomes more like a wedge, thinner in the front than in the back. If compression fractures occur in several vertebrae, the back becomes bent. The posture becomes stooped, making a person shorter.

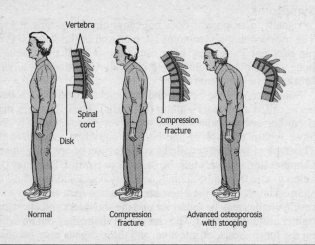

Normal   Compression fracture   Advanced osteoporosis with stooping

Screening and Diagnosis

Screening involves measuring bone density before symptoms occur. All women over 65 should be screened for osteoporosis. Men over 65 who have low testosterone levels should also be screened for osteoporosis. Diagnosis involves checking for osteoporosis when doctors have a reason to think that it is present. For example, doctors should check for osteoporosis whenever an older person breaks a bone.

The most common and most useful test for measuring bone density is dual-energy x-ray absorptiometry (DEXA) scanning. It is used for screening and diagnosis. DEXA scanning is a safe, painless test that uses x-rays to measure bone density. Exposure to radiation is much less than that with a chest x-ray. The test takes about 15 minutes.

DEXA scanning provides two measures of how dense bone is: the T score and the Z score. The T score compares the person's bone density with the average bone density of 25- to 30-year-olds of the same sex. This age group is used because bone density is at its highest then. A T score of 0 means that bone density is the same as the average bone density of 25- to 30-year-olds. A score above 0 (a positive score) means that bones are more dense than the average. A score below 0 (a negative score) means that bones are less dense than the average.

The Z score compares a person's bone density with that of people of the same age, sex, and weight. Because bone density decreases with aging, bone density may be low in older people even when their Z score is average. Thus, this score is not as useful as T scores in determining the likelihood of breaking a bone and in making decisions about treatment.

DEXA scanning is usually used to measure bone density in the lower spine and hip and sometimes the wrist and forearm. Doctors measure bone density in more than one site because scores may vary from site to site. For example, a T score may be normal at the spine but low at the hip, or vice versa.

Ultrasonography (ultrasound) and computed tomography (CT) can also determine bone density. Ultrasonography is used primarily for screening. For example, portable ultrasound devices may be used at health fairs to scan the wrist, forearm, or heel. Special types of ultrasonography can be used to diagnose osteoporosis.

Computed tomography (CT) is used primarily for diagnosis. CT is particularly useful when changes in bone due to arthritis or old fractures make the results of DEXA scanning hard to interpret. Also, CT can help doctors identify or rule out other disorders (such as cancer) that can result in a broken bone.

After osteoporosis is diagnosed, blood and urine tests may be done. They can sometimes help determine how rapidly bone is being broken down and whether osteoporosis is due to another disorder.

Treatment

Ideally, early in life, people should make lifestyle choices to help keep bone density from decreasing and possibly to increase it. Making these choices early is important because bone

INTERPRETING T SCORES

T Score	Bone Density	Chance of Breaking a Bone	Need for Treatment
−1 to 0 or above	Adequate or better	Unlikely (unless substantial stress or force is applied)	None
−1 to −2.5	Low but not low enough to indicate osteoporosis	More likely	Possibly, to prevent further decreases in bone density
Below −2.5	Osteoporosis	Much more likely	Recommended

density starts decreasing to some degree when people are in their 30s. These choices are particularly important for older people whether osteoporosis has been diagnosed or not.

Weight-bearing exercise done regularly may be the most important. Examples are walking, stair climbing, dancing, and weight training. In weight-bearing exercise, people support their entire body weight. The physical stress put on bones during this exercise stimulates bone formation and thus helps maintain or increase bone density. Usually, 30 minutes of weight-bearing exercise each day is recommended. Exercise that does not involve weight bearing, such as bicycle riding and swimming, does little to stimulate bone formation. However, exercise of any type improves muscle strength and balance, which can help prevent falls and the fractures that may result.

Consuming enough calcium and vitamin D helps maintain bone density. Older people should consume 1,200 to 1,500 milligrams (mg) of calcium and 600 to 800 international units (IU) of vitamin D every day—the amounts supplied by about four 8-ounce glasses of milk. Good sources of calcium include dairy products, tofu, broccoli, turnip greens, collard greens, and calcium-fortified juices. If a person does not consume enough calcium and vitamin D in foods and beverages, calcium and vitamin D supplements can be taken. Supplements are safe and inexpensive.

Spending time outside in the sun is another way to get vitamin D (because vitamin D is formed when the skin is exposed to sunlight). But older people cannot get enough vitamin D this way no matter how long they stay in the sun. Also, spending time in the sun becomes harder if older people have problems with walking.

Because smoking makes loss of bone density more likely, quitting or never smoking can help maintain bone density.

Drug treatment: For people who have low bone density or who have broken a bone, drugs that can prevent further decreases in density (and fractures) may be recommended.

A bisphosphonate (such as alendronate, etidronate, pamidronate, or risedronate) is the drug of choice for people who have low bone density. Bisphosphonates decrease the amount of bone being broken down. Men and women who take a bisphosphonate have fewer fractures of the vertebrae, hips, and wrists. These drugs are taken as tablets usually once a week but sometimes once a day. New bisphosphonates that can be given intravenously once or twice a year are being studied.

Foods and other substances in the digestive tract can prevent the body from absorbing bisphosphonates taken as tablets. So a person must take this drug with a full glass of water (6 to 8 ounces) on an empty stomach first thing in the morning. For the next 30 minutes, no other food, drink, or drug should be consumed. Also, bisphosphonates can irritate the lining of the esophagus. So after taking the drug, the person must sit up or stand for the next 30 minutes. People with disorders of the esophagus or a low calcium level in the blood should not take bisphosphonates by mouth.

Estrogen used to be widely prescribed to help maintain bone density in women after menopause and to treat women with low bone density. Estrogen prevents decreases in bone density and, in many women, increases bone density. Nonetheless, long-term use of estrogen for these purposes is no longer routinely recommended because such use has risks.

Because taking estrogen has risks, decisions about whether to use estrogen are complex. Use of estrogen alone increases the risk of cancer of the uterus (endometrial cancer) and may increase the risk of breast cancer. The risk of endometrial cancer can be reduced by taking a progestin with estrogen (hormone replacement therapy, sometimes called HRT). Progestins are

℞ DRUGS USED TO TREAT OSTEOPOROSIS

Drug	Possible Side Effects	Comments
Calcium	Constipation, diarrhea, and upset stomach In some people who are prone to develop kidney stones, an increased risk of kidney stones	Given as tablets Better taken in several small amounts than in one large one Available as supplements and in antacids Best used with at least one other drug for osteoporosis
Bisphosphonates	Irritation of the lining of the esophagus	Usually given as tablets (for specific instructions, see text)
Estrogen	Monthly menstrual bleeding or irregular vaginal bleeding Breast tenderness, fluid retention, migraine headaches, and mood changes Increased risk of cancer of the uterus (endometrial cancer) when not taken with a progestin Increased risk of breast cancer, coronary artery disease, stroke, and dementia when taken with a progestin Increased risk of blood clots Increased risk of gallstones during the first year of use	No longer routinely recommended for long-term use to maintain density or treat low bone density Given as tablets or patches Used only for women
Raloxifene	Hot flashes and leg cramps Increased risk of blood clots	Given as tablets Used as an alternative for women who cannot or do not wish to take a bisphosphonate or estrogen

Drug	Possible Side Effects	Comments
Testosterone	Enlarged prostate, baldness, acne, painful erections, liver inflammation, and fluid retention	Given as patches, tablets, or injections Used in men who have low testosterone levels
Calcitonin	Nausea, flushing, diarrhea, and nasal irritation	Given as injections or a nasal spray Not as effective as other drugs
Teriparatide (a synthetic version of parathyroid hormone)	Nausea, headache, and high calcium levels	Self-administered by injection daily Usually used for people who continue to break bones or whose bone density continues to decrease while they are taking another drug for osteoporosis

drugs related to the female hormone progesterone. However, taking a combination of a progestin and estrogen increases the risk of breast cancer, coronary artery disease, stroke, and dementia. Estrogen, with or without a progestin, also increases the risk of blood clots, particularly for people who are already prone to developing clots, such as people who are temporarily or permanently confined to bed.

If treatment with estrogen is being considered, a woman should talk with her doctor, weigh the benefits and risks of estrogen, and compare all available options for maintaining bone density or treating low bone density.

Raloxifene belongs to a group of drugs called selective estrogen receptor modifiers (SERMs). Raloxifene resembles estrogen in some ways. Like estrogen, raloxifene prevents further decreases in bone density and, in some women, increases bone density. Women who take it have fewer fractures of the vertebrae. But raloxifene has not been shown to reduce the risk of hip or wrist fractures. Like estrogen, raloxifene has side effects and can increase the risk of blood clots. It has some advantages over estrogen because it does not affect the uterus or breasts. Raloxifene is prescribed for women who cannot or do not wish to take a bisphosphonate or estrogen.

Testosterone is used in men who have low testosterone levels. Testosterone can maintain or increase bone density.

Calcitonin, a hormone, can decrease the amount of bone being broken down. Calcitonin also seems to decrease pain due to fractures. But it is not as effective as bisphosphonates and other drugs for treating osteoporosis.

Teriparatide is a synthetic version of parathyroid hormone. The effects of teriparatide differ from those of parathyroid hormone. The continuous production of parathyroid hormone by the body helps balance the normal breaking down and reforming of bone. Because teriparatide is injected once a day, it stimulates the formation of bone more than the breakdown. Thus, it can help new bone form, increase bone density, and reduce the risk of fractures. The main disadvantage of this drug is that it must be injected. Its long-term effects are unknown.

Fluoride supplements should not be used to treat osteoporosis. They may increase bone density, but the resulting bone tends to be fragile. Fluoride supplements do not reduce the risk of fractures.

Treatment of fractures: [1] Treatment of a fracture due to osteoporosis depends on the location of the fracture. Treatments include splints, casts, and surgery (such as insertion of pins or replacement of a joint). If a person has severe pain due to a collapsed vertebra, vertebroplasty or kyphoplasty may be done. In these procedures, a needle is used to inject plastic cement into a collapsed vertebra.

Outlook

Treating osteoporosis can help prevent fractures. However, treatment does not reverse the changes in appearance (such as loss of height) due to previous fractures.

Treatment of osteoporosis is not always effective. In up to 1 out of 6 people who take drugs for osteoporosis, bone density continues to decrease. Doctors periodically check to determine how well a drug is working. Several months after the start of treatment, blood and urine tests may be repeated to determine whether less bone is being broken down. DEXA scanning or an-

1. see page 314

other test to measure bone density may be repeated after 1 to 2 years. If bone density is continuing to decrease, doctors may recommend that the person take a higher dose of the drug, a different drug, or an additional drug. Changing treatment may be effective.

I am still a professional aviator at age 98, actively flying since 1923. I take no medications, have no aches or pains, and my weight and blood pressure are the same as eight decades ago. I take vigorous walks to counteract the effects on my legs and heart of long sittings in airplanes and cars. How did I succeed in preserving my health and vigor?

Listen well, my friends, and you shall learn how to delay the ravages of aging.

From age $4\frac{1}{2}$ I was unalterably determined to be an aviator and was therefore eager to keep my health. Having such a definite goal seems to me to be important. My mother, a nurse, told me when I was 11 that overweight people did not achieve long lives, so I said that I would avoid eating fats, and from then on I rigidly did so. I would not eat butter, bacon, sausage, or any fatty meat. Of course, we know a lot more about diet now than in 1916, but that gave me a head start on practically everybody, so evidently my arteries are not clogged. I have never had a drop of alcohol, a cup of coffee, or a cigarette. I could see that they were addictive and detrimental.

I eat quantities of vegetables, especially green leafy things. I've avoided breads and other starchy foods. I have taken a multiple vitamin each day for decades and extra vitamin E. I avoided junk foods. For breakfasts and lunches I have an orange, a ripened banana, a leaf of romaine lettuce, milk powder, and a slice of red bell pepper, all blended with grape juice, and drink it, plus a little granola-type cereal and chew it dry. For dinner, I eat seafood, except about once a month when I have some white meat of chicken or turkey, and green, red, or orange vegetables. I keep a daily record of my weight, so I can see trends and avoid gain. It takes determination and will power. Walk right past that refrigerator!

My whole program is simple. Stick to it and you will win. No snacks!

John M. Miller

23

Fractures

Fractures and broken bones are the same thing. A fracture may be a crack as thin as a hair, a severing of bone into two or more separate pieces, or a shattering of bone into many small, scattered pieces. A fracture may cause discomfort so slight that the person does not think the bone is broken. Or a fracture may cause extreme pain. In older people, a fracture may have long-lasting effects, because recovery after an injury is slow.

In older people, the most common fractures involve the hip, bones of the spine (vertebrae), shoulder, and wrist. But any bone can be fractured. Fractures that make walking impossible, usually hip fractures, are the most serious.

Causes

A bone breaks when the amount of force placed on the bone is greater than the strength of the bone. A large force can break even the strongest bone. But very slight force can break a weak bone.

In older people, most fractures result from a fall.[1] Fractures may result from fainting or an injury, as may occur in a motor vehicle accident.

As people age, bones become less dense and thus become weaker. A large decrease in bone density is called osteoporosis.[2] In people with osteoporosis, a fracture may result from a fall (even when gentle) or from the moderate stress of ordinary movement (as when getting out of a chair).

Other disorders weaken bones and thus make fractures more likely. Paget's disease and overactive parathyroid glands (hyper-

1. see page 287
2. see page 295

parathyroidism) weaken bones throughout the body. These disorders may also cause a bone to heal more slowly after a fracture or to shorten as it heals. Other disorders, such as infections and cancer, may weaken bones in specific places. These disorders can prevent a bone from healing or from healing as quickly after a fracture.

Symptoms

Most fractures cause pain immediately. They usually continue to hurt, especially when a person uses the injured body part. The area around the fracture is often tender to the touch. When the fracture occurs, a snap is sometimes heard. A limb or joint may be obviously out of place.

Moving the injured part may cause a painful, grating sensation. Movement may be limited or impossible. If a bone in the leg breaks, standing is usually painful or impossible. Injured tissues around the fracture begin to swell. Bruises appear, usually a few days afterward but sometimes within several hours.

Swelling often damages the skin. It can cause itching, flaking, scaling, or blisters. Sometimes swelling in a broken limb continues to worsen. Swelling can become so severe that it prevents blood from flowing out of the limb to the heart. Then, blood flow to the skin of the limb is reduced. As a result, pressure sores may develop and may take weeks or months to heal.

If swelling becomes so severe that it also cuts off blood flow to the limb, the pain in a broken limb suddenly becomes much worse. The limb may feel numb or cool. These symptoms should be reported to a health care practitioner immediately. This disorder is called compartment syndrome. Older people are more likely to have severe swelling after a fracture.

Some symptoms develop later. Some result from the treatment of fractures, for example, from immobilization with casts or other devices or from bed rest.[1] An immobilized limb becomes weak and usually loses muscle tissue. If a joint is not moved for a long time, it may become permanently tight and stiff. This condition is called a contracture.

If people are confined to bed after a fracture, they may develop difficulty breathing and chest pain. These symptoms may result from a blood clot that has formed in a vein of the leg, bro-

1. see page 148

ken off, traveled through the bloodstream, and blocked an artery that carries blood to the lungs. This blockage, called pulmonary embolism, is life threatening.

Pain may persist when the pieces of a broken bone do not grow back together (a condition called nonunion). Pain may also persist when the bone grows back crooked or incompletely (a condition called malunion). Fractures may extend into a joint, often resulting in permanent arthritis and stiffness in the joint. These problems are more common among older people.

Diagnosis

Doctors examine the injured area and the area around it to check whether bones are out of place and whether the person can move nearby joints normally. They also look for swelling, changes in color or temperature of the limb, tenderness, and skin damage.

X-rays are taken. They can detect most fractures. X-rays taken several days later may detect a fracture that could not be seen earlier. If x-rays do not detect a fracture but a fracture seems likely, computed tomography (CT) or magnetic resonance imaging (MRI) may be done. These procedures can detect a less obvious fracture and can usually provide more information about a fracture.

If the diagnosis is still unclear or cancer is suspected, bone scanning is done several days after the fracture. This procedure involves injecting a small amount of a radioactive substance, which can be detected by a special scanner. This substance collects in bone that is starting to heal and thus can identify a fracture.

Doctors ask questions to determine what caused the fracture—a fall, fainting, or an injury. They also ask whether the person has any disorders that can weaken bone. Tests to determine the strength and density of bone (such as dual-energy x-ray absorptiometry, or DEXA) are often done. With this information, doctors may be able to recommend ways to help prevent other fractures.

Prevention

One important way to prevent fractures is to prevent falls.[1] Wearing appropriate shoes (with firm, nonslip soles and low

1. see page 291

heels) may help prevent falls. Exercising to improve balance and muscle strength, having vision checked regularly, and modifying the home to make falls less likely can also help. Treating disorders that can cause fainting[1] and preventing accidents may help prevent fractures. For example, people should always wear a seat belt whether they are driving or riding in a car. Older people can also learn techniques to improve their driving.[2]

Another way to prevent fractures is to keep bones strong.[3] Consuming enough calcium (in foods or in supplements), regularly doing weight-bearing exercises (such as walking or playing tennis), and not smoking can help keep bones strong.

Treatment

If a person may have a broken bone, a doctor should be called so that treatment can be arranged. If possible, first aid techniques are then used to prevent movement of (immobilize) the injured part. Immobilization helps prevent the ends of the broken bone from moving and causing further injury and pain.

For most bones, a splint or sling may be used. A splint consists of a firm object strapped to an arm or a leg. For example, a magazine or stack of newspapers could be wrapped around the arm with ribbon or tape. A sling is a bandage or any piece of cloth used to support the forearm. The bandage is wrapped under the arm and tied behind the neck. Most fractures involving a wrist, an arm, or a shoulder can be immobilized with a sling. Usually, a person with one of these fractures can be taken by car to a hospital. For a person with a fracture of a hip or leg, an ambulance is usually called.

Before and after treatment by a doctor, pain and swelling can be reduced by keeping the injured limb above the level of the heart and by applying ice. These measures are particularly important during the first 2 days after the injury. An ice pack or a bag of crushed or chipped ice can be placed in a plastic bag on a thin towel over the injured part. Ice can be applied every hour while the person is awake. The skin should be checked regularly for numbness, swelling, and redness to make sure the cold is

1. see page 278
2. see page 929
3. see page 303

not damaging the skin. Elevating the limb can also help reduce swelling.

Longer-term immobilization: For most fractures, doctors immobilize the injured part for several weeks or months to give the fracture time to heal. Some fractures (such as rib fractures) cannot and do not need to be immobilized.

Before immobilization, doctors sometimes need to align fragments of broken bone (a procedure called reduction). This procedure helps prevent angled bone fragments from pressing against the skin and improves blood flow to the hands or feet. Also, precisely aligning fragments of broken bone within a joint helps prevent arthritis from developing in the joint. Before the procedure, measures are taken to relieve pain: A local anesthetic is injected near the injury, pain relievers are given intravenously, or a general anesthetic is used, depending on the location and severity of the fracture.

A cast, splint, brace, or sling can be used to immobilize the injured part. Sometimes surgery is needed. The goal is to sufficiently support and immobilize a broken limb while enabling the limb to be used as much as possible.

Casts are the strongest and most rigid devices. They are used when fragments of broken bone might move around. Casts may be made of plaster or fiberglass. All casts are lined with soft cottony material to protect the skin from pressure and rubbing. Because older people take longer to recover from an injury, they may have to wear a cast longer than younger people.

After bone fragments start to grow together, a cast may be replaced with a removable splint or brace. Or the cast may be split into two pieces, re-lined, and fitted with Velcro straps so that the cast may be taken on and off. Removable devices make bathing and skin care easier. Also, the joint can then be stretched and moved periodically so that it is less likely to become stiff.

Using the least restrictive and shortest cast or splint and being able to put it on and take it off as soon as possible are particularly important for older people. The skin of older people is more likely to be damaged by casts and nonremovable devices. Older people are encouraged to regularly check their skin near the ends of the casts or other devices. Also, immobilization is more likely to cause joints to stiffen and muscles to weaken in older people. As soon as possible, older people should take the cast or splint off for a short time each day so that they can move the joint.

If a cast cannot prevent the broken bone fragments in a wrist, forearm, or lower leg from shifting or collapsing, a technique called external fixation is often used. Strong metal pins are inserted into the normal, unbroken bone on either side of the fracture. The pins protrude through the skin. They are clamped to a frame of rods outside the arm or leg. External fixation holds the broken bone fragments securely. It makes skin care possible and enables the person to move and use the rest of the arm or leg. After the bone heals, the rods are unclamped and the pins are removed.

If a broken arm or leg is immobilized with a cast or with pins and rods, many daily activities (especially walking) are difficult. The immobilized limb feels heavy and awkward. It can in-

---

CARING FOR A CAST

• When bathing, do not let the cast get wet. The cast can be enclosed in a plastic bag. The top of the bag should be carefully sealed with rubber bands or tape. However, specially designed waterproof cast covers are easier to use and more effective.

• If a cast gets wet, try using a hair dryer, and ask the doctor whether the cast needs to be changed. The cast may be changed because the underlying padding can retain moisture. Moisture can weaken the cast, damage the skin, and make infections more likely.

• Do not push a sharp or pointed object inside the cast (for example, to scratch the skin). Doing so may damage the skin under the cast, and the cast may have to be removed to treat the injury.

• Check the skin around the cast every day and apply lotion to any red or sore areas.

• Rest the affected limb in an el-

evated position, as needed, to control swelling.

• Do not push or lean on the cast. It may break.

• Pad the edge of the cast with soft adhesive tape, moleskin, tissues, or cloth if the edge of the cast feels rough. The edge of the cast may chafe the skin or cause sores to form.

• When resting, position the cast carefully to prevent the cast's edge from pinching or digging into the skin. A small pillow or pad can be used.

• Immediately contact a doctor if the cast causes persistent pain or feels excessively tight. If swelling is excessive or an odor emanates from under the cast, the cast may have to be removed within hours.

• To decrease swelling and prevent stiffness, periodically move fingers or toes that stick out from the cast.

terfere with balance or get in the way. Some people with an immobilized leg need to use a walker. Most people with an immobilized leg need the help of a physical therapist to learn to walk safely and comfortably.

If the part of the limb below the fracture becomes unexpectedly painful, numb, or cool (possibly indicating compartment syndrome), immediate treatment is needed to prevent tissues from being damaged. Usually, the cast is split open and removed. In severe cases, external fixation may be needed temporarily to immobilize the fracture. Once the swelling goes down and tissues heal, a new cast is applied.

Traction: Traction is rarely used. It requires bed rest for a long time, which can cause many problems.[1] Traction is used only when other treatments, including surgery, are not possible or are too risky. For example, traction is used when a person is too frail to undergo surgery safely or when there are too many bone fragments for a cast. Traction involves applying a gentle, steady pulling action, which may align bone fragments. Traction is done with adjustable bands wrapped carefully around the limb, cords, a pulley (with not more than a 5-pound weight attached), and a metal frame placed over or on the bed.

Surgery: For some fractures, surgery is best. When possible, surgery is done within a day or two. With surgery, broken bones can be precisely aligned and metal implants (such as rods and pins) can be inserted, usually permanently, to hold the broken fragments securely together. Metal rods may be inserted into the broken bone. Or metal plates may be attached to the side of the broken bone with screws. These procedures are called internal fixation, because all of the metal implants used are inserted within the body. Metal implants made in the last 15 years do not interfere with magnetic resonance imaging (MRI). Most do not set off security devices at airports. Some large implants near the skin's surface set them off.

If the upper arm bone (humerus) breaks at the shoulder joint or the thighbone (femur) breaks at the hip joint, repair is often impossible. In these cases, surgery is needed to replace the broken part of the bone that is part of the joint.[2]

Surgery is needed for hip fractures, which otherwise would

1. see page 148
2. see page 323

require months of bed rest and traction to heal. Surgery may enable people to walk within a few days. Surgery also results in a better recovery. Surgery may also be needed for fractures that have not healed after many months of treatment and for fractures in bone weakened by cancer, which heal poorly.

Some circumstances make surgery inadvisable. If osteoporosis has greatly weakened the bones, metal implants may slip out of position. For people who have certain disorders, especially heart, lung, kidney, or liver disorders, surgery may need to be delayed. People who take a drug that makes the blood less likely to clot (anticoagulant) may need to discontinue the drug and delay surgery until the drug's effects wear off and blood can clot normally.

Prevention of problems after treatment: Drugs may be used to control pain during the several weeks needed for healing. For most fractures of the vertebrae or pelvis, treatment includes bed rest for a short time. Reduced activity and bed rest can cause problems, particularly for older people. Problems include loss of muscle tone and tissue, stiff joints, pulmonary embolism, urinary tract infections, pressure sores, confusion, and depression. Hospital staff members take steps to prevent these problems.[1] To the injured person, these steps may seem bothersome or too demanding, but they are necessary for a good recovery. For example, to prevent pressure sores, staff members may periodically change the person's position in bed. Areas of skin that are in contact with the cast, especially areas in which bones are close to the skin (such as the heels), are padded and inspected frequently for any sign of pressure sores.

Rehabilitation: Rehabilitation, particularly physical therapy, may help a person regain the ability to function or to compensate for abilities that were lost.[2] For most fractures, rehabilitation should begin immediately. Doing range-of-motion and muscle-strengthening exercises daily helps keep joints flexible and increase strength. Range-of-motion exercises involve moving a joint in all directions possible. Diligently doing the recommended exercises leads to a better recovery. Family members and caregivers can provide encouragement. If muscles are too weak for the person to move them or if bone fragments could be

1. see page 148
2. see page 167

easily displaced, a therapist moves the muscle. However, ultimately, the person must move muscles against gravity or resistance (using weights) to regain full strength of an injured limb.

While the fracture is healing, a person should also exercise the uninjured joints, particularly other joints in the injured limb. A joint within the cast cannot be exercised until the fracture has healed sufficiently and the cast is removed. When exercising the injured joint, the person should pay attention to how it feels and avoid exercising too forcefully. Also, the person should avoid staying in one position too long.

How long rehabilitation is continued depends on the type and location of the fracture and on the person's general condition. Rehabilitation may take only a few days or require weeks of intensive rehabilitation. Some people need only a few visits for rehabilitation. People who need intensive rehabilitation may have to stay in a rehabilitation facility or nursing home.

Outlook

Fractures heal in stages. How quickly a fracture heals depends on how severe and how large it is, where it occurs, how the broken bone is used, and how strong the bone was before the fracture. Some small fractures in the hands heal in a few weeks. But large fractures in the legs may take many months to heal (partly because leg bones must bear the person's weight).

In older people, bones heal about as quickly as they do in younger adults. However, older people often have weaker muscles, less dexterity, and poorer balance. Also, in older people, stiffness tends to develop after an injury. As a result, many older people have difficulty making the needed adjustments after a fracture. For example, they may be unable to use crutches, so they must wait until a broken leg is healed enough to bear full weight before they can walk. Thus, older people often take longer to return to their daily activities than younger people.

For a while after a fracture has healed, some discomfort may be felt when the injured part is used. For example, after a wrist fracture, gripping forcefully may be painful for up to 1 year, even though the person may be able to use the hand after about

2 months. Also, when the weather is damp, cold, or stormy, the injured part may ache and feel stiff.

After a fracture heals, most people can function reasonably well. However, some older people never recover strength and flexibility in the injured part. For them, daily activities, such as eating, dressing, bathing, and walking, may continue to be difficult or impossible.

HIP FRACTURES

Many older people worry about fracturing a hip. Hip fractures can have serious consequences. A person may be unable to do daily activities, may be unable to live independently, or may develop a serious disorder leading to death. To help prevent hip fractures, people can become or continue to be active. Being active strengthens muscles and bones. It also improves the chances of a good recovery if a hip fracture occurs. Other precautions can also help.[1]

In the United States, about 350,000 people fracture a hip each year. About 9 out of 10 hip fractures occur in people over 60. Hip fractures are much more common among women.

Types and Causes

Most hip fractures occur at or near the upper end (head) of the thighbone (femur). (The head of the thighbone fits into the pelvic bone to form the hip joint—a ball-and-socket joint.) There are two common types of hip fractures. Femoral neck (subcapital) hip fractures occur just below the thighbone's head, in the neck of the thighbone. Intertrochanteric hip fractures occur in the area just below the neck, where the thighbone broadens. There are two large bumps (called trochanters) in this area. They provide a sturdy place for the muscles of the legs and buttocks to be attached to.

The bones may be broken in different ways. The broken bone may remain in place (aligned or nondisplaced) even if the bone is cracked all the way through. The ends of the broken bone may be separated (displaced). Or one end may be jammed (impacted) into the other.

Most hip fractures result from a fall. However, when osteo-

1. see page 313

porosis or another disorder has weakened the bone, a hip fracture may result from the stresses of ordinary activity (such as getting in and out of a chair).

Symptoms and Diagnosis

Hip fractures almost always cause pain, weakness in the affected leg, or both. Pain occurs partly because the ends of the broken bone move around, injuring the surrounding tissue. Most people with a displaced hip fracture cannot walk or stand. When they are lying on their back, the affected leg may appear shorter than the other leg, and the foot of the affected leg turns out (rather than pointing straight up). Some people with an impacted hip fracture can walk, although with pain.

People with an intertrochanteric hip fracture may become light-headed or weak or even go into shock. These symptoms indicate that blood pressure has fallen: Blood pressure falls if a fracture damages blood vessels and causes bleeding inside the hip. Large bruises may develop around the hip.

The stress of having a hip fracture can lead to other problems. Pain due to a hip fracture, the drugs used to control pain, and the experience of hospitalization and surgery may cause an older person to become confused, disoriented, forgetful, and anxious.[1] A change in living arrangements, if needed, can be upsetting. A person may become depressed, especially if a fracture disrupts normal activities and requires a lot of time and adjustments while healing. Family members should report changes in mental function after a hip fracture to a health care practitioner.

After a femoral neck hip fracture, severe, painful arthritis may develop. Arthritis can develop if the fracture disrupts the blood supply to the head of the thighbone. Without a good blood supply, the bone heals slowly or incompletely, and it may eventually die and collapse.

Most hip fractures can be seen on x-rays. However, if the fracture is small, a second x-ray (taken a day or two later), computed tomography (CT), or magnetic resonance imaging (MRI) may be needed to detect it.

1. see page 346

Prevention and Treatment

Preventing hip fractures involves preventing falls,[1] strengthening bones to prevent osteoporosis,[2] and protecting bones. One way to protect bones is to wear a specially designed hip protector (a thigh-length undergarment with padding along its sides). Many hip protectors can be worn comfortably under clothing.

Treatment usually consists of surgery. Surgery prevents the ends of the broken bones from moving and thus relieves pain. Surgery also enables most people to get out of bed and begin to walk again almost immediately. At first, almost everyone uses a walker. For people who have a serious disorder, such as a recent heart attack, surgery may be too risky. For these people, bed rest is continued until they recover enough for surgery to be safe. Rarely, surgery is not done—for example, for people who were permanently unable to walk before the fracture and who are not experiencing pain.

The type of surgery depends on the type and severity of the fracture and on the person's activity level.

For some femoral neck hip fractures, metal pins can be inserted surgically to hold the bone together. For intertrochanteric hip fractures, a different type of metal implant is used. A plate is attached to the top part of the thighbone with compression screws. The screws allow the fragments to move closer to each other and grow together. These procedures, which are types of internal fixation, preserve the person's own hip joint.

For more severe femoral neck hip fractures, the head and neck of the thighbone are removed and replaced in a procedure called partial hip replacement (hemiarthroplasty). They are replaced with a smooth metal sphere on a metal stem. The stem is inserted into the center of the thighbone's shaft and usually cemented in place. The sphere is made to fit into the person's hip socket.

Sometimes, especially if arthritis has damaged the hip socket, total hip replacement is necessary. In this operation, the hip socket is replaced as well as the head and neck of the thighbone. The pelvic bone around the socket is shaped so that a metal cup can be inserted to replace the opening of the socket.

1. see page 291
2. see page 303

REPAIRING A BROKEN HIP

There are two common types of hip fractures. Femoral neck (subcapital) fractures occur in the neck of the thighbone (femur). Intertrochanteric fractures occur in the large bony bumps (trochanters) where the powerful muscles of the buttocks and legs are attached. When a fracture is not too severe, the hip can be repaired. For femoral neck fractures, metal pins may be inserted surgically to support the femoral head. For intertrochanteric fractures, compression screws and a metal plate may be used. These procedures, called internal fixation, preserve the person's own hip joint.

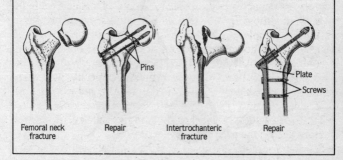

Femoral neck   Repair   Intertrochanteric   Repair
fracture   fracture

Traditionally, hip surgery involves a 9-inch incision at the hip joint. Afterward, people must stay in the hospital 3 to 5 days. They may be able to put full weight on the hip in a few days, or they may have to wait up to 6 weeks. New techniques that cause less pain, involve much smaller incisions (about $2\frac{1}{2}$ to 3 inches), and result in a quicker recovery are being developed. However, whether the new techniques are as safe and effective as traditional surgery is not yet known.

After surgery for a hip fracture, rehabilitation is begun in the hospital as soon as possible.[1]

Outlook

Many people recover reasonably well after a hip fracture. But full recovery may take up to a year. Being healthy, able to move (mobile), and active before the fracture makes a good recovery more likely. However, hip fractures may lead to serious problems, primarily because they limit a person's mobility. Only

1. see page 182

REPLACING A HIP

When the upper end (head) of the thighbone (femur) is badly damaged, it may be replaced with an artificial part (prosthesis), made of metal. This procedure is called partial hip replacement, or hemiarthroplasty. Very rarely, the socket into which the femoral head fits (forming the hip joint) must also be replaced. The part used is a metal shell lined with durable plastic. This procedure is called total hip replacement.

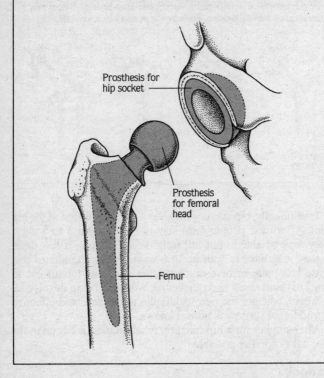

Prosthesis for hip socket

Prosthesis for femoral head

Femur

about one third of people regain the same amount of mobility they had before the fracture. After a hip fracture, about 2 out of 5 people 65 and over need to stay in a nursing home for at least a while. Some of them stay there indefinitely. A year after a hip fracture, some older people still need a walker or another aid to walk. Some people need home care. During the year after they have a hip fracture, about 1 out of 4 people aged 50 and over die. Most of the people who die are over 80.

COMPRESSION FRACTURES OF THE SPINE

In older people with osteoporosis, the bones of the spine (vertebrae) may collapse within themselves and become squashed (compressed). These fractures are called vertebral compression (crush) fractures. Bones affected by osteoporosis are less dense and weaker. Consequently, vertebral fractures can result from very slight force—for example, from turning, bending, or standing. Sometimes they occur for no apparent reason. Vertebral compression fractures are more likely to occur in the middle to lower back.

Symptoms and Diagnosis

When vertebral compression fractures occur, they may cause sudden, sharp pain or no pain. Pain may gradually develop. It may be mild to very severe. Sitting for a long time, standing, bending forward, twisting, carrying heavy objects, and walking usually make the pain worse. Sneezing and coughing may cause pain.

People with many large vertebral compression fractures can lose height, and the back may become rounded and bent. This condition is sometimes called a dowager's hump (kyphosis).[1] Standing up straight may be impossible. Some people have difficulty bending, reaching, lifting, climbing steps, and walking.

Rarely, vertebral compression fractures damage the spinal cord or spinal nerves. In such cases, symptoms include weakness in the leg, numbness, paralysis, and loss of control of the bowels or bladder (fecal or urinary incontinence).

Doctors suspect a vertebral compression fracture on the basis of symptoms: pain in the middle to lower back that is worsened by sitting or standing, loss of height, and a rounded back. X-rays are usually taken. If osteoporosis is suspected, bone density is measured,[2] and blood tests may be done.

1. see page 301
2. see page 302

Treatment

The goals of treatment are to relieve pain, to enable the person to function normally again, and to prevent other fractures. Pain relievers, such as aspirin and other nonsteroidal anti-inflammatory drugs (NSAIDs), can be taken. Sometimes the pain is so severe that opioids are needed. If the fracture is located in the lower back, wearing a brace may make walking less painful. Sometimes a few days of bed rest may be needed to relieve pain. But walking as soon as possible can help people recover more quickly. Walking helps prevent loss of muscle tone and additional loss of bone density. Some people need physical therapy to help them walk and to strengthen muscles.

An experimental procedure to reinforce vertebrae (called vertebroplasty) is sometimes tried. After a local anesthetic is injected near the fractured vertebra, cement is injected into a vertebra through a needle. The cement hardens in about 2 hours and stabilizes the vertebra. The person can go home the same day. This operation may effectively relieve pain, sometimes immediately, and may improve quality of life. Kyphoplasty is a similar procedure. It uses a balloon to expand the compressed vertebra before the cement is injected. The long-term consequences and safety of these treatments are still being studied.

When a fracture is putting pressure on spinal nerves, surgery to relieve the pressure is done within hours if possible. Prompt treatment is necessary to prevent injury to the spinal nerves from becoming permanent.

Outlook

Usually, vertebral compression fractures eventually heal on their own. Pain rarely lasts more than a few months before it gradually subsides. However, a few people, usually those who have many large vertebral compression fractures, need help with daily activities indefinitely. Also, people who have had a vertebral compression fracture are likely to have osteoporosis and thus are likely to have other, sometimes more serious, fractures.

SHOULDER FRACTURES

Falling on an outstretched arm can fracture the collarbone (clavicle) or the upper arm bone (humerus) near the shoulder. In addition to feeling pain, people with a shoulder fracture may be unable to move the arm.

Treatment

For most shoulder fractures, the shoulder is immobilized with a removable device, such as a sling. A removable device is chosen because the shoulder can become permanently stiff within a few days if it is not moved periodically.

If the shoulder is badly out of line or if structures that hold the joint together (such as ligaments, bones, or other tissue) are damaged, surgery is usually needed. Surgery (called internal fixation) often involves wires, pins, or screws inserted into the broken bone. If the shoulder joint is damaged too badly, it is replaced with an artificial joint, similar to that used for the hip.

After all shoulder fractures, the hand and wrist can and should be used immediately. If a removable device is used, range-of-motion exercises for the shoulder and elbow on the affected side are begun within about a week, sometimes sooner. A physical therapist teaches the person how to do these exercises. After 3 weeks, most people can begin exercises that involve raising the arm. However, the person may not be able to raise the arm overhead to do a task (such as comb the hair) for several months. Arthritis can make rehabilitation more difficult, and people who have it may recover more slowly. Problems such as a frozen shoulder or a tear in the muscles and tendons that hold the shoulder in place (rotator cuff) can also slow recovery.

WRIST FRACTURES

Wrist fractures are common among older people. These fractures often result from a fall on an outstretched arm. The most common wrist fracture, called Colles' fracture, occurs near the wrist in one of the arm bones (radius). Osteoporosis increases the likelihood of a wrist fracture.

Symptoms include pain, swelling, and tenderness. Often after a fracture, the wrist is obviously out of line.

HOLDING THE WRIST TOGETHER: EXTERNAL FIXATION

When fragments of bone in the wrist need to be held together, pins may be inserted through the skin into the unbroken bones above and below the fracture. Usually for a wrist fracture, metal pins are inserted into the larger bone in the forearm (radius) and into the bone at the bottom of the index finger. The pins protrude through the skin and are clamped to a frame of rods outside the arm. This technique is called external fixation.

Pins sticking out of the body may look more like a device of torture than one of healing. However, once in place, the pins are painless. With this technique, the broken limb can be used for light activities within a few days. To avoid infection, people with external pins must keep the area around the pins clean. They must also be careful not to injure themselves or other people with the pins. Avoiding such injury may be a particular problem for people with dementia. Sometimes the frame and pins are wrapped with removable protective padding to help prevent injury.

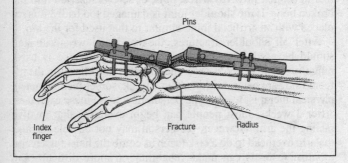

Pins

Index finger   Fracture   Radius

Treatment

A splint or cast is often used to immobilize the wrist. If the fracture is badly out of line, bone fragments are put back in place first. A local anesthetic is usually needed. If the fragments are unlikely to stay in place, metal pins, wires, or screws may be inserted to hold the bone fragments together. External fixation (with a metal frame and pins extending outside the body) or internal fixation (with screws attached to a metal plate inside the body) may be used for the most severe fractures. After either procedure, a splint may be used to provide additional support. The pins or screws used for external or internal fixation are painless once inserted. They may be left in place for weeks. In older people, the plate used for internal fixation may be left in place permanently.

A cast is usually worn for 3 to 8 weeks. The fingers, elbow (if free), and shoulder on the affected side should be moved daily to prevent stiffness. The hand should be rested in an elevated position to control swelling.

A cast or metal frame with pins can be awkward and throw a person off balance. These devices can interfere with sleep. Special foam pillows to elevate the arm may help a person sleep more comfortably. With one arm immobilized, some activities are impossible.

Physical therapy can speed recovery. Comfort, flexibility, and strength of the wrist continue to improve for 6 to 12 months after the fracture. However, older people may not regain full mobility of the wrist joint. Some people develop carpal tunnel syndrome after a wrist fracture.

24

Pain

Some people may think that English novelist Daniel Defoe should have included pain alongside death and taxes on his list of unavoidable evils. However, including pain would have been a mistake: Pain is not an unavoidable consequence of aging.

Almost every older person has pain now and then, and some are unfortunate enough to have pain almost every waking minute. Some older people assume that pain is a normal part of old age and do not seek treatment. Or they may think that admitting to pain is a sign of weakness. Others fear the side effects of drugs used to treat pain.

Feeling pain is bad enough, but pain can also wreak havoc on a person's quality of life and ability to function. Older people with pain may lose sleep and become exhausted. Pain may affect appetite, which can then result in undernutrition. Pain may prevent people from interacting with others, causing them to become isolated and depressed. Some people become so irritable because of pain that they alienate others. When pain interferes with the ability to carry out daily activities, older people become more dependent on others.

Sometimes pain is severe enough to confine a person to a chair or bed, increasing the risk of problems such as pressure sores. The risk of falls may also increase: a chair- or bed-bound person grows progressively weaker, creating a potential hazard when trying to get up.

Causes

The causes of pain are almost limitless. Finding the specific cause of pain in older people often proves to be particularly difficult. Sometimes pain has more than one possible cause. And sometimes no cause can be identified.

To make thinking about possible causes easier, doctors often describe pain as acute or chronic. Acute pain develops suddenly and does not last very long. Acute pain is often caused by an event that has a clear beginning and end, such as an accident or surgery. Chronic pain develops gradually and lasts a long time. Chronic pain often has no clear beginning or end, especially when the cause is a chronic disease (for example, arthritis or diabetes mellitus).

Pain is sometimes felt in one area of the body when the problem causing it is located in another area. This type of pain is called referred pain. For example, pain due to infection and inflammation in the gallbladder may be felt in the shoulder. Referred pain happens because messages from several areas of the body often travel along the same nerves going to the spinal cord and brain.

ADDITIONAL DETAIL

Pain may be caused by an injury that stimulates pain receptors. Pain receptors, located on the tips of nerve cells, recognize and react to pressure, extreme temperatures (hot or cold), or substances released by other cells. This type of pain, called nociceptive pain, may be accompanied by inflammation. Infections, burns, cuts, a severe lack of oxygen in the blood, and stretching of or pressure within an organ can injure tissues and cause nociceptive pain.

Abnormal nerve activity can cause another type of pain, called neuropathic pain. Shingles and diabetes mellitus are examples of disorders that can produce abnormal nerve activity (with shingles, the pain is called postherpetic neuralgia). Sometimes, after a nerve is injured, abnormal nerve activity causes pain to persist long past the time expected for healing of the injury.

Occasionally, pain is attributed—at least in part—to a psychologic disorder, such as depression. Pain attributed to a psychologic cause when no physical cause can be found is called psychogenic pain.

Symptoms and Diagnosis

Pain is described in many different ways: aching, throbbing, squeezing, burning, shooting, and stabbing. Pain can range in severity from mild or annoying to severe or excruciating.

Because pain is so common, many doctors routinely question people about it regardless of the reason for their office visit. Neither examinations nor tests can prove that a person is in pain. Instead, the doctor asks a series of questions. The person's answers can indicate whether the pain is acute or chronic and possibly help identify any causes of the pain.

Questions the doctor might ask can include the following:

• When and how did the pain start? Did it begin suddenly or gradually? Was there a specific event that seemed to trigger the pain?

• What is the pain like? Is there a pattern (for example, steadily worsening, always present, comes and goes, only after meals, or never disrupts sleep)?

• How intense is the pain?

• Where is the pain?

• What makes the pain worse? What makes the pain better?

• Does pain affect the ability to carry out daily activities? How are sleep, appetite, and bowel and bladder function affected?

• Does pain affect mood and sense of well-being? Is the pain accompanied by feelings of depression or anxiety?

Questions also focus on past and present medical problems that might have a role in causing or worsening the pain. Questions are also posed about current and prior drug use, including pain relievers (analgesics).

Other kinds of questions help the doctor gather more information. For example, the person may be asked to rate the intensity of the pain on a scale of 1 to 10, with 1 representing a very small amount of pain and 10 representing the worst pain imaginable. Some doctors ask people to respond to a set of questions developed by experts (a pain assessment tool).

Sometimes obtaining information by asking questions is difficult or even impossible. For example, an older person who has

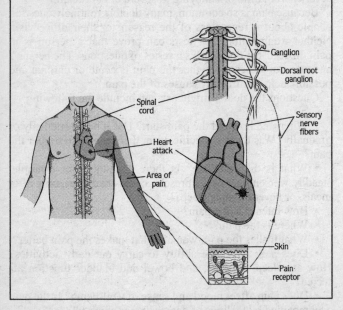

WHAT IS REFERRED PAIN?

Pain that is felt in one area of the body but is caused by a problem in another area is called referred pain. For example, pain produced by a heart attack may feel as if it is coming from the arm because messages from the heart and from the arm travel through the same nerves in the spinal cord.

QUANTIFYING PAIN

To determine how intense pain is, a doctor may show a person pictures of faces with different expressions that might represent different amounts of pain experienced. The person can then point to the face that best represents the amount of pain experienced. Or a doctor may ask the person to rate how intense the pain is on a scale of 0 to 10.

On a scale of 0 to 10, with 0 meaning no pain and 10 meaning the worst pain you can imagine, how much pain are you having now?

had a stroke may be unable to answer because of damage to parts of the brain that control speech. The person may be able to answer "yes" or "no" by making sounds, blinking, or raising a finger or hand. The doctor may show the person a series of pictures depicting faces a person might make when experiencing different amounts of pain. The person can then point to the face that best represents the amount of pain experienced.

In some cases, a person cannot understand questions about pain and cannot describe the pain, even with a tool that uses pictures. For example, a person with dementia or someone who has had a massive stroke may have no way to understand the questions or to communicate. The doctor may have to rely on observations from caregivers. A caregiver may have noticed a change in behavior (for example, a normally outgoing person who withdraws or a calm person who becomes disruptive or aggressive). Changes in sleep patterns or a decrease in appetite may also indicate pain.

A physical examination can provide useful information. Facial expressions can suggest or hint at pain—for example, when a person frowns frequently or seems frightened. Grimacing, tight wrinkling of the forehead, and rapid blinking or eye closing may suggest pain. The person may hold his body rigid or seem to withdraw or guard a painful area when the doctor tries to examine it.

Pale skin, sweating, and a fast heart rate may indicate acute pain. The doctor feels for trigger points, which produce pain when touched. Joints are checked for swelling and inflammation. The doctor also moves the person's arms and legs through their normal range of motion to see if these motions produce pain. The skin may be touched with a variety of objects (for example, soft objects versus sharp objects), to check for abnormal nerve activity.

Treatment

Often, pain goes away by itself. When pain worsens or persists, people usually seek relief.

Treatment begins with a discussion between the person, if able, and the doctor. The discussion is an opportunity to review goals of treatment, expectations, and possible benefits as well as risks and side effects of each treatment choice.

Pain is most often treated with drugs, but there are many effective nondrug treatments. Drugs combined with nondrug treatment can result in better pain control than either method used alone.

Nondrug treatments: Muscle and joint pain may respond to gentle stretching of muscles and movement of joints through their normal range of motion. Massaging painful muscles may also be helpful.

Applying ice, a cold pack, or cold compresses to a painful area may help reduce discomfort that accompanies swelling and inflammation when muscles, ligaments, or tendons are injured. Cold therapy also helps relieve discomfort due to muscle spasms.

Heating pads, warm compresses, hot packs, infrared heat, and hydrotherapy (whirlpool with warm water) can relieve pain on or just below the skin. Heat generated with electrical current (diathermy) or high-frequency sound waves (ultrasound) relieves pain in deeper tissues. Applying heat to painful strained muscles may reduce discomfort. Heat also helps relieve pain in stiff joints affected by arthritis and pain due to sprained ligaments.

Transcutaneous electrical nerve stimulation (TENS) can help relieve pain by applying a gentle electrical current through electrodes placed on the skin's surface. TENS seems to work best when combined with drugs that relieve pain (analgesics).

Acupuncture, which involves inserting hair-thin needles into specific areas of the body, may help relieve pain in some people.[1] Chiropractic therapy may relieve some types of discomfort, such as low back pain.[2]

Cognitive therapy attempts to improve the person's ability to cope with pain and works best when combined with other types of treatment. Types of cognitive therapy include relaxation training, biofeedback, and hypnosis.

Psychologic support can be very helpful for people who live with chronic pain that is not completely relieved.

Drug therapy: Many drugs to relieve pain (analgesics) are available. Unfortunately, older people are more likely than younger people to experience side effects of some analgesics. Doctors "start low and go slow" when deciding how big a dose to start with and how often to increase the dose. In other words, doctors use the lowest dose that provides relief and change doses slowly and cautiously. This approach usually enables older people to safely obtain relief from pain.

Generally, chronic pain is best treated with long-acting or sustained-release drugs that provide steady relief over many hours. Short-acting drugs, which work quickly, may be used while waiting for a long-acting drug to take effect. Relying solely on short-acting drugs may result in peaks of relief alternating with valleys when the pain is poorly controlled.

Under most circumstances, analgesics are taken by mouth. Certain analgesics can be taken under the tongue, as skin patches, or as suppositories inserted into the rectum. Such dosage forms are helpful for people who have trouble swallowing. When rapid action is needed, some opioid analgesics (such as morphine) can be injected directly into a vein (intravenously). If a doctor prescribes patient-controlled analgesia (PCA), the person has some control over the timing and dose of intravenous opioid analgesics.

Analgesics can be divided into three main categories: nonopioids, opioids, and adjuvants (auxiliary drugs).

Nonopioids include nonsteroidal anti-inflammatory drugs (NSAIDs) and acetaminophen. NSAIDs and acetaminophen are equally effective for relieving pain and are commonly used

1. see page 87
2. see page 86

to treat headaches and muscle and joint pain. Unlike acetaminophen, NSAIDs also reduce inflammation. Reducing inflammation often directly treats the cause of pain, thus providing a cure or control rather than simply relief of pain. Some NSAIDs, such as aspirin and low doses of ibuprofen, are available without a prescription.

Aspirin, one type of NSAID, is a tried and true pain reliever. It is relatively safe, although it can irritate the stomach and increase the risk of bleeding. Taking an antacid along with the aspirin (as in buffered aspirin) decreases the likelihood of stomach irritation. Aspirin increases the risk of bleeding because it interferes with the function of platelets, cell-like microscopic particles in the blood that help the blood clot. Taken regularly and at high doses, aspirin may interfere with breathing or produce ringing or other abnormal noises in the ear (tinnitus).

NSAIDs other than aspirin, such as ibuprofen and naproxen, are about equal to aspirin for pain relief. Which NSAID will relieve pain most effectively is impossible to predict. Like aspirin, ibuprofen and naproxen can irritate the stomach and cause bleeding. The risk of side effects, especially the risk of bleeding in the digestive tract, is very high among older people.

Taking NSAIDs with food or liquids reduces the risk of bleeding. Taking other drugs that help protect the digestive tract at the same time, such as misoprostol, histamine-2 (H_2) receptor blockers, and proton pump inhibitors, can also reduce the risk of bleeding.

Coxibs, or COX-2 inhibitors, are another type of NSAID. Celecoxib, rofecoxib, and valdecoxib are examples of coxibs. Compared with other NSAIDs, coxibs provide similar pain relief and are less likely to irritate the stomach or cause bleeding in the digestive tract. However, there is some concern that they may slightly increase the risk of heart attack in some people.

With all NSAIDs, including coxibs, there is a risk of kidney damage. NSAIDs can also cause the body to retain salt (sodium), which may in turn lead to swelling (especially in the feet and ankles) and sometimes an increase in blood pressure. Someone who has had bleeding in the digestive tract or kidney damage should not use NSAIDs.

Acetaminophen, available in several forms and dosages, is a nonprescription drug. Although safer than most other analgesics,

℞ OPIOID ANALGESICS

Drug	Length of Effectiveness	Comments
Codeine	*By mouth*: 3 to 4 hours	Codeine is usually taken with aspirin or acetaminophen
Fentanyl	*By mouth*: 3 to 4 hours *By patch*: 72 hours, sometimes longer in older people	Fentanyl is available as a lozenge that is dissolved in the mouth; it is used to treat pain that is not controlled by the longer-acting patch form of fentanyl or longer-acting forms of other analgesics. The patch is often used to treat chronic pain. A disadvantage of fentanyl patches is that the body takes a long time to eliminate the drug when side effects require that it be stopped
Hydromorphone	*By injection*: 2 to 4 hours *By mouth*: 2 to 4 hours *By rectal suppository*: 4 hours	Hydromorphone begins to work quickly. It can be used instead of morphine
Levorphanol	*By injection*: 4 hours *By mouth*: about 4 hours, sometimes longer in older people	Levorphanol can be used instead of morphine
Methadone	*By mouth*: 4 to 6 hours, often much longer in older people	Methadone is also used for treating dependence on other opioids, but in older people, balancing benefits and side effects can be very difficult
Morphine	*By injection*: 2 to 3 hours, often	Morphine in the injectable or immediate-release

Table continues on the following page.

Drug	Length of Effectiveness	Comments
	longer in older people *By mouth* (immediate-release form): 3 to 4 hours *By mouth* (sustained-release form): 8 to 24 hours	forms starts to work quickly. The oral form can be very effective for chronic pain
Oxycodone	*By mouth*: 3 to 4 hours *By mouth* (sustained-release form): 12 hours	Oxycodone can be used instead of morphine to treat chronic pain. It is usually combined with aspirin or acetaminophen
Oxymorphone	*By injection*: 3 to 4 hours *By rectal suppository*: 4 hours	Oxymorphone starts to work quickly

Note: Other opioid analgesics include meperidine, pentazocine, and propoxyphene, but these drugs are not recommended for use in older people.

acetaminophen can cause dangerous side effects when it is used in large amounts or for a long time. For example, more than 12 regular-strength or 8 extra-strength tablets taken in a single day may damage the liver. In some cases, the damage can cause death. A person with liver disease should not use acetaminophen. More than 12 regular-strength or 8 extra-strength tablets taken daily or almost daily for many years can damage the kidneys.

Opioids are the most powerful analgesics. They are used most often for severe acute pain (such as pain after surgery) and for chronic pain that occurs with cancer. The ability to relieve pain varies widely among different opioids.

With prolonged use of opioids, some people need higher doses because the body sometimes adapts to and responds less well to the drug—a phenomenon called tolerance. People who take opioids for a long time may become dependent on them; that is, they experience symptoms of withdrawal if the drug is discontinued abruptly. These symptoms may include confusion, sweating, and nausea. When opioids are discontinued after long-term use, doctors slowly and steadily reduce the dose to minimize the risk of withdrawal symptoms.

Opioids have many side effects. Many people who take opioids for acute pain become drowsy at first. For some people, this drowsiness may not be a side effect. Rather, it may represent the ability to finally rest as pain is relieved. Many people find the drowsiness a welcome respite; others do not. When opioids are taken regularly, most people stop feeling drowsy. Similarly, many other undesirable side effects diminish. Constipation is an exception.

Almost every older person who takes opioids becomes constipated. Constipation continues to be a problem as long as the opioid is taken. Consequently, some people who take opioids regularly must prevent constipation by increasing their activity, increasing their intake of fluids, and taking laxatives. Laxatives that stimulate the large intestine, such as bisacodyl, cascara, and senna, are often used to treat the constipation caused by opioids. Others such as lactulose or sorbitol may be used over a longer period of time without damaging the digestive tract.

Opioids can cause confusion, especially in older people. This side effect may diminish, but often the amount of the drug or the frequency at which it is taken must be decreased. If confusion persists, some people may need to be switched to a different drug.

Opioids can also make urination (voiding) more difficult, causing urine to remain in the bladder after urinating. One way a person can try to overcome this problem is by urinating again almost immediately after urinating (double voiding).

Opioids can sometimes affect appetite. They may also cause nausea—a particularly troubling problem when a person is already experiencing nausea as a result of the pain. Antiemetic drugs (such as metoclopramide, hydroxyzine, ondansetron, and prochlorperazine) can help prevent or relieve nausea.

Taking too much of an opioid can cause a dangerous slowing of breathing, coma, and even death. These effects can be reversed with naloxone, an antidote given intravenously.

Adjuvants are drugs that are not usually given to treat pain but that may relieve pain in certain circumstances. Antidepressants, anticonvulsants, and oral and topical local anesthetics are adjuvants. When used to relieve pain, adjuvants are usually combined with other analgesics or nondrug pain treatments.

Antidepressants can help relieve pain in people who do not have depression. Tricyclic antidepressants (such as nortriptyline) have been used for many years for this purpose. Selective serotonin reuptake inhibitors (SSRIs), another type of antidepressant that includes fluoxetine and sertraline, can be used.

Anticonvulsants can be used to help relieve pain caused by abnormal nerve activity (neuropathic pain). Gabapentin is commonly used, but others (such as carbamazepine) may be tried.

Anesthetics are sometimes injected directly in or near a sore area or trigger point to help reduce pain. Occasionally, severe long-lasting pain related to nerve injury can be treated by injecting a chemical into the nerve to destroy it.

Some anesthetic drugs can be applied to the skin as a lotion or ointment or in a patch to control pain resulting from problems on or just below the skin. For example, a lidocaine patch can be used to relieve the pain that sometimes follows shingles (postherpetic neuralgia).

A cream containing capsaicin, a substance found in hot peppers, sometimes helps reduce the pain caused by such disorders as shingles and osteoarthritis. This cream must be applied several times a day.

Retirement can become one's golden years of living—relaxed leisure hours for savoring happy experiences and maintaining a balanced program of good, healthy habits of physical exercise, which helps stimulate alertness. Continue to grow and change, engaging with life and those around you.

In recalling significant events from the past, I believe many are worth recording, for mere oral accounts grow dim and are too easily forgotten. Written memories leave a richer, lasting heritage for family and future generations.

During my high school years, I discovered the delight of "making word pictures." When you feel deeply about something, search for the best words to give it expression. There will be a rhythm and flow to the lines, and perhaps even rhyme—and you have written a poem. Perhaps you would like a pattern to follow. A haiku (15 words in three lines of 5–7–5 syllables) is fun and surprisingly easy to write:

Every morning   Take some time this day
Offers us fresh adventures   For "making memories" to
In daily living.   Cherish tomorrow.

Each fresh new day is
A one-time gift from heaven
Sent by God above.

Try writing some of your own to share with others.

I find my volunteer visits to nursing homes are a great joy, and I always look forward to returning. Both residents and staff are so appreciative and responsive to my "readings" each week. The verses seem to open windows of communication—encouraging hearers to compare experiences and listen to others share their thoughts and feelings. My life has been enriched with new friendships and fresh purpose, realizing that sharing one's talents can truly make a difference, bringing pleasure for others. Becoming a **R**etired **S**enior **V**olunteer **P**erson is one way of expressing thanks for the countless blessings in my life.

Iona Patch

25

Confusion

The prospect of becoming confused strikes fear in the hearts of many older people. Older people fear that confusion will cause them to lose their identity and independence. They also fear that once they become confused, they will always be confused. However, confusion is not inevitable, and if it occurs, it is not necessarily permanent. Confusion has many causes. If the cause can be eliminated or treated, the confusion may disappear or lessen. Understanding what confusion is and what can cause it can help reduce the risk of becoming confused.

As people age, many changes occur in the brain.[1] These changes make older people more susceptible than younger people to conditions that can disturb mental function. When mental function is disturbed in older people, they usually become confused.

Confusion has different meanings. But generally, it means that people cannot process information correctly. They cannot

- Follow a conversation
- Answer questions appropriately
- Pay attention to and understand what is going on around them
- Keep track of information
- Remember

Two disorders are characterized by confusion: delirium and dementia. They are very different and have very different causes. However, delirium and dementia may occur together.

Delirium occurs suddenly, typically over a period of hours to-days.[2] It is usually caused by the recent development of a condi-

1. see page 16
2. see page 346

COMPARING TWO DISORDERS OF CONFUSION

Feature	Delirium	Dementia
Development	Sudden, with a definite beginning point	Slow and gradual, with an uncertain beginning point
Duration	Days to weeks, although it may be permanent	Usually permanent
Cause	Almost always another condition, such as infection, dehydration, or use or withdrawal of certain drugs	Usually a chronic brain disorder, such as Alzheimer's disease, Lewy body dementia (which has symptoms similar to those of Parkinson's disease), or vascular dementia (multi-infarct dementia, which results from strokes)
Effect at night	Almost always worse	Often worse
Effect on attention	Greatly impaired	No effect until dementia has become very severe
Effect on alertness	Varies, ranging from sluggishness to alertness	No effect
Orientation to time and place	Varies	Impaired
Use of language	Slow, often incoherent, and inappropriate	Sometimes have difficulty finding the right word
Memory	Varies	Lost, especially for recent events
Need for medical attention	Immediate	Required but less urgently

tion that affects the brain's ability to function. The most obvious symptom of delirium is the inability to pay attention. How well people with delirium are able to pay attention may change over time. They may appear sluggish one moment and alert the next. Often, confusion is worse at night. People with delirium may be calm and focused one moment, then agitated and distracted the next. They cannot think clearly and thus cannot speak coherently. If the disorder causing delirium is quickly identified and successfully treated, confusion may disappear or lessen. Then, most people can function as well as they did before delirium developed.

Dementia develops slowly.[1] It is usually caused by a chronic brain disorder. When dementia first develops, it, unlike delirium, does not interfere with the ability to pay attention. At first, the most obvious symptom is loss of memory. However, all aspects of mental function slowly and steadily deteriorate. Usually, dementia cannot be cured. Eventually, mental function is severely and permanently impaired. The development of a disorder or use of a new drug is more likely to lead to delirium in people with dementia than in those without dementia.

Confusion is always serious. People who suddenly become confused or whose confusion suddenly worsens may have delirium. Consequently, they need medical attention immediately. People with sudden confusion are often hospitalized to be evaluated and treated. People who gradually become more and more confused may have dementia. They also need medical attention but not so urgently. Such people rarely need to be hospitalized, but they need to be evaluated. For them, confusion can be evaluated over a period of days or weeks during a series of visits to the doctor's office. However, people who have dementia that suddenly worsens need to be evaluated more quickly.

Diagnosis

The first thing doctors need to know about the confused person is whether the confusion occurred suddenly or developed gradually. This information helps doctors determine whether the cause of confusion is delirium or dementia. To be sure of the diagnosis, doctors ask the person a standard series of questions called a mental status test. These questions help doctors identify which mental functions are not working normally and to what degree.

1. see page 354

WHAT IS MENTAL STATUS TESTING?

Area of Mental Function Evaluated	Things People May Be Asked to Do
Orientation to time and place	State the current date and place
Attention and immediate recall	Repeat a short list of objects
Recent memory	Recall the short list of objects after 3 to 5 minutes
Abstract thinking	Interpret a proverb (such as "a rolling stone gathers no moss"), or explain a particular analogy (such as "why the brain is like a computer")
Insight into illness	Describe feelings and opinions about the illness
Mood	Tell how they feel on this day and how they usually feel
Ability to follow simple commands	Follow a simple command that involves three different body parts and requires distinguishing right from left (such as "put your right thumb over your left ear and stick out your tongue")
Ability to use language	Name simple objects and body parts, repeat certain phrases, read a simple instruction and do it, and write a sentence of the person's choice
Ability to understand spatial relationships	Copy simple and complex structures (for example, using building blocks) or finger positions, and draw a clock, cube, or house
Ability to solve math problems	Subtract 7 from 100 and continue to subtract 7 from the remainder (93, 86, 79, 72, and so on)

Doctors also talk with a family member or another person who knows the confused person. Such a person can describe how the confused person used to be—days, weeks, and months ago—and exactly what has changed. Doctors may ask to see documents that can indicate a change in mental function, such as a checkbook, recent letters, or notification of unpaid bills or missed appointments. For example, a checkbook shows whether the person's writing has changed over a period of time, as well as how well the person can record entries and do math. Letters can indicate whether a person's thinking is confused.

Doctors ask other questions to help them identify the cause of the confusion. They ask about the disorders the confused person has and the drugs (including nonprescription drugs) and dietary supplements the person has been taking. Doctors may also ask whether the person is taking an illicit drug or consuming a substantial amount of alcohol.

Doctors ask detailed questions about the person's emotional health. This information is helpful because depression may be causing or contributing to confusion.

Evaluation of confusion always includes a complete physical examination and may include blood and other laboratory tests.

26

Delirium

Delirium is confusion that begins suddenly and may vary from slight to severe within hours. People who have delirium cannot pay attention or think clearly.

Delirium is common among older people. About 10 to 20% of older people who are admitted to the hospital already have delirium. People over 85 are the most susceptible. Delirium is a common reason that family members of older people seek help from a doctor or at a hospital.

Delirium is never normal and always indicates a serious problem. People who have delirium need immediate medical attention. If the cause of delirium is identified and corrected quickly, delirium can usually be cured.

DRUGS THAT CAN CAUSE DELIRIUM

Drug	Use
Dopamine agonists	To treat Parkinson's disease
Antiemetics	To prevent or relieve nausea and vomiting
Antihistamines	To relieve allergy or cold symptoms and sometimes to promote sleep
Some antihypertensive drugs	To lower blood pressure
Antipsychotic drugs	To treat loss of contact with reality (psychosis)
Antispasmodic drugs	To treat an overactive bladder
Digoxin	To treat heart failure
Histamine-2 (H_2) blockers such as cimetidine	To treat ulcers in the digestive tract
Muscle relaxants	To relieve muscle spasms
Opioids	To relieve pain
Sedatives, especially benzodiazepines	To produce drowsiness or to calm
Tricyclic antidepressants	To treat depression

Causes

Delirium can be caused by many disorders and drugs and by stressful situations. These causes are especially likely to lead to delirium in people who have dementia.

Severe disorders can cause delirium in any person—young or old. Examples are infections, strokes, seizures, heart disorders (such as heart attack, abnormal heart rhythms, and heart failure), and diabetes that is poorly controlled. But in older people, relatively less severe disorders can cause delirium. For example, urinary tract infections are a common cause. Other examples are dehydration, a deficiency of vitamin B_1 or B_{12}, retention of urine, and constipation.

Certain drugs can cause delirium in any person. But older people are much more sensitive to many drugs. The list of drugs that can cause delirium in older people is long. The drugs that most commonly cause delirium are those that affect the way the brain functions, such as sedatives. Many nonprescription (over-the-counter) drugs, especially antihistamines, can also cause delirium in older people.

Delirium may result from withdrawal of sedatives that have been taken for a long time. Alcoholics may develop delirium if they suddenly stop drinking alcohol. This type of delirium is called delirium tremens (DT).

Stressful situations may be enough to cause delirium. When a stressful situation is combined with drugs or disorders, delirium is more likely to develop. For example, delirium is common after surgery (a stressful situation). The drugs used during surgery, the pain relievers used after surgery, and complications related to surgery make delirium even more likely.

People in intensive care units (ICUs) are particularly likely to develop delirium, mainly because the conditions there are stressful. In an ICU, hospital staff members must awaken people during the night to check vital signs or monitors and to give treatments. People in ICUs are usually able to sleep for only short periods of time. Loud beeping monitors, intercoms, voices in the hallway, or alarms may disturb sleep. People in ICUs must be isolated. Typically, the rooms have no windows or clocks to help people orient themselves. Thus, people in ICUs often cannot distinguish between night and day. Furthermore, most people in ICUs have serious disorders that require drugs, which can make delirium even more likely. The delirium that may develop in these people is sometimes called ICU psychosis.

ADDITIONAL DETAIL

Why disorders, drugs, and some stressful situations so easily cause delirium in older people is not known. However, there are some theories. One theory involves a chemical called acetylcholine, a type of neurotransmitter. Neurotransmitters are chemicals that enable brain cells to communicate with one another. The level of acetylcholine decreases when the body is stressed, as it is by a disorder, drug, or stressful situation. The brain does not function well without enough acetylcholine. As people age, the brain produces less acetylcholine. Thus, older people are more vulnerable to conditions that cause the level of acetylcholine to decrease further.

Another theory involves chemicals that can harm the brain (toxins). Toxins may be produced when a person has a disorder, or toxins may be ingested, for example, in contaminated food. Certain drugs are toxic if the level of the drug in the blood is high enough. These toxins can circulate in the blood. Normally, the body blocks many of these toxins from entering the brain. But as people age, the body is less able to do so. In older people, toxins may accumulate in the brain and prevent it from functioning normally, making delirium more likely.

Symptoms

Delirium begins suddenly. Usually, family members or friends notice that the person has become mildly or severely confused over a period of hours or a few days.

The level of confusion may vary. Often, confusion is worse at night. Confusion may worsen, then clear up during the next few hours, only to worsen again. A person may be sluggish one moment and alert the next. A person may be calm and focused, then agitated and distracted. Some people with delirium tend to be anxious and agitated. Very old people with delirium tend to become quiet and withdrawn. In them, confusion is only apparent when someone tries to rouse or talk with them.

People with delirium cannot pay attention, and their ability to do so may vary over minutes or hours. Thus, they do not understand what is happening around them. They become disoriented. They sometimes lose track of who they are, where they are, or what time or day it is. People with delirium cannot concentrate and have difficulty remembering. In conversation, they wander from topic to topic. Their speech may be slurred, rambling, or incoherent.

Many people with delirium do not sleep normally. They may fall asleep during the day, even in noisy places, and stay awake at night. If delirium becomes severe, people may see or hear things that are not there (hallucinate).

Diagnosis

When confusion begins suddenly, it is almost always delirium. Therefore, people who have recently become confused should be evaluated immediately for delirium. Such people are usually hospitalized so that the cause can be quickly identified and treatment can be started promptly.

Often, health care practitioners have trouble recognizing delirium. Delirium is especially hard to recognize in people who withdraw and thus do not communicate. Delirium is hard to recognize in people who have dementia because dementia can also cause confusion. In people with dementia, confusion develops over a period of months or years and slowly worsens. If a person with dementia develops delirium, the delirium is identified only if someone notices that the confusion has become decidedly worse over a period of hours to days.

Family members and caregivers can help by providing doctors with details about the person's change in mental function—how the confusion began and how quickly it progressed. The most important information a doctor can obtain is the perspective of someone who has known the person over time and who can describe the recent changes.

Family members and caregivers should also tell doctors about all the drugs and any other substances that the confused person may have taken. This list should include all nonprescription drugs and dietary supplements as well as any alcohol or illicit drugs used.

Doctors perform a physical examination. As part of the examination, the person may be asked questions to determine whether the main problem is an inability to pay attention, with the disorientation that results from it.

Samples of blood and urine are taken. Analysis of these samples may help doctors identify the cause of delirium. Sometimes more complex tests are needed. Computed tomography (CT) or magnetic resonance imaging (MRI) may be used to obtain images of the brain. A spinal tap (lumbar puncture) may be done to obtain a sample of the fluid that surrounds the brain and spinal cord (cerebrospinal fluid). Analysis of this fluid helps doctors rule out infections and bleeding. If the cause is thought to be a lung or heart disorder, a chest x-ray may be taken or electrocardiography (ECG) may be done to record the electrical activity of the heart.

While the person is hospitalized, doctors and other staff members watch for signs of withdrawal from alcohol and other drugs.

Prevention

When an older person is hospitalized, family members can talk to hospital staff members about what measures can help prevent delirium. The following measures may help:

- **Keeping the person mobile:** Getting the person out of bed and walking regularly is important. If the person cannot get out of bed, a physical therapist can help the person exercise or move in other ways.
- **Keeping the person's mind active:** Asking questions about the person's life, talking about current events, or reading to the person can help.
- **Keeping the person oriented:** People who wear glasses or use a hearing aid should have access to these items. Placing a clock and calendar in the room is useful. Explaining tests and treatments reminds people of where they are and why.
- **Encouraging the person to do as many normal daily tasks** (such as dressing) **as possible:** Doing daily tasks helps keep the person active and aware of the time of day and makes life seem more normal.
- **Helping the person get a good night's sleep and making sure that light in the room is adequate during the day:** Thus, the person can stay on a normal sleep cycle, get more restful sleep, and be better able to distinguish between night and day. Family members can talk to nurses about trying to reduce the number of loud noises (such as loud beeping monitors) and disruptions (such as giving drugs and checking blood pressure and heart rate) at night.
- **Making sure the person drinks enough fluids and eats enough food:** The person may need encouragement or help with drinking and eating.
- **Asking staff members which drugs are being used and why:** For example, family members can ask whether any of the drugs being used could make the confusion worse. If a sedative is being given to help the person sleep, family members can ask about using approaches that have worked at home, such as a glass of warm milk or a cup of herbal tea. If the person is in pain, family members should ask about more effective pain treatments.

Treatment

Once identified, the disorder causing delirium is treated. Prompt treatment of the disorder causing delirium usually prevents permanent brain damage and may result in a complete recovery.

During treatment, people with delirium may injure themselves, especially if they become very agitated or confused or if they hallucinate. Therefore, they should not be left alone. In the hospital, a full-time attendant may be needed to keep people with delirium safe and to care for them. People with delirium may need help and encouragement with getting in and out of bed, feeding themselves, and using the toilet. They may need someone to accompany them when they walk in the hallway. They may need reassurance because they are frightened. Family members may choose to provide this care, and nurses can help with it. Nurses can also notice signs of pain, the worsening of any other disorders, and other needs that may be hard to recognize because of the confusion.

At every opportunity, staff and family members should help orient a person with delirium to time and place. They should also explain what is going on around the person, including tests or treatments the person is about to receive.

Padded restraints are a last resort. Whenever possible, hospital staff members, with the help of family members, closely monitor the person instead of using restraints. However, restraints may be necessary to prevent falls or to prevent the person from pulling out medical devices, such as an intravenous line (IV), a catheter that drains urine from the bladder, or a feeding tube. Restraints are applied carefully, used only for a short time, and released at frequent intervals. But even then, restraints increase the likelihood that the person will be injured. Restraints can also upset the person and make the person more agitated. Health care practitioners constantly reevaluate the need for restraints. Then they can remove the restraints as soon as possible.

If a person with delirium has been taking drugs that may be making the delirium worse, doctors discontinue them if possible.

Sometimes a person is so confused, agitated, and frightened that a drug is needed. In such cases, antipsychotics are considered the best choice. These drugs help calm the person. Small doses are often effective. For some people, newer antipsychotics (such as olanzapine and quetiapine) are preferred to older antipsychotics (such as haloperidol). The newer antipsychotics have fewer side effects, such as muscle stiffness. When a person cannot tolerate the side effects of antipsychotics or when antipsychotics do not work, benzodiazepines, which are sedatives, may be used. Benzodiazepines sometimes used include midazolam and lorazepam. Although benzodiazepines can calm an agitated person, they cannot cure delirium and can make confusion worse. Therefore, doctors give the lowest possible dose and discontinue the drugs as soon as possible.

Outlook

If the disorder causing delirium is quickly identified and successfully treated, most people recover and can function as well as they did before delirium developed. However, any delay greatly decreases the chance of a full recovery. Even with prompt treatment, delirium may persist for many weeks or months, particularly in people who have dementia to some degree. Improvement may occur slowly. In some people, delirium persists and develops into a chronic disorder that resembles dementia.

People who develop delirium while in the hospital tend to stay in the hospital longer than those who do not develop delirium. They are also more likely to develop complications (such as pressure sores, urinary tract infections, and incontinence) and to fall and be injured.

27

Dementia

Dementia is a disorder that gradually robs people of their ability to remember, think, understand, communicate, and control behavior (mental function).

There are many types of dementia, including Alzheimer's disease. Different types affect different mental abilities and progress at different rates. Therein lies the anguish of dementia: Dementia progresses. It cannot be cured. At some point, people with dementia need complete care. Eventually, dementia results in death.

Dementia may develop at any age but is much more common among older people. About 6 to 8% of people over 65 have dementia. And the older people become, the more common dementia becomes. About 35% of people 85 or over have dementia. Nonetheless, dementia is not an inevitable part of aging. Many people over 100 do not have dementia.

When older people start forgetting or misplacing things more often, they may worry that this forgetfulness is the first sign of dementia, particularly Alzheimer's disease. This forgetfulness is not always dementia, but in about half of these people, dementia sooner or later becomes apparent.

Types and Causes

The most common type of dementia is Alzheimer's disease. Other common types are vascular (multi-infarct) dementia, which is caused by strokes, and Lewy body dementia. Many people have more than one of these dementias (mixed dementia). Several less common types of dementia result from another brain disorder (such as Parkinson's disease or a tumor) or from normal-pressure hydrocephalus.

IS IT DEMENTIA?

Forgetfulness: Some older people become very forgetful. But other mental functions (thinking, understanding, communicating, and controlling behavior) seem unaffected. This type of memory loss is sometimes called mild cognitive impairment or benign senescent forgetfulness. People who have it often worry that this forgetfulness is the first sign of dementia, particularly Alzheimer's disease. For about half of them, their worst fears come to pass, as other signs of Alzheimer's disease very slowly develop over the next 3 to 5 years.

Many other older people have only a very slight problem remembering things, but they also have slight problems with other mental functions. In these people, the problems are often so slight that they are not noticed, and the problems do not seem to worsen. This condition is called age-related cognitive impairment. Its effects are much less drastic than those of dementia. And unlike dementia, it does not affect the ability to function.

Depression: Some older people become forgetful, confused, disoriented, and distracted because they are depressed. In such cases, depression may be mistaken for dementia. Often, people who are depressed are bothered by their forgetfulness. In contrast, people who have true dementia often deny any forgetfulness. Treating depression usually restores mental function. However, some people have dementia and depression. For them, treating the depression may improve (but not restore) mental function.

Other disorders: Several disorders can cause some of the symptoms of dementia. These disorders are sometimes mistaken for dementia. Examples are delirium, vitamin deficiencies (especially vitamin B_{12} deficiency), and an underactive thyroid gland (hypothyroidism)—disorders that are common among older people. Treating these disorders may partly or completely restore mental function.

In some disorders, brain tissue is damaged, sometimes resulting in symptoms similar to those of dementia. But symptoms do not worsen as they do in dementia. These disorders include head injuries and sudden stopping of the heart's pumping (cardiac arrest), which deprives the brain of oxygen. Radiation therapy to the head as treatment for a brain tumor may damage brain tissue and impair mental functions, especially memory. Many months or years after treatment, radiation therapy occasionally results in symptoms that resemble those of dementia.

In some types of dementia (such as Alzheimer's disease), the level of acetylcholine in the brain is low. Acetylcholine is a chemical messenger (called a neurotransmitter) that helps nerve cells communicate with one another. Acetylcholine helps with memory, learning, and concentration and helps control the functioning of many organs. Other changes occur in the brain, but whether they cause or result from dementia is unclear.

Certain disorders, if inadequately treated, can make dementia worse. Examples are diabetes, chronic obstructive pulmonary disease (COPD), and heart failure. Many people improve substantially when these disorders are treated.

Many drugs may temporarily cause or worsen the symptoms of dementia. Common offenders include drugs used to promote sleep (sleep aids or sedatives), cold remedies, and some drugs used to treat anxiety and depression. Some of these drugs can be purchased without a prescription (over the counter). Drinking alcohol, even in moderate amounts, may also make dementia worse.

Some disorders (such as delirium) cause symptoms that resemble those of dementia. These disorders are not considered dementia because treatment can restore all or part of mental function.

Symptoms

Symptoms of most dementias are similar. But different symptoms occur first, and each type of dementia progresses in a different way. Generally, dementia causes the following:

- Memory loss
- Problems using language
- Changes in personality
- Disorientation
- Problems doing usual daily activities
- Disruptive or inappropriate behavior

Some people with dementia also have psychotic symptoms, such as hallucinations, delusions, or paranoia.

Memory loss often begins with forgetting recent events. People with dementia may ask the same questions over and over and constantly forget where they put things. They may forget entire events. Important tasks may be forgotten or done incorrectly. For example, people may forget to pay a bill, pay it several times, send the wrong amount, or forget to sign the check. Forgetting may frustrate them. Learning and remembering new information is also difficult.

LESS COMMON CAUSES OF DEMENTIA

Brain tumors can cause dementia if they are located in areas that control thinking or memory. If the tumor cannot be removed surgically and cannot be shrunk by radiation therapy or drugs, it can cause a progressive decline in mental function.

Parkinson's disease results in dementia in some people. This dementia is a mixed dementia with symptoms similar to those of Alzheimer's disease, vascular dementia, and Lewy body dementia. **Progressive supranuclear palsy** may result in a similar dementia.

In **AIDS** (usually in the late stages), the human immunodeficiency virus (HIV) may infect the brain. Dementia then develops gradually and progresses steadily, usually over a few months or years. Early, continuing treatment of HIV infection can usually prevent dementia.

Rarely, **Lyme disease** or **syphilis** causes dementia. Early treatment of these infections can prevent dementia. Once dementia has developed, treating the infection does not lessen the dementia or restore mental function.

In **normal-pressure hydrocephalus**, the fluid that normally surrounds the brain (cerebrospinal fluid) is not reabsorbed normally. Fluid accumulates and puts pressure on brain tissue, resulting in dementia. Normal-pressure hydrocephalus also causes urinary incontinence and problems with walking. The feet seem stuck to the floor, so taking a first step is hard. Walking is unsteady. If normal-pressure hydrocephalus is diagnosed early, it can sometimes be treated by draining the excess fluid within the brain through a drainage tube (shunt).

Pick's disease, a rare disease, causes a dementia that resembles Alzheimer's disease. However, the dementia progresses more rapidly. The cause is unknown. People with Pick's disease cannot take the initiative, even to do familiar tasks.

In **Creutzfeldt-Jakob disease,** also a rare disease, abnormal proteins called prions damage the brain. The resulting dementia progresses rapidly. It often becomes severe and leads to death within a year. A variant of Creutzfeldt-Jakob disease (so-called mad cow disease) is thought to be acquired from eating contaminated beef.

Rarely, **chronic subdural hematoma** results in dementia. In this disorder, blood accumulates between the outer and middle layers of tissue covering the brain. The blood may put more and more pressure on surrounding brain tissue, progressively impairing mental function. Even soft falls or slight head injuries can cause hematomas, particularly in people who take anticoagulants (which make blood less likely to clot).

Alcohol dementia may result from drinking large amounts of alcohol for many years. Memory is usually affected more than other areas of mental function.

Early in dementia, using language becomes more difficult. People with dementia may use words incorrectly or be unable to find the right word. They may use a general word or many words rather than the specific word. For example, "that thing around the collar" may be used for "necktie." Using numbers (for example, adding and subtracting) and handling money become more difficult.

Personality may change markedly. People with dementia may become depressed, fearful, anxious, or emotionally unresponsive. A particular personality trait may become more and more extreme. People who were always concerned with money become obsessed with it. Emotions may change unpredictably and rapidly. People may be euphorically happy one moment and, without any reason, become inconsolably sad the next. If changes in their personality or mental function are mentioned, people with dementia may become irritable, hostile, or agitated.

People with dementia may misinterpret what they see and hear and become disoriented easily. Disorientation can interfere with doing daily activities. However, some people hide their deficiencies well. They follow established routines at home and avoid activities that have become difficult for them. Early in dementia, people may be able to continue driving, but they become confused in congested traffic or get lost more easily. As dementia progresses, making the quick decisions and coordinating the many manual skills needed in driving become more and more difficult. People may not remember where they are going. They may be unable to make sense of what they see and hear.

As the dementia progresses, people may act disruptively and become less and less able to control their behavior. They may yell, throw, hit, wander, or act in socially inappropriate ways. They may become physically aggressive and more easily agitated. Usually, people with dementia act this way because they have difficulty communicating. Behavior is used to express feelings or needs that they cannot describe in words. They may wander because they are hungry or frightened, because they need to use the toilet, or because they are looking for something or someone. They may yell continuously because they are in pain.

Disruptive behavior may also result from being disoriented.

People with dementia have difficulty understanding what they see and hear, so they may misinterpret an offer of help as a threat and lash out. For example, when someone tries to help them undress, they may interpret it as an attack and try to protect themselves, sometimes by hitting. Because their short-term memory is impaired, they cannot keep track of what is happening to and around them. They may repeatedly demand things (such as meals) that they have already received and become agitated and upset when they do not get them.

People with dementia may act in socially inappropriate ways because they have forgotten how to behave appropriately. When hot, they may undress in public. When they have sexual impulses, they may masturbate in public, use off-color or lewd language, or make sexual demands, sometimes aggressively.

Sleep problems are common. Most people with dementia sleep an appropriate amount, but they spend less time in deep sleep. As a result, they may become restless at night. Problems falling or staying asleep are common. If people do not exercise enough or do not participate in many activities, they may sleep too much during the day. Then they do not sleep well at night. When people with dementia cannot sleep, they may wander, yell, or call out.

Depression and anxiety are common and are understandable reactions to developing dementia. But they may be hard to recognize because people with dementia may not be able to express their feelings. Depression may be expressed by a sad facial expression, crying episodes, loss of interest, apathy, withdrawal, loss of appetite and weight, problems sleeping, or complaints about physical pain. People with dementia may become nervous or worried about making mistakes or forgetting things. Anxiety may become worse when people are separated from their caregivers or their schedules are changed.

Symptoms, including sleep problems and disruptive behavior, may worsen when people with dementia are moved to a nursing home or another institution. They may even try to return home. Symptoms worsen partly because adjusting to changes and remembering new routines are difficult. Symptoms may also worsen when physical problems, such as pain, shortness of breath, retention of urine, and constipation, develop. These problems may cause delirium with rapidly worsening confusion.[1] If the problem is corrected, people may eventually return to the level of functioning they had before the problem.

As dementia progresses, people may need help with eating, dressing, bathing, or going to the toilet. They may not be able to recognize people, places, and things. People with dementia may not even recognize their own face in a mirror. When they see themselves in a mirror, they may think strangers are in the house—a thought that frightens and upsets them. Their increasing confusion and disorientation makes falling more likely. For example, they may not step high or soon enough to clear an obstacle in their path. Many of them become incontinent.

Eventually, memory is completely lost. When dementia is advanced, people cannot follow conversations or recognize close family members.

Advanced dementia may interfere with the control of muscles. Movements may become slow and less coordinated, and muscles may become weak. Speaking may become impossible. Swallowing may be difficult, and choking may occur, leading to undernutrition and dehydration. Walking or getting out of bed may be very difficult, even with help. As a result, pressure sores and infections, such as pneumonia, are more likely to develop. People with advanced dementia may have seizures.

People with dementia become totally dependent on others. Some people become totally unresponsive. Usually, death results from an infection, such as pneumonia, rather than from dementia itself.

Diagnosis

Family members or doctors may first suspect dementia when a person becomes unusually forgetful. Doctors or other health care practitioners can usually diagnose dementia by asking the person and family members questions.

Typically, the person is given a mental status test.[2] This test consists of questions and tasks, such as naming objects, recalling short lists, writing sentences, and copying shapes. Sometimes more detailed testing (called neuropsychologic testing) is needed, usually when the diagnosis is still unclear. This testing is similar but covers more areas of mental function: learning,

1. see page 346
2. see table on page 345

memory, problem-solving, abstract reasoning, orientation in time and space, attention, language, behavior, and mood. Neuropsychologic testing usually takes 1 to 3 hours. When evaluating the results of testing, doctors consider the person's age and educational level.

Family members are asked when the symptoms started, how symptoms developed, and how the person has changed—for example, has the person given up hobbies or stopped doing usual activities. Questions include what drugs the person is taking because a drug may be contributing to the dementia. Questions are asked about the person's emotional health because depression could be causing the symptoms or making them worse.

The diagnosis of dementia is based mainly on symptoms and the results of mental status testing. Dementia is diagnosed only if memory and at least one other area of mental function are impaired enough to affect daily activities.

Doctors usually perform a physical examination and order tests to check for disorders that may be causing the dementia or making it worse. For example, blood and urine tests are done to check for infections, vitamin deficiencies, and diabetes. If the symptoms or results of the physical examination suggest that the cause is a brain tumor, normal-pressure hydrocephalus, or a stroke, computed tomography (CT) or magnetic resonance imaging (MRI) may be done. However, the cause of the dementia can be confirmed definitively only when a sample of brain tissue is removed and examined under a microscope. This procedure is rarely done until after death (during an autopsy).

Treatment

For most people with dementia, no treatment can restore mental function. Correcting conditions that may contribute to dementia and providing a supportive environment can sometimes help slow the mental decline and maintain the person's quality of life. Certain drugs sometimes help. The person with dementia, family members, other caregivers, and the health care practitioners involved should discuss these measures and decide which measures seem most appropriate.

Correcting conditions that may contribute to dementia: Treating disorders that are contributing to dementia sometimes slows mental decline. For people who have dementia and depression, antidepressants and counseling may help, at least temporarily.[1] Abstaining from alcohol can result in long-term improvement. Drugs that may be making the dementia worse are discontinued if possible.

Providing a supportive environment: People with dementia benefit from an environment that is familiar, safe, and stable. But it should not be boring. Some stimulation is important. The environment should also be designed to help with orientation. For example, windows enable people to know generally what time of day it is.

Usually at first, people with dementia function best in a familiar environment and can remain at home. Moving to a new home, rearranging furniture, or even repainting rooms can be disruptive and cause symptoms to worsen.

Extra safety measures are usually needed. Homes can be evaluated for safety by a home health agency, which can suggest needed changes. For example, lighting should be relatively bright. In dim light, people with dementia are more likely to misinterpret what they see, become disoriented, and possibly fall. Leaving a night-light on or installing motion sensor lights may also help. Items that could be dangerous (such as guns, drugs, bleach, paint, and sharp knives) should be kept in locked cabinets.

Certain measures help people do daily activities safely. For example, safety reminders (such as "remember to turn the stove off") can be posted, or timers can be installed on stoves or electrical equipment. Placing detectors on doors may help prevent people from wandering and having accidents. If wandering is a problem, an identification bracelet or necklace is essential.

At some point, people with dementia can no longer drive safely.[2] Some people decide on their own to stop driving. But others need to be persuaded or convinced. Health care practitioners may be able to help. Sometimes measures, such as removing the car keys or the car, must be taken to prevent people with dementia from continuing to drive.

Following a daily routine for such activities as bathing, eating, and sleeping helps people with dementia remember. A routine also gives them a sense of security and stability. The routine

1. see pages 448 to 452
2. see page 927

should be as simple and stress-free as possible. However, the routine should include pleasurable and useful activities, such as listening to music, walking, folding laundry, making the bed, and interacting with other people. Such activities can help people feel independent and needed, enhancing self-esteem. Mental activities can help keep people alert and interested in life and help relieve depression. Physical activities and exercise help relieve stress and frustration.[1] Physically active people are less likely to become agitated, to wander, and to have problems sleeping.

Activities related to the person's interests before dementia began are good choices. Activities should provide some stimulation but should not involve too many choices or challenges. Short activities are best. They should be enjoyable and not be used as tests of mental function. Activities should be modified as the dementia worsens. People with dementia can continue to do familiar activities when caregivers divide the activity into small, simple parts.

Measures that help orient people include a daily calendar, a clock with numbers that are easy to read, and good lighting. Also, family members or caregivers can make frequent comments that remind people with dementia of where they are and what is going on.

Providing a supportive environment at home for a demented person may involve getting extra help. Family members can get a list of available services from health care practitioners, social or human services (listed in the telephone book), or the Internet (through Eldercare Locator). Services may include housekeeping, respite care, meals brought to the home, and daycare programs and activities designed for people with dementia. Around-the-clock care can be arranged but is expensive.

Because dementia is progressive, people with dementia may not be able to remain at home indefinitely. Long before a person with dementia needs to be moved to a more supportive and structured environment, family members should plan for this move and evaluate the options for long-term care.[2] Deciding when the move is necessary is difficult. Family members may want to maintain the person's sense of independence and keep

1. see page 910
2. see page 190

the person in a familiar environment as long as possible. When making decisions about long-term care, family members must consider many factors, including the severity of the person's symptoms, the home environment, the availability of family members and caregivers, financial resources, and the presence of other disorders and needs. Doctors, social workers, nurses, and lawyers can help with these decisions.

Some long-term care facilities, including assisted living facilities and nursing homes, specialize in caring for people with dementia. Staff members are trained to understand how people with dementia think and act and how to respond to them. Staff members get to know the residents and their needs. These facilities have routines that make the residents feel secure and provide appropriate activities that help them feel productive and involved in life. Most facilities have safety features appropriate for people with dementia. For example, signs are posted to help residents find their way, and certain doors have locks or alarms to prevent residents from wandering.

Some people with dementia worsen when they are moved from their home to a long-term care facility. However, after a short time, most people adjust and function better in the more supportive environment.

Slowing the progression of dementia: A group of drugs called cholinesterase inhibitors (such as donepezil, galantamine, and rivastigmine) may stabilize or improve mental function. They may slow the progression of dementia, but they cannot stop it. These drugs were developed to treat Alzheimer's disease but may be useful for other dementias. Cholinesterase inhibitors prevent acetylcholine (which helps nerve cells communicate) from breaking down. As a result, the level of acetylcholine in the brain increases. Cholinesterase inhibitors are most useful early in dementia. Their effectiveness varies considerably from person to person. About one third of people do not benefit. About one third improve slightly for a few months. The rest improve considerably for a longer time, but the dementia eventually progresses. If one cholinesterase inhibitor is ineffective or has side effects, another should be tried. If the ones tried are ineffective or have side effects, they should be discontinued. The most common side effects include nausea, vomiting, weight loss, and abdominal pain or cramps. Tacrine, the first cholinesterase inhibitor developed for treating dementia, is rarely used anymore because of its side effects. Donepezil, galantamine, and rivastigmine are less likely to have side effects.

A new drug called memantine is being studied. It slows the progression of dementia, but it cannot stop it. Memantine works differently from cholinesterase inhibitors and may be used with them. The combination may be more effective than a cholinesterase inhibitor alone.

Ergoloid mesylates, such as dihydroergotoxine, used to be given to prevent mental function from declining. However, they do not help.

An extract of ginkgo biloba (called EGb) is a dietary supplement claimed to enhance memory.[1] Ginkgo has stabilized or improved mental and social function in some people with dementia in its early stages. However, studies of ginkgo have had inconsistent results, and high doses may have side effects. Other dietary supplements have been tried but have generally proved of little value in treating dementia. They include acetyl-L carnitine, choline, and lecithin.

Certain vitamins are also sometimes prescribed for dementia. In one large study, use of vitamin E, an antioxidant, resulted in modest improvements in mental function. Vitamin C and folic acid are sometimes used, but the evidence of their benefit is less conclusive.

Managing symptoms: Agitation or disruptive behavior is best managed by understanding how people with dementia view the world and modifying their environment accordingly. For example, when being given a bath, a person with dementia may not understand what is being done and may feel under attack. Taking time to explain exactly what is being done can help prevent a fight. Caregivers can learn how to respond to disruptive behavior and thus calm the person more quickly and sometimes prevent the behavior. Such information can be obtained from health care practitioners, health organizations, the Internet, and support groups.

Drugs are usually not the best way to manage disruptive behavior. But drugs are often used to reduce the agitation and outbursts that may accompany advanced dementia. They are also

1. see page 78

sometimes used when efforts to calm and reassure (including changes in the environment) do not prevent unwanted behavior. These drugs include those used to prevent seizures (anticonvulsants, such as valproate) and those used to treat loss of contact with reality (antipsychotic drugs). Antipsychotic drugs are most effective in people who have hallucinations, delusions, or paranoia in addition to agitation. Antipsychotic drugs often cause serious side effects, such as drowsiness, shakiness, and falls. They can also worsen confusion. If antipsychotic drugs are used, family members should talk with the doctor about whether the drugs are really helping. Family members may also ask whether newer antipsychotic drugs (such as olanzapine and quetiapine) are being used. These drugs are as effective as older antipsychotic drugs (such as haloperidol or thioridazine) but have fewer side effects. Cholinesterase inhibitors, used to improve mental function and slow the progression of dementia, may also help control disruptive behavior.

For people who have problems sleeping, changes in daily routines can often help.[1] For example, people should be encouraged and helped to exercise regularly and to participate in more activities. Thus, they may sleep less during the day and more at night. Following a regular routine at bedtime may also help. Foods and beverages that contain caffeine should not be consumed late in the day.

If changes in daily routines are ineffective, doctors may consider using a drug to promote sleep (a sleep aid or a sedative). Any of these drugs can impair mental function, make a person more confused, and increase the risk of falling and fractures. So if used, these drugs are given in low doses and discontinued as soon as possible. For older people, some sedatives, such as trazodone (also an antidepressant), may be safer than others. Benzodiazepines (such as flurazepam and temazepam), a type of sedative, are usually not a good choice. Benzodiazepines are more likely than other types of sedatives to impair mental function, cause sleepiness the next day, and lead to falls.

Treating pain and other unrelated disorders may also help. However, health care practitioners may have difficulty identifying pain or other disorders because people with dementia may not be able to report symptoms. An abrupt change in behavior,

1. see page 426

such as increased agitation, may indicate development of pain or a disorder, such as a urinary tract infection or constipation, and should be reported to a health care practitioner.

End-of-life issues: Before dementia becomes severe, decisions should be made about medical care and finances. People with dementia, if able, should appoint a health care proxy, who is legally authorized to make treatment decisions on their behalf. They should discuss their health care wishes with their proxy and doctor, then decide on and write down advance directives.[1] For example, while still able, people with dementia should decide whether they want artificial feeding or antibiotics to treat infections (such as pneumonia) when dementia is very advanced.

As dementia worsens, treatment tends to be directed at comfort rather than at attempts to prolong life. Often, aggressive treatments, such as artificial feeding, increase discomfort. In contrast, less drastic treatments can relieve discomfort. These treatments include adequate control of pain, skin care (to prevent pressure sores),[2] and attentive nursing care. Nursing care is most helpful when it is provided by one caregiver (or a few) who develops a consistent relationship with the person. A comforting, reassuring voice and soothing music may also help.

ALZHEIMER'S DISEASE

In Alzheimer's disease, the ability to remember, think, understand, communicate, and control behavior progressively declines because brain tissue degenerates.

Alzheimer's disease accounts for most dementias in older people. It is very rare among people under 60. Alzheimer's disease becomes more common as people age. It affects only about 1 to 3% of people aged 60 to 64 but up to 30% of those over 85. In the United States, about 4 million people have Alzheimer's disease.

In Alzheimer's disease, brain tissue degenerates in a particular way. Nerve cells are lost. Tangles (neurofibrillary tangles) form in nerve cells, and clumps (senile or amyloid plaques)

---

1. see page 953
2. see page 506

TANGLES AND PLAQUES

Neurofibrillary tangles are proteins that have deteriorated and become twisted in nerve cells. These tangles look like knots in a rope. Senile (amyloid) plaques form when nerve cells die, and an abnormal form of a protein called amyloid collects on the clumps of dead cells. Tangles and plaques interfere with the communication between functioning nerve cells in the brain. They may also cause the death of nearby nerve cells. Such abnormalities develop to some degree in all people as they age but are much more numerous in people with Alzheimer's disease.

Tangles and plaques first appear in a memory processing center deep within the temporal lobe of the brain. This center helps the brain form new memories and retrieve old ones. As Alzheimer's disease progresses, tangles and plaques form in other areas. These areas help the brain form and retrieve complex memories and are involved in the production and expression of emotions. Eventually, tangles and plaques form in the outer layer of the brain (cerebral cortex). This area is involved in many mental functions, including reasoning, memory, language, and interpretation of perceptions.

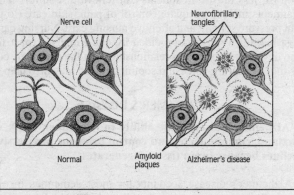

Nerve cell

Neurofibrillary tangles

Normal

Amyloid plaques

Alzheimer's disease

form between nerve cells. People with Alzheimer's disease also have a low level of acetylcholine in the brain. Acetylcholine is a chemical that helps nerve cells communicate with one another.

Some people with Alzheimer's disease also have atherosclerosis. Atherosclerosis can lead to strokes, which sometimes result in vascular dementia. Thus, such people may have two types of dementia (mixed dementia).

Causes

What causes degeneration of brain tissue in Alzheimer's disease is unknown. For most people, the cause seems to be a combination of genes and environment. But the environmental factors involved are not yet known. For some people, genes appear to be more important. The disease seems to run in some families, particularly when it develops at an early age.

ADDITIONAL DETAIL

One of the genes involved in Alzheimer's disease affects a protein called apolipoprotein E (apo E). This protein is one part of lipoproteins, which transport cholesterol through the bloodstream. The gene determines which type of apo E a person has: ∈ 2, ∈ 3, or ∈ 4. People with the ∈ 4 type are more likely to develop Alzheimer's disease than other people. In contrast, people with the ∈ 2 type may have some protection against Alzheimer's disease. People with the ∈ 3 type are neither protected nor more likely to develop the disease. (These associations have been studied primarily in white people and may not apply to other races.) Genetic testing for apo E type cannot definitively determine whether a person will develop Alzheimer's disease. Therefore, this testing is not routinely recommended.

Symptoms

The symptoms of Alzheimer's disease are similar to those of other dementias.[1] They include memory loss, changes in personality, problems using language, disorientation, difficulty doing daily activities, and disruptive behavior. A person with Alzheimer's disease may not have all the symptoms.

Symptoms usually begin subtly. People may not notice any changes at first, depending on what activities they are involved in. At some point, people with Alzheimer's disease may notice they are not doing their job or activities quite as well as in the past.

In most people with Alzheimer's disease, the first sign is forgetting recent events. But the disease may begin with changes in personality. For example, people may become emotionally unresponsive, depressed, or unusually fearful or anxious. Or

1. see pages 356 to 360

emotions may rapidly and unpredictably change from one extreme to another. Early in the disease, people have difficulty using language. They may use a general word or many words rather than a specific word, use words incorrectly, or be unable to find the right word. They become less able to use good judgment and think abstractly.

Disruptive or inappropriate behavior is common. People with Alzheimer's disease may become agitated, irritable, hostile, and physically aggressive. Many of them wander.

Many people with Alzheimer's disease have insomnia. They have trouble falling or staying asleep. Some people become confused about day and night. Thinking it is day, they may get up and get dressed in the middle of the night.

As Alzheimer's disease progresses, some people have psychotic symptoms, such as hallucinations, delusions, or paranoia.

Progression is unpredictable. After symptoms begin, people live, on average, 8 to 10 years. During a good part of this time, many people continue to enjoy much of what they enjoyed before developing Alzheimer's disease. But eventually, as in all dementias, memory is completely lost, and people with Alzheimer's disease become totally dependent on others. Once people can no longer walk, they live, on average, about 6 months. However, there is considerable variation, and some bed-bound people live for several years.

Diagnosis

If dementia is diagnosed in an older person and the person's memory has gradually deteriorated, doctors suspect Alzheimer's disease. The diagnosis is based partly on symptoms, which are identified by asking the person and family members or other caregivers questions. The diagnosis is also based on a physical examination and the results of tests, such as mental status tests, blood and urine tests, and computed tomography (CT) or magnetic resonance imaging (MRI). This information helps doctors exclude other types and causes of dementia. Such a diagnosis is correct most of the time.

The diagnosis of Alzheimer's disease can be confirmed only when a sample of brain tissue is removed (rarely done until after death) and examined under a microscope. Then, the characteristic loss of nerve cells, neurofibrillary tangles, and senile plaques can be seen throughout the brain. Positron emission tomography (PET) and analysis of spinal fluid have been suggested as ways to diagnose Alzheimer's disease. However, these tests are not yet accurate enough for widespread use.

Treatment

Generally, treatment of Alzheimer's disease is the same as that of all dementias.[1] Cholinesterase inhibitors may stabilize or slightly improve mental function (including memory). But they cannot stop the progression of Alzheimer's disease. Ginkgo biloba is sometimes used. Evidence of its effectiveness is inconclusive.

Researchers continue to study drugs that may prevent or slow the progression of Alzheimer's disease. Nonsteroidal anti-inflammatory drugs (NSAIDs), commonly used to treat arthritis, are an example. Vitamin E may also help prevent and slow progression of the disease, although study results are unclear. Before any of these substances are taken, their risks and benefits should be discussed with a doctor.

If people with Alzheimer's disease also have atherosclerosis, conditions that make atherosclerosis worse (and thus stroke more likely) are corrected or eliminated.[2]

VASCULAR DEMENTIA

In vascular dementia (multi-infarct dementia), the ability to remember, think, understand, communicate, and control behavior declines because of brain damage due to strokes.

Abilities often decline in steps (after each stroke), but they can decline more gradually. Unlike other types of dementia, vascular dementia can sometimes be prevented by correcting or eliminating the risk factors for strokes.[3]

Vascular dementia often occurs with Alzheimer's disease (as mixed dementia). The strokes that cause vascular dementia are more common among men and usually begin after age 70. Risk

1. see page 361
2. see pages 384 and 628
3. see page 375

factors for vascular dementia include high blood pressure, abnormal heart rhythms, diabetes, and atherosclerosis. These disorders damage blood vessels in or leading to the brain. People who smoke or have smoked are also at increased risk.

In a stroke, the blood supply to an area of the brain is blocked, causing brain tissue in that area to die.[1] The dead tissue is called an infarct. Dementia may result from a few large strokes or from many small strokes (a disorder called Binswanger's disease).

Symptoms

Unlike Alzheimer's disease, vascular dementia may progress in steps. Symptoms may worsen suddenly, then remain the same (plateau). Months or years later when another stroke occurs, symptoms worsen again. Dementia that results from many small strokes progresses more gradually than that due to a few large strokes.

Symptoms are similar to those of other dementias.[2] They include memory loss, difficulty doing usual daily activities, and a tendency to wander. Vascular dementia may affect judgment and personality less than Alzheimer's disease does. Also, symptoms can vary depending on what area of the brain is affected. Usually, some aspects of mental function are not affected, because the strokes destroy tissue in only part of the brain. People with vascular dementia are thought to be more aware of their losses and more prone to depression than people with Alzheimer's disease. Death usually occurs about 5 years after symptoms begin. Death is often due to a stroke or heart attack.

Diagnosis and Treatment

Once dementia is diagnosed, doctors suspect vascular dementia if a person has risk factors for a stroke or symptoms of a stroke. These symptoms include partial loss of sight, slow and slurred speech, weakness or paralysis of one leg, and difficulty walking. Computed tomography (CT) or magnetic resonance imaging (MRI) may be done. Results of these tests can support the diagnosis but are not definitive.

Generally, treatment of vascular dementia is the same as that

1. see page 374
2. see pages 356 to 360

for all dementias.[1] Treatment also includes measures to prevent more strokes.[2] For example, treating disorders that increase the risk of a stroke, such as atherosclerosis, coronary artery disease, high blood pressure, diabetes, and abnormal heart rhythms, may help prevent vascular dementia or slow or stop its progression. Modifying other risk factors for stroke is also recommended. For example, people who smoke should stop.

Many strokes are caused by blood clots. Therefore, anticoagulants, which make blood less likely to clot, are given to some people who are at risk of developing clots. Taking aspirin can also help prevent blood clots. Warfarin, a strong anticoagulant, is given to some people who have an abnormal heart rhythm (particularly atrial fibrillation), which can lead to stroke.

LEWY BODY DEMENTIA

In Lewy body dementia, mental abilities decline because abnormal round deposits of protein (called Lewy bodies) develop in nerve cells throughout the brain.

Lewy bodies result in the death of nerve cells. Lewy bodies also develop in people with Parkinson's disease but only in one part of the brain.

Lewy body dementia is a relatively common dementia. It usually affects people over 65 and affects more men than women. Its cause is unknown.

Symptoms

The symptoms of Lewy body dementia are similar to those of Alzheimer's disease. They include memory loss, disorientation, and problems remembering, thinking, understanding, communicating, and controlling behavior. However, Lewy body dementia is more likely to cause psychotic symptoms, such as paranoia, delusions, and hallucinations. Hallucinations tend to develop earlier than in Alzheimer's disease. They are usually visual and often complex and detailed (including recognizable people and animals). They may be pleasant.

In the early stages of Lewy body dementia (unlike Alzheimer's

1. see page 361
2. see page 384

disease), mental function varies from day to day, often dramatically. One day, people may be able to converse coherently. The next day, they may be inattentive, drowsy, and almost mute. Fainting is common.

People with Lewy body dementia, like those with Parkinson's disease, move slowly and sluggishly, shuffle when they walk, stoop over, and have stiff muscles. Consequently, the risk of falling is increased. Trembling (tremors) occurs in a few people, but it is milder than that in Parkinson's disease. After symptoms begin, people live about 6 to 12 years.

Diagnosis and Treatment

Once dementia is diagnosed, doctors suspect Lewy body dementia if the symptoms fluctuate and if the person has visual hallucinations and symptoms of Parkinson's disease.

Generally, treatment of Lewy body dementia is the same as that for all dementias.[1] The same drugs used to treat Alzheimer's disease, particularly rivastigmine, may be helpful.

Using antipsychotic drugs to treat psychotic symptoms may make the tremors and other symptoms of Parkinson's disease much worse, sometimes resulting in death. Using drugs to treat the symptoms of Parkinson's disease may make the psychotic symptoms worse.

28

Stroke

A stroke occurs when part of the brain is deprived of blood for too long a time. That part of the brain dies because the brain cannot survive for long without oxygen and nutrients, which are supplied by blood. A stroke causes permanent brain damage.

A stroke can strike with the suddenness and devastation of a

1. see page 361

lightning bolt, sometimes permanently disabling a person. Thus, stroke is one of the most feared disorders, particularly by older people.

Stroke is a leading cause of disability and death worldwide. For people over 55, the risk of stroke more than doubles every 10 years. Most people who die of a stroke are over 65. Stroke affects women and men, and more than half of people who die of a stroke are women.

Even though a stroke causes permanent brain damage, most people recover. How well they recover varies, depending largely on how severe the stroke was. People may recover fully or be disabled slightly, severely, or anywhere in between. Early treatment may result in less brain damage and a better recovery. Consequently, knowing the early symptoms of stroke is important. Then people can seek treatment right away.

There are two types of strokes: ischemic and hemorrhagic. In ischemic stroke, something prevents blood from reaching part of the brain. The most common cause is blockage of an artery. About 85% of strokes are ischemic strokes.

In hemorrhagic stroke, a blood vessel bursts. As a result, blood escapes into or around brain tissue. This blood can irritate brain tissue and can rapidly accumulate. The accumulating blood causes swelling, putting pressure on and damaging brain tissue. The accumulating blood also interferes with the blood supply to brain tissue. Hemorrhagic strokes usually involve bleeding within the brain (intracerebral hemorrhage) or bleeding between two of the layers of tissue covering the brain (subarachnoid hemorrhage). Among people over 60, intracerebral hemorrhage is more common than subarachnoid hemorrhage.

Causes

Certain conditions (called risk factors) make a person more likely to have a stroke. They include abnormal cholesterol levels, atherosclerosis (sometimes called hardening of the arteries), some heart disorders (such as abnormal heart rhythms, heart valve disorders, and heart attacks), high blood pressure, and diabetes. Smoking cigarettes, being physically inactive, being overweight, and drinking large amounts of alcohol also increase the risk of stroke.

CLOGS AND CLOTS: CAUSES OF ISCHEMIC STROKES

When an artery that carries blood to the brain becomes clogged or blocked, an ischemic stroke can occur. Arteries may be blocked by accumulations of materials (plaques) due to atherosclerosis. Arteries in the neck, particularly the carotid arteries, are a common site for plaques. Arteries may also be blocked by a blood clot (thrombus). Blood clots may form on a plaque in an artery. Clots may also form in the heart of people with a heart disorder. Part of a clot may break off and travel through the bloodstream to block an artery that supplies blood to the brain, such as one of the cerebral arteries.

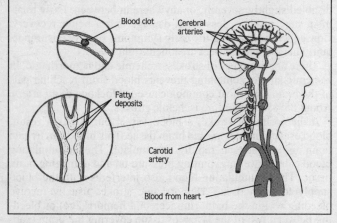

Blood clot
Cerebral arteries
Fatty deposits
Carotid artery
Blood from heart

People who have had a transient ischemic attack (TIA) are more likely to have a stroke—most commonly within the next month and often within 2 days. In a TIA, something temporarily interrupts the blood supply to the brain. The risk factors for a TIA are the same as those for stroke.

Other conditions may increase the risk of stroke, but the connection is less clear. They include inflammation (such as that in periodontal disease or rheumatoid arthritis), a tendency for blood to clot too easily, and a high level of homocysteine in the blood (hyperhomocysteinemia). A high level of homocysteine, an amino acid, may increase the risk of stroke by increasing the risk of atherosclerosis and by making blood more likely to clot. As people age, the homocysteine level increases.

The risk factors for ischemic and some types of hemorrhagic strokes can overlap.

BURSTS AND BREAKS: CAUSES OF HEMORRHAGIC STROKES

When blood vessels of the brain are weak, abnormal, or under unusual pressure, a hemorrhagic stroke can occur. In hemorrhagic strokes, bleeding may occur within the brain (as an intracerebral hemorrhage). Or bleeding may occur between the inner and middle layers of tissue covering the brain (as a subarachnoid hemorrhage). The brain is covered by three layers of tissue: an outer layer (dura mater), a middle layer (arachnoid mater), and an inner layer (pia mater).

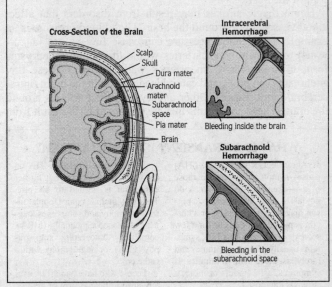

Cross-Section of the Brain

Scalp
Skull
Dura mater
Arachnoid mater
Subarachnoid space
Pia mater
Brain

Intracerebral Hemorrhage

Bleeding inside the brain

Subarachnoid Hemorrhage

Bleeding in the subarachnoid space

ADDITIONAL DETAIL

Ischemic strokes may result from disorders in which arteries can become blocked by accumulation of material or by a blood clot (thrombus). For example, in atherosclerosis, fatty material, calcium, and other materials gradually accumulate in the walls of arteries, forming a plaque (atheroma). Eventually, the plaque may completely block an artery that carries blood to the brain, often the carotid artery (in the neck). Also, blood clots can develop on a plaque, blocking even more of the artery. Part of the blood clot may break off, travel through the bloodstream (becoming an embolus), and eventually block an artery that carries blood to the brain.

An ischemic stroke may result from heart disorders that can cause blood clots to form in the heart. The clots may break off and eventually block an artery that carries blood to the brain. These disorders include abnormal heart rhythms (arrhythmias) such as atrial fibrillation, heart valve disorders, heart attacks (due to coronary artery disease), and bulges (aneurysms) in the wall of the heart.

Hemorrhagic strokes may result from disorders that affect blood vessels in or around the brain. High blood pressure is an example. High blood pressure can cause tiny bulges (aneurysms) to form in small arteries within the brain. (Aneurysms form in areas where an artery's wall is weak.) These tiny aneurysms can break and cause bleeding within the brain (intracerebral hemorrhage). Other aneurysms affect arteries around the brain. These aneurysms may be present at birth, result from

WHAT IS A TRANSIENT ISCHEMIC ATTACK?

A transient ischemic attack (TIA) causes symptoms similar to those of a stroke, but the symptoms do not last as long. For example, a person may feel as if a shade or a curtain is pulled over one eye for a few seconds or minutes. In a TIA, symptoms usually resolve in minutes and rarely last more than 90 minutes. If symptoms last 24 hours or more, a stroke is diagnosed.

A TIA is sometimes mistakenly called a ministroke. However, there is nothing "mini" about it. A TIA is a sign that a stroke may occur soon. The risk of having a stroke is greatest during the next month, but a stroke often follows within 2 days. People who have had a TIA need to see a doctor immediately.

Doctors may suspect a TIA on the basis of symptoms, but further evaluation is needed to be sure. Tests may include color Doppler ultrasonography and sometimes magnetic resonance angiography (MRA), computed tomography angiography (CTA), or angiography with a catheter.

People who have had a TIA usually need to take aspirin or another antiplatelet drug as directed by their doctor. Anticoagulants may be used if the TIA resulted from temporary blockage by part of a blood clot (embolus) that traveled from the heart. Sometimes a surgical procedure called endarterectomy or one called angioplasty is done to open the partially blocked artery.

an injury, or develop over time. They can break and cause bleeding between two of the layers of tissue covering the brain (subarachnoid hemorrhage). The affected arteries may contract (constrict) several days later, cutting off the blood supply, and thus cause an ischemic stroke as well.

Some older people have amyloid angiopathy. It causes blood vessels to become more fragile and thus increases the risk of hemorrhagic stroke. Amyloid angiopathy is especially common among people with Alzheimer's disease.

Infrequently, a hemorrhagic stroke results from an abnormal connection between an artery and a vein (arteriovenous malformation) in or around the brain. The abnormal blood vessels can break, causing a subarachnoid or an intracerebral hemorrhage. Arteriovenous malformations may be present at birth or develop over time.

A hemorrhagic stroke may result from an ischemic stroke. The lack of blood and oxygen resulting from the ischemic stroke damages blood vessels, weakening their walls.

A high level of total cholesterol, low-density lipoprotein cholesterol (LDL, the "bad" cholesterol), or triglycerides (another fat in the blood) increases the risk of stroke. A low level of high-density lipoprotein cholesterol (HDL, the "good" cholesterol) also increases the risk.

Symptoms

Symptoms of a stroke occur suddenly, sometimes instantaneously. They may worsen over a period of hours or sometimes days.

Symptoms of a stroke last for at least 24 hours. If symptoms do not last that long and if bleeding is not the cause, the disorder is considered a transient ischemic attack, not a stroke. Most transient ischemic attacks last less than 90 minutes.

Everyone should know what the common early symptoms of a stroke are. Most strokes, whether ischemic or hemorrhagic, cause one or more of the following early symptoms:

• **Sudden difficulty moving or sudden abnormal sensations on one side of the body.** The affected part may feel weak or be unable to move (paralyzed). Or it may tingle, feel prickly, or be numb. One arm or leg, half of the face, or all of one side of the body may be affected.

• **Sudden difficulty speaking or understanding speech.** Speech may be slurred, or a person may suddenly become confused.

• **Sudden changes in vision, particularly in one eye.** Vision may be dim, blurred, double, or lost.

• **Sudden loss of balance and coordination or sudden dizziness.** Dizziness may involve unsteadiness or a sensation of spinning (vertigo). Falls may result.

• **Sudden, severe headache with no apparent cause.** A hemorrhagic stroke due to a subarachnoid hemorrhage typically begins with a sudden, severe headache.

Other symptoms may occur early or later. They include difficulty swallowing, difficulty walking, partial loss of hearing, uncontrollable leakage of urine (urinary incontinence), and loss of control of bowel movements (fecal incontinence). Remembering, perceiving, understanding, and learning things may be difficult. People may have difficulty remembering where they are, what time it is, and who other people are (orientation problems). They may be unable to pay attention and concentrate. Their thoughts may be disorganized. Some people cannot recognize parts of their body. They may be unaware of the stroke's effects.

Many people have problems with speech and language. For example, they may have difficulty expressing themselves or understanding other people (aphasia) or difficulty physically forming words (dysarthria).[1] A stroke can cause depression or an inability to control emotions. People may cry or laugh at inappropriate times. Some people continue to have these symptoms, even after treatment and rehabilitation.

Strokes, particularly hemorrhagic strokes, can cause nausea, vomiting, and drowsiness. Sometimes a stroke results in a coma. People may suddenly go into a coma. Or they may become progressively drowsy and unresponsive until they cannot be aroused. Some strokes cause blood pressure to go up and down erratically and cause breathing and heart rate to become irregular.

1. see page 186

WHY STROKES AFFECT ONLY ONE SIDE OF THE BODY

Most commonly, strokes damage only one part of the brain at a time. Often, part of the cerebrum is damaged. The cerebrum, the largest part of the brain, consists of two halves: the right and left hemispheres. The right hemisphere controls the left side of the body, and vice versa. Because most strokes damage only one side of the brain, they affect only one side of the body—the side opposite the stroke damage. The opposite side is affected because nerves from one side of the brain cross over to the other side of the body.

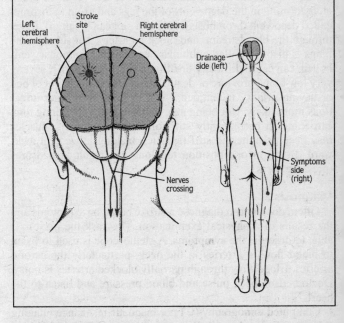

Which symptoms occur and how serious they are depend not only on how much of the brain is affected but also on which part of the brain is affected. Some small strokes cause more devastating symptoms than some large strokes. How many strokes occur also affects symptoms. People who have one stroke may have problems with memory or thinking. If they continue to have strokes, dementia may result.

With some strokes, symptoms are most severe immediately

after the stroke occurs. With other strokes, symptoms become progressively worse, causing the greatest loss of function after a few hours up to a day or two. This type of stroke is called an evolving stroke, a progressing stroke, or a stroke in evolution.

Sometimes a stroke leads to other problems. For example, immediately after a stroke, an arm may be weak, numb, or paralyzed and thus be more easily injured. If swallowing is difficult (whether a person notices it or not), food or saliva may be inhaled into the windpipe and reach the lungs. Aspiration pneumonia may result. Being unable to move can result in blood clots forming in the deep veins of the legs and groin (a disorder called deep vein thrombosis). Part of a clot can break off, travel through the bloodstream, and block an artery that supplies the lungs (a disorder called pulmonary embolism). Pulmonary embolism can cause difficulty breathing, chest pain, and, if severe, very low blood pressure or death. Being unable to get out of bed or having urinary incontinence can make urinary tract infections more likely. Not being able to move joints for a long time can result in permanently stiff joints (contractures). Muscles may become tight and stiff (spastic), making movement awkward. Being in one position too long can result in bedsores (pressure sores).

Diagnosis

Often, doctors can diagnose a stroke based on symptoms and the results of a physical examination. They ask the person, if able, to describe the symptoms. A stethoscope is used to listen to blood flow in arteries in the neck, particularly the carotid arteries. Blood flow through partially blocked arteries is noisy. Doctors also check pulse and blood pressure and listen to the heart.

Computed tomography (CT) or magnetic resonance imaging (MRI) of the head is usually promptly done. CT and MRI help doctors determine whether symptoms are caused by a stroke or another brain disorder, such as a brain tumor or traumatic injury. These tests also help doctors distinguish a hemorrhagic stroke from an ischemic stroke. They can show how much and which part of the brain is affected.

Blood tests can also help doctors determine whether symptoms are caused by a stroke or another disorder. For example, the level of sugar is measured, because a low blood sugar level can cause symptoms similar to those of a stroke. Blood tests are also useful in identifying the cause of the stroke. For example, cholesterol levels are measured because abnormal levels can lead to a stroke. To determine whether the blood clots more easily than normal, doctors measure how long blood takes to clot.

Other tests are often done to identify the cause of the stroke, usually within the first few days. Identifying (and treating) the disorder that caused the stroke can help prevent later strokes. Which tests are done depends on the area of the brain affected, the type of stroke, and the person's medical history.

If an ischemic stroke is suspected, tests are done to check for blockages in arteries. Doctors often use Doppler ultrasonography first because it is painless and safe. Other tests, such as magnetic resonance angiography (MRA) and computed tomography angiography (CTA) may also be done. Magnetic resonance angiography uses radiofrequency waves produced in a magnetic field, and computed tomography angiography uses x-rays. Both tests can provide images of the arteries. In both tests, a substance may be injected into a blood vessel to outline the arteries.

Angiography with a catheter is the most accurate way to detect blockages.[1] However, angiography is an invasive test and is usually unnecessary. (Invasive tests involve cutting into or inserting instruments into the body.) Consequently, particularly for older people, angiography is done only when other tests have not provided enough information for a diagnosis or to help doctors decide on treatment. People with atherosclerosis are more likely to have problems after angiography. For this test, a thin, flexible tube (catheter) is inserted into an artery and threaded into the arteries that supply blood to the brain.

Rarely, a spinal tap (lumbar puncture) is needed to help diagnose a subarachnoid hemorrhage. A spinal tap can detect blood in the spinal fluid, which surrounds the spinal cord. If a subarachnoid hemorrhage occurs, blood almost always appears in the spinal fluid. For this test, a needle is inserted in the lower back to withdraw a sample of spinal fluid, and the fluid is analyzed.

1. see page 132

Electrocardiography (ECG) may be done to check for abnormal heart rhythms and evidence of a recent heart attack.[1] A person may be asked to wear a portable ECG device that records heart rhythms continuously (Holter monitor). The monitor is usually worn for 24 hours or more.

Echocardiography (ultrasonography of the heart) may be done to check for blood clots, a heart valve disorder, or other structural abnormalities of the heart. For this test, a hand-held device that emits and records ultrasound waves is placed on the chest. Sometimes, to get a better view of the heart, doctors pass the device down the person's throat into the esophagus and behind the heart. This method is called transesophageal echocardiography. This test is generally safe but can cause gagging and anxiety. Therefore, doctors usually give the person a sedative beforehand.

Prevention

For strokes, an ounce of prevention is worth a pound of cure. Modifying—eliminating or controlling—risk factors for stroke can often help prevent strokes from occurring and from recurring.

Changes in lifestyle can modify many risk factors.[2] For example, people who smoke cigarettes can stop. After people stop smoking, their risk of having a stroke decreases to that of nonsmokers in about 2 to 5 years. People can increase their physical activity and, after checking with their doctor, start a regular exercise program. People who are overweight can lose weight. For people who drink alcoholic beverages, drinking in moderation (no more than 1 or 2 drinks a day for men and 1 drink a day for women) is recommended.

Sometimes modifying one risk factor modifies another. Stopping smoking, exercising, and losing weight help lower high blood pressure and high cholesterol levels as well as help control diabetes.

Eating a healthy, low-fat diet, including lots of fruits and vegetables,[3] can help reduce the risk of stroke in several ways. It helps people control their weight and keep their cholesterol

1. see page 661
2. see page 35
3. see page 41

levels in a healthy range. It also helps prevent or control diabetes. Limiting the amount of salt in the diet can help prevent or lower high blood pressure.

Having regular checkups is important. Doctors can then identify disorders that may lead to a stroke so that treatment can be started early. People should have their blood pressure checked at least twice a year.

If needed, disorders that can lead to a stroke are treated. High blood pressure can be lowered with antihypertensive drugs.[1] Diabetes can be controlled well with diet, drugs that are taken by mouth to lower blood sugar levels, and, if necessary, insulin injections.[2] High cholesterol levels can be lowered with cholesterol-lowering drugs, such as statins.[3] For people with coronary artery disease, taking a statin may reduce their risk of stroke.

For most people who are at risk of having a stroke or who have had a TIA or stroke, doctors recommend taking an antiplatelet drug such as aspirin to help prevent strokes. Platelets are particles in the blood that help blood clot when an injury occurs. Antiplatelet drugs make platelets less likely to clump and blood clots less likely to form. Other antiplatelet drugs, such as dipyridamole, clopidogrel, or ticlopidine, are sometimes used instead of or in addition to aspirin.

Warfarin (an anticoagulant) can help some people who have a heart disorder that can lead to a stroke, particularly atrial fibrillation. Anticoagulants (commonly called blood thinners) make blood less likely to clot. However, people who take warfarin must have blood tests periodically to check on how the anticoagulant, other drugs, diet, and other conditions are affecting the blood's ability to clot. If blood is taking too long to clot, excessive bleeding can occur.

If a blockage is detected in an artery in the neck (usually a carotid artery), surgery to remove the blockage may be done. This procedure, called an endarterectomy, may reduce the risk of ischemic stroke. However, the effectiveness and safety of the surgery depend on the skill of the surgeon and the resources of the hospital. Furthermore, any major surgery has risks. Angioplasty may be done instead. In angioplasty, a catheter with a

1. see table on page 618
2. see page 480
3. see table on page 630

balloon at its tip is threaded into the blocked artery. The balloon is then inflated to open the artery. To keep the artery open, doctors often insert a tube made of wire mesh (a stent) into the artery. Angioplasty with a stent is still considered experimental as a treatment of blocked carotid arteries.

Treatment

A person with any symptom suggesting a stroke should go to a hospital immediately, even if the symptom goes away quickly or does not cause pain. An ambulance should be called because the person may need emergency care as soon as possible. A person having a stroke may not know a stroke is occurring or may be unable to communicate. So anyone who suspects another person is having a stroke should call an emergency telephone number (usually 911) for help. Treatment is most likely to be effective when given soon after symptoms begin.

When a person who has had a stroke arrives at the hospital, the person's breathing, heart rate, and temperature are restored to normal if necessary. An intravenous line is inserted so that fluids and drugs can be given as needed. If the person has difficulty breathing, supplemental oxygen can be given. Sometimes a breathing tube is needed to help with breathing. If the person has a fever, it may be lowered using drugs (such as acetaminophen) or a cooling blanket. Tests are done to identify the cause of the stroke.

Specific treatment varies depending on the type of stroke.

Ischemic strokes: A drug called tissue plasminogen activator (tPA, or alteplase), which breaks up clots, is sometimes used. This drug must be given intravenously within 3 hours of the first symptoms. Because tPA helps restore blood flow, it may help limit the amount of brain damage. However, tPA can increase the risk of bleeding in or around the brain. Most people who have had an ischemic stroke cannot be given tPA, usually because they arrive at the emergency department too late or because they have a condition that makes tPA too risky. Risky conditions include very high blood pressure, a severe stroke, swelling in or around the brain, a head injury, recent surgery, and bleeding in the digestive tract.

If a stroke is worsening, heparin (an anticoagulant) is sometimes given to reduce the risk of blood clots. However, there is no evidence that heparin is beneficial in this situation.

In some specially equipped hospitals, other treatments for is-chemic strokes are being tried. For example, if people arrive at the hospital too late to be given tPA intravenously, they may be given this or a similar drug in another way. The drug is applied directly to the clot through a flexible tube (called a catheter) that is inserted in an artery and threaded to the clot.

Hemorrhagic strokes: After a hemorrhagic stroke, control-ling blood pressure—preventing it from becoming too high or too low—is important. Drugs such as mannitol may be given to decrease swelling in the brain and thus decrease pressure there. Occasionally, a drainage tube is placed in the brain to decrease pressure. Some people benefit from using a machine that helps them breathe (mechanical ventilation). For subarachnoid hem-orrhage, surgery or another procedure (with a catheter) may be done to repair an aneurysm or another abnormality and thus prevent bleeding from continuing or recurring.

Control of problems after a stroke: People who have had a stroke usually stay in the hospital for at least a few days. They are closely monitored. Tests such as x-rays may be done to check whether swallowing and certain other body functions are impaired. The disorder that caused or contributed to the stroke is treated as needed.

Some hospitals have specialized units that provide stroke care (stroke units). In stroke units, care is focused on prevention of the problems stroke can lead to and on rehabilitation.

Measures to prevent problems are started early. For example, a person is not given food or drink until doctors make sure the person can swallow well enough. This precaution helps prevent aspiration pneumonia. If a person has had an ischemic stroke, heparin or a similar drug may be injected under the skin to prevent blood clots from forming in the veins of the legs. Pneu-matic stockings may also be used to help prevent clots, particu-larly in people who have had a hemorrhagic stroke or who have a problem with blood clotting. Usually made of plastic, pneu-matic stockings are automatically pumped up and emptied by an electric pump. They repeatedly squeeze the calves and empty the veins. Thus, they help keep blood moving. They are worn as long as the person must remain in bed. If a person cannot turn over in bed, staff members turn the person frequently, and mat-tresses designed to minimize pressure on the skin are used. These measures help prevent pressure sores.

Rehabilitation, including physical therapy, is started in the hospital as soon as a person is physically able—usually within 1 or 2 days of admission.[1] Staying in bed for a long time can cause many problems,[2] so the person is encouraged to get up as soon as possible.

Because a stroke often causes mood changes (especially depression), staff members, family members, and friends should be on the lookout for signs of depression. They should tell the doctor if the person seems depressed. Depression can and should be treated.[3]

Long-term treatment: After the person is discharged from the hospital, rehabilitation can be continued in a rehabilitation center, at the hospital, in a nursing home, or at home. Rehabilitation can help many people regain some of their lost abilities. Rehabilitation helps people maintain and improve physical condition as well as relearn old skills and learn new ones.

Specific therapy is available for people who have difficulty walking, paralysis of one side, spastic muscles, lack of coordination, vision problems, problems with thinking (cognitive problems), and speech or language problems. Speech therapists can help people with language problems communicate more effectively. They may also help people who have problems swallowing learn to eat more safely.

Occupational and physical therapists can suggest ways to make life easier and the home safer. For example, they may suggest certain helpful devices.[4] There are devices to help with walking (such as canes, walkers, or braces), to help with daily activities (such as utensils with built-up grips and electric can openers), and to help with communication (such as picture boards or electronic communication devices).

Getting back to daily activities as much as possible helps people recover. Living on the first floor and having access to a car or a driver can help. The home may need to be modified to help a person function better. For example, grab bars may be installed in the bathroom, or a chair lift or glide may be attached to a rail that runs the length of the stairs. Having support from other people and being active can help prevent or lessen de-

1. see page 180
2. see page 148
3. see page 448
4. see box on page 177

pression. Depression can make people less interested in trying to regain lost abilities, doing daily activities, and spending time with people. Exercise helps preserve gains achieved during rehabilitation.[1]

Adjusting to life after a stroke is challenging for family members, other caregivers, and friends as well as for the person who had the stroke. Learning what effects the stroke has had (emotionally and physically) can help family members determine what kind of help is needed. For example, a person who has had a stroke may become angry or upset more easily. Knowing that strokes have this effect can help family members be patient and calm. People who have had a stroke, their family members, and other caregivers can also get help from support groups.

For people whose quality of life remains very poor despite treatment, care focuses on controlling pain, keeping the person comfortable, and providing fluids and nourishment. Many people with severe disabilities need care in a nursing home because their care is so demanding. However, some can remain at home if home health care or hospice care can be arranged.[2]

Outlook

A stroke may result in disability that is slight, severe, or anywhere in between. Some people need help at home. A few need care at a nursing home or another facility. Some people are never able to move, speak, or eat normally again. Some eventually recover completely. However, others die immediately or within days or weeks.

People recover most rapidly during the first 30 days after the stroke. Over the next 2 months, many people continue to recover, although somewhat less rapidly. Some people continue to recover for longer periods after the stroke.

Hemorrhagic strokes, particularly intracerebral hemorrhages, result in death more often than ischemic strokes. Intracerebral hemorrhages due to high blood pressure can be extensive and devastating. However, people who survive a hemorrhagic stroke may also recover. If the hemorrhage is small, people can recover to a remarkable degree. If a subarachnoid hemorrhage is treated before much brain damage occurs (that is, when the only

1. see page 913
2. see page 110

symptom is a headache), complete recovery may be possible. People who have had a hemorrhagic stroke may continue to improve for months, even years.

How well a person who has had a stroke can eventually function depends partly on the location and extent of brain damage and on the type of stroke. Rehabilitation is also important.

People who have had a stroke are at risk of having more strokes. Because strokes recur and progress unpredictably, people who have had a stroke should prepare advance directives[1] as soon as possible. People at risk of having a stroke should also do so. Advance directives help a health care practitioner determine what kind of medical care people want if they become unable to make these decisions. For example, whether to use treatments that sustain life artificially may have to be decided.

At age 69, I realize aging is a process of growth and deterioration of body and mind. At an early age my passion was to become a major league baseball player. Unfortunately, my love of baseball was not matched by my talent. All those years I loved baseball, I hated school. Then, at age 24, acquiring knowledge became my passion. The learning process became part of the aging process. Every waking hour that I wasn't working I was reading.

The more inquisitive I became, the more I wanted to write down my thoughts. Then at age 50, with great trepidation, I started to write in a journal. My fear was that I wouldn't have something worthwhile to write about every day. Today I'm into my 19th year writing in the journal, having missed only a few days. Every day I have the opportunity to be creative without having fear of criticism and rejection rearing its ugly head. I have completed my autobiography. I can't think of a better legacy to leave my kids and grandkids.

For me there is no greater passion than everlasting curiosity of how the world operates. It keeps my mind active. My love for learning provides me the highest level of serenity.

I believe mind and body will atrophy if I don't exercise them. We think of aging in negative terms. We see it as degradation. With people living longer the process is dragged out. However, I see "older" people staying involved with the world. Instead of accepting their fate, they recognize that life offers more when they challenge their minds.

Aging begins at birth. It is not only physical but mental. The aging process needs nurturing throughout one's life. Aging enables us to become the creative, imaginative human beings we were meant to be. Aging has allowed me to enjoy the miracles of the universe. There is such incredible beauty around us and within ourselves that we seem to take for granted. The real beauty is in the mysterious and unknown. The older I get the more opportunities I have to say, "Ah ha, I got it!"

There is no greater love than the love of learning.

Benny Wasserman

29

Nerve Disorders

In nerve disorders, the sense of touch (sensation) may be abnormal or lost. Or, weakness or paralysis may occur. Some nerve disorders cause pain or other unusual, often unpleasant sensations.

Billions of nerves connect the brain and spinal cord with the rest of the body. Some nerves, called sensory nerves, relay information to the brain from the rest of the body about what is happening inside and outside the body. Other nerves, called motor nerves, relay information to the rest of the body from the brain about how to respond to what is happening. Information is sent through nerves by electrical signals. When nerves are damaged, information is distorted or is not sent. Nerves may be damaged by pressure, injury, an inadequate blood supply, toxic substances, autoimmune disorders, or infections. Sometimes the cause is unknown.

Two terms commonly used to describe nerve disorders are "neuralgia" and "neuropathy." "Neuralgia" refers to pain that does not necessarily involve damage to nerves. "Neuropathy" refers to nerve damage that does not necessarily cause pain. One or more nerves may be damaged. A neuropathy may cause pain, abnormal sensations, loss of sensation, weakness, or a combination of these symptoms. Less commonly, a neuropathy affects body functions, such as blood pressure or sweating. The line between neuralgia and neuropathy is sometimes blurred, so some doctors do not distinguish between them.

TRIGEMINAL NEURALGIA

Trigeminal neuralgia (tic douloureux) is an intense, stabbing pain in the face. The pain results from a problem with

the nerve that connects parts of the face to the brain (the 5th cranial nerve, or trigeminal nerve).

Trigeminal neuralgia usually occurs in people over 50, particularly women.

Causes

The cause is often unknown. A common identifiable cause is a blood vessel (artery or vein) in an abnormal position. The blood vessel presses on the trigeminal nerve near the brain, where the nerve originates. Rarely, trigeminal neuralgia results from pressure due to a tumor or develops after an episode of shingles that affects the trigeminal nerve.

Symptoms and Diagnosis

Often, the pain is triggered by touching a particular spot (called a trigger point) on the face, lips, or tongue or by an activity such as brushing the teeth, shaving, talking, or chewing. But the pain may occur spontaneously.

Excruciating, stabbing pain occurs in repeated short, lightning-like bursts. Sometimes the disorder causes a dull, constant burning or aching, with occasional bursts of stabbing pain. The bursts of pain typically last seconds, but they may last up to 15 minutes. The pain may recur as often as 100 times a day. It can be incapacitating. Because the pain is intense, people tend to wince. Thus, the disorder is sometimes called a tic.

The pain is most often felt in the cheek next to the nose or in the jaw. But it can occur in any part of the forehead or lower face. Usually, only one side of the face is affected. When both sides are affected, they rarely hurt at the same time.

Doctors can usually diagnose trigeminal neuralgia based on its characteristic pain. Some tests may be done to determine what is causing the pain. For example, magnetic resonance imaging (MRI) or magnetic resonance angiography (MRA) may be done to check for a blood vessel in an abnormal position or a tumor.

Treatment and Outlook

Usually, typical pain relievers (analgesics) do not help. Gabapentin, a drug used to prevent seizures (anticonvulsant), may help. If gabapentin is ineffective or has intolerable side ef-

TAKING THE PRESSURE OFF A NERVE

When a blood vessel in an abnormal position presses on the trigeminal nerve, a surgical procedure called vascular decompression can relieve the pain. After a general anesthetic is given, an area on the back of the head is shaved, and an incision is made. The surgeon cuts a small hole in the skull and lifts the edge of the brain to expose the nerve. Then the surgeon separates the blood vessel from the nerve and places a small sponge between them.

The procedure is unlikely to cause problems. Problems that can occur include numbness and weakness of the face, double vision, infection, bleeding, changes in hearing and balance, and paralysis. Usually, the procedure relieves the pain, but in about 15% of people, pain recurs.

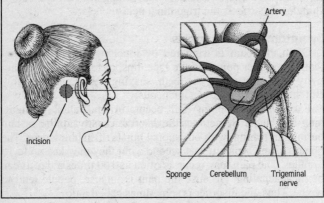

Artery

Incision

Sponge   Cerebellum   Trigeminal nerve

fects, other anticonvulsants, such as carbamazepine, phenytoin, or valproate, may be prescribed. Baclofen (a drug used to reduce muscle spasms) or a tricyclic antidepressant[1] may be used instead.

If the cause is a blood vessel in an abnormal position, surgery may be done. The blood vessel is separated from the nerve, and a small sponge is placed between them. This procedure usually relieves the pain for many years. If the cause is a tumor, the tumor can be surgically removed.

If drugs are ineffective and surgery to take pressure off the nerve is not possible, a test may be done to determine whether other treatments would help. For the test, an anesthetic is in-

1. see table on page 450

jected into the nerve to temporarily prevent the nerve from functioning. If the pain is relieved, a drug such as glycerol may be injected into the nerve through a needle inserted through the skin in the cheek. This treatment, called a nerve block, often provides relief for a few months to a few years. When discomfort in the face returns, another injection can be given. However, injections may become less effective as they are repeated.

Another option is cutting the nerve. The nerve can be cut surgically or with heat (applied by inserting a needle). This procedure relieves the pain permanently. But afterward, the face is likely to be numb.

Trigeminal neuralgia occurs in bouts or episodes. There may be long intervals without any episodes. How long these intervals will last cannot be predicted, and what makes the episodes stop and start is unknown.

POSTHERPETIC NEURALGIA

Postherpetic neuralgia is pain that persists after an episode of shingles (herpes zoster) has resolved. Usually, the pain develops during an episode and continues. But occasionally, the pain starts 4 months or more after an episode has resolved.

Shingles is a painful skin rash caused by reactivation of the virus that causes chickenpox (the varicella-zoster virus).[1] In many people, the pain of shingles gradually goes away over a period of a few weeks to a few months. But shingles leads to postherpetic neuralgia in up to half of people over 60 and up to three fourths of people over 70.

Postherpetic neuralgia lasts longer and is more severe in older people. It is more likely to develop if pain occurred before the skin rash of shingles appeared, if pain was severe while the rash was present, or if shingles affected the eyes (causing a rash on the tip of the nose or making the eyes inflamed and red). Postherpetic neuralgia is also more likely to occur if the immune system is weakened. Taking chemotherapy drugs or drugs that suppress the immune system (immunosuppressants), such

1. see page 499

as cyclosporine and corticosteroids, can weaken the immune system.

Symptoms and Diagnosis

Postherpetic neuralgia may be a constant deep aching or brief bouts of burning, excruciatingly sharp pain. The pain may feel like an electric shock. Pain may come and go. It may be easily triggered, for example, by a light touch or a change in skin temperature.

Constant or unpredictable pain can be very disruptive, affecting nearly everything a person does. Wearing clothing, particularly fitted clothing, or taking a bath can cause agonizing pain. The pain may interfere with sleeping. Some people stop driving because they fear an attack of pain might occur and cause an accident. Thus, postherpetic neuralgia can sometimes lead to social isolation or depression.

The diagnosis is based on symptoms and a history of having had shingles. Doctors ask what the pain feels like, where it occurs, and when it started (particularly in relation to having a skin rash).

Treatment and Outlook

Relieving the pain of postherpetic neuralgia is difficult. Typical pain relievers, such as acetaminophen or ibuprofen, may be tried, but they usually do not provide enough relief. Creams or lotions containing capsaicin (a substance in hot red peppers) are often used to relieve pain and are often effective. Lidocaine, a type of anesthetic, can be applied to the skin as a gel. It usually helps. Gabapentin (an anticonvulsant) may effectively relieve pain.

Postherpetic neuralgia often disappears, even without treatment, within a year. However, in up to half of people over 70, it persists.

NEUROPATHIES

Neuropathy is damage to one or more nerves.

Neuropathies can cause abnormal sensations (paresthesias), pain, loss of sensation, and weakness. Sometimes body functions are impaired. These neuropathies are called autonomic neuropathies because body functions are controlled by nerves that operate without conscious effort (autonomic nerves).

As many as one fifth of older people have some sort of neuropathy. The effects of a neuropathy range from slight to disabling. They may be temporary or permanent.

Causes

Physical injury can damage a nerve. Often, the injury is caused by prolonged pressure on a nerve that runs close to the surface of the body near a prominent bone. Examples are nerves in the knees, elbows, shoulders, or wrists. Pressure on a nerve during a long, sound sleep or after sitting too long with the legs crossed may be enough to cause damage. Such damage is usually only temporary. Repeated pressure on the nerve that supplies the fingers (due to habitually using the hands in the same way) can result in carpal tunnel syndrome.

Diabetes and excessive use of alcohol are common causes of neuropathies. Other common causes are nutritional deficiencies (particularly of vitamin B_{12}), kidney disorders, cancer (such as multiple myeloma), and the use of certain drugs. These drugs include amiodarone (used to treat abnormal heart rhythms), colchicine (used to treat gout), and vincristine (used to treat cancer).

Less commonly, neuropathies result from infections (such as Lyme disease) and radiation therapy for cancer. Rare causes include exposure to toxic substances (such as lead, mercury, arsenic, or gold) and amyloidosis, which is a little known disorder.

Symptoms

Neuropathies may cause a pins-and-needles feeling, burning pain, numbness, or weakness in the affected part. If the neuropathy is severe, muscles may waste away (atrophy). Muscles are affected (even though they are not directly damaged) because healthy nerves are needed to keep muscles healthy.

Some people lose the abilities to feel vibrations (vibratory sense) and to know where their arms and legs are (position sense). If position sense is lost, walking and even standing may become unsteady. Consequently, muscles may not be used and may eventually weaken and waste away.

CARPAL TUNNEL SYNDROME: NUMB HANDS

Hands that are used over and over in the same way can start to feel tingly, numb, and painful. These symptoms may result from carpal tunnel syndrome.

Carpal tunnel syndrome can be caused by any repeated forceful movements made when the wrist is extended. Examples are using a walker or using a badly positioned computer keyboard. Having diabetes, an underactive thyroid gland, gout, or rheumatoid arthritis increases the risk of developing carpal tunnel syndrome. Being obese or using tobacco products may also increase the risk.

Repeated use of the hands can cause inflammation and swelling in the wrist. Such swelling can put pressure on the nerve in the wrist (median nerve). This nerve enters the hand through a narrow opening—the carpal tunnel—that is formed by bones and ligaments of the wrist.

The thumb, index finger, and middle finger or the whole hand can be affected. Sometimes both hands are affected. Numbness may begin while writing, driving, sewing, holding a book, or typing. Typically, people are awakened during the night because their hands are burning or aching and tingle or feel numb. Numbness may come and go or be constant. People may have trouble gripping objects and may drop them.

Doctors can usually diagnose carpal tunnel syndrome by examining the affected hand and wrist and testing reflexes with a small hammer. Tests to measure how quickly nerve signals travel along nerves may be done to confirm the diagnosis.

The disorder is best treated by avoiding positions that overextend the wrist or put extra pressure on the median nerve. Keeping the wrist in a neutral position—bent neither up nor down too much—can help. Adjusting the angle of a computer keyboard may help keep the wrist in a neutral position. A person may need to get a walker that is the right height and has arm rests. Varying movements and taking breaks during repetitive activities can help.

Injections of a corticosteroid into the carpal tunnel occasionally bring long-lasting relief. If pain is severe or if the muscles atrophy or weaken, surgery may be done to relieve pressure on the median nerve.

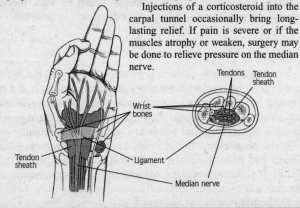

Tendons
Tendon sheath
Wrist bones
Tendon sheath
Ligament
Median nerve

WHAT IS AMYLOIDOSIS?

Sometimes a nerve disorder develops because amyloid, an abnormal protein, accumulates in and around nerves and interferes with their functioning. This disorder, called amyloid neuropathy, is a form of amyloidosis. Amyloid can accumulate in almost any tissue or organ, including the heart, lungs, liver, skin, tongue, thyroid gland, intestines, kidneys, spleen, and blood vessels. Amyloidosis is rare but is more common among older people. Amyloidosis is twice as common among men.

What causes amyloid to accumulate is unknown. Amyloid may accumulate in people who have certain disorders, such as arthritis, a kidney disorder, or multiple myeloma (cancer of the bone marrow). It accumulates in the brain of people with Alzheimer's disease and may play a role in causing the disease. Sometimes amyloidosis runs in families.

The symptoms depend on where and how much amyloid accumulates. When amyloid accumulates in and around nerves, it often causes numbness, tingling, and pain in the hands and feet. If amyloidosis affects nerves in the hands and arms,

carpal tunnel syndrome may result. Sometimes nerves are damaged. Then, people may lose sensation or become very sensitive to changes in temperature. If enough amyloid accumulates in a vital organ, the consequences may be serious. For example, heart or kidney failure may result. The only way to diagnose amyloidosis is a biopsy. Depending on the symptoms, a sample of nerve tissue, fat in the abdomen, or other tissue is removed and examined under a microscope.

No treatment cures amyloidosis. But treating other disorders the person has may help. For most people, treatments to control symptoms (such as prednisone) are only moderately effective. Sometimes surgery to remove the amyloid is done. The outlook for people with amyloidosis depends on where and how much amyloid accumulates. If amyloid affects only nerves in the arms and legs, life expectancy is not shortened. But if amyloidosis causes heart failure, as many as half of the people die within 6 months. The outlook also depends on other disorders present. Most people with amyloidosis and multiple myeloma die within 1 to 2 years.

Other people lose the ability to feel temperature and pain. Consequently, they often burn themselves. Open sores may develop because these people are unaware of prolonged pressure or other injuries. Without pain as a warning of too much stress, joints are susceptible to injuries. This type of injury is called Charcot's joint. The affected joint becomes stiff, painful, and swollen. Without treatment, the joint may be permanently damaged.

Diabetes or a kidney disorder can damage the nerves that

control body functions, such as salivation, digestion, urination, heart rate, blood pressure, and sweating (causing an autonomic neuropathy). Such damage can result in constipation, loss of bowel or bladder control (leading to fecal or urinary incontinence), sexual dysfunction, and changes in blood pressure. Blood pressure may suddenly fall when a person stands up (a disorder called orthostatic hypotension). The skin may become pale and dry, and less sweat may be produced.

Diagnosis

Doctors can often identify the cause of a neuropathy on the basis of symptoms and the results of a physical examination. Certain tests can help locate the damaged nerve and provide additional information. They include electromyography (which records electrical activity in muscles) and nerve conduction velocity studies (which measure how quickly nerve signals travel along nerves).[1]

Doctors try to identify the disorder causing symptoms so that it can be treated. Blood and urine tests may be done to check for diabetes or a kidney disorder. Occasionally, a nerve biopsy is necessary. For this procedure, a small piece of a nerve, usually one near the surface, is removed through a small incision and examined under a microscope.

Treatment and Outlook

Specific treatment depends on the cause. If the cause is a disorder, it is treated. For example, vitamin B_{12} deficiency may be treated with vitamin B_{12} supplements. If a drug is the cause, it is discontinued if possible.

If the cause is exposure to a toxic substance, exposure to the substance is stopped. Doctors may give the person a drug that binds with the substance, causing it to pass out of the body in the urine. This treatment is called chelation therapy. Chelation drugs remove the substance slowly. These drugs can have serious side effects.

If pressure is causing the problem, avoiding the pressure may relieve symptoms. For example, sitting without crossing the legs may help. Moving the affected part can relieve the pressure. Then nerves can function normally again, and the symptoms may stop.

1. see page 139

For pain, anticonvulsants, such as gabapentin, phenytoin, or carbamazepine, are sometimes useful. Other drugs that may help include some antidepressants, such as tricyclic antidepressants and selective serotonin reuptake inhibitors (SSRIs),[1] and creams containing capsaicin (a substance in hot red peppers).

Physical therapy sometimes reduces muscle weakness.

The outlook for people with a neuropathy depends on the cause. Some neuropathies, such as carpal tunnel syndrome, resolve completely with treatment. Other neuropathies become progressively worse. An example is the neuropathy that causes numbness in the hands and feet of people with diabetes.

POSTPOLIO SYNDROME

Postpolio syndrome is the development of tired, painful, and weak muscles 15 years or more after recovery from polio.

In most people who have had polio, such symptoms are not due to postpolio syndrome but to the development of a new disorder, such as diabetes, a slipped (herniated) disk, or osteoarthritis. However, sometimes muscle tissue also wastes away, suggesting postpolio syndrome.

Doctors suspect postpolio syndrome when muscles become progressively weaker but sensation is not lost. Muscle weakness can have many causes, so tests, such as electromyography,[2] are needed.

No specific drugs are available. Physical therapy and exercise help people maintain muscle strength and help prevent permanent stiffening of the muscles (contractures). People should pace their physical activities so that they do not become tired.

1. see table on page 450
2. see page 139

As we walk hand-in-hand into our favorite restaurant after 5 years of marriage, we are amazed how blessed we are. Both of us were married to the love of our lives for over 40 years, but early deaths took our spouses. Although we had families and friends, there were empty places in our hearts. Fortunately, we found that love the second time around can be as sweet as the first.

The vows the second time take on new meanings as we age. In youth we didn't dissect the vows but took them as a singular commitment that we would stay together and work things out forever. After 40 plus years we knew there was so much more to those vows.

Take the vow "in sickness and in health." As we age our sicknesses are commonly greater than a cold or flu. We have been through hospitalizations that have resulted in our health never quite being the same. We will face other medical crises, but our commitments of support will remain. Retirement enables us to have time to help each other heal.

"For richer and for poorer" has also taken on a different meaning. When we were young, we worked to pay the bills and raise our families. Since retirement, we live in comfort but are concerned about rising health care costs and the amount our prescriptions cost. The cost of living is rising quite a bit faster than our pensions. We are grateful that we are not facing the expenses of raising a family.

"For better or worse" is our favorite. We have lived through the worst with the loss of our first spouses, and are eternally grateful for the better we have found in each other. Since we are retired, we are able to spend our days and nights together. We are able to enjoy things we like to do and places we cherish going and do them on our schedule.

We were both married the first time "until death do us part" and that vow has not and will not change. Indeed, love the second time around can be and IS as sweet as the first, and we have again made the commitment "until death do us part."

Virgil and Penny Lawson

30

Movement Disorders

Normally, most movements are intentional (voluntary). That is, people will a movement or decide to move, even though these decisions are usually made automatically. In movement disorders, people no longer have control because areas of the brain that control movement malfunction or become damaged. Movements may occur unintentionally (involuntarily) or voluntary movements may not be made as intended. As a result, daily activities can become frustratingly difficult or impossible. Many movement disorders are progressive, eventually resulting in disability. However, they progress at different speeds, and treatments can often relieve symptoms, sometimes for a long time.

The types of movements affected and the severity of the involuntary movements depend on the disorder causing them. Some disorders cause quick jerking of muscles (myoclonus). Others cause muscles to contract and stay contracted for several minutes, forcing the person into an abnormal position (a condition called dystonia). Certain drugs have side effects that can cause repeated muscle contractions (dyskinesia) or a general restlessness (akinesia), making a person unable to be still. Some disorders, such as Parkinson's disease, cause shaking (tremors).

MYOCLONUS

Myoclonus refers to unintentional, quick, lightning-like jerks (contractions) of muscles. Although not life-threatening, myoclonus can interfere with daily activities.

Myoclonus may occur normally. For example, it often occurs when a leg jerks as a person is falling asleep. But it may result from a disorder, such as liver or kidney failure. Myoclonus may

WHERE DAMAGE OCCURS IN MOVEMENT DISORDERS

Certain areas of the brain control the way a person moves. Damage to these areas may result in a movement disorder. These areas include clusters of nerve cells deep within the brain (basal ganglia) and the cerebellum.

The basal ganglia help coordinate and smooth out movements. Damage to the basal ganglia can cause involuntary or decreased movements. Such damage does not cause muscle weakness or change the reflexes.

The cerebellum coordinates the body's movements. It constantly adjusts muscle tone and posture and helps maintain balance. The cerebellum also stores memories of complex movements that have been learned by practice, such as a ballroom dance step. The cerebellum enables people to perform such movements with speed and balance. Damage to the cerebellum causes incoordination.

Movement disorders sometimes also affect the brain stem. The brain stem controls internal body functions (such as blood pressure control, breathing, heart rate, and swallowing) and helps adjust posture. Clusters of nerve cells (nuclei) in the brain stem control eye movements. When these areas are damaged, internal functions are disrupted, and the eyes cannot move normally.

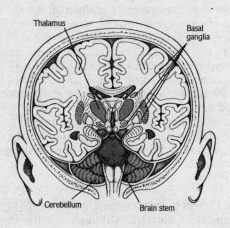

Thalamus

Basal ganglia

Cerebellum

Brain stem

occur after cardiac arrest—when the heart's pumping stops suddenly—or after taking high doses of certain drugs such as levodopa or bismuth. It may be caused by seizure disorders, Parkinson's disease, Alzheimer's disease, other dementias, head injuries, or heatstroke.

Myoclonus may affect only one hand, a group of muscles in the upper arm or leg, or a group of facial muscles. Hiccups are a type of myoclonus that involves only the diaphragm, the muscle that separates the chest from the abdomen. Myoclonus may also affect many muscles at the same time.

One type of myoclonus is called flapping tremor (asterixis). Flapping tremor occurs when a person stretches out the arms and extends the hands. One or both hands quickly drop, then return to their original position. That is, they flap. Flapping occurs because the muscle tone is lost briefly, then returns. Flapping

---

HICCUPS: SPASMS OF THE DIAPHRAGM

Almost everyone, regardless of age, has had hiccups, so hiccups are hardly thought of as a movement disorder. But they are. They occur when there are spasms of the diaphragm, followed by quick, noisy closings of the glottis. (The diaphragm, a muscle that separates the chest from the abdomen, is responsible for each breath. The glottis is the opening between the vocal cords that closes to stop the flow of air to the lungs.) Although not life threatening, hiccups are annoying and can disrupt daily activities.

Usually, hiccups have no obvious cause. But they may be triggered by laughing, talking, eating, or drinking. Less commonly, hiccups result from a serious disorder, such as pneumonia or a stroke, or from abdominal surgery.

Hiccups usually begin suddenly and stop after several seconds or minutes. Occasionally, they persist for a longer time, even in healthy people. When due to a serious cause, hiccups tend to persist until the cause is corrected. Older people are more likely to have persistent hiccups, which may become exhausting.

Many home remedies have been used to cure hiccups. Holding the breath is the simplest way. Breathing into a paper (not plastic) bag, drinking water quickly, or swallowing dry bread or crushed ice may stop hiccups. Other remedies include gently pulling on the tongue and gently rubbing the eyeballs. For most people with hiccups, any one of these remedies works.

For persistent hiccups, treatment is needed, particularly when the cause cannot easily be corrected. Several drugs have been used with varying success. They include scopolamine, prochlor-perazine, chlorpromazine, baclofen, metoclopramide, and valproate.

tremor commonly results from liver failure and so has been called liver flap. However, it may also result from kidney failure or brain damage that results from lack of oxygen (for example, because blood flow is blocked) or from a low blood sugar level (hypoglycemia).

Myoclonus may vary in severity and frequency. It may be triggered by sudden noise, movement, or light. If severe, myoclonus can interfere with walking, talking, and eating. Thus, severe myoclonus can worsen an older person's quality of life and lead to undernutrition.

Diagnosis and Treatment

The diagnosis is based on symptoms and the results of a physical examination. Certain tests may be done to identify the cause of myoclonus. They include electroencephalography (EEG—which records electrical activity in the brain), electromyography (EMG—which records electrical activity in muscles), magnetic resonance imaging (MRI), and computed tomography (CT). For flapping tremor, blood tests are done to evaluate liver and kidney function.

If possible, the disorder causing myoclonus is treated. For flapping tremor, the underlying liver or kidney disorder is treated if possible. The tremor may then resolve. If myoclonus is severe, the same drugs used to prevent seizures (anticonvulsants), such as clonazepam or valproate, are sometimes helpful.

DYSTONIA

In dystonia, prolonged muscle contractions (spasms) force the body into abnormal, sometimes painful positions or movements.

Part or all of the body may twist or turn: the eyelids, neck, mouth, tongue, arms, legs, or trunk. The movements are usually slow and repetitive. Dystonia does not affect mental function, muscle strength, vision, or hearing. Dystonia may cause few problems or greatly interfere with functioning. It is usually chronic (that is, people continue to have spasms).

Causes

Dystonia may occur because the basal ganglia are overactive. The basal ganglia, which are clusters of nerve cells deep within the brain, help coordinate muscle movements. Dystonia may occur in people with Parkinson's disease or stroke. Drugs used to treat loss of contact with reality (antipsychotic drugs) and drugs used to treat Parkinson's disease can cause dystonia. Dystonia that affects the whole body often has a genetic cause.

Types and Symptoms

Dystonia may affect most of the muscles in the body or only one or two groups of muscles. **Writer's cramp** is dystonia that affects only the hand muscles, causing muscle spasms in the fingers. These spasms make holding and writing with a pen or pencil difficult.

Blepharospasm is repeated spasms of the muscles around the eyes, forcing the eyelids shut. The eyes may remain shut for seconds to minutes. Usually, both eyes are affected. Blepharospasm usually begins gradually with excessive blinking. These spasms may be triggered by bright light, fatigue, or stress. Many people with blepharospasm find ways to keep their eyes open, such as yawning, singing, or opening the mouth wide. These techniques become less effective as the disorder progresses. When blepharospasm is very severe, the eyes may be forced closed for hours, making the person effectively blind for that time. However, blepharospasm is not painful.

Spasmodic torticollis involves spasms of the neck muscles, causing the head to twist forward, backward, or sideways. The spasms may be sustained or jerky. They can be painful. The abnormal positions sometimes cause nerves in the neck to be pinched. Touching the face gently may relieve the spasm. In about one fourth of people, the spasms spread to the face, jaw, or arms. The spasms may remain stable for years or may become progressively more severe. A few people have symptom-free periods (remissions), but symptoms eventually return.

Spasmodic dysphonia involves spasms of the muscles of the vocal cords that interfere with speech. Speech may sound strained, quavery, hoarse, whispery, jerky, staccato, or garbled and be difficult to understand. Sometimes speech is impossible.

Diagnosis and Treatment

The diagnosis is based on symptoms and results of a physical examination. Examination by a specialist, such as a neurologist or speech pathologist, may be needed. No test can confirm the diagnosis.

Correcting or eliminating the cause of dystonia, if known, usually reduces its frequency and severity. For example, if a drug is causing dystonia, the drug is discontinued. The dystonia may then lessen. If dystonia persists after an antipsychotic drug is discontinued, pimozide (used to lessen involuntary movements) may help.

If the cause of dystonia is unknown, the effectiveness of treatment varies. Injecting botulinum toxin (which can paralyze muscles) into the overactive muscle is usually effective. The injections reduce the activity of the muscle enough to relieve the spasm but not enough to cause paralysis. These injections are useful when only part of the body is affected, as in blepharospasm, spasmodic torticollis, and spasmodic dysphonia. Injections are repeated every few months.

If the whole body is affected or if botulinum injections are not effective, certain drugs may be given by mouth. However, side effects of the drugs may limit the dose that can be given. Some people benefit from baclofen, a muscle relaxant. However, this drug can cause excessive drowsiness, confusion, and hallucinations. Drugs with anticholinergic effects,[1] such as trihexyphenidyl and diphenhydramine, are sometimes helpful. However, these drugs can cause drowsiness, confusion, blurred vision, constipation, dry mouth, light-headedness, difficulty starting and continuing urination, and loss of bladder control (urinary incontinence), especially in older people. Benzodiazepines (a type of sedative, used to calm, relieve anxiety, or aid sleep) may be used. Some people improve dramatically when treated with levodopa, a drug often used to treat Parkinson's disease.[2] The antipsychotic drugs clozapine and olanzapine may be useful.

If drugs are ineffective and symptoms are severe, surgery may be recommended. Surgery may consist of destroying a tiny area in one basal ganglion (a procedure called pallidotomy) or

1. see box on page 58
2. see page 412

implanting electrodes to stimulate the same area of the brain (deep brain stimulation).

Physical therapy helps some people, especially those who are treated with botulin injections. Exercises to stretch muscles or maintain a joint's range of motion may be recommended.

TARDIVE DYSKINESIA AND AKATHISIA

Tardive dyskinesia is involuntary, repetitive movements of muscles. Akathisia is a feeling of restlessness. People with akathisia cannot sit still.

Tardive dyskinesia and akathisia are often caused by antipsychotic drugs or related drugs. Certain antidepressants (tricyclic antidepressants) can cause tardive dyskinesia.

Symptoms

In tardive dyskinesia, the muscles of the face are affected most often. Typically, people grimace, chew, stick their tongue out, and pucker or smack their lips. The muscles of the arms, legs, or trunk may also be affected. People with the disorder may rock back and forth or rotate their ankles. They may march in place. Their fingers may seem to be playing an invisible guitar or piano.

People with akathisia feel restless and anxious when they are not moving. They may repeatedly stroke parts of their body or pick at their clothes. They may cross and uncross arms and legs, pace, or march in place. They may moan, groan, or shout.

Diagnosis and Treatment

Diagnosis is based on symptoms and a history of taking an antipsychotic, a related drug, or a tricyclic antidepressant for a long time.

Treatment begins with discontinuing the drug or lowering the dose if possible. Sometimes a different drug can be substituted. After the drug is discontinued, symptoms may lessen, sometimes after worsening temporarily. But they may persist.

If the drug that may be causing tardive dyskinesia or akathisia cannot be discontinued, certain other drugs may help. They include benzodiazepines (a type of sedative), opioids (narcotics), and reserpine or propranolol (a beta-blocker, a type of drug used to treat high blood pressure).

ESSENTIAL TREMOR

A tremor is unintentional, rhythmic shaking or trembling. Essential tremor is a tremor whose cause is unknown. However, some evidence suggests the cause could be an abnormality of the cerebellum.

This tremor, once called benign or senile tremor, affects up to 1 out of 5 people over 65. The tremor often begins in young adulthood and slowly becomes more obvious as people age. However, the tremor may begin much later in life. Some forms of essential tremor run in families and are sometimes called familial tremor.

In many people, essential tremor remains mild, although it may be troublesome and embarrassing. However, the tremor often gradually worsens over time, eventually resulting in disability.

Essential tremor affects the arms most often and the legs rarely. Because it occurs during movement, such as writing or using eating utensils, it is considered an action tremor. Essential tremor also occurs when the limbs are held out from the side. The tremor usually stops when the arms or legs are at rest. Usually, essential tremor affects both sides of the body, but one side is affected more than the other.

Sometimes essential tremor affects the head, causing it to tremble and bob, and the vocal cords, causing the voice to shake.

Diagnosis

The diagnosis is usually based on characteristics of the tremor. Doctors ask the person to describe the tremor, including when it started, when it usually occurs, which parts of the body it affects, and whether other symptoms also occur. Doctors observe the person while moving, resting, and holding different positions. Sometimes if the diagnosis is uncertain, electromyography (EMG, which records electrical activity in muscles)[1] is done. Or the speed and range of the tremor may be measured with a device called an accelerometer, which is attached to the finger.

1. see page 139

WHEN PEOPLE TREMBLE

At some time, everyone unintentionally shakes or trembles (has a tremor). Such tremors are normal (physiologic). In most people, they are too slight to be noticed. But some things cause normal tremors to become noticeable—for example, holding the arms out from the side, consuming foods or beverages with caffeine, or feeling stressed, anxious, or tired. When people who are used to consuming caffeine or alcohol suddenly stop, a normal tremor may become more noticeable. An overactive thyroid gland (hyperthyroidism) may also make a normal tremor more noticeable.

Most tremors are not serious, although they may be troublesome. Some tremors are symptoms of disorders. For example, they may indicate brain damage, as occurs in Parkinson's disease, or a problem with the nerves that supply certain muscles.

Tremors that are caused by disorders or drugs are classified by when they occur: when resting, when moving, when performing a precise and purposeful action, or when holding a position for a long time. These tremors may be fast or slow (frequency). Their range of movement may be narrow (fine) or wide (coarse). Tremors may be constant or occur once in a while.

Resting tremor is a slow, coarse tremor that occurs when the muscles are at rest. An arm or a leg shakes even when the person is completely relaxed. Resting tremor may be caused by Parkinson's disease or certain drugs, such as lithium (used to treat mood disorders) or antipsychotic drugs (used to treat loss of contact with reality). Resting tremor, although sometimes embarrassing, usually interferes slightly if at all with movements, such as drinking a glass of water or eating soup.

Action tremor occurs during movement, such as writing or using utensils. It usually stops when the movement is stopped. Action tremor may be caused by using certain drugs, such as prednisone and some drugs used to treat asthma (beta-adrenergic agonists), or by disorders, such as essential tremor.

Intention tremor is a relatively slow, broad tremor that occurs at the end of a precise, purposeful movement, such as trying to press a button or put a key in a lock. Intention tremor may result from malfunction of or damage to areas of the brain that coordinate movements (the cerebellum or clusters of nerve cells connected with the cerebellum). Excessive use of alcohol can cause intention tremor.

Postural tremor occurs when part of the body is held in one position, for example, when an arm is held out from the side. The tremor usually stops when the body is relaxed. It may be caused by using certain drugs (such as lithium or thyroid hormones).

Any tremor that is easily noticed should be evaluated by doctors. Doctors can usually identify the type of tremor by its characteristics, including when it occurs. Tests done to identify the cause depend on the type of tremor, and treatment depends on the cause.

Usually, blood tests are done to determine whether the tremor is caused by an overactive thyroid gland (hyperthyroidism) rather than essential tremor.

Treatment

Treatment depends on how troublesome the tremor is. Certain simple precautions can enable many people to continue their normal daily activities. For example, objects should be grasped firmly but comfortably and held close to the body. Specially designed utensils (such as rocker knives and utensils with large handles) and electrical appliances (such as can openers and toothbrushes) can make daily activities easier. Cylinders of foam can be placed around handles to make them easier to hold. Other helpful measures include using straws, button hooks, Velcro fasteners, zipper pulls, and shoe horns.

Drinking small amounts of alcohol may reduce the tremor. But stopping drinking can make the tremor worse. Avoiding caffeine may help.

If the tremor interferes with daily activities or work, drugs may help. A beta-blocker (used to treat high blood pressure), such as propranolol, is most commonly prescribed. If a beta-blocker does not help, primidone, an anticonvulsant, is often tried. However, this drug may cause confusion, nausea, unsteadiness, and excessive drowsiness in older people. Other choices include gabapentin and topiramate (anticonvulsants) and clozapine (a sedative and an antipsychotic).

If a tremor is severe and disabling and drugs are ineffective, brain surgery may be done. There are two types of surgery. In a thalamotomy, parts of the thalamus are destroyed. The thalamus, a cluster of nerve cells, relays nerve signals through the brain. Thus, the pathways that produce the tremor are interrupted. In thalamic stimulation, an electrical probe is placed inside the thalamus. The probe continuously stimulates the thalamus. The tremor is usually reduced. Such procedures are available only at special centers.

PARKINSON'S DISEASE

In Parkinson's disease, some parts of the nervous system slowly and progressively degenerate.

The disease causes a tremor when muscles are at rest (resting tremor). Movements become slow and uncoordinated, and muscles become tight and rigid. The disease inevitably progresses, usually slowly.

Parkinson's disease affects about 1 out of 100 people over 65. It commonly begins between the ages of 50 and 79. It is twice as common among whites as among blacks.

In Parkinson's disease, the basal ganglia degenerate. The basal ganglia are clusters of nerve cells located at the base of the cerebrum, deep within the brain. They help make muscle movements smooth and coordinated. Like all nerve cells, those in the basal ganglia communicate with other nerve cells by releasing chemical messengers (neurotransmitters). The main neurotransmitter in the basal ganglia is dopamine. When nerve cells in the basal ganglia degenerate, less dopamine is produced. As a result, the basal ganglia cannot smooth out movements as they normally do. Tremor is thought to result from an imbalance: having too little dopamine and too much acetylcholine, another neurotransmitter.

Causes

Why brain cells in the basal ganglia degenerate is unknown. In only a few cases, the disease seems to run in families.

Other conditions that affect the basal ganglia can cause symptoms similar to those of Parkinson's disease. Any condition that causes these symptoms is considered parkinsonism.

Symptoms

Usually, Parkinson's disease begins subtly and progresses gradually. In many people, it begins with a coarse, rhythmic tremor in the hand while the hand is at rest. Typically, the fingers move as if rolling pills. The tremor decreases when the hand is moving purposefully and disappears completely during sleep. Emotional stress or fatigue may worsen the tremor. The tremor may eventually progress to the other hand, the arms, and the legs. The jaws may also be affected. The tremor may become less obvious as the disease progresses. In about one third of people with Parkinson's disease, a tremor is not the first symptom. In some people, a tremor never develops.

Early in Parkinson's disease, people may not be able to smell as well. Part of the reason may be that they have difficulty sniffing or taking a deep breath. Parkinson's disease affects muscles, including those used in breathing. Cells in the areas of the brain involved in smell may degenerate, affecting the brain's ability to identify smells. Although a reduced sense of smell may seem a minor problem, it can dampen the appetite, contributing to undernutrition.

Early in the disease, muscles become rigid. If the forearm is straightened out by another person, the movement may feel stiff or the forearm may move in jerks, like a ratchet. At first, one side of the body is often affected more.

People with Parkinson's disease move slowly and have difficulty starting movements. Gradually, walking becomes impaired. Taking the first step in walking becomes difficult. Once started, people with Parkinson's disease often shuffle and take short steps without swinging their arms as they walk. Some people have difficulty stopping or turning while walking. Sometimes people are in the middle of a movement, then suddenly and unpredictably freeze in place. As they walk, they may suddenly feel as if their feet are glued to the ground, and they cannot take another step. Because movement is difficult, people with Parkinson's disease move around less. Lack of movement makes muscles even stiffer. Muscles may ache and feel tired.

Often, the small muscles of the hands do not function normally. Thus, daily tasks, such as buttoning a shirt and tying shoelaces, become increasingly harder. Most people with Parkinson's disease have shaky, tiny handwriting (micrographia), because initiating and sustaining each stroke of the pen is difficult.

Sometimes movements become faster. For example, when walking, people may unintentionally quicken their steps, breaking into a short-stepped, stumbling run to avoid falling. They may talk faster, running words together in a mumble.

Posture becomes stooped, and the head tends to droop forward and rest on the chest. Balance becomes difficult to maintain, so that falling becomes more likely. When balance is lost, people often cannot move their feet or hands quickly enough to prevent or break a fall.

The face becomes less expressive because the facial muscles that control expression do not move. This lack of expression

WHAT IS PARKINSONISM?

Parkinsonism is any condition that causes symptoms similar to those of Parkinson's disease. Any condition that affects the basal ganglia can cause these symptoms. Parkinsonism may be a side effect of certain drugs, especially antipsychotic drugs. These drugs interfere with or block the action of dopamine, the main chemical messenger (neurotransmitter) in the basal ganglia. Disorders that can cause parkinsonism include other degenerative brain disorders, viral encephalitis (a rare disorder that follows a flu-like infection), brain tumors, strokes, and head injury (particularly the repeated injury that occurs in boxing).

Levodopa, which can often cause people with Parkinson's disease to improve dramatically, is often less helpful to people who have parkinsonism.

may be mistaken for depression. Or it may cause depression to be overlooked. Depression is common among people with Parkinson's disease. Eventually, the face can take on a blank stare with the mouth open, and the eyes may not blink often. People with Parkinson's disease often speak softly in a monotone and may stutter because they have difficulty articulating words. They may whisper.

Often, people with Parkinson's disease drool or choke because the muscles of the face and throat have become rigid or move slowly, making swallowing difficult. They may become malnourished and dehydrated. As the disease progresses, swallowing becomes increasingly difficult. Thus, aspiration pneumonia, which can be fatal, is more likely to develop.

Constipation and insomnia are common. In many people with Parkinson's disease, mental functions remain normal. But dementia develops in about half of people with Parkinson's disease.

Diagnosis

Doctors usually diagnose Parkinson's disease based on symptoms and the results of a physical examination. Mild disease may be difficult to diagnose, because it usually begins subtly. Also, older people may have parkinsonism or other problems that cause some of the same symptoms as Parkinson's disease, such as loss of balance, slow movements, muscle stiffness, and stooped posture.

Tests are rarely needed. However, when the diagnosis is unclear, positron emission tomography (PET) may help. This imaging procedure can often detect abnormalities in the brain that are characteristic of Parkinson's disease. Computed tomography (CT) and magnetic resonance imaging (MRI) cannot detect these abnormalities, but they may be done to look for another disorder that could be causing the symptoms. Sometimes, if the diagnosis is unclear, a person is given levodopa (commonly used to treat Parkinson's disease) for a brief time. The diagnosis of Parkinson's disease is likely if treatment with this drug results in improvement.

Treatment

Parkinson's disease cannot be cured. But drugs can usually control symptoms effectively for many years.

If another disorder or a drug is causing the symptoms, treating the disorder or discontinuing the drug is more effective than taking additional drugs.

General measures: Continuing to do as many daily activities as possible and following a program of regular exercise, such as walking, can help people stay mobile.[1] Physical and occupational therapy[2] can help people maintain or regain muscle tone and maintain range of motion. Therapists can also teach new ways to do activities that have become difficult (adaptive techniques). Therapists can teach ways to manage the unpredictable episodes of freezing when walking. They may recommend installing grab bars and railings to help prevent falls or using mechanical aids, such as a wheeled walker or a cane.

Eating fiber-rich foods (such as prunes), drinking plenty of fluids (particularly prune juice and other juices), and taking stool softeners (such as senna) can help keep bowel movements regular. These things should be done daily before constipation develops or becomes severe. Eating a nutritious diet is important.

Simple changes around the home can make the home safer. For example, removing throw rugs can prevent tripping. Installing railings in bathrooms, hallways, and other locations reduces the risk of falling. Daily tasks can be simplified, for

1. see page 912
2. see pages 171 and 177

℞ DRUGS USED TO TREAT PARKINSON'S DISEASE

Type	Drug	Possible Side Effects	Comments
Dopamine precursor (a substance that can be converted to dopamine)	Levodopa	Involuntary movements, nightmares, changes in blood pressure, constipation, nausea, insomnia, palpitations, and flushing	Levodopa given in combination with carbidopa is the mainstay of treatment. Carbidopa helps increase the effectiveness of levodopa and helps reduce its side effects. After several years, the effectiveness of the combination may lessen
Dopamine agonists (drugs that mimic the action of dopamine)	Bromocriptine Pergolide Pramipexole Ropinirole	Drowsiness, nausea, changes in blood pressure, and hallucinations When the drug is suddenly withdrawn, neuroleptic malignant syndrome (a rare, sometimes fatal disorder)	These drugs may be used alone in the early stages of the disease. Early use may delay the development of levodopa's side effects
MAO inhibitor (a type of antidepressant)	Selegiline	Nausea, dizziness, confusion, insomnia, dry mouth, and abdominal pain	Selegiline can be used alone but is often given as a supplement to levodopa. At best, selegiline is mildly effective

Table continues on the following page.

Type	Drug	Possible Side Effects	Comments
COMT inhibitors (drugs that block an enzyme that breaks down levodopa)	Entacapone Tolcapone	Nausea, abnormal involuntary movements, diarrhea, back pain, and discoloration of the urine	Either of these drugs can be used to supplement levodopa late in the disease. They are not useful taken alone
Drugs with anticholinergic effects	Benztropine Trihexyphenidyl	Excessive drowsiness, confusion, blurred vision, constipation, dry mouth, lightheadedness, difficulty starting and continuing urination, and loss of bladder control	These drugs may be given alone in the early stages of the disease and with levodopa in the later stages. They can reduce the tremor
Antiviral drug	Amantadine	Nausea, dizziness, insomnia, anxiety, and confusion When the drug is withdrawn or the dose is reduced, life-threatening high fever with disturbances in internal functions	Amantadine is used alone in the early stages for mild disease and in later stages to enhance levodopa's effects. If used alone, this drug may become ineffective after several months Amantadine is thought to work by causing dopamine to be released

MAO-B = monoamine oxidase, type B; COMT = catechol O-methyltransferase.

example, by having buttons on clothing replaced with Velcro fasteners or buying shoes with such fasteners.

Drugs: No drug can cure Parkinson's disease or stop its progression. However, many drugs can make movement easier and enable people to function effectively for many years. Two or more drugs may be needed. People with Parkinson's disease must take these drugs for the rest of their life.

Taking levodopa can produce dramatic improvement in people with Parkinson's disease. This drug is taken by mouth and is most effective in reducing tremor and muscle rigidity. The drug enables many people with mild Parkinson's disease to return to a nearly normal level of activity and enables some people who are bedridden to walk again.

Levodopa is converted to dopamine in the basal ganglia. Thus, this drug partially compensates for the decrease in dopamine production. Levodopa is almost always given with carbidopa. Carbidopa prevents levodopa from being converted to dopamine before it reaches the brain. When the two drugs are given together, a lower dose of levodopa can be used, and some side effects of levodopa (nausea and flushing) are reduced.

To determine the best dose of levodopa for a particular person, doctors must balance control of the disease with the development of certain side effects, which may limit the amount of levodopa the person can tolerate. Side effects include involuntary movements of the mouth, face, and limbs and sometimes difficulty sleeping and nightmares.

After taking levodopa for 5 or more years, more than half of the people begin to have problems. These people alternate rapidly between responding well to the drug and not responding. This effect is called the on-off phenomenon. Within seconds, a person may change from being able to move (mobile) fairly well to being almost unable to move. Also, the period of improved mobility after a dose becomes shorter over time and may be accompanied by an increase in involuntary movements, such as writhing. Taking lower, more frequent doses controls these effects at first, but after several more years, these effects become hard to avoid.

Other drugs may benefit some people, particularly if levodopa is not tolerated or does not control symptoms well. Drugs that mimic the actions of dopamine (dopamine agonists), such as bromocriptine, pramipexole, and ropinirole, may be useful and are often used before levodopa. Selegiline, a type of antidepressant called a monoamine oxidase inhibitor (MAOI), prevents the breakdown of dopamine, thereby prolonging dopamine's action in the body. Tolcapone and entacapone appear to be useful as supplements to levodopa, but they are not helpful when taken alone. They also prevent the breakdown of dopamine.

Some drugs with anticholinergic effects,[1] such as benztropine and trihexyphenidyl, can reduce the severity of tremors. These drugs can be used early in Parkinson's disease. They can also be used later to supplement levodopa. But these drugs can cause many troublesome side effects in older people.

Amantadine, a drug sometimes used to treat influenza, may be used as a supplement to levodopa or alone.

If depression develops, antidepressants are usually used.

Surgery: When symptoms are severe (late in the disease), surgery is sometimes done. In a pallidotomy, a tiny area in one of the basal ganglia on one side of the brain is surgically destroyed. This procedure can greatly reduce the "off" part of the on-off phenomenon and the involuntary movements due to years of levodopa therapy. In deep brain stimulation, tiny electrodes are implanted in the basal ganglia. They stimulate the area, often producing similar improvements.

Several experimental procedures are being studied. In one, nerve cells that produce dopamine are taken from human fetal tissue and implanted in the brain of a person with Parkinson's disease. These cells form connections with other nerve cells and produce dopamine, thus supplying the missing neurotransmitter.

Outlook

Usually, Parkinson's disease progresses slowly, and people can function for many years. But Parkinson's disease is progressive, and people eventually need help with normal daily activities, such as eating, bathing, dressing, and going to the toilet. Some people are incapacitated within 5 years. Caregivers can benefit from learning about the physical and psychologic effects of Parkinson's disease and about ways to enable people to func-

1. see box on page 58

tion as well as possible. Because such care is tiring and stressful, caregivers may benefit from support groups.

Eventually, most people with Parkinson's disease become severely disabled and immobile. They may be unable to eat, even with help. If dementia develops, the situation is more difficult. Before people with Parkinson's disease are incapacitated, they should prepare advance directives, indicating what kind of medical care they want at the end of life.[1] For example, they should state whether they want tube feedings or aggressive treatment for common problems that develop, such as aspiration pneumonia.

PROGRESSIVE SUPRANUCLEAR PALSY

In progressive supranuclear palsy, muscles become stiff (rigid), the eyes become unable to move, and the throat muscles become weak. Usually, this incurable disorder progresses rapidly.

Progressive supranuclear palsy is similar to Parkinson's disease, but it is much rarer. Progressive supranuclear palsy usually begins after age 50. The cause is unknown.

Progressive supranuclear palsy destroys parts of the basal ganglia and the brain stem. The basal ganglia help coordinate and smooth out movements. The brain stem controls vital body functions (such as breathing, heart rate, and swallowing). Clusters of nerve cells in the brain stem control eye movements.

Symptoms

Usually, the most obvious symptoms are vision problems. People with progressive supranuclear palsy cannot roll their eyes downward. They have difficulty focusing on a stationary object or following a moving object. Because they cannot move their eyes normally, reading is difficult. The upper eyelids may pull back, making people with the disorder look astonished. People may have difficulty opening and closing their eyes. They may blink less often, resulting in dry eyes. The neck tends to arch backward. Muscles become very rigid, and movements are slow. Steps become wider, and walking becomes unsteady. Falls, particularly backward, are more likely.

1. see page 953

Speaking becomes slurred and guttural. Swallowing becomes increasingly difficult. As a result, aspiration pneumonia is likely to develop.

As the disorder progresses, people may have insomnia. They become irritable and agitated easily. Emotions may change rapidly. They may laugh one moment and cry the next. They may become apathetic. Late in the disorder, depression and confusion due to dementia are common.

Diagnosis and Treatment

The diagnosis is based on symptoms, particularly vision problems and the tendency to fall backward. Progressive supranuclear palsy is sometimes mistaken for Parkinson's disease because the symptoms of the two disorders are similar. However, noticeable tremors are less common than in Parkinson's disease. No tests can directly confirm the diagnosis.

No effective treatment exists. But the drugs used to treat Parkinson's disease, such as levodopa and pramipexole, may provide some relief for rigid muscles. Antidepressants may help relieve symptoms of depression and reduce the rapid changes in emotion.

People may use weighted walking aids or even a wheelchair to help prevent falls. Bifocals and special glasses with prisms or tinted lenses may help with vision problems.

People may be evaluated periodically to determine how well they swallow. If swallowing becomes difficult, health care practitioners may recommend eating certain foods that are more easily swallowed. Swallowing may become so difficult late in the disorder that practitioners recommend placing a tube directly into the stomach (a procedure called gastrostomy).

Outlook

Progressive supranuclear palsy results in disability, usually within 3 to 5 years. Usually, death, often due to infection, occurs within 10 years after symptoms begin.

People with progressive supranuclear palsy should prepare advance directives, indicating what kind of medical care they want at the end of life.[1]

1. see page 953

SHY-DRAGER SYNDROME

Shy-Drager syndrome, like Parkinson's disease, causes tremors when muscles are at rest (resting tremor). It also causes internal body processes, such as blood pressure control, to malfunction.

Shy-Drager syndrome usually develops between the ages of 37 and 75. It is more common among men. The cause is unknown. This syndrome progresses, eventually resulting in death.

Shy-Drager syndrome results from deterioration of the parts of the brain that control internal body functions. These parts include nerve cells of the brain stem and spinal cord. They control such functions as heart rate, blood pressure, breathing rate, the amount of stomach acid secreted, and the speed at which food passes through the digestive tract.

Symptoms

Like Parkinson's disease, Shy-Drager syndrome causes tremors, rigid muscles, and problems with movements. Walking and speaking become slow. Like people with Parkinson's disease, people with Shy-Drager syndrome may shuffle, have difficulty taking a first step, freeze in the middle of a movement, and have to take many small, quick steps to prevent a fall. Speech may become slurred.

In addition, Shy-Drager syndrome interferes with the regulation of blood pressure, heart rate, bladder and bowel function, body temperature, and focusing of the eyes. When people with this disorder stand up, blood pressure falls dramatically. They then feel dizzy, light-headed, or faint. This disorder is called orthostatic hypotension. Blood pressure may increase when they lie down.

Less sweat, tears, and saliva are produced. So people do not tolerate heat well, and their eyes and mouth are dry. People may have difficulty urinating or become constipated, sometimes severely. Uncontrollable loss of urine (urinary incontinence) or loss of control of bowels with leakage and soiling (fecal incontinence) may develop. In men, erectile dysfunction (impotence) may develop. Walking may become unsteady, and movements may become uncoordinated.

Late in the disorder, people may become confused and have difficulty controlling their emotions. Mental function may decline slightly. Breathing and swallowing become difficult, and the heart beats irregularly.

Diagnosis and Treatment

Doctors suspect Shy-Drager syndrome on the basis of symptoms. No tests can directly confirm the diagnosis. However, a tilt table test[1] may be done to determine whether the body's control of blood pressure is abnormal. For the test, a person is strapped to a motorized table, which tilts the person who is lying flat to an almost standing position. Blood pressure and heart rate are continuously monitored during the test.

No treatment can cure the disorder, but some symptoms can be relieved. Usually, the drugs used to relieve the symptoms of Parkinson's disease are less effective in treating Shy-Drager syndrome. However, different people respond differently.

Several measures can help relieve the symptoms resulting from a fall in blood pressure when a person stands up.

- Consuming more salt and drinking a lot of water (which may increase the volume of blood and thus help increase blood pressure)
- Drinking caffeinated beverages early in the day (which may increase blood pressure slightly)
- Wearing fitted elastic stockings up to the waist
- Raising the head of the bed (which can help prevent blood pressure from increasing too much when a person lies down)
- Avoiding extreme heat
- Abstaining from alcoholic beverages
- Eating small meals
- Getting up slowly
- Not straining during a bowel movement

The drug fludrocortisone can help prevent blood pressure from becoming too low. This drug increases blood pressure because it causes the body to retain salt and water. Midodrine may help prevent blood pressure from decreasing too much when a person stands. Taking propranolol at night can help prevent

1. see page 282

blood pressure from increasing too much when a person lies down.

Outlook

Shy-Drager syndrome results in death, usually due to pneumonia, 7 to 10 years after symptoms begin. People with Shy-Drager syndrome should prepare advance directives,[1] indicating what kind of medical care they want at the end of life.

31

Sleep

Many people envision the "golden years" not only as a time to reap the rewards of life's labors but also as a time to catch up on years of missed sleep. However, for many older people, labor's rewards come more easily than does sleep: Up to half say that they do not sleep as well as they would like.

Sleep is important for health and a long life, but why sleep is necessary and what benefits it provides are not known.

Two of the main disturbances of sleep experienced by older people are insomnia during the night and excessive daytime sleepiness. These disturbances often result from poor sleep habits (for example, going to bed at different times on different nights) or changes in the brain that occur with aging. Insomnia and daytime sleepiness can also be symptoms of specific sleep disorders or other physical or mental health disorders. Sleep disorders that can cause insomnia or daytime sleepiness include limb movement disorders (which involve leg symptoms and movements while sleeping or trying to sleep), sleep apnea, circadian rhythm disorders, and REM sleep behavior disorder (which involves REM sleep, a deep stage of sleep characterized by dreams and rapid eye movements). In addition, physical de-

1. see page 953

pendence on others, lack of social stimulation, and loss of control over physical surroundings, as can occur with a move to a nursing home, can all affect the quality of sleep.

For older people who sleep together, sleep problems can be extremely "catching"; one sleepless person can quickly turn a restful night into a sleepless one for the other person.

Changes in Sleep Patterns With Aging

As people age, their sleep patterns almost always change. Older people tend to get sleepy earlier in the evening and wake up earlier in the morning. They may take a bit longer to get to sleep once they are in bed. Additionally, the brain changes the way it "organizes" sleep. Older people seem to spend less time in the deep sleep stages (which help the body recover from daytime activities) and more time in light sleep stages. Once asleep, they then wake up easily and frequently. As a result, they feel less rested and less alert than they might expect after a full night's sleep. The bottom line is that older people spend more time in bed getting less sleep than they did when they were younger.

ADDITIONAL DETAIL

There are two main kinds of sleep: nonrapid eye movement (NREM) sleep and rapid eye movement (REM) sleep. NREM sleep is divided into four stages, based on the amount and frequency of different types of brain waves (electrical activity of the brain). Stage 1 occurs as people become drowsy and fall into light sleep. Stage 2, where most sleep time is spent, is a continuation of light sleep. Stages 3 and 4 are the deepest levels of sleep and are necessary for feeling rested.

REM sleep is a very deep but active stage of sleep in which people dream, their heart rate and breathing speed up and slow down, and their eyes move rapidly. In younger people, REM sleep usually follows stage 4 sleep, then alternates with NREM sleep through the night. Many older people reach the deepest sleep (stage 4) slowly, if at all, and spend less time in REM sleep.

Physical and Mental Health Disorders Affecting Sleep

Dementia can cause confusion, paranoia, agitation, wandering, and disruptive behavior. For unknown reasons, these symptoms are often more intense in the evening and at night (an effect called "sun-downing"). People with dementia spend less time in deep and REM sleep, but whether this change explains why they become restless at night is unclear. Often, the effects of sleep disruptions on households compel family members to move their relatives to assisted living facilities or nursing homes. However, sleep problems may worsen in a nursing home, where residents have little control over noise, light, temperature, privacy, use of certain drugs, and nighttime interruptions.

Diagnosis of sleep disturbance in a person with dementia is usually obvious from family or caregiver reports. Behavioral strategies, such as encouraging daytime exercise and discouraging napping, are the safest and usually the most effective treatment. But drugs are sometimes needed temporarily. Benzodiazepines may help nighttime sleep and reduce anxiety. Certain antidepressants that cause sleepiness, such as trazodone or mirtazapine, may help, especially when dementia is accompanied by symptoms of depression.

Sensory loss, particularly vision and hearing loss, causes some older people to become confused at bedtime. No one knows why, but one possibility is that hearing or vision loss makes people feel disoriented in the dark and quiet of nighttime. Some people who have lost their vision fall asleep and wake up on an unpredictable cycle independent of night and day. Low nighttime doses of melatonin may help such people resume a normal day-night schedule.

Other physical disorders (such as arthritis and gastroesophageal reflux disease) can keep people from falling asleep or cause them to wake up several hours into their sleep. Sleep may also be disrupted by nocturia (excessive urination during nighttime). Nocturia can be caused by a variety of disorders (such as benign prostatic hyperplasia, diabetes, and heart failure), or it can be a side effect of certain drugs (such as diuretics). Many other drugs can interfere with sleep or cause excessive daytime sleepiness.

Mental health disorders, such as anxiety, posttraumatic stress disorder, and depression, can have a severe impact on sleep. Bereavement also affects sleep.

SOME STRATEGIES FOR IMPROVING SLEEP

- Get regular daytime exercise and exposure to sunlight
- Avoid smoking
- Avoid alcohol in the evening and excessive drinking at any time of day
- Avoid caffeinated coffee, tea, and soda and possibly chocolate during late afternoon or the evening, and consume only limited amounts earlier in the day
- Avoid daytime napping, or if napping is unavoidable, sleep no more than 15 to 30 minutes
- If diuretics, decongestants, and other drugs that disturb sleep are needed, take them early in the day
- Keep the bedroom at a comfortable temperature and shield it from light
- Limit bedroom use for activities associated with being awake; use the bedroom only for relaxing activities that induce sleep
- Wear comfortable bedclothes, use comfortable blankets and pillows, and use a mattress that is neither too firm nor too soft
- Go to bed at the same time each night and get up at the same time each morning, including weekends
- Encourage a restless or noisy bed partner to see a doctor
- Perform bedtime rituals (brushing teeth, washing up) at the same time every evening whether at home or away
- Urinate before going to bed
- Keep eyeglasses, canes, walkers, hearing aids, and telephone where they can be found without difficulty in the dark

INSOMNIA

Insomnia is the inability to fall or remain asleep when a person wants to be sleeping.

Insomnia can lead to restlessness and anxiety, which make sleep even more difficult. Insomnia can interfere with the ability to function at other times of the day. It is extremely common among older people.

Causes

Insomnia may be due in part to changes in sleep patterns that occur with aging. Certain behaviors can also cause or contribute to insomnia. Examples are drinking a large amount of any fluids during evening hours, drinking even a little alcohol or caffeinated beverages during evening hours, taking drugs that can have a stimulating effect (such as decongestants), and smoking. Exercise has many health benefits for older people and may promote a good night's rest, but exercising vigorously too close to bedtime can also cause insomnia.

Insomnia is sometimes a symptom of a physical disorder (such as heart failure, gastroesophageal reflux disease, or hyperthyroidism), a mental health disorder (such as depression or anxiety), or a sleep disorder (such as sleep apnea or restless legs syndrome). Insomnia sometimes occurs as a normal response to stress or to a change in surroundings. It can also occur for no apparent reason.

DISORDERS AND SITUATIONS THAT DISTURB SLEEP

Types	Examples	Sleep-Related Symptoms	Treatment
Physical disorders	Dementia	Confusion, paranoia, agitation, and wandering	Improving sleep behaviors (getting regular exercise during the day and developing a regular bedtime routine) or taking sleep aids
	Sensory loss	Confusion, paranoia, agitation, and wandering	Possibly taking melatonin for people with complete vision loss or correcting sensory problems
	Osteoarthritis	Low back or hip pain	Exercising during the day or, when sleeping, using pillows under the knees or hips
	Gastro-esophageal reflux disease	Chest pain and heartburn	Avoiding meals and snacks 4 to 6 hours before bedtime, putting the

Table continues on the following page.

Types	Examples	Sleep-Related Symptoms	Treatment
			head of the bed at an angle above floor, or taking antacids
	Benign prostatic hyperplasia and urinary incontinence	Urge to urinate and loss of urine onto bedclothes or bed	Emptying the bladder and avoiding drinking fluids 2 to 4 hours before bedtime, using absorbent pads during sleep, or taking alpha-blocker or antispasmodic drugs
	Heart failure	Cough, shortness of breath, palpitations, and chest tightness or pain	Using more than one pillow under the head or trunk or taking heart failure drugs
Mental health disorders	Anxiety	Nighttime worrying and agitation	Going to counseling or taking antianxiety drugs
	Depression and bereavement	Excessive sleepiness, insomnia, or early morning wakening	Going to counseling or taking antidepressants
	Post-traumatic stress disorder	Nighttime panic and nightmares	Going to counseling or taking sleep aids
Social conditions	Isolation	Frequent daytime napping, fear of falling asleep, and inability to fully	Getting stimulation by spending time with other

Types	Examples	Sleep-Related Symptoms	Treatment
		prepare self for bed	people and arranging for supervision during the evenings
	Change in surroundings, such as a move to an assisted living facility or nursing home	Insomnia and nighttime worrying	Using a "white noise" machine, low-level night-lights, personal linens and blankets, and a mattress pad; eliminating unnecessary nighttime light and noise; and decreasing daytime napping and excessive daytime hours spent in bed

Diagnosis

Determining that a person has insomnia is simple: The doctor relies on the person's report of a problem falling or remaining asleep. Determining the causes or the severity of insomnia is less straightforward.

Causes of insomnia are identified by looking closely at a person's sleep patterns, habits around bedtime, use of drugs, use of cigarettes and alcohol, physical activity, and medical history. This evaluation along with a few common blood tests usually provides all the information the doctor needs. However, if the insomnia continues for more than 6 months and does not improve with treatment, a person may be referred to a sleep laboratory. The person's brain waves, heart rate, and breathing may be monitored while he or she sleeps. This test, called polysomnography,[1] can help a doctor determine whether a specific sleep dis-

1. see page 137

order (such as periodic limb movements or sleep apnea) is causing the insomnia.

Treatment

Adopting proper sleep habits is the most important thing a person can do to relieve insomnia. For people with insomnia, trying to refrain from napping during the day is essential. They should also eat dinner at least 2 to 3 hours before going to bed and avoid beverages containing caffeine (such as cola, coffee, and tea) during the late afternoon or evening.

Relaxation techniques, such as controlled breathing to relieve tension and meditation to relieve worry, are useful and safe for inducing sleep. Limiting the amount of time a person spends lying awake in bed when he is having trouble falling asleep may help. Instead, the person should get out of bed and engage in relaxing activities (for example, reading or listening to soothing music). Time spent in bed can be gradually increased as sleep improves. Learning about sleep from a therapist or another source can also be helpful.

When these measures are ineffective, drugs used appropriately can help a person sleep. Drugs that cause sleepiness (sleep aids, sometimes also referred to as hypnotics, sedatives, or tranquilizers) are generally safe and effective when used in low doses and for very short periods. However, most require a doctor's prescription because they can become habit-forming when used for longer periods or in higher doses. Also, some sleep aids can produce dangerous effects when taken with alcohol and opioid analgesics, such as morphine.

Sleep aids can cause daytime sleepiness and confusion in older people. Insomnia can recur as sleep aids wear off (an effect called rebound insomnia). When used for a long time on a nightly basis, sleep aids become less effective or not effective at all. Prolonged use of sleep aids can cause a person to depend on them for sleep.

Benzodiazepines are the most commonly used sleep aids. Short-acting preparations (such as temazepam, estazolam, and lorazepam) are safer than long-acting preparations. The longer-acting benzodiazepines (such as diazepam and flurazepam) stay in the body past nighttime, causing daytime sleepiness, forgetfulness, and confusion. Older people who use longer-acting benzodiazepines can become unsteady on their feet, increasing the risk of falls (which can lead to hip fractures and other broken bones). Paradoxically, benzodiazepines can directly stimulate the brain, causing agitation and worsening insomnia in some older people. This effect is often worse when the drug is first started or when the dose is increased.

Zolpidem and zaleplon are also effective sleep aids for older people. However, these drugs can cause confusion and disorientation. Their long-term effects in older people are not known, and their effectiveness may lessen if used for long periods.

Certain antidepressant drugs (such as trazodone, nefazodone, and mirtazapine) cause sleepiness and may be effective for depressed people who cannot sleep. Antidepressants that cause sleepiness may also be effective for people without depression if insomnia has not responded to other treatment. However, each of these drugs can cause side effects. Trazodone can lower blood pressure when a person stands up, leading to falls when getting up at night or in the morning. Nefazodone has less effect on blood pressure, but it has caused life-threatening liver failure. Thus, it should be avoided by people with liver disease. Mirtazapine can cause weight gain.

Several sleep aids are available without a prescription. Many antihistamines (such as diphenhydramine) contained in cold and allergy remedies cause sleepiness. But they also cause impaired thinking and balance, dry eyes and mouth, and urinary problems and should be avoided. They are far less safe for older people than sleep aids available with a prescription.

Melatonin is a hormone in the brain that naturally sets the body's sleep cycles. It is sold as a supplement in some drug stores and alternative health stores.[1] It may help some people, and it causes few side effects. However, the manufacture and marketing of melatonin supplements is unregulated, so the amount and quality of melatonin in supplements made by different manufacturers may not be the same. Consequently, most doctors do not prescribe or recommend melatonin. Little is known about its effects in older people.

1. see page 84

NAPPING

Older people tend to nap more than younger people do because they are less physically active and less stimulated. Napping may also help older people compensate for the changes in sleep that come with aging and for interruptions in nighttime sleep caused by sleep disorders.

An additional reason older people nap relates to changes in blood supply to the brain. In younger people, blood vessels widen and narrow, keeping blood pressure in the brain constant even when blood pressure in the rest of the body is changing. In older people, blood vessels are less able to compensate for changes in blood pressure in the body. When blood pressure in the body decreases, as occurs after eating, blood pressure in the brain is more likely to decrease as well, possibly leading to sleepiness. The decrease in blood pressure in the brain is one reason older people may fall asleep after eating a big meal, even in a room filled with noise and commotion.

Napping is generally healthy if it provides needed rest, is kept short, and does not interfere with nighttime sleeping. However, napping should be avoided if it makes a person less able to fall asleep at night.

Outlook

The outlook for people with insomnia is good if they receive treatment for any disorders causing or contributing to insomnia and they adopt healthy sleep behaviors.

EXCESSIVE DAYTIME SLEEPINESS

The feeling of being tired or of wanting to nap often through the day is extremely common in older people.

Excessive daytime sleepiness often accompanies insomnia, but many people who do not describe insomnia do describe excessive daytime sleepiness.

Often, excessive daytime sleepiness has more than one cause. In addition to insomnia, a sedentary lifestyle and overall lack of physical fitness are common reasons older people feel sleepy during the day. Isolation and depression are also causes. Drugs are a common but under-recognized cause of excessive daytime sleepiness, as are cigarettes and alcohol.

Excessive daytime sleepiness can be caused by other sleep disorders, such as sleep apnea and restless legs syndrome.

Excessive daytime sleepiness can also be a symptom of a physical disorder (such as anemia, kidney failure, or hypothyroidism).

An increase in social contacts and exercise during the day may keep an older person stimulated and less bothered by excessive daytime sleepiness. Treatment for insomnia can help those bothered by both sleep disorders. Sometimes methylphenidate or modafinil, drugs used to treat narcolepsy, is tried as treatment for excessive daytime sleepiness.

LIMB MOVEMENT DISORDERS

Restless legs syndrome, periodic limb movements of sleep, and leg cramps are disorders in which a person experiences leg symptoms and movements while sleeping or trying to sleep.

The movements are usually involuntary, and they can keep older people from falling asleep or cause them to wake up once they have been asleep. The disorders are not a problem in themselves, but they require attention if they cause insomnia or daytime sleepiness.

Restless legs syndrome is an uncomfortable sensation in the legs (often described as a pulling, drawing up, or crawling of the legs) that seems to be relieved only by rubbing or moving the legs. It occurs while the person is awake, usually in the evening.

Periodic limb movements of sleep produces quick twitches or kicks of the leg that occur repeatedly during but not before sleep. The limb movements interfere with deep sleep, though the person may not be aware of it and simply feels unrested the next day.

Leg cramps are muscle spasms ("charley horses") that are temporarily relieved by moving the legs. Leg cramps can keep people from falling asleep or can wake them up at night.

Causes

Restless legs syndrome may occur because of iron deficiency, an imbalance of chemicals in the brain, or some unknown cause. Most people with restless legs syndrome also have periodic limb movements of sleep. The causes are unknown but may be the same. Restless legs syndrome and periodic limb movements of sleep can be worsened by drugs, such as lithium or certain antidepressants. These two disorders can also be worsened when people discontinue taking certain drugs, such as anticonvulsants or benzodiazepines.

Leg cramps may be caused by dehydration, abnormal electrolyte levels in the blood, and diuretics, but mostly they occur for no apparent reason.

Diagnosis

People with restless legs syndrome are aware of the disorder. Periodic limb movements of sleep may be suspected when a person's bed partner reports kicking but may be discovered in a laboratory sleep evaluation conducted for other reasons. People with leg cramps diagnose the disorder themselves, although a doctor may order blood tests to check for a cause.

Treatment

Daily exercise, including leg stretches, helps people with restless legs syndrome; hot baths or hot soaking of the legs may also help. People with iron deficiency may get relief with iron supplements. If these treatments are ineffective or if restless legs syndrome is severe, prescription drugs may be needed. Most commonly used are nighttime doses of antiparkinson drugs (such as levodopa with carbidopa, pramipexole, or ropinirole), anticonvulsants (such as carbamazepine or gabapentin), and benzodiazepines (such as clonazepam).

Treatment for periodic limb movements of sleep is similar to that for restless legs syndrome. Antiparkinson drugs are usually effective in low doses.

Leg cramps can be relieved by doing stretching exercises before bedtime. Keeping well hydrated is also important. Taking a hot bath or soaking the legs may help. In the past, some older people believed that taking quinine tablets relieved leg cramps. But quinine is no longer widely available in drug form because of uncertainty about its safety and benefits.

Outlook

The outlook for people with any of these disorders is good. Restless legs syndrome sometimes worsens with age but gener-

STRETCHING EXERCISES FOR LEG CRAMPS

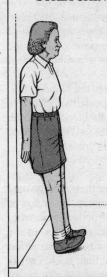

Stretching before bedtime can help prevent leg cramps during the night.

Toe Raises

Stand with the back to the wall and the feet about 1 foot from it. The feet should be a few inches apart. With the arms slightly bent, place both palms against the wall at about upper thigh level. Slowly raise the toes of both feet as high as is comfortable. Hold the position for several seconds, then lower the toes to the floor. Repeat 10 times.

ally responds to treatment. Periodic limb movements of sleep can often be treated if recognized, but treatment may need to continue indefinitely. Leg cramps frequently resolve by themselves, but they may reappear again periodically for no apparent reason.

SLEEP APNEA

Sleep apnea is a temporary interruption of breathing that happens repeatedly during sleep.

Many people think they have sleep apnea because they snore when sleeping. However, snoring is much more common than sleep apnea.

Obstructive sleep apnea is the most common type of sleep apnea. In obstructive sleep apnea, the body's effort to breathe is normal, but the passageway for air (airway) through the mouth and the throat is partially or completely obstructed during sleep, so that breathing is interrupted.

Another type of apnea is called central sleep apnea. In central sleep apnea, although the airway is open, changes in the part of the brain that controls breathing bring a temporary halt to the body's effort to breathe. Rarely, people have a combination of obstructive and central sleep apnea.

Sleep apnea can cause the level of oxygen in the blood to fall, and it interferes with sleep. Sleep apnea, especially obstructive sleep apnea, may increase the risk of high blood pressure, strokes, heart attacks, confusion, and depression, but whether sleep apnea actually causes these problems is unclear.

Causes and Symptoms

People who have an airway that is narrower than average may be more likely to develop obstructive sleep apnea. Disorders or drugs may cause or contribute to airway obstruction in obstructive sleep apnea. Overweight people have increased fat in the wall of the throat. The increased fat makes airway obstruction more likely, especially when people sleep on their back. Drinking alcohol or taking sleep aids regularly may add to airway obstruction, possibly by relaxing muscles in the throat.

Obstructive sleep apnea leads to loud snoring, grunting, and restlessness. A bed partner may notice periods of shallow breathing or periods when breathing appears to stop. To overcome the obstruction and low oxygen level, people with obstructive sleep apnea frequently move from deeper to lighter stages of sleep. As a result, they are irritable and feel poorly rested and sleepy the following day.

Central sleep apnea may result from disorders such as strokes, heart failure, and kidney failure, which can interfere with the brain's control of breathing. People with central sleep apnea experience repeated, prolonged periods of nonbreathing during sleep, often followed by periods of rapid breathing (Cheyne-Stokes breathing). This pattern occurs in cycles through the night.

Diagnosis

Doctors suspect obstructive sleep apnea in older people who feel excessively sleepy during the day. The combination of obesity, a thick neck, and high blood pressure increases the doctor's suspicion. Central sleep apnea is suspected if a pattern of non-breathing alternating with rapid breathing is witnessed.

To confirm the diagnosis of either type of sleep apnea, the doctor needs to detect a fall in the level of oxygen in the blood during sleep. The diagnosis can be confirmed only by having the person undergo a specific type of test, called polysomnography,[1] in a sleep laboratory.

Treatment

Mild obstructive sleep apnea is best treated by losing weight, eliminating excessive alcohol intake, and discontinuing use of sleep aids.

When these measures are not successful, obstructive sleep apnea is sometimes treated with mechanical devices. An orthodontic device can keep the lower jaw or tongue in a position that prevents obstruction of the airway. Most people, particularly those with moderate or severe sleep apnea, instead need a nighttime breathing apparatus that uses pressurized air to keep the airway open (continuous positive airway pressure [CPAP] or bi-level positive airway pressure [Bi-PAP]). Both CPAP and Bi-PAP are safe and effective but must be used indefinitely. Bi-PAP is used only in people who cannot tolerate CPAP. Some people find it difficult to sleep with a CPAP or Bi-PAP apparatus, but adjustments to the apparatus that improve comfort are sometimes possible.

People who have an underlying abnormality in their airway or who do not improve with a CPAP or Bi-PAP apparatus may be candidates for traditional or laser surgery to remove throat tissue that obstructs the airway (uvulopalatopharyngoplasty). But the long-term benefit of surgery is unproved.

Treatment of central sleep apnea involves treating the disorder causing it, but oxygen and drugs such as theophylline (which is used to treat asthma or chronic obstructive pulmonary disease—COPD), acetazolamide (a diuretic), and progesterone (a hormone used in women after menopause) may be of some benefit.

1. see page 137

Outlook

Obstructive sleep apnea may cause daytime confusion, high blood pressure, strokes, and heart attacks. But adequate treatment of sleep apnea may prevent these conditions or control symptoms. Because treatment rarely cures the causes of central sleep apnea, the outlook for people with this type of apnea is not as good.

REM SLEEP BEHAVIOR DISORDER

REM sleep behavior disorder is one of the most dramatic sleep disorders. People with the disorder thrash around in bed, responding physically and sometimes violently to their dreams.

Normally, people in REM sleep do not move their arms and legs. People with REM sleep behavior disorder can harm themselves or their bed partner by flinging their arms and legs about.

When REM sleep behavior disorder occurs suddenly, it is usually caused by intoxication with or withdrawal from alcohol or a prescription drug. Long-term REM sleep behavior disorder can be caused by drugs (such as fluoxetine or venlafaxine), stroke, tumor, Parkinson's disease, dementia, and other serious brain disorders. Sometimes the cause is unknown.

Treatment consists of identifying and treating the cause, if there is one. A low dose of a benzodiazepine, usually clonazepam, taken at bedtime can be very effective.

CIRCADIAN RHYTHM DISORDERS

Circadian rhythm disorders are disruptions of the natural biological cycles that control how people are attuned to night and day.

Most people function on a circadian rhythm of about 24 hours, which is controlled by the internal biological clock in the brain. Shifting into or out of daylight savings time, traveling across time zones (which can cause jet lag), or working at a job that involves late evening or nighttime work can affect the body's circadian rhythm. However, factors outside the body, especially bright light, help to set the internal clock to the day cycle or time schedule appropriate to where the person is.

In a person with a circadian rhythm disorder, the body is unable to maintain its normal rhythm. The natural sleep schedule changes so that the person is out of phase with day and night.

Advanced sleep phase syndrome is a circadian rhythm disorder in which people fall asleep earlier in the evening and wake up earlier in the morning than they would like; it is common among older people. In delayed sleep phase syndrome, people fall asleep later at night and wake up later in the morning.

Less commonly, older people can have such a severe circadian rhythm disorder that they seem to be on no schedule at all, falling asleep and waking up unpredictably. These changes may be caused by aging. Visual loss and changes in hormones and surroundings may also contribute.

Diagnosis and Treatment

A doctor diagnoses a circadian rhythm disorder by looking closely at the timing of a person's sleep. Good sleeping habits are essential to restoring desirable sleep schedules.

Bright light therapy, in which a person is exposed during the day to sunlight or bright light from special light sources, may reinforce the body's natural responses to light. Bright light therapy may be effective for advanced or delayed sleep phase syndrome. Usually, the bright light is used in the evening for an advanced sleep phase and in the morning for a delayed sleep phase.

Short-term treatment with a sleep aid may help reset the circadian rhythm. Melatonin taken an hour before a person's regularly scheduled sleep time may be effective for preventing jet lag, especially when traveling east across more than three time zones. Melatonin has also been used to establish regular sleep-wake cycles in people with unpredictable rhythms.

OTHER SLEEP DISORDERS

Other sleep disorders can occur in older people but are rare. These disorders include sleepwalking, sudden collapse into sleep (narcolepsy), and night terrors. People who had these disorders as children may continue to experience them as they age. Night terrors in older people may be a sign of emotional difficulties that require assessment by a psychiatrist. Treatment for narcolepsy may require drugs that stimulate the brain, such as methylphenidate or modafinil.

32

Mental Health Disorders

Many people harbor worries about developing debilitating chronic physical disorders, such as arthritis, in their old age. Few give a thought, however, to the possibility of developing mental health disorders, such as depression. But mental health disorders can rob an older person of the ability to function and enjoy life just as surely as any physical disorder can.

The realization that mental health disorders can greatly impair the ability to function comes at a time when experts are discovering that many so-called physical disorders can directly affect mental health and many so-called mental disorders can directly affect physical health. The lines that used to divide physical and mental disorders have become very blurry.

Depression, anxiety, and psychosis are three of the most common mental health disorders that affect older people. Fortunately, these disorders, like most mental health disorders, can be effectively treated.

DEPRESSION

Depression is extraordinary sadness that interferes with the ability to function.

Everyone feels sad from time to time as a natural response to disappointment and loss. Like ordinary sadness, depression may develop after a sad event or may develop for no apparent reason. Depression can also occur with many physical disorders. But depression differs from ordinary sadness in several ways. For some, depression involves a nagging sense of feeling blue that drags on as they try to perform daily activities. For others, it is a heavy shroud of despair or emotional emptiness that becomes incapacitating. And depression can and often does become life threatening when a person has a deep sense of hopelessness or worthlessness and stops eating or turns to suicide for relief.

Depression affects about 1 out of every 6 older people. Some older people have had depression earlier in their lives, whereas others develop it for the first time during old age.

Doctors have identified several types of depression. However, the symptoms that some people experience may not easily fit into any one type.

Major depression lasts at least 2 weeks, although it often lasts much longer. Some people have brief episodes of depression in reaction to certain holidays (holiday blues) or anniversaries, such as the anniversary of a loved one's death. These brief episodes are similar to major depression, but they may last only a few days.

Psychotic depression, a more severe form of major depression, is complicated by a loss of contact with reality (psychosis), which usually includes harboring false beliefs (delusions).

Seasonal affective disorder (also called a mood disability with a seasonal pattern) is depression that recurs at a certain time of the year. It typically begins in October or November and ends by February or March; thus it is sometimes referred to as autumn-winter depression. Because this type of depression usually occurs in geographic locations in which the winter is longer and harsher, experts think that a lack of sunlight may play a role.

Dysthymic disorder is a less severe type of depression that smolders and persists for at least 2 years, though often much longer. Most older people who experience dysthymic disorder do not experience major depression.

Bipolar disorder is sometimes called manic depression. Bipolar disorder involves not only depression but also periods of mania—intense joyousness and elation. Unlike younger people with bipolar disorder, in whom periods of mania tend to be more frequent and more intense than periods of depression, most older people with bipolar disorder have long periods of depression and infrequent, subtler episodes of mania. During

WHEN ALCOHOL IS A PROBLEM

Older people are less likely than younger people to drink heavily or to be alcoholics. This observation seems reassuring. However, there is no doubt that alcohol is a problem for many older people. In fact, more older people are hospitalized for alcohol-related problems than for heart attacks.

When is alcohol considered a problem? It is a problem when people need to drink more and more alcohol to get the same effect and have withdrawal symptoms if they stop drinking. Such people have alcohol dependence. Drinking is also a problem if it causes physical, social, or psychologic harm. In such cases, alcohol abuse is diagnosed. Alcohol dependence or abuse is sometimes called alcoholism.

For older people, formal definitions of dependence or abuse are less meaningful—for them, drinking any amount of alcohol can interfere with functioning. The aging body processes alcohol differently. As a result, alcohol has a greater effect. So after drinking the same amount, older people are more impaired than when they were younger. Drinking even a small amount can make them sleepy, confused, uncoordinated, and unsteady.

The more alcohol consumed and the more often it is consumed, the greater the risk of more serious problems, such as hip fractures. Heavy drinking can cause or worsen urinary incontinence, problems with walking, depression, sleep disturbances, memory loss, dementia, delirium, high blood pressure, and bleeding in the digestive tract. Nutritional deficiencies, particularly deficiencies of thiamin, folate, vitamin B_6, niacin, and vitamin A, are more likely in heavy drinkers. Regularly consuming more than two drinks a day increases the risk of certain cancers (particularly those of the head, neck, and esophagus) and liver disorders.

Alcohol can interact with many drugs. When alcohol and drugs used to calm, relieve anxiety, or aid sleep (such as benzodiazepines) are combined, loss of balance, falls, and sleepiness are more likely, and reaction times are slower. Alcohol plus nonsteroidal anti-inflammatory drugs (NSAIDs) irritates the stomach and makes bleeding more likely. Aspirin increases the effects of alcohol in women, but not in men. Alcohol plus acetaminophen may lead to liver failure. So people who take acetaminophen daily are advised not to drink any alcohol.

How many alcoholic drinks are safe? Answers continue to be debated. A drink is considered to be 12 ounces of beer, 5 ounces of wine, and 1 1/2 ounces of liquor (such as whiskey). Most experts agree that older women should not drink more than 1 drink a day. For older men, the safe limit is thought to be 1 or 2 drinks. Adding to the confusion is evidence that drinking 1 or 2 drinks a day has some health benefits, such as a reducing the risk of coronary artery disease. With alcohol consumption, only a thin line separates potential health benefits from potential harm. For older people, less alcohol is definitely more in terms of health benefits.

these periods of mania, older people are often more likely to be irritable than elated.

Causes

The exact cause of depression is unknown, although imbalances of certain substances that carry messages between nerves (neurotransmitters) in the brain play an important role. An emotionally stressful life-changing event or experience precedes depression in some people. These events or experiences may include the death of a loved one, the ending of a significant relationship, or a loss of familiar surroundings, as when moving away from a long-time neighborhood. More persistent, smoldering sources of stress, such as ongoing poverty, a worsening chronic illness, a gradual loss of independence, or a lack of social support, may also contribute.

Depression sometimes develops during or soon after a person develops a physical disorder. Depression is common among people with cancer, heart attack, heart failure, hypothyroidism, or hyperthyroidism. Depression often occurs in people with nervous system and brain disorders, such as stroke, dementia, and Parkinson's disease. Depression also occurs in combination with other mental health disorders, such as anxiety.

Some drugs that older people take for physical disorders can cause symptoms of depression. These drugs include corticosteroids, digoxin, opioid analgesics, and certain drugs used to treat high blood pressure (antihypertensives), such as methyldopa and reserpine.

Abuse of alcohol or drugs, including prescription and illegal drugs, may contribute to the development of depression in some older people.

Symptoms

Extraordinary sadness is at the core of depression for many people. For others, a feeling of emptiness or absence of emotion may be the primary symptom. Many other symptoms may be present as well. Absence of pleasure or of interest in activities is often noticeable. Some depressed older people stop performing daily activities at work or at home, and they may simply stop making any effort to care for themselves. Many depressed people have trouble falling asleep and staying asleep. Early awak-

SUICIDE AND SUICIDAL BEHAVIOR

Suicidal behavior is a successful or unsuccessful attempt to kill oneself. It is an unmistakable proclamation of a person's feelings of desperation and hopelessness.

Suicidal behavior includes attempted suicide, suicide gestures, and completed suicide. An attempted suicide does not result in the person's death. A suicide gesture is a suicide attempt that has almost no potential of being fatal (for example, ingesting six acetaminophen tablets). A person taking such an action is usually making a plea for help without intending to actually end his life. A completed suicide results in death.

Married people of either sex have a much lower suicide rate than single people. People who live alone because of separation, divorce, or a spouse's death have higher rates of attempted and completed suicides. Men over age 70 (especially white men) have the highest rate of completed suicide, compared with younger men and with women of any age.

Suicidal behaviors usually result from the interaction of several factors, the most common of which is depression. In fact, depression is involved in more than half of attempted suicides. Marital problems or the recent loss of a loved one may precipitate the depression. Depression associated with a physical disorder is frequently a factor in suicide attempts among older people. People whose depression includes anxiety or psychosis may be at higher risk of suicide than people whose depression does not include these features.

Depression may be intensified by the use of alcohol, which in turn makes suicidal behavior more likely. Because persistent and excessive drinking often leaves a person with deep feelings of remorse during dry periods, suicidal behavior is common even when heavy drinkers are sober.

Although suicide threats or suicide attempts often come as a shock, clear warnings are given in many cases. Any suicide threat or suicide attempt is a plea for help and must be taken seriously. If the threat or attempt is ignored, a life may be lost. If a person is threatening or has already attempted suicide, the police should be contacted immediately so that emergency services can arrive as soon as possible. Until help arrives, the person should be spoken to in a calm, supportive manner.

After a completed suicide, family, friends, and health care practitioners may feel guilt, shame, and remorse at not having prevented it. They may even feel angry toward the person. Eventually, many of them realize that they could not have prevented the suicide. Sometimes a grief counselor or a self-help group, such as Survivors of Suicide, can help family and friends deal with their feelings of guilt and sorrow. The primary care doctor or local mental health services (for example, at the county or state level) can often help locate these resources. In addition, national organizations, such as the American Foundation for Suicide Prevention, often maintain directories of local support groups.

ening in the morning is especially common. Appetite is often decreased or lost altogether.

Depression may slow thinking and interfere with concentration and memory. Some depressed older people are mistakenly thought to have dementia because of confusion, forgetfulness, and disorientation (a condition often called pseudodementia). Feelings of hopelessness, worthlessness, and guilt are common in people with pseudodementia.

Some depressed people are restless, wringing their hands and talking continuously. In contrast, other people with depression are withdrawn, seem tired all the time, move slowly, and gain weight. Symptoms may be worse at a certain time of the day, usually in the morning. Thoughts about death and suicide often surface. Many depressed people want to die or feel that they should die.

Loss of contact with reality (psychosis) develops in some severely depressed people. When this occurs, it usually involves false ideas or beliefs (delusions). For example, people with psychotic depression may become convinced that they are worthless or sinful or that they are impoverished. Some may become convinced that they hear or see people or things that no one else hears or sees (hallucinations).

People with symptoms of depression may also develop episodes of intense joyousness or elation if they have bipolar disorder. During such episodes, they may also be very restless, distracted, and irritable.

Screening and Diagnosis

Depression is often difficult to diagnose among older people, for several reasons:

• The symptoms may be less noticeable because older people may not work or may have less social interaction.

• Some people believe that depression is a weakness and are reluctant to tell anyone that they are experiencing sadness or other symptoms.

• The absence of emotion may not be interpreted as depression, but rather, as indifference.

• Family and friends may regard a depressed person's symptoms simply as evidence that the person is getting older.

• The symptoms may be attributed to another disorder.

Because recognition and diagnosis of depression can be challenging and because depression threatens a person's quality of life and ability to perform daily activities, some experts recommend screening. Screening involves asking a person a series of questions that help identify symptoms of depression. Screening for depression is offered at many community health fairs and through doctors' offices, clinics, and hospitals.

A doctor diagnoses depression by thoroughly reviewing a person's symptoms. But a physical examination and medical tests are performed to determine whether a physical disorder is causing or contributing to the person's symptoms of depression. Hypothyroidism is one of the most common of the physical disorders that causes depression. Therefore, a blood test to assess thyroid function is particularly useful.

Treatment

When a physical disorder or a drug is thought to be causing or contributing to depression, treating the disorder or reducing or stopping the offending drug may relieve the depression. However, in most instances, other treatment is needed for depression.

Depressed older people are commonly treated with drug therapy. Other treatments include counseling, electroconvulsive therapy, phototherapy, and exercise. Often a combination of therapies is best.

Drug therapy: Drug treatment with antidepressants is effective in about two thirds of depressed older people. The three types of antidepressants are selective serotonin reuptake inhibitors (SSRIs), tricyclic antidepressants, and monoamine oxidase inhibitors (MAOIs). Other types of drugs, including psychostimulants, antipsychotics, and mood stabilizers, are available to treat certain symptoms of depression.

No one antidepressant has been found to be consistently more effective than another, although the side effects of the different types of antidepressants vary widely. Therefore, doctors usually recommend an antidepressant that is least likely to cause side effects for the person taking it.

Antidepressants usually must be taken for at least 4 weeks before they help. Occasionally, however, people respond to an antidepressant in as little as 2 weeks. If the initial dosage does

DETECTING DEPRESSION OR ANXIETY: AT A LOSS FOR WORDS

Depression or anxiety can be challenging enough, but some people have the additional challenge of being unable to tell anyone how they are feeling. For example, a person with dementia or a stroke may be unable to express the very kinds of feelings that indicate to others that they may be experiencing depression or anxiety. In such cases, other clues may become important.

Family members, friends, and caregivers may begin to suspect depression or anxiety if they note changes in the older person's behavior. If a person has become depressed, closer observation may reveal that the person no longer seems to derive pleasure from or take interest in activities that were once pleasurable or interesting. A person who normally enjoys being with others may begin to give signals of wanting to be left alone (such as frowning, ignoring others,

or pushing others away), which may indicate depression. A person who normally has a good appetite may start picking at his food or ignore it completely, which also may indicate depression. A person who normally seems relaxed and calm under most circumstances may have developed anxiety if he seems to have tense muscles, an inability to remain seated for very long, or the appearance of being afraid for no apparent reason.

Anxiety symptoms are common in people with dementia and may develop in combination with impaired memory and thinking. However, anxiety symptoms in someone with dementia may also indicate that the person is experiencing pain; hunger, thirst, or other unmet needs; new medical problems; or side effects of prescription or nonprescription drugs.

not help, the doctor gradually increases the amount. If no benefit results after about 12 weeks and the dosage is as high as it can be safely increased, the doctor usually adds another drug or discontinues the first drug and switches to another.

Selective serotonin reuptake inhibitors (SSRIs) are the type of antidepressants used most often in older people. SSRIs have fewer side effects than other types of drugs used for depression. However, some SSRIs, especially fluoxetine and paroxetine, may interact with other drugs. Citalopram and escitalopram may be the least likely to cause side effects and may relieve symptoms of depression more rapidly than most other antidepressants.

Other antidepressants similar to SSRIs (both in effectiveness and side effects), such as venlafaxine, mirtazapine, and bupropion, are also often used.

℞ DRUGS USED TO TREAT DEPRESSION

Type	Drug	Side Effects	Comments
Selective serotonin reuptake inhibitors (SSRIs)	Citalopram Escitalopram Fluoxetine Fluvoxamine Paroxetine Sertraline	Restlessness and jitteriness (akathisia), difficulty falling or staying asleep (insomnia), nausea, diarrhea, sexual dysfunction (decreased desire, diminished arousal, delayed orgasm)	Cause fewer side effects than other drugs used to treat depression
Tricyclics	Amitriptyline Desipramine Doxepin Imipramine Nortriptyline	Light-headedness and low blood pressure, dry mouth, blurred vision, difficulty beginning or continuing urination, constipation, confusion, memory loss, involuntary repetitive movements of muscles (tardive dyskinesia), restlessness and jitteriness (akathisia)	Many experts recommend against use of amitriptyline, doxepin, and imipramine among older people because of their common and serious side effects
Psychostimulants	Dextroamphetamine Methylphenidate	Nervousness, tremor, insomnia, dry mouth	Not as effective as antidepressants when used alone. Often used in combination with antidepressants, especially to improve appetite and energy level

Type	Drug	Side Effects	Comments
Other drugs	Bupropion	Seizures (rare), mild headache, insomnia, weight loss	Least likely of the antidepressants to cause sexual dysfunction
	Mirtazapine	Sleepiness, increased appetite, weight gain, dry mouth	
	Nefazodone	Dry mouth, constipation, sleepiness, dizziness, liver damage (rare)	
	Trazodone	Sleepiness, light-headedness when standing, irregular heart rhythms (rare), persistent erection in men	May be less effective than other antidepressants
	Venlafaxine	Nausea, dizziness, insomnia, constipation, increased blood pressure	

Tricyclic antidepressants are used much less often for older people. Although they are effective in treating depression, they more often cause disturbing and disabling side effects.

Monoamine oxidase inhibitors (MAOIs) are a type of antidepressant that is rarely used for depressed older people because of a risk of severe side effects. Certain foods and drugs interact with MAOIs, causing high blood pressure, dizziness, headache, and fatigue.

Psychostimulants, such as methylphenidate, are an effective treatment for some symptoms of depression. If these drugs are going to work, they take effect within days rather than weeks. They are generally reserved for depressed people who are endangering themselves by not eating or drinking, because these drugs often greatly stimulate appetite. Psychostimulants may also be used to stimulate the level of energy and activity in depressed people who move very slowly and who are extremely withdrawn.

Antipsychotics are drugs that help eliminate or control symptoms of psychosis, such as delusions or hallucinations, that occur in some people with depression. Antipsychotics may be given in combination with an antidepressant, but they are typically discontinued once the antidepressant has started to take effect.

Mood stabilizers are used to treat people with bipolar disorder. These drugs help to calm some of the intense elation as well as the restlessness and irritability that occur during episodes of mania. Lithium is one such drug, but it can cause many side effects in older people. Drugs used for treating seizures, such as divalproex and gabapentin, are often better tolerated and also help stabilize mood. Tremor is a side effect of many mood stabilizers.

Counseling: Counseling (psychotherapy) is an effective treatment for mild depression. It is also effective when combined with drug therapy for more severe depression. Counseling may focus on helping the depressed person change unrealistic expectations, reduce tendencies to self-criticize, and avoid automatic reactions to negative, distorted thoughts. Counseling may also help the person use insight to distinguish between life problems that are most important and those that are minor. Problem-solving strategies may be taught so that the person is better able to cope with everyday stress. Counseling may take place in group or individual sessions. Visits are usually once a week for 12 to 20 sessions. Counseling may be performed by a specially trained social worker, a psychologist, or a psychiatrist.

Electroconvulsive therapy: Electroconvulsive therapy consists of passing an electrical current through the brain so that a seizure results. The seizure may help relieve depression by causing a release of neurotransmitters in the brain. Electroconvulsive therapy is used for people who are severely depressed, including those who have lost contact with reality (psychotic depression) and those who are a threat to themselves. Electroconvulsive therapy is also useful for people whose condition has not been helped by drug therapy. Before receiving the treatment, the person is given a drug that induces sleep (an anesthetic) and a muscle-relaxing drug to reduce the risk of injury during the seizure. Results of electroconvulsive therapy are usually felt within days. It often needs to be repeated several times.

Phototherapy: Phototherapy is the use of bright light for people with seasonal affective disorder. Phototherapy consists of sitting daily for brief periods in a room lit by a special lighting device (sometimes called a light box). Increasing the time spent outdoors may also help.

Exercise: A number of studies have pointed out the beneficial effects of exercise, particularly aerobic exercise, on mood. This may in part be due to the role of exercise in elevating the level of a type of neurotransmitter called endorphins. Endorphins are small proteins that produce a feeling of well-being and tolerance to pain by stimulating certain sites in the brain. Therefore, a supervised exercise program, perhaps combined with psychotherapy, antidepressants, or both, may be recommended.

Outlook

People with depression usually respond to treatment. However, only about one third remain free of symptoms indefinitely. Another third experience improvement with treatment but have relapses. About one third do not respond well or at all to initial treatment. Changing treatment or adding additional treatment helps some of these people. Even among those who do not respond well to treatment, the ability to function and perform daily activities usually improves somewhat.

ANXIETY

Anxiety is intense nervousness or worrying that interferes with the ability to function.

Nervousness or worrying is a normal response to a threat or to stress. Everyone experiences nervousness or worrying occasionally. But anxiety is intense nervousness or worrying. Anxiety may develop for no apparent reason. Anxiety can occur with many physical disorders, or it can be a side effect of certain drugs. Anxiety may also be a symptom of an anxiety disorder that requires treatment. Anxiety disorders often are chronic, but the symptoms fluctuate. Therefore, the person may be calm at times and overwhelmingly nervous at other times. Anxiety disorders can interfere greatly with an older person's quality of life and ability to perform daily activities.

Anxiety disorders are common in older people. Many anxious older people have had anxiety disorders earlier in their lives, whereas others develop an anxiety disorder for the first time during old age.

The most common anxiety disorder in older people is generalized anxiety disorder. People with this disorder have at least 6 months of almost daily nervousness and worry about activities or events. Generalized anxiety disorder affects at least 1 out of every 30 older people. Women are more likely than men to experience generalized anxiety disorder.

Other anxiety disorders, including obsessive-compulsive disorder and phobic disorders, are also quite common among older people. Posttraumatic stress disorder and panic disorder are much less common among older people.

ADDITIONAL DETAIL

Obsessive-compulsive disorder is characterized by obsessions, which are ideas, images, or impulses that intrude into a person's thinking (for example, fear of contamination). The obsessions may seem silly, weird, nasty, or horrible and may be accompanied by compulsions, which are repetitive, even ritualistic urges (for example, ritualistic hand washing) to do something that will lessen the discomfort that they cause. People with this disorder are aware that their obsessions are not actual risks or threats, so they have not lost touch with reality (which would be called psychosis). Obsessive-compulsive disorder is common among older people but usually begins in earlier life. Women are more likely than men to be affected.

Phobic disorders involve persistent, unrealistic, yet intense anxiety brought on by certain situations. Examples include fear of public places (agoraphobia) and fear of confinement (claustrophobia). Phobic disorders are more common among children and younger adults than they are among older people, though they are not rare among older people. Phobic disorders can severely inhibit social interactions, though most phobias are not disabling.

Posttraumatic stress disorder involves the re-experiencing or replaying of an overwhelmingly disturbing event, resulting in intense fear, a sense of helplessness, horror, and an urge to avoid things associated with the disturbing trauma. The re-experiencing or replaying of the event usually takes the form of a nightmare or flashback. The event may have occurred long ago: The effects of severe stress during childhood or young adulthood on the way some people function later in life are widely recognized. Disturbing, traumatic events can certainly occur in middle or old age as well.

Panic disorder is characterized by recurrent, brief periods of intense fear or nervous discomfort. These periods, or panic attacks, are rare in older people and when they occur tend to be less severe than those in younger adults.

Causes

The cause of anxiety is usually not determined. However, anxiety can be caused by a variety of physical disorders, such as hyperthyroidism, chronic obstructive pulmonary disease (COPD), and heart failure. Impaired memory and thinking (cognitive impairment), whether it develops suddenly and lasts for a limited period (for example, delirium) or develops gradually and progresses (for example, dementia), is often accompanied by anxiety symptoms. Anxiety can also be a side effect of several drugs taken for physical disorders, including thyroid hormone replacement drugs, corticosteroids, and certain drugs used to treat some lung problems (beta-adrenergic agonists). Drinking excessive amounts of beverages containing caffeine, such as coffee, tea, and certain sodas, can also contribute to anxiety.

The exact cause of anxiety disorders is unclear. Both temporary stressors and ongoing, persistent daily hassles contribute to development of anxiety disorders in some people. Anxiety disorders often develop in people with other mental health disorders, such as a depressive or psychotic disorder. Some experts think that imbalances of certain substances that carry messages between nerves (neurotransmitters) in the brain play an important role.

Symptoms and Diagnosis

Anxiety can develop gradually and continue to worsen. In some, the symptoms occur more suddenly and wax and wane. Symptoms range in intensity from barely noticeable worrying and jitteriness to complete fear or panic.

People with generalized anxiety disorder may feel worried almost all of the time, although brief respites of calmness can occur. Nervousness and worrying often worsen during stressful situations. The focus of the worries among older people is often health, safety, or money. This focus often shifts from one topic to another over time. Difficulty falling and staying asleep (insomnia) is common among people with generalized anxiety disorder. Nervousness and worrying may be accompanied at any time by restlessness, fatigue, difficulty concentrating, irritability, and a sense of increased muscle tension.

Symptoms in people with obsessive-compulsive disorder, phobic disorders, and posttraumatic stress disorder tend to fluctuate and consist mainly of nervousness and worrying. People with panic disorder develop a surge of anxiety that lasts for only a few minutes or hours (panic attacks).

The diagnosis of an anxiety disorder is based largely on symptoms. The ability to tolerate anxiety varies, and determining what constitutes abnormal anxiety can be difficult.

Treatment

When a physical disorder or a drug is thought to be causing or contributing to anxiety, treating the disorder or reducing or stopping the offending drug may relieve the anxiety. If a person is consuming an excessive amount of caffeinated beverages, reducing or eliminating caffeine from the diet may help. However, other treatment is usually needed for anxiety disorders.

Most people with anxiety disorders respond best to a combination of drug therapy and counseling (psychotherapy).

Drug therapy: Several types of drugs are used to treat anxiety disorders. They are similar in effectiveness but differ by the side effects they can cause.

Certain drugs used to treat depression (antidepressants) are used to treat anxiety. These antidepressants are helpful not only in people who have both anxiety and depression, but also in people who do not have depression. The antidepressants used are usually selective serotonin reuptake inhibitors (SSRIs), such as sertraline and paroxetine, or antidepressants that are similar to SSRIs, including venlafaxine and mirtazapine. Antidepressants usually must be taken for a few weeks before they help control anxiety. For this reason, faster-acting drugs, such as benzodiazepines, may be taken along with an antidepressant until the antidepressant takes effect. The benzodiazepine can then be discontinued.

Benzodiazepines are also used to treat anxiety. They begin to work very quickly after they are taken. Thus, they can be used for brief periods when they are most needed to control symptoms. For some older people, however, they are best used regularly. Their use for periods longer than several months is not recommended because of the risk of side effects. Lorazepam, oxazepam, and temazepam are three drugs that may be safer for older people. Older, long-acting benzodiazepines, such as diazepam, chlordiazepoxide, and flurazepam, are best avoided in older people because they cause more side effects. Still, all benzodiazepines, even the safer ones, may cause confusion, poor concentration, sleepiness, and unsteadiness while walking.

Buspirone is another drug used in treatment. In most cases, this drug takes 2 to 4 weeks to take effect. Buspirone has few side effects. However, this drug is not as effective in people who have previously taken benzodiazepines.

Counseling: Counseling may focus on the root of anxiety. Often, however, counseling is not able to uncover a cause and instead focuses on helping the person learn new techniques for relaxation. Some counseling techniques make use of soothing music or visual images. People with anxiety disorders can also be taught to recognize triggers and stimuli that bring on episodes of worsened anxiety. Once the triggers or stimuli are recognized, people can learn new ways to cope and maintain control. Exposure therapy is sometimes used, especially for people with panic disorder and obsessive-compulsive disorder. Exposure therapy involves repeatedly exposing the person to a feared object or situation. This causes the person to experience the anxiety over and over until the feared object or situation loses its effect.

PSYCHOSIS

Psychosis is a loss of contact with reality.

Psychosis often involves harboring false beliefs (delusions) and seeing or hearing things that no one else sees or hears (hallucinations). People with psychosis often become unreasonably fearful or suspicious (paranoid). People with psychosis are sometimes referred to as being psychotic.

Psychosis may develop suddenly or gradually. Psychosis may be a temporary symptom of a physical or mental health disorder or the primary symptom of a chronic disorder (a psychotic disorder). Even when psychosis is part of a chronic disorder, the symptom may fluctuate, so that at times the person seems to have a grasp on reality.

Some older people with a psychotic disorder first developed symptoms as an adolescent or young adult or during middle age as part of a disease called schizophrenia. However, most older people with a psychotic disorder develop symptoms for the first time during old age. Many of them have paraphrenia, which is characterized by paranoid delusions and hallucinations. Psychotic disorders may affect as many as 1 out of every 50 older people.

Psychosis is usually very distressing, both to the person who experiences it and to family and friends who witness the strange behaviors of their loved ones. Fortunately, people with psychosis often respond well to treatment with drugs, especially when accompanied by reassurance and support from family, friends, and health care practitioners.

Causes

Psychosis may occur as part of other mental health disorders. Some older people with severe depression also become psychotic. And some people with dementia have psychosis.

Severe physical illness, such as severe infection, can cause temporary psychosis. Injury to the brain from a stroke or tumor can also lead to psychosis. Even extreme stress can lead to temporary psychosis. When older people are cared for in intensive care units, where they are deprived of sleep and bombarded by tests, psychosis is common.

Certain drugs, such as opioid analgesics, benzodiazepines,

digoxin, and drugs with anticholinergic side effects, can also cause temporary psychosis. Excessive alcohol use can cause temporary psychosis; chronic psychosis can result if the drinking is long-term.

The exact cause of psychotic disorders is unknown. Many experts think that these disorders develop because the brain overreacts to certain substances that carry messages between nerves (neurotransmitters) in the brain. Heredity may play a part as well, because some psychotic disorders, especially schizophrenia, tend to run in families.

Symptoms

Some people with psychosis have false beliefs that can best be described as fearfulness and suspiciousness (paranoia). They may have vague fears or complaints about others controlling their lives, but many describe consistent suspicions of very specific, elaborate, and persistent plots against them. Very often, these beliefs are directed at family members or friends. For example, people with psychosis may believe that their spouse or children have deserted them or that their family or friends are scheming to obtain control of their finances or property.

Hallucinations—seeing or hearing things that no one else sees or hears—are sometimes experienced by people with psychosis. These hallucinations may seem dangerous and threatening to the person, although in some cases they are taken in stride.

People with psychosis may lose the ability to take care of their personal hygiene. They may seem withdrawn and without any emotions. However, when a psychotic disorder, such as paraphrenia, develops during old age, it is common for a person to communicate and function quite well despite delusions or hallucinations.

When psychosis is part of a disorder that impairs memory and the ability to think clearly, such as dementia, the nature of false beliefs often becomes increasingly paranoid. The person may become distraught, accusing others of stealing personal belongings or of attempting poisoning or molestation. The paranoia associated with dementia is usually very unpredictable and changeable. For example, a demented person with paranoia may accuse a particular person of some behavior yet shortly thereafter describe that same person as his best friend. The demented person with paranoia can be very irritable and angry, sometimes even to the point of striking out at others.

Diagnosis

A doctor diagnoses psychosis by reviewing and exploring the person's symptoms. When a person who is dependent on someone else's care strongly and consistently feels endangered and unable to protect himself, the doctor must entertain the possibility that some real danger exists, given how common the problem of mistreatment of older people has become.[1]

After a person has been diagnosed as having psychosis, the doctor focuses on identifying the cause. A review of prescription and nonprescription drugs is important. A physical examination is performed to determine if disorders are present that might be causing or contributing to the psychosis. Similarly, medical tests may be useful. For example, the blood may be tested for evidence of certain drugs that can cause psychosis. Blood tests help exclude many physical disorders as a cause. If any unusual neurologic abnormalities are found, such as weakness of only one side of the body, a computed tomography (CT) or magnetic resonance imaging (MRI) scan of the brain may be performed.

Treatment

When a person develops psychosis as part of another disease, such as depression, appropriate treatment for that disease may lessen or even stop the psychosis. When people are sleep-deprived because they are in intensive care, moving them to a quieter environment, if possible, usually cures the psychosis. Recovery may take time, however; thus, other steps may be needed to treat the psychosis.

Treatment of psychosis involves an effort on the part of health care practitioners, family, and friends to support and reassure the person rather than confront him about delusions or hallucinations. People with psychosis living in long-term care facilities (such as nursing homes) have better control of their symptoms when the staff reminds them of who everyone is and reassures them of their safety. Treatment also usually involves drug therapy.

1. see page 945

℞ DRUGS USED TO TREAT PSYCHOSIS (ANTIPSYCHOTICS)

Type	Drug	Side Effects	Comments
Older antipsychotics	Chlorproma-zine Fluphenazine Haloperidol Loxapine Mesoridazine Molindone Perphenazine Pimozide Thioridazine Thiothixene Trifluopera-zine	Dry mouth, blurred vision, seizures, increased heart rate, decreased blood pressure, constipation, tremor, muscle stiffness that may progress to rigidity, involuntary repetitive movements of muscles (tardive dyskinesia), fever and muscle damage (neuroleptic malignant syndrome)	These drugs usually are not used for people with problems with balance and stability, so that their risk of falls and injuries is not further increased Eye examinations are routinely performed when taking thioridazine Many experts recommend against the use of thioridazine because it may cause life-threatening abnormal heart rhythms
Newer antipsychotics	Aripiprazole Clozapine Olanzapine Quetiapine Risperidone Ziprasidone	Tremor, muscle stiffness that may progress to rigidity, uncontrolled movements of the face and arms (tardive dyskinesia), fever and muscle damage (neuroleptic	Older people tolerate newer antipsychotics much better, because these drugs are less likely to cause tremor, muscle stiffness, uncontrolled movements, and fever and muscle damage Clozapine is not

Table continues on the following page.

Type	Drug	Side Effects	Comments
		malignant syndrome), drowsiness, weight gain, dizziness	used often because it can stop the bone marrow from producing white blood cells that are needed to fight infections and it can also cause seizures However, it is often effective in people who not helped by other drugs Clozapine and ziprasidone may cause abnormal heart rhythms

Drug therapy: Drugs called antipsychotics can be effective in reducing or eliminating symptoms, such as delusions and hallucinations. After the immediate symptoms have subsided with treatment, antipsychotics may need to be continued to help reduce the likelihood of future episodes.

Unfortunately, antipsychotics can have many side effects, including sedation, muscle stiffness, tremors, weight gain, and restlessness. Antipsychotics may also cause tardive dyskinesia, a disorder in which a person has one or more types of involuntary movements.[1] These movements most often involve puckering of the lips and tongue or writhing of the arms or legs. Tardive dyskinesia may not go away, even after the drug that is suspected of causing the problem is discontinued. If tardive dyskinesia persists, no effective treatment is available.

A number of new antipsychotics that cause fewer side effects, such as risperidone, olanzapine, and quetiapine, have become available. However, in people with dementia, risperidone may increase the risk of stroke.

1. see page 409

Outlook

The outlook depends greatly on the cause of psychosis. When psychosis is caused by depression, sleep deprivation, or another treatable disorder, treating the other disorder often cures the psychosis. However, for people whose psychosis is part of dementia and for those whom psychosis is the primary symptom of a chronic disorder (a psychotic disorder), long-term treatment must usually include drug therapy and supportive care if it is to succeed in controlling symptoms and preventing relapses. If the person with psychosis is followed closely by health care practitioners, treated appropriately, and cared for in a supportive environment, then quality of life can improve significantly.

33

Thyroid Disorders

Tucked away at the base of the neck, in front of the windpipe (trachea), just below the Adam's apple, the thyroid gland measures only 2 inches across. It has two lobes connected in the middle, giving it the shape of a bow tie or butterfly. When the thyroid gland is functioning normally, as it does most of the time in most people, there is little reason to give a second thought to its shape or to any of its other characteristics.

The main purpose of the thyroid gland is to make the hormones thyroxine (T_4) and triiodothyronine (T_3). Thyroid hormones control the speed of many vital body functions (the body's metabolism). For example, thyroid hormones make the heart beat faster and cause the body to burn up calories more quickly. T_3 plays a much greater role than T_4 in controlling the speed of body functions.

Aging itself has only minor effects on the thyroid gland and thyroid hormones. As people get older, the thyroid gland

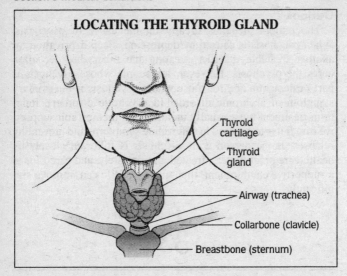

LOCATING THE THYROID GLAND

Thyroid cartilage

Thyroid gland

Airway (trachea)

Collarbone (clavicle)

Breastbone (sternum)

shrinks and shifts lower in the neck. The level of T_3 may fall slightly, but the speed of vital body functions changes very little. However, thyroid disorders become more common with aging.

In some cases, thyroid disorders produce extremely subtle changes in thyroid function. More commonly, however, disorders cause a noticeable change in function, especially underactivity of the thyroid gland and decreased production of thyroid hormones (hypothyroidism). The entire thyroid gland may enlarge, or one or more thyroid nodules may develop. Any enlargement of the thyroid gland—with or without nodules—is called a goiter.

Disorders that affect thyroid function can be thought of as great masqueraders in older people, because these disorders so often cause symptoms that are easily mistaken for symptoms of other conditions or even as signs of getting old. Increased or decreased thyroid function can dramatically worsen the way an older person feels and can greatly diminish the ability to carry out daily activities. For these reasons, the great masqueraders must be unmasked and recognized for what they are so that they can be effectively treated.

ADDITIONAL DETAIL

The thyroid gland concentrates iodine that the body absorbs from various foods to make thyroid hormones. The thyroid gland makes mostly T_4. Very little T_3 is made by the thyroid gland. The liver and other organs convert T_4 into T_3. Certain diseases and drugs can affect the conversion of T_4 into T_3.

Both T_4 and T_3 circulate in the blood, mostly bound to certain proteins. Thyroid hormones become active in their role of controlling the speed of vital body functions when they are freed from protein binding. The body regulates a balance between bound thyroid hormones and free thyroid hormones.

Through a complex interaction between the hypothalamus (a part of the brain) and the pituitary gland (located inside the skull, just underneath the brain), the thyroid gland knows how much of its hormones to produce. The hypothalamus makes thyrotropin-releasing hormone, which then stimulates the pituitary gland. The pituitary gland responds by making another hormone called thyroid-stimulating hormone, or TSH. As the name suggests, thyroid-stimulating hormone stimulates the thyroid gland to make hormones. If the level of thyroid hormones in the blood climbs above what is needed, the pituitary gland makes less thyroid-stimulating hormone. The thyroid gland then cuts back on making thyroid hormones. If the level of thyroid hormones in the blood falls too low, the pituitary gland makes more thyroid-stimulating hormone. In response, the thyroid gland makes and secretes more thyroid hormones. The body adjusts the amount of thyroid hormones to suit its needs in the same way a thermostat adjusts the temperature in a house.

HYPOTHYROIDISM

Hypothyroidism, or an underactive thyroid gland, is a decrease in the production of thyroid hormones, which slows vital body functions.

More than 15% of older people have some degree of hypothyroidism. Women are affected about twice as often as men.

Causes

Hypothyroidism can have several causes, although in many people a specific cause cannot be found. In Hashimoto's thyroiditis, the most common specific cause of hypothyroidism, something triggers the body's immune system to produce cells called lymphocytes that attack the thyroid gland. At first, the gland may enlarge. Eventually, Hashimoto's thyroiditis damages the thyroid gland and can leave it unable to make enough hormones, resulting in hypothyroidism.

Other causes of hypothyroidism include previous radiation to and surgical removal of the thyroid gland. Much less commonly, hypothyroidism results from disorders of the hypothalamus or pituitary gland. Certain drugs, such as lithium (which is used to treat bipolar disease), drugs used to treat overactivity of the thyroid gland, and drugs that contain iodine (such as amiodarone, which is used to treat heart disease), can cause hypothyroidism as well.

Symptoms

In older people, hypothyroidism can cause confusion, decreased appetite, weight loss, sensitivity to cold, constipation, joint stiffness, dizziness, and a tendency to fall. Some people feel tired, weak, or depressed. The skin may become dry and coarse, and the face may become puffy and swollen, especially around the eyes. Muscles and joints may ache. Weakness may progress, interfering with the ability to walk. In its most severe form, hypothyroidism can cause a person to slip into a coma (myxedema coma) and may even be fatal.

Doctors may not recognize these symptoms as being caused by hypothyroidism: the symptoms may be subtle and vague and are common among older people who do not have hypothyroidism. Symptoms of hypothyroidism that are common among younger and middle-aged people, such as weight gain, muscle cramps, tingling, and the inability to tolerate cold, are less common among older people, and when they do occur among older people, they are less obvious.

Diagnosis and Screening

Doctors feel (palpate) the thyroid gland, which may be enlarged. During a physical examination, doctors may find some evidence of hypothyroidism. The area around the eyes is checked for puffiness, and the skin is checked for dryness. Doctors tap the knees, ankles, and elbows to see if reflexes are slow. Body temperature may be slightly decreased. Often, however, the examination findings are normal.

If hypothyroidism is considered a possibility, blood tests are usually done. The level of thyroid-stimulating hormone is measured first. If hypothyroidism is present, the level of thyroid-stimulating hormone is almost always high. In rare instances in which hypothyroidism is due to a disorder that affects the pituitary gland rather than the thyroid gland, the level of thyroid-stimulating hormone is normal or low. If the level of thyroid-stimulating hormone is normal and doctors still suspect hypothyroidism, they measure the level of T_4 hormone. A low level confirms the diagnosis of hypothyroidism. Other tests may be needed to determine the cause.

Screening older people for hypothyroidism is helpful. Many experts recommend measuring the level of thyroid-stimulating hormone in the blood every 5 years. The level should be measured more often in people taking certain drugs (such as lithium or amiodarone), in those who have had a thyroid problem in the past, in those who have a family history of thyroid disorders, and in those who have conditions involving the immune system. Thyroid testing should also be done in people who have high cholesterol levels, which can be caused by an underactive thyroid gland.

Treatment and Outlook

People who have hypothyroidism need to take thyroid hormone to replace the hormones that the thyroid gland is no longer making. Treatment usually begins with a small dose of thyroid hormone. The dose is then slowly increased about every 4 weeks. The body may take that long to fully adapt to each change in dose. To reduce the risk of side effects from treatment, people who have heart disease or other serious disorders begin treatment with yet a smaller dose, which is increased even more slowly.

After about 3 to 4 months, the appropriate dose of thyroid hormone is usually reached. After this point, the dose occasionally needs to be adjusted, depending on weight loss or gain and the use of certain drugs. Sometimes certain drugs (such as iron supplements, calcium carbonate, or aluminum-containing antacids) can interfere with the absorption of thyroid hormone. Certain other drugs (especially drugs used to prevent seizures, such as carbamazepine) increase the body's metabolism of thyroid hormone. When a drug interferes with absorption or speeds up metabolism of thyroid hormone, an alternative drug may be taken or a higher dose of thyroid hormone may be needed. To help determine if the person is responding well to treatment, doctors periodically measure the level of thyroid-stimulating hormone.

Treatment is very successful in eliminating or greatly reducing the symptoms of hypothyroidism. However, treatment with thyroid hormone does not cure the problem that caused the hypothyroidism. For this reason, treatment with thyroid hormone almost always has to be continued for life.

HYPERTHYROIDISM

Hyperthyroidism, or an overactive thyroid gland, is an increase in the production of thyroid hormones, which speeds up vital body functions.

Hyperthyroidism affects about the same percentage of older people as younger people—fewer than 2%. However, hyperthyroidism is often more serious among older people because they tend to have other disorders as well.

Causes

Hyperthyroidism in older people often results from Graves' disease. In Graves' disease, the body makes antibodies that stimulate the thyroid gland, causing it to produce excessive amounts of thyroid hormones.

Almost as often, hyperthyroidism is caused by the gradual growth of many small lumps (nodules) in the thyroid gland. In this condition, called toxic multinodular goiter, the nodules secrete excessive amounts of thyroid hormones. Sometimes a single nodule is the cause of hyperthyroidism.

Some drugs can cause hyperthyroidism as well. The most common is amiodarone, a drug used to treat heart disease that may stimulate or damage the thyroid gland. The potential for amiodarone to cause hypothyroidism in some people and hyperthyroidism in others is a reminder of the unpredictability of the effects of amiodarone on the thyroid gland.

Symptoms

Hyperthyroidism can produce many vague symptoms that can be attributed to other conditions. Typically, the symptoms of hyperthyroidism differ between older and younger people. In younger people, the most common symptoms are an increased heart rate, sensitivity to heat, trembling of the hands, and bulging of the eyes (exophthalmos). In contrast, among older people, the most common symptoms are weight loss and fatigue. The heart rate may or may not be increased, and the eyes usually do not bulge. Older people are also more likely to have abnormal heart rhythms (such as atrial fibrillation), other heart problems (such as angina and heart failure), and constipation. Older people occasionally develop diarrhea, sweat profusely, become nervous and anxious, and experience trembling of the hands.

The thyroid gland is of normal size in almost half of the older people with hyperthyroidism. However, the thyroid gland often enlarges in people with Graves' disease. The gland is enlarged only in the areas in which nodules have formed if people have toxic multinodular goiter.

In very rare instances, the thyroid gland becomes extremely overactive. This life-threatening condition is called thyroid storm. Thyroid storm is usually triggered by a stressful event, such as an infection or surgery. It usually occurs in a person with an overactive thyroid gland who has not been under a doctor's care. Occasionally, thyroid storm is unexpectedly triggered by radioactive iodine given to treat hyperthyroidism. In thyroid storm, fever develops and the heart rate increases greatly. A person may feel nauseated or may vomit. Heart failure may develop. The person may become confused and less alert and may lose consciousness.

Diagnosis

To diagnose hyperthyroidism, doctors usually begin by measuring the level of thyroid-stimulating hormone. If the thyroid gland is overactive, the pituitary gland produces less thyroid-stimulating hormone. The level of thyroid-stimulating hormone in the blood is low, sometimes so low that it cannot be detected. The levels of T_3 and, to a lesser extent, T_4 are increased.

Once hyperthyroidism is diagnosed, other tests may be used to determine the cause. A thyroid scan may be performed. A thyroid scan involves the administration of a small amount of a radioactive material, either iodine by mouth or technetium by injection, into the bloodstream. The radioactive material collects in the thyroid gland, where it gives off small amounts of radiation that can be detected with a special camera that produces images of the thyroid gland.

Treatment and Outlook

Often, doctors can quickly begin treating hyperthyroidism using drugs called beta blockers to slow the heart rate and reduce trembling of the hands. Additional treatment is almost always necessary and depends on the cause.

Drugs that reduce the production of thyroid hormones (propylthiouracil and methimazole) are often used to treat hyperthyroidism due to Graves' disease. Usually, the drug is taken for 1 to 2 years. Unfortunately, hyperthyroidism often returns after the drug is discontinued. If this happens, other treatments, such as radioactive iodine, are used.

Radioactive iodine, which is taken by mouth in one dose, is usually successful in treating people who have Graves' disease. Very little radioactive iodine spreads around the body, because iodine is collected, concentrated, and stored only in the thyroid gland. Unfortunately, radioactive iodine treatment almost always results in an underactive thyroid gland (hypothyroidism). When this occurs, people must then take thyroid hormone for the rest of their lives to replace the hormones that the thyroid gland no longer produces. Radioactive iodine is also used very successfully to treat toxic multinodular goiter. Surgery may be needed to remove most or all of the thyroid gland in some situations, especially when the thyroid is greatly enlarged.

Treatment of hyperthyroidism requires time and patience. In almost all cases, however, the condition can be cured and the symptoms eliminated.

THYROID NODULES

Thyroid nodules are small lumps of abnormal tissue within the thyroid gland.

Thyroid nodules are more common among older people than among younger people. In most cases, the cause of thyroid nodules is unknown. The only known cause is radiation treatments to the neck during childhood. The vast majority of thyroid nodules are noncancerous (benign). However, because thyroid cancer usually begins as a nodule in the gland, each nodule must be examined to ensure that it is not cancerous (malignant).

Nodules vary in their composition and in whether they produce thyroid hormone. One or many nodules may gradually develop. When many nodules develop, the condition is called a multinodular goiter. If many nodules have developed and hyperthyroidism occurs, the condition is called toxic multinodular goiter.

Symptoms and Diagnosis

Some people notice a painless swelling in the front part of their neck. More often, the swelling is not noticeable, and the doctor feels (palpates) the thyroid gland and finds one or more nodules. In some cases, a nodule is found when a person undergoes an ultrasound scan of the carotid arteries or a computed tomography (CT) or magnetic resonance imaging (MRI) scan of the neck or chest for another medical condition.

An ultrasound scan may also be performed to determine the composition of the nodule. Nodules may be solid or partially or completely filled with fluid (in which case they are cysts). The likelihood of a nodule being cancerous is lowest if the nodule is completely filled with fluid. Partially fluid-filled and solid nodules have a higher chance of being cancerous. But the vast majority of nodules are not cancerous. Blood tests are performed to determine whether hypothyroidism or hyperthyroidism is present, but usually the person has normal thyroid function.

Doctors describe nodules as hot or cold: These labels do not refer to temperature, but to how the nodules appear on a radioactive thyroid scan. Hot nodules take up the radioactive material (iodine or technetium) and secrete thyroid hormones. Such nodules may cause hyperthyroidism. Hot nodules are noncancerous. Cold nodules do not take up the radioactive material and do not secrete thyroid hormones. Cold nodules are more likely to be cancerous, although most (95%) are noncancerous.

Most often, a sample of tissue from the nodule is removed through a small needle and examined under a microscope. This procedure is called a fine-needle aspiration biopsy. A biopsy is usually needed to determine whether a nodule is cancerous. The procedure is usually performed in the doctor's office and takes 20 minutes or less. If the nodule is difficult to feel, the biopsy may be done using ultrasound to guide the needle. A local anesthetic is usually used to numb the neck where the needle is inserted.

Treatment and Outlook

Treatment of noncancerous nodules depends on the cause and on the symptoms they produce. Nodules that secrete too much thyroid hormone may produce hyperthyroidism, which requires treatment, usually with radioactive iodine. Noncancerous nodules that do not secrete thyroid hormones usually do not require treatment. If the nodules cause discomfort or are cosmetically displeasing, they can be removed surgically.

Thyroid cancer can almost always be treated and cured: Most people with thyroid cancer are still alive 20 years after the cancer is detected. A few rare types of thyroid cancer, particularly anaplastic thyroid carcinoma and thyroid lymphoma, have a poorer outlook.

If tests suggest or confirm that a nodule is cancerous, surgery is performed to remove as much of the gland as possible. After surgery, radioactive iodine is usually given to destroy any remaining thyroid tissue. Once a person's thyroid gland has been removed or destroyed, treatment with thyroid hormone must continue for life.

34

Diabetes Mellitus

Diabetes mellitus is a disease in which blood sugar (glucose) levels are abnormally high because the body does not produce enough of the hormone insulin or fails to respond to insulin.

Diabetes is extremely common in older people, of whom about 15 to 25% have the disease. Diabetes can lead to such complications as chest pain (angina) and heart attacks, heart failure, stroke, kidney failure, blurred vision and blindness, pain and loss of sensation in the hands and feet, and amputation. Many of these complications arise because diabetes leads to narrowing and leakage of blood vessels, which impairs circulation and damages tissues. These complications are even more likely in people who smoke or have high blood pressure and high cholesterol levels, both of which often accompany diabetes. Fortunately, many complications can be prevented by quitting smoking and by taking steps to control blood pressure and cholesterol levels as well as blood sugar levels.

Causes

Diabetes is categorized as type 1 or type 2, each with a different cause. Type 2 diabetes is the main form of diabetes among older people. Obese older people with a family history of diabetes have the highest risk of developing type 2 diabetes. In type 2 diabetes, the body does not respond normally to the insulin produced. This phenomenon is called insulin resistance. Also, the body may not make enough insulin. Type 1 diabetes is much less common among older people. In type 1 diabetes, the body does not produce any insulin.

When sugar from food is absorbed into the bloodstream, the pancreas responds by producing insulin. Insulin plays a key role in moving sugar from the bloodstream into the cells, where it is then converted into energy. The body uses this energy to function; sugar is the fuel on which the body runs.

If the body cannot adequately produce or respond to insulin, sugar cannot enter the cells. Instead, sugar accumulates in the blood, and the cells must turn to other sources for energy.

ADDITIONAL DETAIL

The main risk factor for type 2 diabetes is obesity: 80 to 90% of people with type 2 diabetes are overweight. Obesity causes insulin resistance, possibly by increasing the blood levels of building blocks of fats (fatty acids) and certain proteins that interfere with the action of insulin. Older people tend to accumulate more body fat as they age, thus their risk of developing diabetes increases. Normal accumulation of fat with aging is a small part of the problem. The lion's share of the problem stems from eating too much and exercising too little.

Muscle mass also decreases in older adults. Muscles use sugar for energy, so less muscle means that less sugar is consumed for energy and more sugar is converted to fat.

Aging itself puts people at higher risk of developing diabetes. As people age, insulin secretion tends to decrease slightly and insulin resistance tends to increase slightly, even among people without obesity or diabetes. Therefore, even older people who do not have diabetes tend to have slightly higher blood sugar levels after eating than do their younger counterparts.

Heredity is a risk factor as well. Diabetes is especially likely to develop among blacks, Hispanics, and American Indians as well as among people whose parents or other close relatives had the disease.

Symptoms

People with type 2 diabetes may have no symptoms for months or even years before the disease is diagnosed. The first symptoms of diabetes, which may be subtle, result from the high level of sugar in the blood. When the blood sugar level rises too high, sugar spills into the urine. The kidneys then must excrete additional water to dilute the sugar. Therefore, a person with diabetes urinates large volumes (polyuria). The loss of water due to excessive urination also creates abnormal thirst (polydipsia). Also, because the body cannot use sugar as energy, a person with diabetes may experience excessive hunger and thus eat more (polyphagia) and yet still lose weight. Other symptoms include blurred vision, drowsiness, decreased endurance during exercise, and light-headedness on standing, a sign of dehydration.

Occasionally, blood sugar levels in people with type 2 diabetes become extremely high. These extremely high levels often result from failing to take drugs to control blood sugar or from stress to the body, such as infection or surgery. When blood sugar levels rise extremely high, the person may become severely dehydrated, which may lead to confusion, drowsiness, seizures, and coma—a condition called nonketotic hyperosmolar (or hyperglycemic hyperosmolar) coma.

Symptoms may result from complications that develop gradually over years, sometimes even before diabetes is diagnosed. Chest pain or heart attack can result from poor blood flow to the heart. Sudden loss of strength, sensation, coordination, speech, or vision can result when poor circulation to the brain causes a stroke. Gradually worsening vision can also occur with damage to blood vessels in the eyes (retinopathy).[1] Decreased urination and swelling in the legs and other parts of the body can occur when poor blood flow results in kidney failure. Pain or numbness and tingling in the hands and feet can occur when nerves are damaged by high blood sugar (diabetic neuropathy). Leg pain with walking (claudication) can be an indication of poor blood flow. Serious foot infections and ulcers can develop when not enough blood reaches the legs and feet. Sudden loss of function in a leg can occur if poor blood flow to a nerve damages the function of the nerve. Skin can be damaged by poor blood flow as well.

Diagnosis and Screening

Health care practitioners perform blood tests to diagnose diabetes. The tests are performed in people with symptoms of high blood sugar or complications of disease. The same tests are often used to screen for diabetes in people without symptoms: many older people have the disease but do not know it.

A simple blood test called a glucose test is most commonly used to make the diagnosis. The level of sugar (glucose) in the blood is measured, usually after the person has fasted for at least 8 hours. Sometimes the blood sugar level is measured randomly, without regard to when the person last ate, but this test is not as accurate. In a person who does not have diabetes, blood sugar levels after fasting range from about 70 to 100 milligrams per deciliter (mg/dL) of blood. The levels may be higher if the person has recently eaten. Diabetes is the likely diagnosis if the blood sugar level is 126 mg/dL or higher if the person fasted before the test or 200 mg/dL or higher if the test was performed at random. But a repeat test must be done if the first result is higher than 100 mg/dL (recently changed from 110 mg/dL at the recommendation of an expert panel). The diagnosis of diabetes mellitus is confirmed if any one of the following results is obtained:

1. see page 522

LONG-TERM COMPLICATIONS OF DIABETES

Tissue or Organ Affected	What Happens	Complications
Large blood vessels	Atherosclerotic plaque builds up and blocks arteries in the heart, brain, and legs	Poor circulation, which can lead to angina, heart attack, heart failure, stroke, leg pain with walking, and gangrene of the feet
Eyes	The small blood vessels of the retina become damaged; fluid leaks into the back of the eyes, and abnormally weak blood vessels grow and can burst	Vision loss and, ultimately, blindness
Kidneys	The small blood vessels in the kidneys become damaged; protein leaks into the urine and the blood is not filtered normally	Poor kidney function; kidney failure and the need for dialysis or kidney transplantation
Nervous system	The small blood vessels that feed nerves in the hands and feet and nerves that control unconscious functions, such as blood pressure, digestive processes, and sexual functioning, become damaged. The nerves function abnormally or stop functioning altogether	Tingling or pain in the hands and feet; reduced sensation, leading to unawareness of injury; sudden or gradual weakness of a leg; weakness of eye or facial muscles; swings in blood pressure; swallowing difficulties and altered digestive function, with nausea, constipation, and diarrhea and erectile dysfunction (impotence)
Skin	The small blood vessels in the skin become damaged	Poorly healing cuts, blisters, sores, and other wounds can lead to deep ulcers (diabetic ulcers) that can become

Tissue or Organ Affected	What Happens	Complications
		infected and sometimes result in amputation of a foot or leg
Blood	White blood cell function is impaired	Increased susceptibility to infection throughout the body, most commonly in the skin, urine, and lung
Connective tissue	Abnormal processing of sugar causes tissues to thicken or shrink (contract)	Carpal tunnel syndrome; Dupuytren's contracture

- Two fasting levels are 126 mg/dL or higher
- Two random levels are 200 mg/dL or higher
- A fasting level is 126 mg/dL or higher and a random level is 200 mg/dL or higher

People who have two or more fasting blood sugar levels between 100 and 125 mg/dL (a condition sometimes called impaired fasting glucose) should have this test repeated every year. People in whom both fasting blood sugar levels are less than 100 mg/dL should have the test repeated at least once every 3 years.

Once diabetes has been diagnosed, the person should be screened for disease complications at least once a year. The eyes should be examined by an eye specialist, who can detect and treat retinopathy before it leads to vision loss. Kidney problems can be detected with urine and blood tests. Blood cholesterol levels should be checked. An electrocardiogram is sometimes used to find evidence of heart damage, although the information that this test provides is limited. In some cases, an exercise (or other form of) stress test is done to find out if blood flow to the heart is poor.

A person's feet should be examined closely once or twice a year by a health care practitioner for poor blood flow, decreased sensation, skin breakdown, and infection. Self-examination of the feet daily or weekly is also important for early detection of skin breakdown. Breakdown, which can involve cuts, blisters, and sores, should receive medical attention.

Prevention

Diabetes often can be prevented, though usually not without some work. Losing weight through dietary changes, increased physical activity, or both is a very effective preventive measure. Brisk walking for 30 minutes a day is one type of beneficial physical activity.[1] Preventive measures are especially important for people whose blood sugar levels are only slightly elevated. Some drugs used to treat diabetes may also be used preventively for people at high risk of developing the disease. However, drugs are no substitute for proper diet, exercise, and weight loss.

Treatment

The goal of treatment is to maintain blood sugar levels within the normal range so as to prevent or control symptoms and reduce the risk of developing complications. However, some people with other diseases, such as advanced cancer, may not benefit from strict control of blood sugar levels if one or more of their other diseases are life threatening. Strict control may also be impossible for people with dementia or poor eyesight.

The focus of diabetes treatment is not limited to control of blood sugar. Management of associated cardiovascular risk factors, such as high blood pressure and elevated cholesterol, are also important. Treatment involves education, diet, exercise, drugs (for most people), and frequent monitoring of blood sugar levels.

Education: Learning about diabetes, understanding how diet and exercise affect blood sugar levels, and knowing how to avoid complications are essential. A nurse trained in diabetes education can provide information. Diabetes education programs are available in many communities, the cost of which is now covered by many health insurance programs, including Medicare.

Diet: Maintaining a healthy diet is extremely important for people with diabetes. Well-balanced, healthy meals that include

1. see page 36

THE FOOT IN DIABETES

Changes in the feet caused by diabetes are common and difficult to treat.

• Neuropathy (damage to the nerves) affects sensation in the feet, so that pain is not felt. Irritation and other forms of injury may go unnoticed; an injury may wear through the skin before any pain is felt.

• Other changes in sensation alter the way people with diabetes carry weight on their feet, concentrating weight in certain areas so that calluses form. Calluses (along with dry skin) increase the risk of skin breakdown and ulcers.

• Diabetes can cause poor circulation in the feet, making it more likely that ulcers will form when the skin is damaged and making the ulcers slower to heal.

In addition to the changes in the foot, diabetes can affect the body's ability to fight infections. Therefore, once an ulcer forms, it becomes infected easily; the infection may become serious and difficult to treat, leading to gangrene. People with diabetes are more than 30 times more likely to require an amputation of a foot or leg than are people without diabetes.

Foot care is critical.[1] The feet should be protected from injury, and the skin should be kept moist with a good moisturizer. Shoes should fit properly and not cause areas of irritation. Shoes should have appropriate cushioning to spread out the pressure caused by standing. Going barefoot is ill advised. Regular care from a podiatrist, such as having toenails cut and calluses removed, may also be helpful. Also, sensation and blood flow to the feet should be regularly evaluated by a doctor.

a variety of foods should be eaten at regular times. Starchy foods (such as bread, pasta, and rice) and sweets (such as fruits and foods with added sugar) are most likely to increase blood sugar levels. Foods with a high sugar content should be eaten sparingly. Because people with diabetes tend to have high blood cholesterol levels, foods containing saturated fats should be eaten sparingly as well.[2]

Dietary measures alone are sometimes enough to maintain a healthy weight and control blood sugar levels. However, many older people have difficulty implementing such measures. In some cases, older people with diabetes who also have other diseases that can be affected by diet may become confused about how to follow recommendations for a healthy diet. Some people

1. see box on page 576
2. see page 44

have difficulty because of long-held food preferences. In addition, they may not have control over what they eat because someone else is cooking for them or because they are living in a nursing home or institution. When people with diabetes do not do their own cooking, those who shop and prepare meals for them must also understand proper diet. Older people and their caregivers generally benefit from meeting with a dietitian to develop an optimal eating plan.

Exercise: People with diabetes should be physically active. Putting extra physical activity into ordinary activities, such as walking instead of driving to a store or taking stairs instead of elevators, can often help. However, formal exercise is often needed.[1] Most people can find some form of exercise they enjoy, such as swimming, playing tennis, riding a stationary bicycle while watching television, walking in a mall, or participating in an exercise program offered by a local community center.

Drug therapy: Drug therapy is started when diet and exercise do not adequately lower blood sugar levels or when a person's living conditions, physical strength, or motivation make proper diet and exercise impossible.

Oral antihyperglycemic drugs are usually the first drugs given. There are many different types of oral antihyperglycemic drugs, including biguanides, sulfonylureas, meglitinides, thiazolidinediones, and glucosidase inhibitors. A doctor may prescribe one of these drugs alone or may combine two or more of them. Some of these drugs work by stimulating the pancreas to produce more insulin, others increase the body's response to the insulin it produces, and still others block the intestines from absorbing sugar.

Insulin is usually given if oral antihyperglycemic drugs alone cannot control blood sugar levels adequately. As many as half of the people with type 2 diabetes eventually require insulin treatment to control blood sugar levels. Temporary insulin treatment is also sometimes necessary during periods of stress, such as illness, surgery, or hospitalization.

Insulin is divided into four basic types based on how quickly it works and how long it lasts. Rapid-acting insulin (such as lispro or aspart) is the fastest and shortest acting. It is taken as

1. see page 910

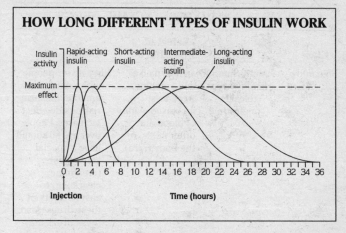

HOW LONG DIFFERENT TYPES OF INSULIN WORK

several daily injections up to 5 minutes before meals or just after eating. Rapid-acting insulin reaches its maximum effect in 45 to 75 minutes and works for 2 to 4 hours. Short-acting insulin (such as regular insulin), which is taken 30 to 60 minutes before a meal, reaches its maximum effect in 2 to 4 hours and works for 6 to 8 hours. Intermediate-acting insulin (such as lente or NPH) starts to work in 2 to 3 hours, reaches its maximum effect in 6 to 10 hours, and works for 18 to 26 hours. It may be used in the morning to control blood sugar levels for the first part of the day or in the evening to control blood sugar levels during the night. Long-acting insulin (such as ultra-lente or glargine) begins to work very slowly but lasts for 24 to 36 hours. Long-acting insulin usually has its maximum effect at 14 to 24 hours. Glargine, unlike other forms of long-acting insulin that reach a maximum effect at a specific time, works continually at about the same level of effectiveness.

The four types of insulin can be taken in a variety of ways. Insulin treatment is tailored to individual needs, often starting with a single daily injection and progressing to a more complicated regimen. For many people, a single daily injection of an intermediate- or long-acting insulin, sometimes combined with oral drugs, may control blood sugar levels. However, for some people this regimen may not prevent high blood sugar levels after meals.

℞ ORAL ANTIHYPERGLYCEMIC DRUGS

Class	Drug	Selected Side Effects	Comments
Biguanide	Metformin Extended-release metformin	Diarrhea, nausea, and vomiting; weakness; increased acidity of blood and other fluids in the body (rare)	Not safe for people with poor kidney function because risk of side effects increases. People over age 80 should have a special kidney test (creatinine clearance) to ensure safety of these drugs. Also, these drugs may not be safe for people with heart failure because of risk of side effects. May help prevent diabetes when taken by people with early-stage disease (impaired fasting glucose)
Sulfonylurea	Chlorpropamide Glimepiride Glipizide Glipizide GITS Glyburide Micronized glyburide Tolazamide Tolbutamide	Weight gain, which may make these drugs less effective; with chlorpropamide, low sodium in blood (hyponatremia)	Low blood sugar (hypoglycemia) can occur, especially with longer-acting drugs (such as chlorpropamide and glyburide)
Meglitinides	Nateglinide Repaglinide	Weight gain, which may make these drugs less effective	Low blood sugar levels can occur

Class	Drug	Selected Side Effects	Comments
Thiazolidine-diones	Pioglitazone Rosiglita-zone	Weight gain, which may make these drugs less effective; fluid retention (edema)	May help prevent diabetes when taken by people with early-stage disease (impaired fasting glucose)
Glucosidase inhibitors	Acarbose Miglitol	Diarrhea; abdominal pain; bloating	May help prevent diabetes when taken by people with early-stage disease (impaired fasting glucose)

Better control can usually be achieved by combining two types of insulin—for example, a rapid-acting and an intermediate-acting insulin—in one or more daily doses. Administering a combination requires more skill, because doses may need to be varied depending on factors such as the size of the meal and the time of day. The best control is often achieved by injecting a rapid-acting insulin at mealtime and an intermediate- or long-acting insulin in the morning and evening.

The types of insulin taken and the frequency with which they are taken may change based on the person's diet, exercise, and blood sugar patterns. In addition, insulin needs may change if a person experiences weight changes, emotional stress, or illness, especially infection.

A doctor considers several factors when choosing insulin therapy, including the person's blood sugar levels, the constancy of those levels from day to day, and the person's ability and willingness to monitor his blood sugar levels and to adjust the insulin dosage.

Some older people may have difficulty injecting insulin because of impaired vision, which may make it hard to prepare an accurate dose in a syringe. Others may have problems manipulating the syringe as a result of arthritis, Parkinson's disease, or stroke. A caregiver can help by preparing the syringes ahead of time and storing them in the refrigerator. Also, magnifying devices may allow a person with limited vision to see the measurements on the syringe more easily. Prefilled insulin pen devices, either disposable or with replaceable cartridges, may be easier for people with physical disabilities to use. Some of these devices have been specially designed with large numbers and easy-to-turn dials.

Sometimes, complications from insulin treatment develop. Insulin injections can affect the skin and underlying tissues. An allergic reaction, which occurs rarely, produces pain and burning, followed by redness, itchiness, and swelling around the injection site for several hours. More commonly, the injections either cause fat deposits, making the skin look lumpy, or destroy fat, causing indentation of the skin. However, these problems are less common with newer insulins and can usually be prevented by rotating the injection site.

Monitoring blood sugar levels: Regardless of whether a person takes insulin or oral antihyperglycemic drugs, monitoring blood sugar levels is essential to the treatment of diabetes. Blood sugar levels can change from hour to hour in response to diet, physical activity, stress, illness, drugs, and site of insulin injection. Blood sugar levels rise in many people in the early morning because of the normal release of hormones (growth hormone and cortisol), a reaction called the dawn phenomenon. Blood sugar levels may also rise if the body releases sugar in response to low blood sugar levels (Somogyi effect).

Monitoring blood sugar levels provides the information needed to detect these changes and to make the necessary adjustments to diet, exercise, and drug regimens. Most people with diabetes should keep a record of their blood sugar levels and report them to their doctor. Many people can learn to adjust their insulin dose on their own as necessary. The number of times per day that blood sugar should be checked depends on many factors, including the type of insulin a person is taking and the way blood sugar levels change in response to meals. Some people check their blood sugar only once or twice a day, whereas others check it more than 4 times a day.

Most blood sugar monitoring devices, especially newer models, use only a tiny drop of blood. The blood sample is obtained by pricking the tip of the finger with a small lancet. Some models allow for testing at sites less painful than the fingertips, like the forearm. The lancet is a tiny needle that can be placed in a spring-loaded device that easily and relatively painlessly pierces the skin. A drop of blood is then placed on a test strip.

MORE ABOUT INSULIN

Insulin is injected, not swallowed, because it is destroyed by acid in the stomach. New forms, such as an insulin nasal spray and a form that can be taken by mouth, are being tested. Insulin is injected under the skin into the fat layer, usually in the arm, thigh, or abdominal wall. Insulin is absorbed fastest from the abdominal wall and slowest from the thigh. A person should use one of these three sites consistently and rotate injections within the site (for example, different areas of the abdominal wall) to avoid complications, such as an allergic reaction, fat deposits, or indentation of the skin.

An air pump device that blows the insulin under the skin can be used for people who cannot tolerate needles, but most people find them more problematic than the tiny needles available today. An insulin pen, which contains a cartridge that holds insulin, is a convenient way for many older people to carry insulin, especially if they cannot see well enough to draw insulin into the syringe.

Insulin preparations generally are stable at room temperature for up to several months, allowing them to be taken outside the home. Insulin should not, however, be exposed to extreme temperatures.

The test strip undergoes a chemical change in response to sugar. A palm-sized machine reads the changes in the test strip and reports the result on a digital display.

Special devices are available for use by people with poor vision or other physical limitations, such as limited manual dexterity due to arthritis, tremor, or stroke. Some devices have large numerical displays that are easier to read. Special devices with audible instructions and results are available as well. A new device reads blood sugar levels through the skin: no blood sample is necessary. The device is worn like a wristwatch and measures the blood sugar level every 15 minutes. Alarms on the device can be set to sound when blood sugar levels drop too low or rise too high. However, results must be compared periodically to those of a blood test. Also, the device may irritate the skin, is somewhat large, and does not work when a person moves a lot or becomes sweaty. This device cannot completely replace the need for blood testing. Because there is a wide variety of meters available, a person with special needs may wish to consult with a diabetes educator to determine which meter is best for him.

Virtually all meters are sufficiently accurate when used properly. Most important is to make sure that test strips have not exceeded the expiration date, that an adequate blood sample is obtained, and that "control solutions" and check strips are used periodically to confirm that the meter is functioning well.

Although urine can also be tested for the presence of sugar, checking urine is not a good way to monitor treatment or to adjust therapy. Urine testing can be misleading, because the level of sugar in the urine may not reflect the level of sugar in the blood. Sugar levels in the blood can get very low or reasonably high without any change in the sugar levels in the urine. People with type 1 diabetes are sometimes asked to check their urine for the presence of ketones, which indicates a severe lack of insulin and a potential health emergency. But for people with type 2 diabetes, urine testing for sugar or ketones is rarely appropriate.

Health care practitioners can monitor blood sugar levels using a blood test called hemoglobin A_{1C}. Most doctors recommend that this test be performed every 3 to 6 months. Unlike blood tests that reveal sugar levels at a particular moment, hemoglobin A_{1C} measurements provide a measure of blood sugar levels over the previous 2 to 3 months. The normal level for hemoglobin A_{1C} is 6% or less. People with diabetes may not be able to achieve normal levels, but good control of blood sugar should bring a person close. The goal in most cases is to achieve a hemoglobin A_{1C} below 7%. Levels above 8% show poor control, and levels above 10% show very poor control.

Prevention and Treatment of Diabetes Complications

Many, if not all, diabetes complications can be prevented by keeping blood sugar levels as close to normal as possible at all times.

The eyes, kidneys, and feet should be examined annually by a doctor to detect complications before they cause permanent damage. Cholesterol levels and blood pressure should be checked every year too. Treatment of high blood pressure and cholesterol levels and attempts to stop smoking can prevent the buildup of plaque (atherosclerosis) in blood vessel walls. Specific treatments may also help prevent complications. Laser surgery can seal leaking blood vessels in the eye and prevent permanent damage to the retina.[1] Progression of kidney compli-

1. see page 523

cations can be slowed or stopped with angiotensin-converting enzyme (ACE) inhibitors or angiotensin II receptor blockers. Indeed, many experts believe that most people with diabetes should receive these drugs to prevent kidney damage from diabetes. Prevention of stroke and coronary artery disease involves daily aspirin, cholesterol-lowering drugs, ACE inhibitors, and other blood pressure–lowering drugs as needed. The treatment of nonketotic hyperosmolar coma involves fluid and electrolyte replacement and insulin injection.

Complications of Treatment

The most common complication of treating high blood sugar levels is low blood sugar levels. Having low blood sugar levels is serious, develops rapidly, and can be life threatening. Older people who are frail, who are sick enough to require frequent hospital admissions, or who are taking multiple drugs are at greatest risk. Of all available treatments for diabetes, sulfonylureas—especially glyburide and glipizide—and insulin injections can cause low blood sugar levels. Drugs such as metformin and the thiazolidinediones rarely, if ever, cause low blood sugar when used alone.

Common symptoms of low blood sugar include sweating, nausea, warmth, anxiety, shakiness, palpitations, hunger, headache, blurred or double vision, confusion, and difficulty speaking. Older people are at greater risk of low blood sugar levels when they use long-acting sulfonylurea drugs. They are also more likely to experience serious symptoms, such as fainting and falling, and to develop stroke as a result of low blood sugar. In the worst cases, low blood sugar can cause coma, permanent brain damage, and even death. For this reason, low blood sugar levels must be treated immediately.

Sugar must get into the body within minutes to relieve symptoms of low blood sugar and prevent harm to the brain. A person with diabetes can usually eat or drink some form of sugar. Fruit juice, milk (which contains lactose, a type of sugar), and regular soda (not diet) are usually effective. So is eating a piece of cake, fruit, or another sweet food. People with diabetes can also carry glucose tablets or gels, which are particularly convenient and easy to transport. Most of the time, 4 to 6 ounces of juice or 4 to 5 glucose tablets are sufficient to correct hypoglycemia. Care should be taken not to overtreat, because an abnormally high blood sugar level will result. When sugar is unavailable or the person is unconscious, emergency medical personnel may have to inject glucose into a vein.

Ideally, blood sugar is tested about 20 to 30 minutes after sugar has been eaten to ensure that the blood sugar level has increased to the normal range.

Another treatment for low blood sugar is glucagon. Glucagon can be injected into the muscle and causes the liver to release large amounts of glucose within minutes. Small transportable kits containing a syringe filled with glucagon are available for use in emergency situations. Glucagon is generally used only if a person is unable to take adequate amounts of sugar by mouth.

Outlook

The outlook is excellent for older people with diabetes who are willing and able to eat a proper diet, exercise, maintain a healthy weight, and take blood sugar—lowering drugs regularly. However, older people who choose not to or who are unable to adhere to recommended treatment measures are at risk of developing the serious complications of diabetes. Most complications of diabetes are progressive and tend to develop after only a few years of having the disease. Fortunately, many complications can be slowed or even prevented with strict control of blood sugar levels.

What are children? They are enthusiastic about life, they love unconditionally, and always are ready for a new adventure. Now, that is how I want to spend the remainder of my life, even if society wants to call it "aging."

Surfing has been one of many passions since moving to Hawaii in 1964 at age 29. There were so few women surfers, I would get strange looks from the men, but after proving myself on big waves, I was accepted.

You see, from a very early age, my knowing I wanted to be a physician was a sign that I would not live by the rules and attitudes of the society and times into which I was born. So, being one of the few female surfers was nothing new. Therefore, as I hit the half-century mark, I never bought into the notion that being old was unfashionable, unattractive, or even frightening. Oh, I stopped surfing some of the really big waves and stopped wearing a bikini. And I use my boogie board more because of inner ear balance problems, but I am in the ocean I love! I cannot imagine never surfing any more than I can imagine not practicing medicine. Medicine has never been just a "job" . . . it is a part of my being. I may hang up my stethoscope, but I am not retiring from "Life"!

My mother and grandmother were amazing role models; they set an example that taught me beautiful lessons about aging: First, each day is a gift . . . choose to celebrate it! Secondly, nothing keeps you young like vigorous activity, whether in the ocean, pool, garden, or gym. And lastly, old age is like a bank account . . . you withdraw from what you've deposited. I learned to deposit many healthy habits, giving to others, and memories from an abundant life well lived. I look forward to the future with enthusiasm and am confident of more time surfing with my 9-year-old granddaughter. To me, success in retirement is wondering when I ever had time to go to work.

So, hey kids, I'll see you on the playgrounds!!!

Shay Bintliff, MD

35

Skin Disorders

When people think about how their skin will change as they age, they are most often concerned about how it will look. They may fear that their skin will be dry, wrinkled, and covered with spots. Undeniably, the appearance of the skin changes as people age. But most unwanted changes in the skin's appearance are due to chronic sun damage, not to aging itself. Avoiding excessive sun exposure can prevent some of these changes or prevent them from worsening.

The skin is much more than just part of a person's appearance. It has many other functions, which can also be affected by aging. They include:

• Protecting internal organs from physical and chemical injuries and from the sun's radiation
• Helping prevent viruses and bacteria from entering the body and helping defend the body against infection (the skin contains cells and substances of the immune system)
• Helping regulate the body's temperature by sweating and by insulating the body
• Helping regulate the body's temperature: tiny blood vessels in the skin expand (dilate) to release heat and narrow (constrict) to retain heat
• Forming vitamin D when the skin is exposed to sunlight
• Regulating the activity of many hormones and thus affecting some of the body's functions
• Regrowing and repairing itself to some degree when damaged
• Enabling people to know when the body touches something
• Enabling people to feel changes in temperature and to feel pain (sometimes warning them of danger)

GETTING INTO THE SKIN

The skin consists of three layers. Beneath the surface of the skin are nerves, nerve endings, glands, hair follicles, and blood vessels.

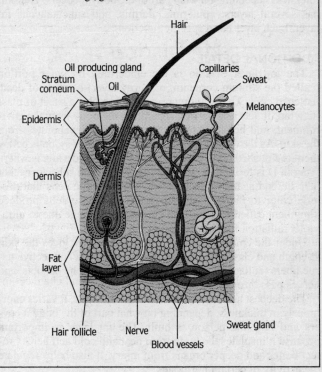

As people age, their skin changes in many ways.[1] On the positive side, the skin tends to become less sensitive to substances that trigger allergic reactions, so allergic rashes become less common. On the negative side, the skin thins and becomes drier, less elastic, and more fragile. The skin gradually functions less well. It becomes less able to form vitamin D and to regulate the activity of hormones. Also, the sense of touch diminishes. For example, regulating body temperature and repair-

1. see page 14

ing damaged skin become more difficult. Thus, as people age, skin disorders become more common and bothersome.

The skin is the largest organ in the body. The skin varies in thickness depending on what part of the body it covers. The skin has several layers: epidermis, dermis, and subcutaneous fat layer. Each layer has a specific function.

ADDITIONAL DETAIL

The top layer of skin is the epidermis. Its outer portion (called the stratum corneum, or horny layer) consists of dead, flattened cells. The stratum corneum resembles a sheet of plastic wrap. It acts as a barrier, separating the body from the environment, and helps control how much water evaporates from the skin. As the dead cells on the surface wear away, cells below them are pushed up to take their place. The epidermis is where vitamin D is formed. It contains many cells and substances that help defend against infection. Melanocytes, the cells that provide color to the skin, are in this layer. These cells produce a pigment called melanin, which reduces damage due to ultraviolet radiation from sunlight.

Under the epidermis is the dermis. This layer gives the skin strength and elasticity. It is composed mostly of connective tissue fibers (collagen fibers). Blood vessels, lymph channels, and nerves pass through these fibers.

The deepest layer is the subcutaneous fat layer. It varies enormously in thickness, depending on what part of the body it covers and how the person is built. The fat layer is important because it insulates the body from heat and cold and helps protect bones and deeper organs from injury. It also helps regulate the activity of certain hormones.

DRY SKIN

As people age, the outer layer of skin (not the inner layers) loses water. As a result, the skin surface often becomes dry or rough. Noticeably dry skin is called xerosis.

Causes and Symptoms

Older people often have xerosis. With aging, the outer layer of skin becomes less able to keep water in. Some drugs can worsen xerosis by changing the chemical composition of the skin's outer layer.

Dry skin, particularly on the forearms, hands, and lower legs, tends to itch and flake (scale). Itching can be distracting and distressing. Symptoms are often worse in winter because low humidity indoors (due to heating) and outdoors (due to cold and wind) dries the skin even more.

Many soaps, detergents, and alcohol (applied to the skin alone or as an ingredient in some skin care products) dry the skin, worsening symptoms. Using hot water during bathing dries the skin. The hotter the water, the drier the skin becomes. Occasionally, dry skin cracks. If irritating substances enter the cracks, the skin may become red, itchy, swollen, or painful. This condition is called eczema craquelé or asteatotic eczema.

Prevention and Treatment

Usually, xerosis cannot be cured. However, people can usually take steps to avoid drying the skin and thus control symptoms. For example, they can bathe or shower only once a day (in warm, not hot, water) and use a mild soap. Patting rather than rubbing dry can help. Clothing made of wool or other potentially irritating materials should not be worn next to the skin. Increasing humidity in the air, for example with a humidifier, relieves xerosis.

Certain moisturizers, such as those that contain lanolin or white petrolatum, trap and hold water in the skin. They can help if applied generously and frequently, particularly after bathing or showering. Many such moisturizers are available without a prescription. Skin care products that contain alcohol should be avoided. Scented products are more likely than unscented products to cause allergic reactions and should be avoided by people prone to allergies.

Occasionally, prescription products are needed. Creams and lotions that contain a high concentration of lactic acid or glycolic acid can help remove scales and keep the skin moist. Some products contain urea, which can help moisturize the driest areas. If the skin becomes temporarily red, swollen, or painful, corticosteroid ointments can be very helpful.

ITCHING

Itching (also called pruritus) is an unpleasant sensation that makes people scratch or rub the skin.

Itching is common among older people. It can be caused or worsened by dry skin. Usually, itching can be treated effectively, but treatment may need to be continued indefinitely.

Causes and Symptoms

Noticeably dry skin (xerosis), which occurs with aging, is the most common cause of itching. Other skin disorders that cause itching include allergic reactions, yeast infections, and infestation with lice (pediculosis) or the scabies mite. These disorders usually produce a rash or other changes in the skin. Disorders that affect other parts of the body can also cause itching but usually do not affect the skin's appearance. These disorders include excess production of red blood cells (polycythemia), infection with the virus that causes AIDS (HIV), infection with intestinal parasites, and liver or kidney disorders. Less commonly, diabetes, thyroid disorders, cancer, or certain drugs cause itching. Sometimes a cause cannot be identified.

Itching can distract or preoccupy a person to the point where living a normal life is difficult. Sometimes scratching makes the skin thick and coarse. Scarring may result.

Diagnosis

Itching is the most common symptom of a skin disorder, and a skin disorder is the most common cause of itching. So to identify the cause of itching, doctors first carefully examine the skin to look for the sometimes subtle evidence of a skin disorder.

If the skin appears normal, tests (such as blood tests, a chest x-ray, or stool sample analysis) may be done to check for other disorders that can cause itching. If there is an abnormality in the skin, doctors sometimes recommend a biopsy. For this procedure, a small piece of the skin, usually ¼ inch or less in diameter, is removed and examined under a microscope.

Treatment and Outlook

Treatment for itching is directed at the cause. Also, treating dry skin can relieve itching, regardless of the cause. Many drugs used to treat itching in younger people (such as antihistamines) can have serious side effects in older people. If symptoms remain bothersome despite treatment, exposing the affected skin to certain types of light (phototherapy) may help.

A person's outlook depends on the disorder that is causing itching. Many of these disorders can be cured. Sometimes itching resolves on its own.

ROSACEA

Rosacea is a persistent inflammatory disorder that can cause several different kinds of rashes, most noticeably on the central part of the face. This disorder is also called acne rosacea, although it is unrelated to acne, which affects mostly adolescents and young adults.

Rosacea usually begins in middle age or later. Fair-skinned people are affected most often. Rosacea varies in severity. Once it develops, it usually persists indefinitely.

Occasionally, rosacea can irritate the eyes or cause gradual but permanent enlargement of the nose (rhinophyma), as it did for comedy actor W.C. Fields. Rhinophyma usually affects men.

Causes and Symptoms

The cause of rosacea is unknown. However, the disorder can run in families. Folk wisdom sometimes associates rosacea with alcohol use, but the cause is probably something else. Hormones, psychologic factors, infections of the digestive tract, or mite infestations may be involved. Sun exposure can worsen the symptoms.

In people with rosacea, the skin of the nose and cheeks becomes chronically red. Blood vessels in the skin expand (dilate) so that more blood flows through them. These blood vessels often become twisted and visible. Acnelike bumps that may contain pus or small solid bumps often appear. The redness may temporarily worsen after drinking alcohol or hot beverages, eating spicy foods, using certain cosmetics, or being exposed to excessive heat or sunlight.

Rosacea can cause the eyes to burn, water, or feel sore or gritty. Commonly, the hair follicles at the base of the eyelashes become red and irritated. The whites of the eyes may become bloodshot.

SKIN GROWTHS: BUMPS AND SPOTS

Skin growths are common among older people. Most are noncancerous (benign). That is, they may enlarge, but they do not spread to other parts of the body. Common noncancerous growths include age spots, most moles, seborrheic warts (seborrheic keratoses), skin tags (acrochordons), and cherry angiomas (hemangiomas). What causes these growths is unclear.

Age spots are light brown, flat spots, similar to freckles. They develop after years and years of exposure to the sunlight. Thus, they appear most often on areas usually exposed to sunlight—the hands, forearms, and face. They are sometimes called liver spots, although they are unrelated to the liver. Dermatologists can recommend creams or ointments that may lighten the spots after several weeks of frequent, regular applications.

Moles are colored (usually dark), painless spots that can be flat or raised. They can appear anywhere on the body. Once formed, moles remain for decades. Most moles are harmless, but some become cancerous.

A **seborrheic wart** is a small, rough, irregularly shaped, flesh-colored or dark bump. The surface is waxy or scaly. It can look pasted or stuck on to the skin. These warts usually appear during middle or old age, usually on the torso and temples.

Skin tags are soft, flesh-colored or dark bumps that may be connected to the skin by a stalk. Most often, they develop on the neck or in the armpit.

Cherry angiomas are overgrowths of blood vessels that form raised red or purple bumps or spots. They are typically no more than $\frac{1}{8}$ inch (3 millimeters) across. They usually appear on the trunk.

Noncancerous skin growths can be removed if they are unattractive or they rub against clothing and become irritated. Usually, they can be removed in a doctor's office with a scalpel, scissors, liquid nitrogen, or a laser. Sometimes a local anesthetic is used.

Some skin growths in older people are cancerous (malignant).[1] That is, they invade other tissues and spread to other parts of the body. Skin cancer usually develops in areas that have been most exposed to the sun. But skin cancer can develop anywhere on the body. Consequently, skin should be checked periodically for changes. Having someone else check areas that are hard to see, such as the back, is useful. Or, a mirror can be used.

Certain changes should be reported to a doctor. They include the following:

• New growths, particularly moles (small, dark growths that develop from melanocytes)
• Moles that have enlarged
• Moles that have developed irregular or jagged edges
• Moles that are several different colors (for example, different shades of tan, brown or black or patches of red, blue or white)

A doctor should thoroughly examine all of the skin once a year to check for new growths or changes in old growths. Sometimes a doctor removes a piece of a growth for examination under a microscope (biopsy).

1. see page 797

Treatment and Outlook

Treatment can usually control symptoms and improve the skin's appearance. But the redness of the face often persists even when the acnelike bumps and eye irritation clear up.

Avoiding things that make the redness worse can help. Examples are alcohol, hot beverages, or spicy foods. Using a sunscreen with a high sun protection factor (SPF) and staying out of the sun can help. Exposure to excessive heat should be avoided. For example, showers or baths should not be too hot. People should not use cosmetics that irritate the skin. Scrubbing or rubbing the face can also irritate the skin.

Applying an antibiotic lotion or gel (a topical antibiotic) to the affected skin can help clear the acnelike bumps. Topical antibiotics that may help include metronidazole, erythromycin, clindamycin, and sulfacetamide. Ketoconazole, an antifungal drug, may also help. If topical antibiotics do not help, azelaic acid, a topical drug also used to treat acne, may be tried.

If the acnelike bumps are severe or if the eyes are affected, antibiotics are taken by mouth, usually for at least a month. Tetracycline, doxycycline, and minocycline are effective. If these drugs are ineffective or if a person cannot tolerate them, erythromycin or metronidazole may be used. Some people need to take antibiotics frequently or continuously. If no other treatment is effective, isotretinoin (a drug used to treat severe acne) may help.

Treatment with lasers (pulsed dye laser therapy) or electric current (electrocautery) may be used to destroy blood vessels that remain dilated. This treatment can be very effective. If rhinophyma develops, treatment with another type of laser may reduce the size of the nose. Certain kinds of makeup can hide redness that persists.

Rosacea is usually chronic. For some people, redness of the face is the only symptom. Often, symptoms are mild for long stretches of time, with periodic flare-ups. For a few people, symptoms worsen steadily and progressively despite treatment.

SEBORRHEIC DERMATITIS

In seborrheic dermatitis, the skin is usually itchy, red, and flaky. It often affects the scalp (causing dandruff) and the

central part of the face or chest. Seborrheic dermatitis can also affect skin on other parts of the body.

Dandruff is common among adults of all ages. Seborrheic dermatitis of the face and chest becomes more common as people age.

Causes and Symptoms

The cause is unknown, but seborrheic dermatitis may be a reaction to an otherwise harmless fungus. Seborrheic dermatitis is more common among people who have certain brain or nerve disorders (such as Parkinson's disease), those whose immune system is weakened (for example, by some cancers or by use of corticosteroids for a long time), and those who take certain drugs (such as chlorpromazine or haloperidol).

In older people, seborrheic dermatitis most commonly affects the scalp, eyebrows, eyelids, the skin between the nose and upper lip, the part of the face where the beard grows, and the area just behind the ears. The disorder can also affect the middle of the chest and the area between the shoulder blades.

Sometimes the eyes burn or become red. These symptoms may indicate conjunctivitis. Scales sometimes accumulate at the base of the eyelashes, plugging the follicles and causing them to become red, painful, or swollen (a disorder called seborrheic blepharitis).

Treatment and Outlook

Dandruff can be treated with shampoos that contain sulfur, zinc pyrithione, salicylic acid, tar, ketoconazole (an antifungal drug), or a combination of these substances. If shampooing is difficult, particularly if scalp symptoms are severe, hydrocortisone (a corticosteroid) can be applied as a lotion.

If the face or body is affected, hydrocortisone cream or creams or lotions containing ketoconazole, sulfacetamide, sulfur, or salicylic acid are effective.

For conjunctivitis, treatment with eye drops or an eye ointment containing a corticosteroid is occasionally needed.

For seborrheic blepharitis, an ointment containing hydrocortisone can be applied to the eyelids. Scales should be removed from the eyelashes. Applying warm compresses or gently cleaning with a cotton-tipped swab dipped in diluted baby shampoo is effective.

Seborrheic dermatitis is usually permanent. However, serious complications are rare, and symptoms can usually be controlled with treatment.

SHINGLES

Shingles (herpes zoster) is an infection caused by the virus that causes chickenpox (varicella-zoster). One or more nerves and the skin over them are affected. Typically, the disorder causes a painful blistering rash, usually limited to one side of the body.

Shingles occurs most often between the ages of 50 and 70, but it can occur at any age. It occurs only in people who have been previously infected with the virus that causes chickenpox.

More than one third of older people with shingles have persistent pain (postherpetic neuralgia). Generally, the older a person is, the greater the chance of developing postherpetic neuralgia. Rarely, shingles leads to other serious problems.

Causes

The virus that causes chickenpox often continues to live in a person after the symptoms of chickenpox disappear. Usually, the virus lives in the part of a nerve near the spinal cord (dorsal root ganglion). Shingles develops when the virus becomes active again (is reactivated) decades later and travels down the nerve to the skin.

Most people who develop shingles have a healthy immune system. But shingles is more likely to occur when the immune system is not functioning well. As people age, the immune system becomes slightly less effective. This slight change may be all that is needed for shingles to develop. Conditions that weaken or suppress the immune system make shingles more likely to develop. These conditions include certain disorders (such as some cancers, diabetes, and HIV infection), use of drugs that suppress the immune system (immunosuppressants, such as cyclosporine and corticosteroids), and inadequate nutrition. Surgery or other trauma can trigger shingles. However, what reactivates the virus in a particular person at a particular time usually cannot be determined.

Symptoms

Usually, shingles causes abnormal sensations in the affected part of the body a few days before the rash appears. The abnormal sensations include deep pain, burning, a "pins and needles" sensation, itching, numbness, and extreme sensitivity to touch. Before the rash appears, some people have symptoms similar to those of influenza (flu), such as fever or muscle aches.

The rash may appear anywhere on the skin over the nerve in which the virus lives. The skin over a nerve is supplied (innervated) by that nerve. This area is called a dermatome. Usually, the rash is limited to an area on the trunk. But the rash can affect an arm or a leg, occasionally even fingertips or toes. In some people, the rash develops on the neck or face instead. Almost always, the rash develops on only one side of the body.

Typically, the rash begins with clusters of red bumps. Over several days, new bumps appear, tending to form a path toward the spine. Within about a day, the bumps usually turn into small, fluid-filled blisters. The skin around the blisters is usually red. The blisters are usually painful, particularly when touched.

The blisters eventually dry and scab, usually about 5 days after they appear. However, if the immune system is weakened, scabs may not develop until much later. After blisters heal, scars may form or the areas of skin may turn brownish.

If the virus spreads through the blood, scattered blisters appear on other parts of the body. Rarely, the rash spreads over much of the body or to the brain or spinal cord. Serious problems, such as confusion and partial paralysis, may result.

Shingles on the face can sometimes spread to one of the eyes. The eye may become red, swollen, painful, and very sensitive to light. Also, it may water easily. Shingles in the eye is very dangerous. Scar tissue may form on the eye. Occasionally, the eye is permanently damaged, and vision is lost.

Some people experience persistent pain (postherpetic neuralgia) for months to years after the rash resolves.[1] The pain may be a constant, deep aching or burning. Or brief bouts of burning, sharp pain may occur. The pain may feel like an electric

1. see page 395

THE PATTERN OF SHINGLES: DERMATOME DRIVEN

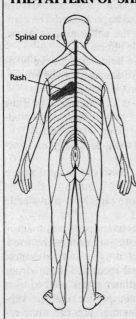

Spinal cord

Rash

Where the rash of shingles appears is determined by the activity of the virus that causes it—the same virus that caused an earlier episode of chickenpox. After chickenpox resolves, the virus travels up a nerve (called a spinal nerve) and lives in the part of the nerve near the spinal cord (dorsal root ganglion). The rash of shingles appears when the virus becomes active again and travels down the nerve. Thus, the rash can appear anywhere on the skin over the nerve or nerves affected by the virus.

The skin over a nerve is called a dermatome. Dermatomes exist in bands. Each begins at the spinal cord and extends across one side of the body. There is a dermatome for every part of the body—from the head to the toes, front and back. Thus, the arrangement of spinal nerves and dermatomes explains the pattern of shingles. The rash of shingles tends to appear within the affected dermatome or dermatomes, often as a continuous band corresponding to the dermatome. The rash appears only on one side of the spinal cord, because the virus travels from the spinal cord down a spinal nerve.

shock. It may be easily triggered by a light touch or a change in skin temperature.

Diagnosis and Treatment

Usually, the diagnosis is based on symptoms and the appearance of the characteristic rash. Doctors use maps of dermatomes to help them determine whether a rash is likely to be shingles. Doctors sometimes puncture one of the blisters and take a sample of the fluid inside to be analyzed in a laboratory.

The goals of treatment are to make the rash disappear quickly, relieve pain, and prevent postherpetic neuralgia and other problems.

If treatment can be started within 3 days of the rash's appearance, doctors prescribe an antiviral drug (such as acyclovir, valacyclovir, or famciclovir), taken by mouth. The antiviral drug must be taken early if it is to make the blistering rash disappear sooner and prevent postherpetic neuralgia. A corticosteroid (such as prednisone), taken by mouth, may also be prescribed. The combination may be more effective than the antiviral drug alone. However, corticosteroids can have side effects.[1]

Antiviral drugs taken by mouth also help when an eye is affected. If the drug is used promptly, eye damage may be less severe. In addition, corticosteroid eye drops sometimes help.

If shingles causes serious problems or is widespread or if the immune system is greatly weakened, a person may be hospitalized and treated with an antiviral drug given intravenously.

Pain is treated with pain relievers (analgesics). If pain is severe, opioids may be needed.

Burow's solution, a powder that is dissolved in cool water, can be used to soak the affected skin. This solution soothes the skin and makes the blisters dry up more rapidly. It is available without a prescription.

For postherpetic neuralgia, the effectiveness of treatment is difficult to predict. Often, several treatments need to be tried. Most people feel better after taking drugs used to control seizures (anticonvulsants, such as gabapentin). These drugs suppress painful nerve activity. Sometimes drugs used to treat depression (antidepressants, such as nortriptyline) can also suppress pain sensation. Strong analgesics may provide some relief. A cream containing capsaicin (a substance in hot red peppers) can be applied to the skin. It deadens nerves temporarily, but it causes a burning sensation that many people will not tolerate. Alternatively, a local anesthetic, such as lidocaine, can be applied to the skin as a cream, lotion, or patch. However, it is poorly absorbed through the skin, limiting its effectiveness.

If other treatments do not work, a doctor may inject a local anesthetic into the affected nerve near the spine to relieve pain. However, relief may be only temporary. Injecting a corticosteroid into the nerve may provide relief for months or longer. Electrical stimulation of nerves may be tried, but relief is often incomplete.

Outlook

The rash usually clears up in a week or two. However, if the immune system is weakened, the rash may last far longer, and

1. see table on page 593

serious problems are more likely. Only 10% of people with shingles develop the disorder again.

Any contact with open blisters on a person with shingles can cause chickenpox—but only in people who have never had chickenpox. If these people also have a weakened immune system, avoiding such contact is crucial. For them, chickenpox can be life threatening. People with shingles should be aware that pregnant women and infants should not come in contact with the open blisters (because the virus can harm unborn children and infants). Whether people who have been vaccinated against chickenpox have lifelong protection is not yet known.

Postherpetic neuralgia persists in about half of people over 70, despite the best treatment. The constant or unpredictable pain can disrupt nearly everything a person does. It can sometimes lead to social isolation or depression. In some people, post-herpetic neuralgia disappears, even without treatment, within a year.

PRESSURE SORES

Pressure sores (also called pressure ulcers, decubitus ulcers, or bedsores) are areas of damaged skin that result from prolonged pressure on the skin. Pressure applied for as little as 2 hours can damage the skin and cause a pressure sore.

Pressure occurs when the skin is pressed between a bone and a hard object, such as a bed, wheelchair, or cast. Pressure prevents blood from reaching the tissues.

Pressure sores are common among people who are confined to bed or a wheelchair, especially those who have reduced sensation or difficulty changing their position. Pressure sores develop in about one fourth of nursing home residents.

Pressure sores develop in stages. They usually start with redness on the surface of the skin and may penetrate through the layers of the skin and eventually reach muscle and bone. Pressure sores can become infected. The infection can spread to nearby skin, bones, and joints. It can also spread through the blood. Serious infections are more likely to develop in deep sores.

Most often, pressure sores develop on skin over a prominent bone (such as the hip, tailbone, elbows, or heels), especially if the layers of muscle and fat between the bone and the skin are thin.

WHERE DO PRESSURE SORES DEVELOP?

Most often, pressure sores develop on the lower back, buttocks, hips, backs of the knees, ankles, and heels. They may also develop on the elbows, back, ears, and back of the head.

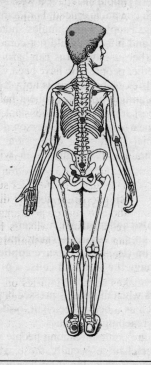

Preventing pressure sores is preferable and usually easier than treating them. Many pressure sores and the infections that result from them can be treated effectively.

Causes

The skin needs a steady supply of blood to stay alive. Pressure can cut off the skin's blood supply or even make blood vessels rupture. If the blood supply is greatly reduced for more than an hour or two, the skin deprived of blood may die.

Aging itself does not cause pressure sores. But it causes changes in tissues that make pressure sores more likely to develop. As people age, the outer layers of the skin thin. Many older people have less fat and muscle, which help absorb pressure. The number of blood vessels decreases, and blood vessels rupture more easily. All wounds, including pressure sores, heal more slowly.

Certain conditions make pressure sores more likely to develop:

• Being unable to move normally (immobility) because of a disorder such as stroke. Such people tend to stay in one position, putting pressure on one area for too long.

• Having to stay in bed for a long time, for example, because of surgery.

• Being excessively sleepy. Such people are less likely to change position or ask someone to reposition them.

• Losing sensation because of a disorder such as nerve damage (neuropathy). Such people do not feel discomfort or pain, which could prompt them to change positions.

• Becoming less responsive to what is happening in and around them, including their own discomfort or pain, because of a disorder such as dementia.

Anything that makes sores or injuries on the skin's surface heal more slowly can contribute to the development of pressure sores. Examples are undernutrition, diabetes, smoking, poor circulation (peripheral arterial disease), and the use of corticosteroids.

Moisture that remains in contact with the skin for a long time can irritate it, sometimes causing it to break down. Then, pressure sores are more likely to develop. People who cannot control bowel movements or urination (are incontinent) are prone to pressure sores, because feces or urine may remain in contact with the skin for a long time.

Pulling or rubbing on the skin excessively can contribute to the development of pressure sores. These actions (which can occur when a person is repositioned) can injure the skin by stretching it or creating friction against it.

Symptoms

Symptoms vary depending on the stage of the pressure sore.

- **Stage 1:** The surface of the skin becomes red.
- **Stage 2:** If pressure continues, a blister or shallow crater forms because the outer layer of skin dies. It dies because it does not get enough blood.
- **Stage 3:** Pressure sores penetrate through the deeper layers of skin.
- **Stage 4:** All of the skin is lost, exposing muscle or bone.

Pressure sores may be painful. But many people who have them may not notice the pain, because they have lost sensation or they no longer respond to what is happening to them.

If pressure sores become infected, they usually have an unpleasant odor. Pus may be visible in or around the sores. The area around the pressure sore may become red or feel warm, and pain may worsen if the infection spreads to the surrounding skin (causing cellulitis). If deep pain lasts several days or longer, the cause may be infection of the bone (osteomyelitis). If a joint swells and becomes painful (particularly when it is moved), the cause may be an infection in the joint (septic arthritis). If a person has fever or shaking chills or suddenly feels ill or weak, an infection may have spread throughout the body via the blood. This infection is called sepsis. Any change suggesting infection requires immediate medical attention.

Diagnosis

A doctor diagnoses pressure sores by their appearance. A nurse or doctor usually measures the size and depth of a sore to determine its stage and to plan treatment. If the pressure sore appears to be infected, a sample of the sore is sometimes taken and cultured so that bacteria can be identified. However, such tests are often unhelpful. Results of cultures taken from the sore's surface are always unhelpful.

Prevention

Usually, pressure sores can be prevented. If a person is likely to develop pressure sores, a concerted effort to prevent them should be made by all caregivers as well as the person (if able).

Changing positions frequently is important. Caregivers should encourage activity. Caregivers should turn or reposition people who cannot move themselves. Such people, whether asleep or awake, should be moved every 2 hours. Moving them less often does not prevent ulcers from forming. Drugs that cause drowsiness and thus make people move less are avoided or used sparingly.

If a person is confined to bed or a wheelchair, closely inspecting the skin each day is important. If the skin is red or discolored, a caregiver should reposition the person more frequently. The person should be kept from lying or sitting on the affected area until it returns to normal.

The skin must be kept clean and dry because moisture irritates the skin, increasing the chance of developing pressure sores. Dry skin is less likely to stick to fabrics (including sheets) and to tear. For people confined to bed, sheets should be changed frequently to make sure they are clean and dry. Applying noncaking body powder to skin in areas where two parts of the body press against each other (such as the buttocks and groin) can help keep the skin in these areas dry.

Pulling and creating friction on the skin should be avoided. One way is for caregivers to learn the safest way to reposition the person. Another is to use sheepskin to cover a bed or chair and thus reduce friction on the skin.

Areas where bones are prominent, such as the heels and elbows, can be cushioned with soft materials, such as cotton or fluffy wool. Special beds, mattresses, and seat cushions that contain water, gel, or air can reduce pressure on areas where pressure sores tend to develop. Foam mattresses and cushions do little to help prevent pressure sores. A doctor or nurse can recommend the most appropriate type of mattress or seat cushion for people who are confined to a bed or a wheelchair. However, these devices do not eliminate pressure. Even when the devices are used, people still need to be repositioned frequently.

Protein and calorie supplements may help prevent pressure sores in undernourished people. With adequate nutrition, the body's ability to heal itself improves. A person may also gain some fat, which can cushion the skin and sometimes help prevent pressure sores.

Treatment and Outlook

Pressure sores on the surface of the skin can heal on their own if the skin is kept dry and is protected from prolonged or intense pressure. Usually, deeper sores require additional treatment. Sores that heal on their own do so very slowly.

The main goals of treatment are to relieve pressure on the pressure sores, keep them clean and free of infection, and provide adequate nutrition. If the person is undernourished, protein, calorie, vitamin C, and zinc supplements may help pressure sores heal more quickly.

Dead tissue must be removed with a scalpel or chemical solution. Removal of dead tissue is usually painless, because pain is not felt in dead tissue. Some pain may be felt because healthy tissue is nearby. Health care practitioners may flood (irrigate) the sore, particularly its deep crevices, with a sterile solution to help clean away hidden debris.

Most pressure sores should be cleaned at least once a day with a sterile solution. The only exceptions are sores covered with a dressing that must remain in place for 3 to 5 days. Such dressings are designed to form tight barriers over sores to keep them from drying out and to keep microorganisms that can cause infection from getting in. Except when cleaning or another treatment is needed, pressure sores should remain covered with special dressings that do not stick to the sores. For a severe pressure sore on a foot or the lower part of a leg, a paste is applied to the foot and leg. The paste hardens and is wrapped with a bandage, forming a soft, castlike boot (Unna boot). The boot provides extra protection.

Sometimes a bed that circulates air (air-fluidized bed) is used in hospitals or nursing homes. This special bed helps deep sores heal more quickly by reducing or redistributing pressure on the body.

Sometimes if a pressure sore is deep, healthy skin is removed from another part of the person's body and applied (transplanted or grafted) over the sore. Skin transplantation or grafting can help prevent infections and speed healing. However, it may be too risky for people who are frail or undernourished.

If all other treatments are ineffective, an area of skin next to the pressure sore is cut and folded over the sore. This procedure is called flap surgery.

Unless the conditions that contributed to the development of pressure sores are corrected, ulcers are likely to recur, even after skin grafting. Flap surgery reduces the likelihood of recurrence but does not eliminate it.

Infections are treated with antibiotics. Some infections, particularly those in the bones, can be difficult to cure and may require weeks of antibiotics. Protein, calorie, vitamin C, and zinc supplements can help the body fight infection.

If a serious infection develops, people often have to stay in a hospital for a long time. Many older people with pressure sores die within a year or two. However, death often results from the disorder that caused the person to become confined to bed or immobile rather than from the pressure sores.

VENOUS ULCERS

Venous ulcers are sores that develop after veins in the legs have been damaged. These ulcers penetrate deep into the skin.

Venous ulcers are relatively common among older people. Venous ulcers become infected easily. Occasionally, if a venous ulcer persists for a long time, skin cancer develops at the edge. Some venous ulcers, particularly large ones, never heal. However, with or without treatment, many venous ulcers heal.

Causes

Venous ulcers form when blood flow through the legs is reduced, causing blood to pool in the leg veins. Then, pressure increases in the veins and capillaries (tiny blood vessels that connect arteries and veins). The increased pressure causes fluid to leak from the blood vessels into surrounding tissue, and swelling develops. Eventually, swelling interferes with the movement of oxygen and nutrients from capillaries into the tissues. Tissues are damaged because they lack oxygen and nutrients and because the fluid that has leaked puts pressure on them. As a result, venous ulcers may form.

Any disorder that causes blood to pool in leg veins can cause a venous ulcer. A varicose vein or a vein blocked by a blood clot (deep vein thrombosis) can become damaged, causing blood to pool. Such damage to leg veins is called chronic venous insufficiency.[1] Heart failure can also cause blood to pool in veins.

Symptoms and Diagnosis

One or more ulcers develop on the leg. The outer layers of skin die and are shed (sloughed), exposing deeper tissues. Spots of white scar tissue may develop in the skin around a venous ulcer.

If venous ulcers result from chronic venous insufficiency, the legs are swollen, and the skin is dark reddish brown and very firm (a condition called stasis dermatitis). The skin may itch, and the ulcers are usually very painful.

Infection of the skin (cellulitis) often develops around a venous ulcer. Typically, the infected skin is red, warm, swollen, and tender. Red streaks occasionally appear. Pus or fluid may leak from the ulcer, especially if infection involves tissues below the skin (such as muscle).

The diagnosis is based on the appearance of ulcers and symptoms.

Prevention and Treatment

The goals of prevention and treatment are to reduce leg swelling and reduce the pressure in veins. If swelling is reduced enough, a venous ulcer may never form or may heal on its own. Often, specially designed bandages and pressure stockings help reduce swelling. Elevating the leg whenever possible reduces swelling and pressure in veins. However, elevating the legs continuously can keep a person in bed, causing other problems.[2] Drugs that remove extra fluid from the body (diuretics) are sometimes used to treat swelling due to heart failure. However, diuretics usually do not help reduce leg swelling in people with venous ulcers. Also, they may cause excessive urination, which can lead to dehydration.

If cellulitis or signs of an infection of deeper tissues (such as pus) are present, antibiotics are taken by mouth or given intravenously.

Drugs, such as nonprescription antibiotics, should not be applied directly to the skin of the leg. These drugs can cause

1. see page 649
2. see page 148

allergic reactions that worsen the problem, particularly when the skin is cracked or there is an open sore. A doctor who specializes in ulcers can prescribe safe dressings that are often helpful.

If a venous ulcer is very deep or does not heal, healthy skin taken from another part of the body may be applied (transplanted or grafted) over it. Sometimes skin taken from another person and grown in the laboratory is used.

For deep or severe venous ulcers on the foot or lower part of the leg, a paste may be applied to the foot and leg. The paste hardens and is wrapped with a bandage, forming a soft, castlike boot (Unna boot). With the extra protection provided by the boot, the ulcer can heal more quickly.

36

Eye Disorders

For most people, eyesight is the most treasured of the senses. People never stop wanting to watch children play, peer at the stars, or gaze into their partner's eyes. Old age should provide an opportunity to relish these experiences, but many older people get shortchanged when their vision becomes impaired by changes due to aging itself as well as a range of disorders.

The eyes undergo many changes with aging.[1] In addition, many eye disorders become more common with aging, so many people experience visual impairment as they get older. They may be able to see everything but much less clearly (decreased visual acuity). They may lose some areas of vision completely (blind spots) while retaining others. Or they may lose most or all of their eyesight.

Most commonly, vision loss among older people is due to clouding of the lens of the eye (cataracts) or to damage to the

1. see page 9

A LOOK AT THE EYE

The eye is one of the most specialized parts of the body. It has many parts that must work well together to do its job.

Light enters the eye through the cornea, a transparent dome on the surface of the eye. The cornea focuses the light toward the lens. Next, the light passes through the anterior chamber, a space behind the cornea. This chamber is filled with fluid that nourishes the front part of the eye (aqueous humor).

The light then passes through the pupil, which is the opening centered in the colored part of the eye (the iris). The lens further focuses the light into a narrow beam. Muscles around the lens enable the lens to change its shape, depending on whether the eye needs to focus on near or far objects. After passing through the transparent gel that fills most of the back part of the eye (vitreous humor), the narrow beam of light falls on the retina.

The retina contains cells that sense light as well as cells that transmit images to the brain (nerve cells). Blood vessels in the retina nourish the nerve cells. The most sensitive part of the retina—the part responsible for detailed vision—is a small area called the macula, which contains millions of light-sensing cells.

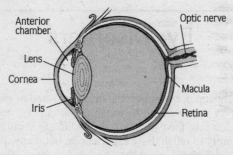

Anterior chamber
Lens
Cornea
Iris
Optic nerve
Macula
Retina

optic nerve (as occurs in glaucoma) or the retina (as occurs in age-related macular degeneration and diabetic retinopathy). A less common cause of vision loss is blockage of the blood supply to the eye. Eyelid disorders mostly change the appearance of the eye, but they can cause discomfort and contribute to vision loss as well.

Whatever the reason for vision loss, any vision change can compromise an older person's quality of life and, indirectly, health. For example, poor eyesight may contribute to a car crash or to a fall. Loss of vision can be especially devastating to older people coping with other problems as well, such as poor bal-

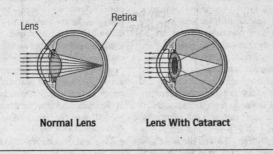

HOW CATARACTS AFFECT VISION

A normal lens receives light and focuses it on the retina. A cataract blocks some light from reaching the retina and distorts the light being focused on the retina.

Normal Lens   **Lens With Cataract**

ance and hearing loss. In such cases, vision loss can contribute to significant injury and can impair a person's ability to perform daily activities.

CATARACT

A cataract is a clouding of the lens of the eye.

A clouded lens blocks light from entering the eye. Most cataracts grow slowly until they cloud the entire lens, causing progressive, painless vision loss.

Cataracts are the most common cause of reversible vision loss among older people in the United States. The likelihood of developing a cataract continues to rise with every passing year—it does not level off. Fortunately, vision loss caused by cataracts is usually reversible with surgery.

Causes

The cause of cataracts among older people is mostly unknown. People with dark eyes, those who have had prolonged exposure to bright sunlight, those with poor nutrition, and past or present smokers are more likely to develop them. Also at increased risk are people with diabetes and those who have had other eye diseases or an eye injury. Long-term use of cortico-

UNDERSTANDING EYE SURGERY

Most eye surgery is done in an operating room or surgery center. Some procedures can be done in a properly equipped doctor's office or clinic. General anesthesia is usually not needed. Instead, anesthetic eye drops or injections into or around the eye are used to prevent pain. Drugs may be given by vein (intravenously), when necessary, to make a person groggy, to ease anxiety and awareness, and to prevent memory.

Common procedures, such as those for cataracts or glaucoma, take 1 to 2 hours, and the person usually can go home the same day. The eye that has been operated on is often patched overnight.

Eye drops are used for several weeks after the procedure. For people undergoing retinal surgery, the head may need to be specially positioned for several weeks. Head positioning is usually done to keep a gas bubble in place against the part of the retina that was detached or torn. For example, after surgery to repair a hole in the macula (center of the retina), a gas bubble may be placed in the eye for days to weeks, depending on the substance that is used. The person is instructed to remain face-down for a specified period immediately after surgery. This allows the bubble to shift upward, which in turn positions the bubble at the macula so that the macula is pushed onto the eye wall to promote closure of the hole. Special pillows and devices are used to assist the person in maintaining eye and head positioning during waking and sleeping hours.

Usually, a person is asked to return to the doctor's office the day after the procedure and again at 1 week and 1 month to ensure that the eye is healing as expected.

steroids and exposure to x-rays (such as with radiation therapy to the eye) increase the risk as well. People who have had a cataract in one eye are more likely to develop one later in the other eye. Sometimes cataracts develop in both eyes at the same time.

Symptoms and Diagnosis

The first symptom of a cataract is often blurred vision. Sometimes glare is the initial symptom. Reading may become difficult because of a worsening ability to distinguish between the light and dark of printed letters on a page. Colors may seem more yellow and less vibrant. The person may see rings of light around objects (halos) or glare or, less commonly, two images of one object (double vision). The way in which vision is changed by a cataract depends on the intensity of light entering the eye and on the location of the cataract. Occasionally, a cataract temporarily refocuses light and improves vision when near objects are viewed. This phenomenon, called second sight, allows some people to read the newspaper without their reading glasses. Eventually, however, the cataract grows denser. It then blocks light from entering the eye and impairs vision.

A general doctor may diagnose a cataract on examining the eye. However an eye doctor (ophthalmologist) must evaluate the cataract to help determine its specific effects on vision and plan treatment.

Prevention

Some evidence suggests that cataracts may be prevented with consistent use of sunglasses that protect the eyes from sunlight and ultraviolet (UV) light. Prevention of cataracts may also be aided by eating a diet rich in carotenoids (which are substances present in vegetables such as spinach and kale), vitamin C, and vitamin A. For people with diabetes, keeping blood sugar (glucose) levels as close to normal as possible helps prevent cataracts. People who are taking corticosteroids for extended periods might discuss with their doctor the possibility of using a different drug.

Treatment

Cataracts usually require no treatment until vision is significantly impaired. Eyeglasses and contact lenses may improve a person's vision, as may wearing sunglasses that block UV light (sunglasses with polarized lenses). Avoiding lighting that shines directly in the eyes and using lighting that brightens without shining in the eyes (for example, using a lamp that provides over-the-shoulder lighting while reading) may help.

Beyond these measures, surgery is the only treatment that provides a cure. However, surgery should be performed only when visual impairment is making the person feel unsafe, uncomfortable, or unable to perform daily tasks. Having cataracts removed sooner usually offers no advantage. Cataracts are sometimes removed earlier if they prevent a doctor from examining the back of the eye in people at risk of vision loss from glaucoma, diabetes, or age-related macular degeneration.[1]

1. see page 520

Cataract surgery can be performed at any age and is generally safe even for people with chronic diseases, such as coronary artery disease and diabetes. During surgery, the doctor usually makes a small incision in the eye, breaks up the lens using ultrasound (phacoemulsification), and removes all of the pieces. The tissue surrounding the lens (the lens capsule) is left in place in the eye. The surgeon usually implants an artificial lens (intraocular lens). The artificial lens, which is supported and held in position by the lens capsule, restores the eye's ability to focus images on the retina. If an artificial lens cannot be implanted safely, the person must wear thick eyeglasses or contact lenses to substitute for the eye's natural lens.

Complications after cataract surgery are infrequent. An infection or serious bleeding may develop in the eye, which can lead to partial or complete vision loss. Eye pressure may become too high (glaucoma), or the lens implant can become displaced. The central and most sensitive part of the retina (macula) can become swollen or detached. Rarely, an existing retinal disorder, such as diabetic retinopathy,[1] may progress after cataract surgery, which can lead to further vision loss.

In about one third of people who have had cataract surgery, the remnants of the lens capsule become cloudy, impairing vision. Vision can be restored with laser therapy.

Outlook

Many people notice improved vision within a few weeks after cataract surgery. Almost everyone who has undergone this surgery needs eyeglasses to see near objects (for example, for reading), and most people need weak eyeglasses to reach their potential for seeing far objects. People with cataracts in both eyes can further improve their vision by having a cataract removed from the other eye several months after the first eye has healed.

GLAUCOMA

Glaucoma is a disorder that damages the optic nerve, leading to progressive, irreversible vision loss.

1. see page 522

Glaucoma is typically associated with high pressure within the eye, although it can occur with normal pressure. How the high pressure damages the cells of the optic nerve is unknown.

Glaucoma is one of the most common causes of vision loss among older people in the United States.

Glaucoma is classified as open-angle (chronic) or closed-angle (acute). Open-angle glaucoma is much more common than is closed-angle glaucoma. In both kinds, people who have had glaucoma in one eye are likely to develop glaucoma in the other eye. And either kind can cause blindness if left untreated. Blindness often can be prevented, however, with the use of eye drops and surgery that decrease eye pressure.

ADDITIONAL DETAIL

Normally, fluid that nourishes the front part of the eye is produced behind the iris, passes into the anterior chamber, and drains into drainage canals (the "angle") in the front of the eye. Balance between fluid production and drainage—like that between an open faucet and a properly draining sink—keeps fluid flowing freely and prevents pressure in the eye from building up.

The drainage canals become partially or completely blocked in some people. Fluid cannot drain normally, and new fluid keeps being produced. In other words, the sink "backs up," while the faucet continues to run. Because the fluid has nowhere else to go, pressure in the eye increases. Glaucoma results when the pressure becomes higher than the optic nerve can tolerate. Sometimes eye pressure rises to levels that are unhealthy for the optic nerve, even though the pressure remains at or below a level that is considered normal for most people (low-tension glaucoma).

In open-angle glaucoma, the optic nerve damage occurs gradually over years. In closed-angle glaucoma, the drainage canals in the eyes become blocked or covered suddenly. Pressure in the eye rises rapidly, often to a much higher level than in open-angle glaucoma, because of the sudden blockage, while fluid production continues. Permanent damage to vision occurs within hours or days.

Causes

In most cases, the underlying cause of glaucoma is unknown, although both open-angle and closed-angle glaucoma tend to run in families. Glaucoma occurs more commonly among older blacks, Asians, and Eskimos (Inuits); people who have difficulty seeing near and far objects (hyperopia); people who have diabetes; and people who have used corticosteroids for a long time.

In rare cases, glaucoma results from damage to the eye caused by infection, inflammation, a tumor, large cataracts or surgery for cataracts, injury, or other conditions that keep fluid from draining freely from the eye, leading to increased eye pressure and optic nerve damage (secondary glaucoma).

Symptoms

Open-angle glaucoma is painless and causes no early symptoms. The most important symptom is the development of blind spots, or areas of vision loss, over months to years. The blind spots slowly grow larger and merge. Vision loss occurs so gradually that it is often not noticed until much of it is lost. Side (peripheral) vision is usually lost first; central vision is lost last. The changes may progress to the point where only a small central island of vision remains, in which the person can see straight ahead perfectly but becomes blind in all other directions (sometimes referred to as tunnel vision). If glaucoma is left untreated, eventually even central vision can be lost, resulting in total blindness.

Closed-angle glaucoma causes abrupt onset of severe pain in and around the eye, headache, redness, blurred vision, rainbow-colored halos around lights, and sudden vision loss. Nausea and vomiting may occur in response to the increased eye pressure. Closed-angle glaucoma is considered a medical emergency, because if left untreated, blindness can occur as quickly as 2 to 3 hours after the start of symptoms.

Diagnosis

An eye doctor performs a complete eye examination, which includes measuring pressure in the eye, inspecting the optic nerve for damage, testing peripheral vision for blind spots, and inspecting drainage canals in the eye. Because older people can develop glaucoma and lose vision without knowing it, they should undergo a comprehensive screening eye examination every 1 to 2 years.

Treatment

The goal of treatment is to prevent the onset of vision loss or to stop its progression.

Eye drops are the primary treatment for open-angle glaucoma. These include beta-blockers, such as betaxolol and timolol; carbonic anhydrase inhibitors, such as brinzolamide and dorzolamide; prostaglandin-like drugs, such as bimatoprost and latanoprost; alpha agonists, such as apraclonidine and brimonidine; and cholinergic drugs, such as carbachol and pilocarpine. They either decrease production or increase drainage of fluid in the eye. Although generally safe, the drops may cause side effects in the eye or throughout the body.

An older person may find it difficult or impossible to self-administer eye drops because of arthritis or a neurologic condition, such as a tremor. In such cases, an alternative device, such as an eyedropper with an oversized bulb, may be necessary. Alternatively, a caregiver can administer the drops. Carbonic anhydrase inhibitors can be taken by mouth to lower eye pressure, but their use is limited because of frequent side effects.

Surgery or laser therapy is almost always needed if the person has closed-angle glaucoma. These treatment methods may also be needed for people with open-angle glaucoma if eye drops cannot effectively control eye pressure, if they cannot be used, or if they cause serious side effects. Surgery and laser therapy aim to improve fluid drainage by opening drainage canals or creating new ones. Although generally safe, surgery or laser therapy may not always achieve the desired level of eye pressure and occasionally causes a temporary increase in eye pressure or inflammation and bleeding within the eye. Surgery or laser therapy may need to be repeated to achieve the desired level of eye pressure. Eye drops to lower eye pressure may be needed even after surgery or laser therapy. Cataracts may develop or progress as a result of surgery for glaucoma.

Treatment of secondary glaucoma may include antibiotic or antiviral eye drops for infection, corticosteroid eye drops for inflammation, and surgery for a tumor or cataract.

Outlook

There is no cure for open-angle glaucoma. Therefore, eye drops must be used for the rest of the person's life. In addition, regular checkups are needed for monitoring eye pressure, optic nerve health, and areas of vision seen out of each eye (visual field testing). Surgery and laser therapy can cure closed-angle glaucoma in many people, but regular checkups for monitoring and eye drops may still be needed in some people.

AGE-RELATED MACULAR DEGENERATION

Age-related macular degeneration is deterioration of the macula, the central and most sensitive area of the retina.

Macular degeneration is the most common cause of irreversible central vision loss among older people. In its early stage, macular degeneration usually does not cause any symptoms. In advanced stages, macular degeneration can lead to distortion of vision, vision loss, and central blind spots.

Macular degeneration is categorized into two types: dry (non-neovascular) and wet (neovascular). In dry macular degeneration, the more common of the two types, the light-sensitive cells of the macula may be lost, and the retina thins (atrophies). In wet macular degeneration, abnormal blood vessels develop beneath the macula. These vessels leak fluid and blood, which results in the formation of scar tissue. Scar tissue can impair vision by causing light-sensitive cells to die. The dry type usually is present in both eyes, whereas the wet type most often affects one eye at a time. Only a few people with dry macular degeneration eventually develop wet macular degeneration. However, once wet macular degeneration develops in one eye, there is a 50% chance that it will develop in the other eye within 5 years. People who smoke or who have high blood pressure may be at higher risk of progression to the wet type.

Causes

The exact cause of age-related macular degeneration is unknown. In general, the disease occurs only in older people. It is also more common among whites, people with a family history of the disease, past or present smokers, and people with low dietary intake of antioxidants. Age-related macular degeneration may also be more common among women, people with fair skin, and people with light-colored eyes.

Symptoms

Most people with the dry type of the disease have no symptoms, although some people experience mild distortion in their vision. Painless progressive loss of central vision and development of a central blind spot can occur with advanced dry macular degeneration as the retina thins (atrophies). In contrast, people with the wet type often experience an abrupt deterioration and distortion of vision over days or weeks.

People who experience distortion in their central vision or the gradual appearance of a blind spot in one eye, either from advanced dry macular degeneration or wet macular degeneration, have difficulty reading, driving, seeing faces, and watching television. Objects may appear washed out, and the ability to distinguish fine detail or to see in the dark may be lost. People retain their peripheral vision, which allows them to perform daily tasks (other than driving and reading) and remain independent. Total blindness is rare, but if both eyes are affected, blindness may result.

Diagnosis

An eye doctor diagnoses macular degeneration by examining the back of the eye after dilating the pupils. Fluorescein angiography—a test in which a dye is injected into an arm vein and photographs are taken of the retina—may be necessary to determine whether new blood vessels are forming. The test can also help the doctor assess whether treatment will benefit a person with the wet type of the disease.

Treatment

Some people with certain forms of dry macular degeneration can slow the rate of further vision loss by taking high-dose supplements of vitamin C, vitamin E, beta-carotene, zinc, and copper. A doctor can inform the person as to whether he has one of the forms that might be helped by vitamin supplements.

People with wet macular degeneration may be candidates for a special type of laser therapy (thermal laser photocoagulation) or photodynamic therapy. Photodynamic therapy has been shown to be effective for people with wet macular degeneration that has certain features. These features can be identified only by fluorescein angiography and a physical examination. Laser and photodynamic therapy either destroy abnormal blood vessels or limit their growth and thereby reduce the likelihood of further vision loss and the rate of progression of any additional loss that does occur.

Low-vision aids may optimize quality of life for people with vision loss.

DIABETIC RETINOPATHY

Diabetic retinopathy is damage to the retina that results from diabetes mellitus.

Diabetic retinopathy is one of the most common causes of blindness in older people in developed countries. Diabetic retinopathy is most common in people with a history of poorly controlled blood sugar levels. The risk is especially high in those people who have had diabetes for many years, high blood pressure, and high blood cholesterol levels.

Causes

Diabetic retinopathy occurs when blood vessels in the retina are damaged over time by high levels of sugar in the blood. At first, high blood sugar levels cause the blood vessels to leak blood and fluid into the retina. Eventually, the blood vessels close, depriving the retina of nutrients and oxygen. This fosters the growth of new blood vessels. The appearance of these vessels indicates the beginning of a phase of proliferative retinopathy, which can lead to blindness through bleeding, retinal detachment, or glaucoma.

Symptoms and Diagnosis

People with diabetic retinopathy may have no symptoms despite extensive growth of new blood vessels. Some people experience gradual vision loss. Others develop blind spots scattered about in their field of vision. More serious symptoms include "floaters" or "flashing lights" due to retinal tears and detachments[1] or abrupt vision loss when newer, weaker blood vessels burst and bleed into the eye.

1. see page 527

WHAT ARE LOW-VISION AIDS?

Aids for coping with vision loss (referred to as low-vision aids) can be an enormous help to older people with only partial vision. Low-vision aids for reading, writing, watching television, and engaging in outdoor activities include the following:

- Large-print books
- Large-numbered telephones, clocks, watches, and thermometers
- Closed-circuit television to magnify objects
- Electronic "talking" clocks and other "talking" devices
- Computer programs that can scan text and then produce larger text or read the text out loud

- Light filters to improve contrast
- Color-coded pill boxes
- Hand-held magnifying glasses
- Glare-reducing sunglasses
- Hand-held binoculars
- Hand-held or eyeglass-mounted telescopes
- Reflective canes and walkers

Eye doctors working with other health care practitioners can usually evaluate how vision loss affects a person. They can then recommend a combination of low-vision aids that they believe would best help the person perform daily tasks.

An eye doctor can diagnose diabetic retinopathy by examining the retina through a dilated pupil. If blood vessels are leaking, the central part of the retina may become swollen (macular edema). Fluorescein angiography may be performed, in which a dye is injected into an arm vein and the retina is photographed.

Treatment

Treatment usually involves using light energy from a laser to seal abnormal blood vessels and decrease leakage. This procedure is called laser photocoagulation. Laser photocoagulation is also used to inhibit new blood vessel growth. Periodic treatments over years may be necessary. Laser photocoagulation prevents further vision loss but rarely improves vision. Vision may improve, however, after surgery is performed to clear blood from the vitreous gel of the eye (vitrectomy) or after repair of retinal detachments.

Prevention

Strictly controlling blood sugar levels, blood pressure, and blood cholesterol levels helps prevent diabetic retinopathy. In addition, an eye doctor should examine the eyes at least annually, because people with diabetes may develop retinopathy without knowing it.

DISRUPTIONS OF BLOOD SUPPLY

The eye is extremely sensitive to any disruption of its blood supply. Disruptions are relatively uncommon but occur more frequently as people get older. Most disruptions of blood supply result at least partly from atherosclerosis, in which cholesterol and fatty material in the blood form deposits (plaques) in the arteries.[1] Less common conditions that disrupt blood flow to the eye include inflammation of the blood vessels (vasculitis, such as temporal arteritis), infection in or around the eye, damage from radiation, and injury to the eye.

When blood flow to the eye is disrupted, the person experiences vision loss, usually in one eye. Vision may disappear completely or in patches. Sometimes vision is lost suddenly and is regained within a few minutes (a phenomenon called amaurosis fugax). This kind of sudden, temporary vision loss requires immediate medical attention, because it may indicate an impending stroke or permanent blindness.

Diagnosis and treatment of vision loss due to impaired blood flow to the eye depend on the cause.

Retinal Vein Blockage
Retinal vein blockage is blockage of a vein that drains blood from the eye.

The blockage can affect the largest vein in the eye (central vein) or a much smaller branch. Retinal vein blockage is the most common cause of blood supply disruption to the eye in older people. It occurs more commonly in people with atherosclerosis and glaucoma. People with leukemia or lymphoma, autoimmune disease, or abnormalities of the blood that cause excessive clotting may also develop retinal vein blockage.

An eye doctor diagnoses retinal vein blockage by examining the back of the eye and by taking pictures of the eye's blood supply (a test called fluorescein angiography). No treatment has been proven effective for the blockage itself. However, compli-

1. see page 624

cations of retinal vein blockage, including swelling of the macula, bleeding into the eye, and glaucoma caused by growth of abnormal blood vessels on the iris, can often be prevented or treated with laser therapy.

Retinal Artery Blockage

Retinal artery blockage is blockage of an artery that supplies blood to the retina.

The blockage can affect the largest artery supplying the retina (central artery) or a much smaller branch. The central artery or its branches most often become blocked because of atherosclerosis or an embolus (a piece from a larger blood clot in some other part of the body that has broken off and traveled through the bloodstream). Less often, people with temporal arteritis,[1] inflammation of the optic nerve, infection around the eye, and clotting disorders develop a blockage. Rarely, increased eye pressure in a person with glaucoma can become high enough to cause blockage of the retinal artery.

An eye doctor diagnoses retinal artery blockage by examining the back of the eye and by performing tests to observe blood flow in the vessels (fluorescein angiography [in which a dye is injected into an arm vein and the retina is photographed] or Doppler ultrasound scanning).

No treatment has been proven effective for retinal artery blockage due to atherosclerosis. However, some doctors try improving oxygen delivery to the tissues by massaging the eyeball, by withdrawing fluid from the eye to lower pressure on the blood vessels, and by promoting dilation of the blood vessels, sometimes by having people breathe a limited amount of carbon dioxide.

If begun early, treatment can be effective for less common causes of retinal artery blockage. Treatment options include corticosteroids for inflammation of the artery or optic nerve; antiviral or antifungal drugs for infection; and anticoagulants for clotting disorders. Anyone without one of these less common causes should be tested for carotid artery disease and treated for any risk factors for atherosclerosis.[2]

1. see page 606
2. see page 624

Retinal Emboli

Emboli are blood clots or clumps of cholesterol and fatty material that break off from atherosclerotic plaques.[1]

When emboli lodge in blood vessels in or close to the eye, the eye's blood supply can be suddenly blocked. Emboli most often come from arteries in the chest or neck, but they can also come from the heart.

Emboli are a common cause of sudden but temporary vision loss; they can also cause permanent vision loss. Vision loss from emboli is sometimes described as a slow dimming of light or as a window shade being pulled down or up over the eye. When emboli travel to the brain and the eye at the same time, vision loss may be accompanied by loss of speech or weakness in an arm and leg. If these symptoms last more than a day, they indicate that the person has had a stroke.

A doctor diagnoses the source of retinal emboli using ultrasonography or magnetic resonance angiography. Echocardiography and recordings of heart rhythm may be performed to determine if the person is at risk for further emboli.

Treatment may involve surgery (carotid endarterectomy) if test results show that the emboli may have come from the arteries in the neck and if the arteries are significantly narrowed. Otherwise, aspirin or other anticoagulants (sometimes called blood thinners) are used. Warfarin is given if test results show that emboli may have come from the heart. Treatment of atherosclerosis is important as well.[2]

Ischemic Optic Neuropathy

Ischemic optic neuropathy is a sudden painless loss of vision in one eye from insufficient blood flow to the optic nerve.

The cause is unknown. Atherosclerosis, diabetes, and high blood pressure may increase the risk of developing ischemic optic neuropathy. Temporal arteritis is a treatable form of ischemic optic neuropathy.[3]

Some people have pain or discomfort around the eye. An eye

1. see page 624
2. see page 628
3. see page 606

doctor diagnoses the condition by examining the eye. No proven treatments are available for most forms of ischemic optic neuropathy. For some people, vision improves without treatment. Only a small percentage of people experience the same symptoms in the other eye. Control of risk factors for atherosclerosis may help prevent ischemic optic neuropathy.

People with optic neuropathy due to temporal arteritis experience vision loss, which may be sudden in one eye.[1] They may also experience headache, scalp tenderness at the temple, fever, and jaw pain when chewing. A doctor diagnoses the condition by examining the eye, performing blood tests, and performing a biopsy of the temporal artery. Treatment involves use of corticosteroids, mainly to prevent occurrence of disease in the other eye, but also to reduce risk of further vision loss in the affected eye.

Occipital Lobe Stroke

An occipital lobe stroke involves loss of blood flow to the part of the brain that receives images from the eye.

Causes are the same as those for other strokes.[2] Partial vision loss occurs in both eyes and involves the same area of vision. For example, both eyes can see to the right side but lose vision on the left side. Generally, 50% or less of the area of vision is impaired. Diagnosis and treatment are the same as for other types of stroke.

RETINAL TEARS AND DETACHMENT

A retinal tear is an irregularly shaped break in the retina. A retinal detachment is separation of the retina from the eye wall and supporting tissues.

The retina can tear or detach when the gel that fills the eye (vitreous humor) pulls away from the retina (posterior vitreous detachment). Separation of the gel from the retina is a normal change that occurs with aging. But when parts of the gel are stuck to the retina (adhesions), the pulling away can lead to tearing of the retina. The person may see flashes or sparkling lights. When fluid from the eye gel leaks through the tear, the retina itself can lift off the eye wall or become detached, causing partial or complete loss of vision.

An eye doctor diagnoses retinal tears and detachment by examining the eye through a dilated pupil or by using ultrasound.

It is essential to get treatment for a retinal tear or detachment as quickly as possible to decrease the likelihood of permanent damage. Treatment usually involves using surgery or laser therapy to repair the tear and seal the retina to the back of the eye. Surgery may involve injecting gas into the eye to flatten the retina, applying gentle pressure to the side of the eye (buckling) to repair the detachment, or removing all of the gel that fills the eye (vitrectomy).

DISORDERS OF TEAR PRODUCTION

Tears aid normal vision, provide a smooth surface on the outside of the eye that helps clear debris while blinking, and nourish the eye surface. Tears normally drain or evaporate at the same rate at which they are produced; thus people are unaware of the tears in their eyes. But when production and elimination of tears are not in balance, dry eyes or excessive tearing can result. Both conditions are common in older people. Tearing is also a reflex to dryness of the surface and can actually be an indication that the eye is dry.

Dry Eyes

Dry eyes are common among older people because tear production decreases with aging, especially among women. Exposure to a dry climate or to cigarette smoke can worsen the condition. Drugs are a common cause of dry eyes, as are eyelid disorders, especially blepharitis.[1] Less common causes include eye infection and, in developing countries, vitamin A deficiency. The most serious cause of dry eyes is Sjögren's syndrome, an uncommon autoimmune disease that also causes dry mouth and sometimes arthritis.

A doctor diagnoses dry eyes by collecting tears with a special paper strip placed next to the eyeball. Sjögren's syndrome is diag-

1. see page 530

nosed with the use of blood tests and possibly a biopsy. Regardless of the cause, treatment is with artificial tears. Other treatments, such as the surgical placement of plugs in the drainage canals to decrease tear drainage, are needed only if artificial tears do not relieve symptoms or maintain the health of the eye surface.

Excessive Tearing

Excessive tearing can be caused by impaired drainage of tears or as a reflex when the eye surface is dry. An improperly positioned lower eyelid or an obstruction of the drainage ducts in the eyes or nose can impair drainage. The doctor probes and irrigates the drainage ducts if obstruction is suspected; otherwise, no tests are necessary. Treatment usually involves treating the underlying cause.

EYELID DISORDERS

The eyelids play a key role in protecting the eyes. They sweep away debris when the eyes close and help spread moisture (tears) over the surface of the eyes when the eyes open. Some eyelid disorders and eyelid growths in older people are common and have only cosmetic significance. But others, like skin cancers on the eyelid, are more serious.

Ectropion

In ectropion, the lower eyelid grows lax and droops. The edge of the eyelid often turns outward (becomes everted).

Because the lower eyelid can no longer distribute tears across the eyeball or drain tears, tears fall onto the face instead. In addition, the lower eyelid may not close completely, thus the eye is exposed to the air and may become dry, red, and irritated. Artificial tears and ointments used at night may help the irritation, but most people need surgery.

Entropion

In entropion, the lower eyelid turns inward into the eye.

The lower eyelashes may rub against the eyeball, which in turn can cause tearing, irritation, infection, ulceration of the cornea, and scarring. Carefully placed stitches can pull the eyelid outward when scar tissue develops along the stitch. Botulinum toxin can pull the eyelid outward by paralyzing the muscle around the eye. However, these procedures offer only temporary solutions to the problem, and entropion eventually recurs. Correction with surgery offers the best hope of a permanent cure.

Eyelid Droop

Eyelid droop (ptosis) has several causes. The nerve that supplies the muscle of the upper eyelid may be paralyzed (this paralysis is often caused by diabetes). The cause can also be other neurologic diseases, such as Horner's syndrome and myasthenia gravis. Separation or stretching of the eyelid muscle where it connects to the eyelid can also result in eyelid droop. Surgery and injury to the eye are additional causes.

Eyelid droop usually causes no symptoms, although some people experience obstruction of vision as well as headache and fatigue from using their brow muscles while attempting to elevate their eyelids. Surgery is the only treatment available for eyelid droop and is necessary only if a person has symptoms. Complications of surgery include difficulty closing the eyes, dry eyes, and ulcers on the cornea.

Blepharitis
Blepharitis is inflammation of the edges of the eyelids.

It is sometimes caused by staphylococcal infection, and people with rosacea and seborrheic dermatitis are more likely to develop the condition. However, older people without these disorders frequently develop blepharitis for no apparent reason.

Blepharitis produces a range of symptoms, including a sensation of having something in the eye; itching, burning, swelling, and redness of the eyelid edges; watery eyes and sensitivity to bright light; and loss of eyelashes. Dried secretions may make the eyelids sticky after sleep.

Diagnosis is usually based on symptoms and on the appearance of the eyelids. Treatment consists of three measures: warm compresses, gently washing the eyelashes and eyelid edges with a dilute solution of baby shampoo, and use of antibiotic ointment or drops. Blepharitis is a chronic condition and can only be controlled, not cured. However, although blepharitis may be inconvenient or unattractive, it usually does not damage the eye.

Blepharospasm
Blepharospasm is a spasm of the muscles around the eye, causing involuntary blinking and closing of the eyes.

In severe cases, people with blepharospasm cannot open their eyes. Blepharospasm can occur as a result of other eye diseases, but its cause is more often unknown. It affects women more than men and tends to occur within families. Blepharospasm may also be more common in people with thyroid disease.

Spasms are often made worse by fatigue, bright light, and anxiety. Treatment involves injecting botulinum toxin into the muscles. Antianxiety drugs may also be of use. Surgery to cut the muscles is also effective but causes more complications than botulinum toxin. Sunglasses help decrease the light sensitivity that may cause or accompany blepharospasm.

Chalazion
Chalazion is a swelling of oil glands in the eyelid, usually because of a blocked duct.

The disorder occurs for unknown reasons and is most common in people with rosacea and blepharitis.

A person notices a chalazion when the eyelid becomes swollen, irritated, or red or when a painless swelling develops on or under the eyelid. A chalazion that is large enough can rub against the eyeball, causing irritation or, rarely, vision changes.

Treatment involves applying a warm compress to the eyelid several times a day. Even without treatment, a chalazion usually disappears after several months. If it persists, a doctor can inject a corticosteroid or drain the chalazion using a special spoon-shaped instrument (curettage).

Stye
A stye is an infected eyelid gland that is often difficult to distinguish from a chalazion.

Styes look like small, round swellings of the eyelid that may have a pinpoint yellow or white spot where the duct of the gland is blocked. Styes often accompany blepharitis and cause redness, tenderness at the edge of the eyelid, and a sensation that something is in the eye.

Warm compresses can open the infected gland. Antibiotic drops or ointments may also be useful. Surgery may be necessary for styes that do not respond to compresses or antibiotics.

Xanthelasmas
Xanthelasmas are flat yellow or white growths of the upper eyelid that appear thick and fatty.

Xanthelasmas in older people can occasionally be a sign of high cholesterol levels and therefore warrant a blood test.

37

Hearing and the Ear

Hearing is easy to take for granted. But appreciation for normal hearing usually grows when hearing loss occurs. The importance of hearing, however, goes beyond the mere perception of sound. It also affects a person's interactions, thoughts, and skills. Several common expressions, with their emphasis on the ear as symbolic of hearing, give hearing its due. They describe attention ("lend an ear"), the ability to play a song after only having heard it ("playing by ear"), the act of willfully ignoring ("turn a deaf ear"), forgetfulness ("in one ear and out the other"), and suspicion and deceit ("the walls have ears").

The ear is a complex organ capable of perceiving the minute changes in air pressure that make up sound. The ear has three parts: the outer ear, the middle ear, and the inner ear. The outer ear consists of the external ear (pinna) and the ear canal. The external ear focuses sound waves into the ear canal, which boosts the volume of frequencies critical to human hearing. The ear canal leads to the eardrum, which separates the external ear

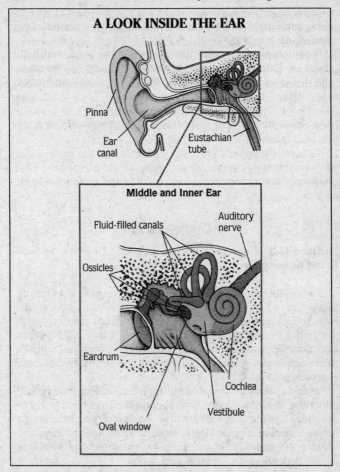

A LOOK INSIDE THE EAR

Pinna

Ear canal

Eustachian tube

Middle and Inner Ear

Fluid-filled canals

Auditory nerve

Ossicles

Eardrum

Cochlea

Vestibule

Oval window

from the middle ear. The eardrum vibrates in response to sound waves and transmits the vibrations to three tiny bones in the middle ear called ossicles. The ossicles amplify the vibrations and transmit them to the cochlea. Within the cochlea—a fluid-filled structure in the inner ear—small hairlike projections (cilia) conduct electrical current when moved by sound vibrations. The signal is then transmitted by the auditory nerve to the brain.

The eustachian tube connects the back of the pharynx (throat and nose) with the middle ear. It functions like a safety valve, allowing fluid that accumulates in the middle ear (for example, from ear infections) to drain into the throat. The eustachian tube allows air pressure in the middle ear to balance, or equalize, with the air pressure in the throat. When the nose is stuffy because of an allergy, a viral illness, sinusitis, a large adenoid (common in children), or a tumor, the eustachian tube may not open normally. Without this equalization of pressure, hearing loss may result.

Numerous disorders can affect hearing and the ears. Older people commonly experience some degree of hearing loss. Also common among older people are tinnitus and accumulation of earwax.

HEARING LOSS

Hearing loss is deterioration in hearing. Deafness is profound hearing loss.

Among the older population, 29% have significant hearing loss by age 65 and 50% by age 80. Hearing loss can have a profound effect on quality of life, especially when it interferes with the ability to hear and understand speech. Many older people who develop hearing loss also have impaired vision, and the combination can greatly interfere with the ability to carry out everyday activities.

Several characteristics of sound, including loudness and pitch, affect the ability to understand sounds created by speech. For example, hearing loss may involve the inability to hear words below a certain threshold of loudness. Hearing loss may also involve the inability to discriminate among similar-sounding words, depending on loudness and pitch.

Even mild hearing loss makes understanding speech difficult. As a result, an older person with mild hearing loss may avoid conversations. Understanding speech may be particularly difficult if there is background noise or more than one person is talking, such as in a restaurant or at a family gathering. Thus, hearing loss can lead to social isolation, inactivity, loss of social support, and depression. In a person with dementia, hearing loss can make communicating even more difficult. Hearing loss can cause both emotional and physical harm. A person who has trouble hearing, for example, may not hear a fire alarm, a smoke detector, or an automobile horn.

Hearing aids can improve quality of life for about 95% of older people with hearing loss. However, only 30 to 40% of older people with hearing loss in the United States use hearing aids. Those people who cannot benefit from hearing aids may be helped by a cochlear implant.

One of the important barriers to coping with hearing loss is overcoming the embarrassment that some older people experience. Wearing a hearing aid or letting someone know that they are "hard of hearing" makes some older people feel old. Hearing loss, however, is a medical condition and is nothing to be ashamed of. By facing the reality of hearing loss, people can do so much to improve their lives.

Causes

The gradual loss of hearing that affects many older people is called presbycusis. Presbycusis may begin in a person's 20s but go unnoticed until the person reaches his 50s or 60s.

Aging itself plays a role in the development of presbycusis,[1] but noise is probably the most common cause. Noise destroys the small hairlike projections in the cochlea that conduct sound. Both the loudness and duration of noise exposure are important. A single exposure to a very loud noise can cause hearing loss, but such hearing loss is usually temporary. However, repeated exposure to loud noises usually causes permanent hearing loss. Millions of people in the United States are repeatedly exposed to levels of noise that can damage hearing. Typically, each exposure causes hearing loss that is so subtle as to be imperceptible. Only after decades of cumulative noise exposure and damage does hearing loss become noticeable.

Some drugs, including gentamicin and related antibiotics (aminoglycoside antibiotics), cisplatin (a chemotherapy drug), aspirin and related drugs (salicylates), and furosemide and related diuretics (loop diuretics), can cause hearing loss. Aspirin can cause ringing in the ears (tinnitus); this is generally temporary and occurs only at high doses. Quinine occasionally causes similar symptoms.

1. see page 12

Blockage of the ear canal by earwax[1] is a common cause of mild hearing loss among older people. People who swim in cold water for many years may develop blockages due to bony projections in the ear canal (exostoses). Although usually of little significance, these bony projections can cause wax and dead skin to accumulate. Less often, the ear canal is partly or completely blocked by changes in the skull due to abnormal bone growth (Paget's disease).

Much less common causes of hearing loss include rupture of the eardrum; infection or allergy that causes fluid to develop behind the eardrum; blockage of the ear canal by a foreign object; a tumor of the auditory nerve, brain, or eustachian tube; strokes; and disorders in which a person's own immune system turns against the body in some way (autoimmune disorders).

ADDITIONAL DETAIL

Doctors divide the causes of hearing loss into two categories: conductive hearing loss and sensorineural hearing loss.

Conductive hearing loss is reduced conduction (transmission) of the vibrations of sound waves to the inner ear. It generally results from a problem with the outer or middle ear. Typical causes of conductive hearing loss among adults are blockage of the ear canal by earwax, stiffening of the ossicles by scar tissue that results from middle ear infection or surgery, and fluid accumulation in the middle ear due to a blocked eustachian tube.

Sensorineural hearing loss is an inability to sense sounds once they have reached the cochlea. It can result from disorders that damage the hairlike projections in the inner ear, the auditory nerve, or parts of the brain that decode and interpret sounds. In addition to aging itself, nerve damage due to tumors or strokes can cause sensorineural hearing loss.

Very often, hearing loss is both conductive and sensorineural. Otosclerosis is a condition in which one of the ossicles stiffens, causing conductive hearing loss. But otosclerosis may also cause sensorineural hearing loss by affecting the bone of the cochlea. Changes in the skull and temporal bone due to Paget's disease can cause both conductive and sensorineural hearing loss.

1. see page 544

Symptoms

Hearing loss due to aging itself usually develops so gradually that people may not notice the first symptoms. High-pitched sounds are affected more than low-pitched sounds. The voices of women and children, therefore, which are higher in pitch than those of men, become particularly difficult to understand. High-pitched musical instruments, such as violins, may sound dull. In addition, certain consonants, such as C, D, F, K, P, S, and T, become hard to distinguish. An inability to hear the sounds of some consonants may make it sound as if a speaker is mumbling. Words can be misinterpreted. For example, a person may hear "bone" when the speaker said "stone."

Conversations become difficult to follow, particularly in crowded or noisy areas. Constantly asking others to talk louder can frustrate both the listener and the speaker. People with hearing loss may misunderstand a question and give an apparently bizarre answer, leading others to believe they are confused. They may misjudge the loudness of their own speech and thus shout, discouraging others from conversing with them.

Background noise tends to mask high frequencies and blur sounds, making speech more difficult to understand even for older people who hear normally. To compensate for background noise, many older people develop an ability to watch a person's lips for clues about what is being said.

Diagnosis

During an examination, a doctor may test a person's hearing by whispering or by using a hand-held sound generator. In addition, the doctor may place a vibrating tuning fork near the person's ear, on the top part of the skull, or on the bone behind the ear. A person's symptoms and the results of the examination can be important in establishing the diagnosis. However, special diagnostic tests usually are performed as well.

• **Audiometry** is the first hearing test performed. In this test, a person wears headphones that play tones of different pitch and loudness. The person signals when he hears a tone, usually by raising his hand or pressing a button on the side that he heard the tone. For each pitch, the test identifies the quietest tone the person can hear in each ear.

PREVENTING NOISE-INDUCED HEARING LOSS

Loudness is measured in decibels on a logarithmic scale. This means that 10 decibels represents a 10-fold difference in sound intensity. That is, 20 decibels is 10 times as loud as 10 decibels, and 30 decibels is 100 times as loud as 10 decibels. Interestingly, although an increase in volume of 10 decibels represents a 10-fold increase in volume, it seems only twice as loud to the person hearing it.

Glycerin-filled earmuffs, headphones, or plastic or foam rubber earplugs can be used to protect the ears from noise that can cause hearing loss. Such protection is recommended if exposure exceeds the following durations and noise levels: 8 hours at 85 decibels; 2 hours at 100 decibels; 15 minutes at 115 decibels; any exposure that exceeds 115 decibels. In addition, music should be played at moderate or low volume levels, particularly when headphones are used.

Decibels	Example
30	Whisper, quiet library
60	Normal conversation, sewing machine, typewriter
90	Lawnmower, truck traffic
100	Chainsaw, snowmobile
115	Automobile horn
140	Gun muzzle blast, jet engine

• **Speech threshold testing** measures how loudly words have to be spoken to be understood. A person listens to a series of two-syllable, equally accented words, such as "railroad," "stairway," and "baseball," presented at different volumes.

• **Speech discrimination testing** assesses the ability to hear differences between words that sound similar. Pairs of similar one-syllable words are presented, such as "snake" and "flake."

Other tests are less commonly done. They include tests (1) to measure nerve impulses in the brain produced by sound vibrations in the ears; (2) to measure the ability to interpret and understand distorted speech; (3) to understand a message presented to one ear when a different, competing message is presented to the other ear; (4) to combine incomplete messages to each ear into a meaningful message; and (5) to determine where a sound is coming from.

If a person has fluid in the ear, the doctor examines the back of the throat with a mirror or viewing tube (endoscope). Occasionally, imaging studies (such as computed tomography [CT] or magnetic resonance imaging [MRI]) are done to check for sinusitis or a tumor, especially when a person has significantly greater hearing loss in one ear along with dizziness or ringing in the ears.

Treatment

Unfortunately, most hearing loss in older people cannot be cured. However, some treatments can compensate for hearing loss and improve quality of life. Hearing aids, for example, can benefit most people with mild to moderate hearing loss. Cochlear implants can benefit people with severe or profound hearing loss.

Hearing aids: Hearing aids increase the volume of sound reaching the eardrum. They are helpful regardless of the cause of hearing loss and significantly improve a person's ability to communicate. If hearing loss occurs in both ears, as is the case with most older people, wearing a hearing aid in each ear achieves the best results. However, if hearing loss is much greater in one ear than in the other, a single hearing aid worn in the more impaired ear may work best.

Hearing aid technology continues to improve. People who have been dissatisfied with older models may be pleasantly surprised by more recently developed hearing aids. A comprehensive hearing aid center can help people choose a hearing aid that best meets their specific needs. A 30-day trial period is usually offered at such centers.

All hearing aids have a microphone that picks up sounds, a battery-powered amplifier that amplifies sounds, and a means of transmitting the sounds to the person. Some recent hearing aids have several microphones. Most hearing aids transmit the sounds through a small speaker placed in the ear canal. Much less common are hearing aids that require surgical implantation, allowing sounds to be transmitted directly to the tiny bones of the middle ear or to the skull instead of through a speaker. Implanted devices eliminate feedback (squealing), which is common in conventional hearing aids. A person with an implanted device also feels less of a sense that the ear is plugged.

Hearing aids differ in size and in where they are worn. Small hearing aids fit entirely or almost entirely in the ear canal. They generally are more attractive because they are less noticeable. However, their small size may limit the number of features they

HEARING AIDS AND THE TELEPHONE

Many older people with hearing loss have difficulty using the telephone even when they use a hearing aid. Holding the phone's headpiece close to the ear often causes squealing. However, there is a solution.

Some hearing aids have a switch that converts the hearing aid to "phone mode." In phone mode, the aid's microphone is turned off and a special magnetic coil is turned on. Meanwhile, the speaker in the phone's headset has been replaced with a magnetic coil (in most cases the phone company can provide this service). This replacement does not interfere with normal operation of the phone. When the person with this type of hearing aid places his ear close to the phone headset and the coils from each of these devices are in close proximity, the coils act like a direct plug-in connection. As a result, sound clarity is vastly improved and squealing is eliminated.

offer and the ease with which their controls can be adjusted or batteries replaced.

Hearing aids also have different electronic characteristics to suit a person's particular needs. For example, people whose hearing loss affects mainly higher frequencies do not benefit from amplification of all sound frequencies, which merely makes the mumbled speech they hear louder. Hearing aids that selectively amplify the high frequencies markedly improve speech recognition and sound clarity. Most older people need this type of hearing aid, which must be adjusted for a person's specific hearing deficits. Other hearing aids contain vents in the ear mold, which increase the passage of high-frequency sound waves into the ear. As a result, high-frequency sounds become clearer.

Some digital hearing aids can match amplification even more precisely with the person's hearing loss. People who cannot tolerate loud sounds may need hearing aids with special electronic circuitry that keeps the maximum volume of sound at a tolerable level. Hearing aids with complex features tend to be the most expensive but are often essential.

People with dementia may fare best with a simple style of hearing aid that resembles a portable radio that can be worn on a belt buckle or tucked into a pocket. The device consists of a box containing an amplifier, a microphone or microphone jack, a headphone jack, and a volume control. The wearer plugs a conventional headphone into the amplifier. Compared with con-

HEARING AIDS: AMPLIFYING THE SOUND

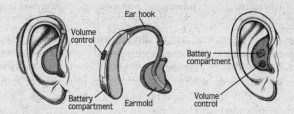

Behind-the-Ear Hearing Aid
- Best choice for severe hearing loss
- Most powerful but least attractive

In-the-Ear Hearing Aid
- Used for mild to moderate hearing loss
- Easy to adjust but hard to use with telephones

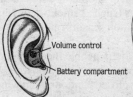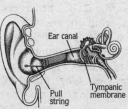

In-the-Canal Hearing Aid
- Used for mild to moderate hearing loss
- Relatively inconspicuous but hard to use with telephones

Completely-in-the-Canal Hearing Aid
- Used for mild to moderate hearing loss
- Good sound, nearly invisible, and easily used with telephones
- Most expensive and hard to adjust
- Not a good choice for people who have trouble using their hands

ventional hearing aids, this device is relatively inexpensive, easily repaired if broken, and more difficult to lose.

Cochlear implants: People with severe or profound hearing loss who cannot benefit from hearing aids may benefit from a cochlear implant. Cochlear implants combine an external microphone, external processor, and external coil with electrodes inserted surgically into the cochlea and a coil inserted surgically into the skull above and behind the ear. Cochlear implants provide electrical signals directly into the auditory nerve. Cochlear implants do not restore normal hearing. However, they do help almost everyone who gets them to better distinguish spoken words, with or without reading lips, and, for some, a greater ability to understand telephone conversations. Cochlear implants also help deaf people hear and distinguish environmental and warning signals, such as doorbells, telephones, and alarms.

Other ways to cope with hearing loss: If hearing cannot be fully restored, a person can adapt in other ways.

Alerting systems that use a flashing light or a wearable vibrating alarm enable people to know when the doorbell or telephone is ringing or when a person in another room is calling out for help. Similarly, safety devices (such as smoke detectors, carbon monoxide detectors, and motion sensors) and timers can be equipped with a flashing light.

Special sound systems can help people hear in theaters, churches, and other places where there is competing noise. Many television programs carry closed captioning, in which the dialog is shown as text. Telephone communication devices, called text telephones (TTY or TTD), display the words of the caller on a screen.

Lip reading (speech reading) and other strategies for coping with hearing loss are part of a program of aural rehabilitation. Lip reading is particularly helpful for people who can hear but who have trouble discriminating certain consonant sounds, as in hearing loss that occurs with aging. Speech comprehension can be significantly improved by observing the position of a speaker's lips.

In addition to training in lip reading, people are taught how to anticipate difficult communication situations and to modify or avoid them. For example, people can visit a restaurant during off-peak hours, when it is quieter. They can ask for a booth, which blocks out some extraneous sounds. They can request that "specials of the day" be written rather than spoken. In direct conversations, people may ask the speaker to face them, to allow for lip reading. At the beginning of a telephone conversation, people can identify themselves as being hearing-impaired.

TINNITUS

Tinnitus is noise originating in the ear rather than in the environment.

Tinnitus is common, affecting 15% of people over 45 and about 25% of people over 65. The distraction created by the noise greatly distresses some people. Fortunately, certain measures can make tinnitus more tolerable.

Causes

Hearing loss is the most common cause of tinnitus. In addition, most disorders that affect hearing can cause tinnitus, including accumulated earwax, Ménière's disease, fluid in the middle ear, and acoustic neuroma (a type of tumor). Disorders that do not involve the ear, for example, anemia, hardening of the arteries (atherosclerosis), and heart murmurs, can also cause tinnitus. Drugs that can cause hearing loss can also cause tinnitus. High doses of aspirin are a common cause of tinnitus.

In many cases, the cause of tinnitus is unknown.

Symptoms and Diagnosis

People with tinnitus use a seemingly endless list of words to describe what they hear. The noise may sound like bells or crickets, or it may be a ringing, a buzzing, a roaring, a whistling, or a hissing sound. Some people hear combinations of sounds. Usually the noise is continuous and affects both ears. The noise may pulsate if it is caused by anemia, atherosclerosis, or heart murmurs. Tinnitus becomes more prominent when surroundings are quiet or when the person is not focusing on something else. Thus, tinnitus tends to be most disturbing when trying to fall asleep.

If the cause of tinnitus is not clear, tests may be needed. Because subtle hearing loss can cause tinnitus, doctors usually perform hearing tests. Magnetic resonance imaging (MRI) of the head or computed tomography (CT) of the area of the skull that contains the ear (temporal bone) is often performed in those who have symptoms in only one ear, who sense a pulsating to their tinnitus, or who also have hearing loss in only one ear. Blood tests may be required, for example, to exclude anemia. Sometimes an ultrasound of the arteries in the neck is performed to find evidence of disorders such as atherosclerosis (narrowing of the arteries).

Outlook and Treatment

Attempts to silence the sounds are often unsuccessful. However, certain techniques can make tinnitus more bearable. Sometimes a cause can be found and tinnitus can be relieved. For example, tinnitus due to hearing loss often subsides if a person uses a hearing aid. Substituting a new drug for one that has been causing tinnitus (such as aspirin) or reducing the dose may relieve the condition as well.

Background sounds often offer temporary distraction from tinnitus. For example, music may help during the waking hours. At night, neutral sounds may help. Neutral sounds are the sounds most easily ignored as background noises. They can be produced by a white-noise generator (a machine that generates noise at every pitch simultaneously) or an FM radio tuned to a frequency between stations. If tinnitus is bothersome constantly, a tinnitus masker may help. This device, which generates neutral sounds, is worn in the ear like a hearing aid.

If none of these measures relieves tinnitus, biofeedback may help. Biofeedback is a technique in which a person learns to gain control over unconscious bodily functions (in this case, the triggers that cause tinnitus). Biofeedback involves a process of trial and error and is taught by a professional.

EARWAX

Earwax (cerumen) is a substance produced by the glands in the ear canal.

Earwax helps protect against ear infections and probably has other functions as well. Normally, the earwax eventually moves out of the canal, often along with skin cells that are shed. However, as a person ages, earwax and the skin become drier, causing the earwax to stick to the canal. As a result, earwax can accumulate, eventually becoming hard, thick, and firmly plugged. Seborrheic dermatitis of the scalp (dandruff) and around the ears, which is common among older people, makes earwax plugs especially likely. Earwax accumulation does not reflect poor personal hygiene.

Symptoms and Diagnosis

If an earwax plug blocks the ear canal or presses against the eardrum, ringing of the ears (tinnitus) or a feeling of fullness may develop. Hearing loss may also occur. If a person does not already have hearing loss caused by something else, the hearing loss caused by earwax plugging usually is barely noticeable. However, many older people, even before they have accumulated an earwax plug, already have lost a small degree of hearing without noticing it. For them, earwax plugs, which worsen hearing only a little bit, can make hearing loss obvious.

A doctor diagnoses earwax accumulation by examining the ear with a viewing tube (otoscope).

Treatment

Sometimes earwax can be softened or dissolved at home with hydrogen peroxide, mineral oil, or baby oil. Alternatively, a nonprescription oil preparation specifically designed to soften and dissolve earwax can be used. Whichever softening liquid is used, several drops should be put in the ear canal and retained there for about 15 minutes by tilting the head to one side. After 15 minutes, the ear is gently rinsed with tap water—for example, in the bathtub or shower. Alternatively, a rubber bulb syringe, available without a prescription, can be used to gently flush the ear with tap water. To remove large amounts of earwax, the person may need to repeat this procedure several times. If earwax remains, a doctor usually can remove it with a small instrument or by flushing the ear with pressurized water.

A person can sometimes prevent accumulation of hard earwax by using softening liquids about once or twice a week as described above. Allowing warm water to flow into the ears while bathing or showering may also help.

Attempting self-treatment by sticking an object (even soft cotton-tipped swabs) into the ear canal can pierce (perforate) the eardrum or cause infection or bleeding. Health care practitioners, however, can usually safely use cleaning tools in the ear canal, often with the aid of an otoscope.

38

Nose and Throat Disorders

Savoring the aroma of a favorite food and belting out a verse from a familiar song are but two examples of how the sense of smell and the ability to use one's voice can add richness to a person's quality of life. The sense of smell and the ability to use one's voice can even be the difference between life and death, as any person knows who has ever smelled smoke in a building and called out to alert others. And any person who has experienced an improperly working nose or sinuses may well know the vexing discomfort and challenges faced in trying to lie down and sleep comfortably. The sense of smell, the proper functioning of the nose and sinuses, and the ability to use one's voice all remain vitally important to older people. Therefore, disorders of the nose and throat, even if they seem minor at first, cannot be considered trivial.

The Nose and Sinuses

The expression "as plain as the nose on your face" does not give the nose its due: There is so much more to the nose than what can be observed in the mirror. The nose can be thought of as having two parts. The visible part consists of bone and cartilage. Hollow passageways extend from the nostrils (nares) upward and inward along the sides of the nose, separated by a thin sheet of cartilage and bone called the nasal septum. The hidden part begins where passageways from the visible part of the nose join a hollow space (nasal cavity) that extends back to the upper part of the throat (nasopharynx), connecting the nose with the airways. Together, the passageways in the visible part of the nose and the nasal cavity in the hidden part of the nose are sometimes called the nasal passages.

Sinuses are smaller hollow spaces in the front portion of the skull. The purpose of the sinuses remains unknown. The paranasal sinuses, of which there are several types, are located around the nose and eyes. The maxillary sinuses are under the cheekbones and just above the upper teeth. The ethmoid sinuses are on the sides of the upper nose and between the eyes. The sphenoid sinuses are behind the ethmoid sinuses. The frontal sinuses are above the eyebrows. All of the paranasal sinuses have passageways that open into the nasal cavity.

The nose plays an important role in breathing and in the sense of smell. It also protects against infection and contributes to a person's appearance and tone of voice. But aging changes the nose. The mucous membranes lining the nasal passages become thinner and drier, which may increase the risk of nosebleeds and impair the sense of smell. Sense of smell is further impaired as the nerves responsible for smell deteriorate with aging. A runny nose and mucus draining into the throat become more common because of changes in the nerves controlling blood vessels in the nasal passages. Cosmetic changes occur as well. Cartilage weakens, causing the tip of the nose to droop. This drooping makes the nose appear longer and more humped. These cosmetic changes also contribute to the sense of nasal obstruction that grows more common with aging.

Chronic disorders of the nose and sinuses can affect a person's appetite and nutrition, sense of smell, breathing, appearance, and sense of well-being. Nasal and sinus congestion, the most common symptoms of nose disorders, frequently cause problems when a person lies down, thus making it difficult to fall and stay asleep. Nasal and sinus congestion usually cause fatigue from both the sleep disturbance and the constant effort to get air through the congested nose.

The Throat

The throat, like the nose, is more complex than its appearance suggests. The throat has three main parts. The upper part (nasopharynx) connects with the nasal passages as they pass

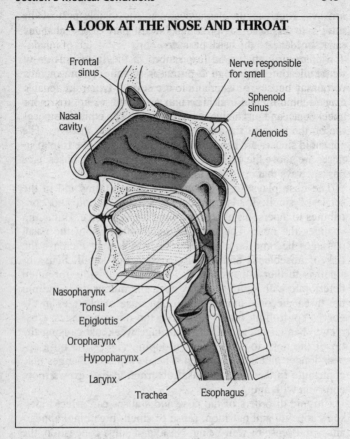

A LOOK AT THE NOSE AND THROAT

Frontal sinus

Nerve responsible for smell

Sphenoid sinus

Nasal cavity

Adenoids

Nasopharynx

Tonsil

Epiglottis

Oropharynx

Hypopharynx

Larynx

Trachea

Esophagus

into the back of the mouth. The middle part (oropharynx) is in the back of the mouth and is visible when the mouth is opened wide. This part of the throat extends to the base of the tongue and assists in swallowing and speech. The lower part (hypopharynx) extends into the windpipe (trachea) in the neck, where the voice box (larynx) is located. The voice box is a complex structure composed of cartilage and muscle. Muscles in the voice box (vocal cords) vibrate and move to produce the basic tone that is shaped by the rest of the throat, mouth, and lips into speech.

With aging, the muscles in and around the tongue weaken, leading to less efficient, prolonged swallowing. These changes can put older people at risk of undernourishment and of inhalation of unswallowed food (aspiration). The vocal cords grow weaker, leading to change in pitch (presbylarynx). A woman's voice may become huskier and lower in pitch, whereas a man's may become thinner and higher in pitch. Hoarseness is more likely to accompany colds or excessive voice use as the vocal cords weaken. Uncommonly, a tremor of the voice develops and grows more pronounced with aging; this voice tremor tends to occur with tremors of the hands. Disorders of the throat can change the sound and volume of a person's voice. Throat disorders can also impair swallowing,[1] thereby adding to the risk of undernutrition and aspiration.

RHINITIS

Rhinitis is inflammation of the mucous membranes of the nose. Rhinitis often occurs with sinusitis.[2]

Rhinitis is commonly caused by a viral infection or allergy. Older people, however, may develop rhinitis in response to aging itself (atrophic rhinitis), irritants and cold temperatures (vasomotor rhinitis), certain foods (gustatory rhinitis), certain drugs (drug-induced rhinitis), low levels of thyroid hormone (hypothyroidism), or fleshy outgrowths in the nose (nasal polyps).

The symptoms of rhinitis are about the same no matter what the cause; the most common symptom among older people is a runny nose. Other symptoms include the following:

- Nasal congestion
- Postnasal drip
- Coughing from postnasal drip, especially upon lying down
- Sneezing
- Itchiness in the nasal passages (itchiness can occur no matter what the cause but is especially common with allergies)

1. see page 822
2. see page 552

A diagnosis of rhinitis is based on the cause and duration of symptoms. The doctor may use a flexible viewing tube (endoscope) to examine the nasal passages, especially if polyps are suspected. Treatment often involves the use of general measures to help alleviate the symptoms of rhinitis, regardless of the cause. However, many causes can be treated specifically. For example, rhinitis caused by nasal polyps can be treated by surgically removing the polyps.

Viral rhinitis: Viral rhinitis is extremely common and is often the most bothersome feature of the common cold. No treatment is completely effective. Nonprescription decongestants taken by mouth in pill or liquid form (pseudoephedrine) or sprayed into the nose (phenylephrine or oxymetazoline) help control congestion. However, symptoms can worsen if decongestant nasal sprays are taken for more than 3 days and then abruptly stopped.

Antihistamines, either alone or combined with other drugs in a cold remedy, should not be taken. They are ineffective against viral rhinitis, and many older antihistamines, such as diphenhydramine and chlorpheniramine, can cause drowsiness, confusion, urinary retention, worsening of glaucoma, and loss of balance in older people.

Antibiotics are ineffective against viruses. Zinc lozenges are probably safe for older people, but their effectiveness is controversial. Receiving the influenza (flu) shot each year can help protect against the most severe viral rhinitis, which is rhinitis associated with the influenza virus.

Allergic rhinitis: Allergic rhinitis is caused by an allergic reaction to dust, molds, animals, foods, the pollens of grasses and trees, or other environmental triggers. Often, the person has a family history of allergies or asthma. Allergic rhinitis may cause itchy, watery eyes in addition to other symptoms. Blood tests or skin testing may help a doctor make the diagnosis.

Treatment involves avoiding substances that trigger the allergy, if possible. If avoidance is impossible, nasal sprays containing corticosteroids, antihistamines, or cromolyn are effective and safe for older people. Certain antihistamines taken by mouth are also effective and safe. Older antihistamines, such as diphenhydramine and chlorpheniramine, which are in most nonprescription products, can cause many side effects in older people. Newer antihistamines, such as fexofenadine, cetirizine, and loratadine, which cause fewer side effects, should be used instead. Leukotriene receptor blockers, such as montelukast, taken by mouth, are also moderately effective and safe. Allergy shots (immunotherapy) can make people less allergic by desensitizing them to the triggering substance. However, allergy shots are usually recommended only for people with severe symptoms that do not respond to drugs.

Atrophic rhinitis: Atrophic rhinitis occurs when the mucous membranes of the nasal passages thin (atrophy) and harden, causing the passages to widen and dry out and become more vulnerable to infection. The nasal bone can also become weakened and is more likely to break. The disorder affects older people worldwide but is growing less common in developing countries. Atrophic rhinitis may result from aging itself or from chronic infection, sinus surgery, radiation therapy, or unusual diseases, such as sarcoidosis.

Symptoms of burning or pain in the nose are common. So is congestion, which in severe cases is accompanied by thick, dry, offensive-smelling crusts in the nasal passages. Nosebleeds occur as well, and a person can lose the sense of smell. The disorder may be confused with sinusitis.

Treatment may involve several approaches. Salt water can be sprayed into the nose to keep the nasal passages moist. Topical antibiotics, such as bacitracin, may be applied directly inside the nose to kill bacteria. If the crusting becomes severe, other antibiotics, given by mouth or intravenously, may help. As a last resort, surgery can be performed to narrow the nasal passages, but severe nasal congestion may result.

Vasomotor rhinitis: Vasomotor rhinitis occurs when blood vessels in the nose widen (dilate) or narrow (constrict) in response to irritants such as perfumes or other odors, cigarette smoke, pollution, or cold, dry air. Avoiding irritants is the primary treatment. Warm humidified air, such as that from a vaporizer, may also help. Ipratropium nasal spray is effective but seems to relieve a runny nose more so than relieving congestion. Azelastine, an antihistamine nasal spray, also works because it dries out the mucus.

Gustatory rhinitis: Gustatory rhinitis may be a form of vasomotor rhinitis. Gustatory rhinitis is triggered by eating. Any type of food can trigger symptoms, although hot, spicy foods and alcohol have been reported to cause the most severe symptoms. Many cold foods can also be culprits. Treatment involves avoiding problematic foods and extremely hot or cold foods.

Drug-induced rhinitis: Drug-induced rhinitis is caused by a variety of drugs, including estrogen supplements; some anti-hypertensive drugs, such as angiotensin-converting enzyme (ACE) inhibitors and beta-blockers; antidepressants; aspirin; and some antianxiety drugs. Using decongestant nasal sprays for more than 3 days at a time can lead to rebound nasal congestion.

Treatment involves discontinuing the drug that causes symptoms. Withdrawal from long-term regular use of a decongestant nasal spray may need to be supervised by a doctor specializing in ear, nose, and throat disorders. Corticosteroid nasal sprays may also help ease symptoms as the body begins to rid itself of the offending drug.

SINUSITIS

Sinusitis is inflammation of the sinuses.

Sinusitis is one of the most common disorders affecting older people. It may last only for a brief period (acute sinusitis) or may persist for 3 months or longer (chronic sinusitis).

Sinusitis is categorized as infectious or allergic. Sinusitis in older people most frequently occurs with rhinitis as part of the common cold and so is caused by a virus. The nasal congestion that results blocks the sinuses, preventing drainage of mucus into the nose and mouth. The sinus mucus then builds up and thickens, and infection in the sinuses becomes more likely. Infectious sinusitis can also be caused by a bacterial infection or sometimes by a fungal infection (particularly in people with poor immune functioning, such as those receiving chemotherapy for cancer or those with diabetes).

Allergic sinusitis is caused by an allergic reaction to dust, mold, pollen, or another substance in the environment. Some people develop an allergic reaction to harmless fungi that can grow in their sinuses if they have fleshy growths (polyps) or other obstructions in the nose (allergic fungal sinusitis).

Sinusitis does not become more common with aging because of aging itself but rather because the conditions that predispose a person to sinusitis increase with aging. For example, older people are more likely to develop sinusitis because of tooth or gum infections, nosebleeds, nasal polyps, an aging immune system, or dryer nasal secretions that do not drain well.

Symptoms and Diagnosis

Sinusitis causes nasal and sinus congestion, nasal discharge, sinus pain or pressure, headache, and sometimes pain or tingling in the upper teeth. Fever may occur if an infection is present. Bacterial sinusitis sometimes causes a foul smell or bad breath due to pus draining down the back of the throat.

A diagnosis of sinusitis is usually made on the basis of symptoms. Computed tomography (CT) can be used when sinusitis is not relieved by the use of appropriate drugs or is relieved but keeps recurring after treatment. A doctor can also diagnose sinusitis by inserting an endoscope (a flexible viewing tube) into the nose to inspect the sinus openings and to obtain samples of sinus drainage to detect and identify bacteria. This procedure is useful when the diagnosis of sinusitis is uncertain, when the type of infection must be identified, or when sinusitis recurs.

Treatment

Infectious sinusitis is treated according to the type of infection believed to be causing it. Often, antibiotics are needed.

Viral sinusitis, which doctors typically assume is the cause, does not respond to antibiotics. Salt water may be sprayed into the nose to improve drainage of the thick mucus. A nasal rinse may be used: A solution containing salt water, with or without other additives, is irrigated into the nose until the solution begins to run down the back of the throat. Although some people find this process unnerving, most people tolerate it well and obtain considerable relief. Decongestant nasal sprays or pills may be taken to lessen congestion. Acetaminophen or a nonsteroidal anti-inflammatory drug (NSAID), such as ibuprofen, may be taken by mouth to lessen pain. Guaifenesin may be taken by mouth to thin mucus secretions. Drinking fluids, which keeps secretions thin, is encouraged.

When symptoms do not subside after 5 to 7 days despite treatment, doctors suspect a bacterial infection and may prescribe antibiotics. People whose condition does not improve after taking antibiotics may be given stronger antibiotics or corticosteroid nasal sprays. They may undergo a sinus x-ray to help doctors identify the precise problem. Sinusitis involving the maxillary sinus may, on rare occasions, require puncturing of the sinus wall to allow for drainage.

Invasive fungal sinusitis is treated with antifungal drugs given intravenously and by surgery that opens existing passageways or that creates new passageways that allow sinuses to drain (surgical drainage).

Allergic sinusitis is treated with corticosteroid sprays or antihistamines taken by mouth. Newer antihistamines, such as fexofenadine, cetirizine, and loratadine, should be used. Older antihistamines, such as diphenhydramine and chlorpheniramine, can cause many side effects and should not be taken. Antihistamines taken as sprays are also effective. Guaifenesin, which is taken by mouth, can thin secretions and thereby improve drainage. Allergic fungal sinusitis is treated surgically. Fungal material and any obstruction caused by nasal polyps are removed. Treatment may also involve the use of corticosteroid sprays or, sometimes, pills. Allergy shots may help. Antifungal drugs given as mist treatments may also be of use but are unproven.

Outlook

The outlook for most kinds of sinusitis is generally good. Bacteria can occasionally cause chronic infection that is not easily treated with antibiotics. Although uncommon, a bacterial infection can spread from the sinuses to the orbit around the eye, causing pain, difficulty moving the eye, and even vision loss and blindness. Rarely, a bacterial infection can spread into the central nervous system, causing meningitis or clotting of blood vessels in the brain (cavernous sinus thrombosis). Fungal infections can be difficult to treat and require long-term treatment with corticosteroid and antifungal drugs, which sometimes requires that the person continue to receive the drug intravenously at home for a while.

VOICE DISORDERS

Voice disorders produce involuntary (uncontrollable) changes of voice. The two voice disorders that commonly affect older people are vocal cord atrophy and laryngitis.

Vocal Cord Atrophy

Vocal cord atrophy is weakening or abnormal movement of the vocal cords. The difference between the normal changes in voice that occur with aging (presbylarynx) and vocal cord atrophy is one of degree.

Other than aging itself, the cause of vocal cord atrophy is unknown. As atrophy occurs, muscle tissue in the vocal cords may be replaced by fibrous connective tissue and fatty tissue.

Dryness of the larynx may worsen the changes in the vocal cords that occur with atrophy. Dryness may be due to decreased salivary gland function; use of certain drugs, such as antidepressants with anticholinergic side effects, diuretics, and antihistamines; and nasal obstruction that causes a person to breathe through the mouth. Vocal cord atrophy may also be aggravated when a person strains the voice to overcome changes in sound that normally occur with aging. Straining typically occurs when a person talks too much at a loud volume.

Vocal cord paralysis may occur when a disease or an injury affects the cords themselves or when a disease or injury affects the nerves that control the vocal cords. Examples of such diseases or injuries are viral infections that cause inflammation (viral laryngitis), injury when a breathing tube is inserted into the throat during surgery or when a person is placed on a ventilator, neurologic diseases (such as Parkinson's disease), and tumors.

Symptoms and Diagnosis

Vocal cord atrophy may make the voice sound weak, thin, hoarse, husky, breathy, or rough. A weak cough or difficulty swallowing (especially fluids) may also develop. Vocal cord atrophy can also cause a "tickle" that gives a person a constant sensation of needing to clear his throat. These symptoms can also signal the presence of laryngeal cancer and should prompt a visit to a doctor if they last more than a week or two. A doctor makes the diagnosis by passing an endoscope (a flexible viewing tube) through the nasal passages and into the throat to observe vocal cord movement. A special type of x-ray may be taken to ensure that the person can swallow safely without inhaling food: A series of x-rays is taken while a person eats food containing material that can be seen on the x-ray.

Treatment

Drinking plenty of fluids and using lozenges, sugarless candy, or chewing gum may help restore the voice by increasing moisture. Resting the voice for a few days can often be helpful. But the main treatment of vocal cord atrophy is speech therapy, in which the person learns how to speak comfortably without straining the vocal cords.[1] Repetition of vocal exercises taught during therapy gradually helps strengthen the voice. Speech therapy is very successful and usually results in a stronger and clearer voice. These methods also help relieve any tickling sensation.

Surgery is effective but is regarded as a last resort. The aim of surgery is to move the weak vocal cord closer to the mobile vocal cord; when the two vocal cords make contact, they produce a stronger and clearer voice.

Laryngitis
Laryngitis is inflammation of the vocal cords.

The most common cause is a viral infection, such as the common cold, with nasal drainage into the throat. Other causes in older people include tobacco use (either smoking or chewing) and damage to the larynx due to regurgitation of stomach acid (reflux laryngitis).[2]

Symptoms and Diagnosis

Symptoms of laryngitis are hoarseness or even loss of voice, sore throat, throat tickling and an urge to clear the throat, and cough. A doctor diagnoses laryngitis and in some cases its cause by asking questions and by examining the throat, either with a light and a mirror or with an endoscope (a flexible viewing tube).

Treatment

For most causes, treatment involves resting the voice by not speaking or singing. Drinking extra fluids helps too. If a person smokes or chews tobacco, quitting helps to cure or relieve the laryngitis. If reflux laryngitis is diagnosed, treatment is the same

1. see page 179
2. see page 831

as that for gastroesophageal reflux.[1] Such treatment includes the following:

- Changing the diet
- Limiting or eliminating certain foods (including fatty foods) or beverages (such as caffeinated beverages and alcohol) that make reflux worse
- Avoiding food or fluids several hours before bedtime
- Elevating the head of the bed while sleeping
- Taking drugs that reduce levels of acid production in the stomach, such as proton pump inhibitors (for example, omeprazole or lansoprazole) and H_2 blockers (for example, ranitidine or famotidine)

1. see page 834

I am a passionate promoter of exercise and I love traveling alone by train. The dining car provides three new acquaintances each meal. After the initial chitchat, I ask about what exercise they do and create an opportunity to talk about the importance of stretching and strengthening exercises.

The response is almost always the same—a confession that they are not doing enough and want to do more. Rarely, someone has started to get into a new routine with a personal trainer because they feel the need. Then I can tell them about my video exercise kits.

As the meal draws to an end, I ask them to guess my age. This is the fun part. They guess 70 and I say 91! The reaction warms my heart and inspires me to keep following my passion.

At 55 I had a painful knee and my hands began to seem arthritic. I needed to consciously keep these moving. In my 70s I began to lose flexibility and strength. Rather than accept this as "part of the aging process," I got into structured exercise. My husband and I moved into a continuing care community where I found a new hobby: promoting exercise and becoming a role model for the community.

My exercise kits came from my desire to make a difference in this supportive community. The funds generated by the kits are returned to the community. One kit is for seated exercise and another for those able to get on the floor.

I am grateful to have a pain-free body with the help of my exercises, a skilled massage therapist, a careful diet, and nutritional supplements, and currently no prescription drugs.

The importance of exercise is not a new idea. We're just slow learners. Hippocrates, who lived more than 2,000 years ago, told us all parts of the body which have a function, if used in moderation and exercised in labors to which each is accustomed, become healthy, well developed, and age slowly. But, if unused and left idle, they become liable to disease, defective in growth, and age quickly.

Marguerite Watson

39

Mouth and Dental Disorders

The mouth does much more than take food in and begin to digest food—two essential and enjoyable functions. The mouth also helps defend the body against invading microorganisms (bacteria, fungi, and viruses), which can cause infections. The mouth prevents microorganisms from entering the throat, which is the gateway to the lungs and stomach. Thus, the mouth helps prevent infections that could develop in these organs. Also, without the mouth, people could not speak. But even without uttering a word, the mouth helps people express emotions—for example, by smiling, grimacing, pursing the lips, or baring the teeth. It comes as no surprise, then, that the mouth has an important say in determining a person's quality of life and ability to do daily activities.

After years of faithful tasting, chewing, and talking, the mouth is often taken for granted. When minor problems develop, people may assume that nothing needs to be done or that seeking help is not worth the trouble. For many older people, going for regular checkups and cleanings falls by the wayside. Some go to a dentist only when something goes seriously wrong. But contrary to what people may think, preventing mouth and dental disorders requires more attention as they age. One reason is that older people develop disorders and take drugs that can worsen the mouth's health or interfere with the way the mouth functions.

For older people, common problems include dry mouth, tooth decay, and periodontal disease. In periodontal disease, the gums may be inflamed and infected (as gingivitis). Or the ligaments and bones that support and anchor the teeth may be inflamed and infected (as periodontitis). Most of these problems can be prevented or treated effectively. Oral cancer is a less common problem.[1] But more than 90% of oral cancers occur in people over 50, and for them, this cancer is fatal about half the time.

TOOTH DECAY

Tooth decay is the gradual destruction of a tooth. Decay begins when acids produced by bacteria in the mouth dissolve the hard surface (outer layer) of the tooth. A cavity is a specific site of tooth decay.

Cavities may start on the tooth's surface above the gum line (in the enamel). These cavities are called coronal cavities. Or they may start on the surface below the gum line (in the cementum). These cavities are called root surface cavities.

Decay can extend into a tooth's interior, which consists of the dentin and pulp. The pulp contains the nerve, artery, and vein of each tooth. If decay extends into the pulp, an infection may develop in the tooth and in nearby gum (gingiva) and bone. A collection of pus (abscess) may form. Rarely, the infection can spread through the bloodstream to other parts of the body.

Cavities can develop in people of all ages. Older people are especially likely to have root surface cavities and decay at or near the edge of a restoration, such as a filling or a crown.

People get two chances with their teeth. During childhood, they learn how to care for 20 baby (deciduous) teeth. The risk of not caring for baby teeth is offset by the reassuring awareness that these teeth will be replaced. The second set, the permanent teeth, is for keeps: They must last for the rest of a person's life. Aging itself does little to interfere with the ability to keep permanent teeth in good repair.

Causes

Bacteria that produce acid cause tooth decay. When brushing and flossing (called oral hygiene) are not done well or not done at all, food debris is left in the mouth. Bacteria thrive on this debris. Food debris, mixed with saliva and dead cells from the inside of the mouth, is deposited in a soft, thin film on teeth every day. This deposit is called dental plaque. The bacteria that cause

1. see page 785

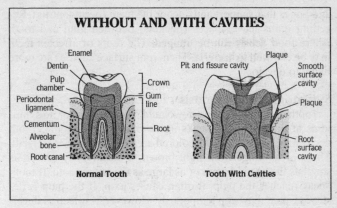

WITHOUT AND WITH CAVITIES

Normal Tooth

Enamel
Dentin
Pulp chamber
Periodontal ligament
Cementum
Alveolar bone
Root canal

Crown
Gum line
Root

Tooth With Cavities

Plaque
Pit and fissure cavity
Smooth surface cavity
Plaque
Root surface cavity

decay accumulate in plaque. When plaque remains on teeth, it can harden to form tartar. Tartar cannot be removed with a toothbrush, so it must be removed by a dentist or dental hygienist. Plaque builds up mainly when oral hygiene is poor. Poor oral hygiene is especially common among older people. It may be poor because a person sees less well, hands are less agile, arms are less flexible and less easy to move, or memory is less reliable.

Having a dry mouth increases the risk of tooth decay. The risk is higher because saliva contains substances that kill certain microorganisms. Saliva also helps wash away food debris. As people age, the mouth may produce slightly less saliva and so may become drier. Dry mouth may also be caused by a disorder or the use of certain drugs. Disorders and certain drugs can change the mouth in ways that make it easier for the bacteria that cause tooth decay to grow. For example, disorders or drugs can change the acidity (pH) of the mouth.

Older people tend to have many restorations, such as fillings or crowns. After many years of use, restorations are more likely to break down, leaving small gaps at the edges. These gaps provide ideal spots for bacteria to accumulate and for decay to begin.

As people age, the enamel on teeth may wear away, the bone that supports teeth may be lost, and gums may recede around and between teeth. Receding gums may result from inflammation and infection of the gums (gingivitis) or of the ligaments and bones that support and anchor the teeth (periodontitis). Receding gums leave spaces (pockets) between gum and tooth where food debris can be trapped. The roots of affected teeth may be exposed to bacteria. Then, root surface cavities are more likely to develop.

Symptoms and Diagnosis

Tooth decay progresses slowly and produces few or no symptoms at first. Thus, it sneaks up on many older people. Tooth decay may be visible as discolored areas on the surface of teeth. These areas range from light brown to black. They can be as small as the head of a pin or as large as the entire tooth. If tooth decay reaches the pulp, it often causes pain. If the pulp is destroyed, pain may stop temporarily. However, if infection develops and results in a collection of pus (abscess), pain is likely to return, especially when food is chewed or the tooth is touched. Swelling may develop around the tooth's root or even in the face or neck. Swelling may indicate that the infection has spread into the jawbone, face, or neck.

Tooth decay is suspected when a dentist or doctor notices a dark brown or black area on a tooth. The diagnosis is confirmed when a dentist closely inspects and probes the surface of the tooth. Dental x-rays can help confirm the diagnosis.

Prevention

People never outlive the need for regular dental examinations. Examinations every 4 to 6 months are recommended. They usually include removing plaque followed by polishing the teeth with fluoride (the entire procedure is called prophylaxis). Sometimes people who cannot get to a dentist's office (whether they live at home or in a long-term care facility) can arrange for a dentist to come to them.

Using a toothbrush and fluoride toothpaste every day can help prevent tooth decay. Brushing after each meal is best. When brushing cannot be done immediately after a meal, rinsing the mouth with a fluoride rinse or even water or chewing sugarless gum helps remove food debris. Brushing cannot remove all the food debris and plaque between teeth. So people should floss their teeth every day as a part of their oral hygiene regimen. Between-the-teeth (proxy) brushes can be very helpful, particularly for people with receding gums or gaps between the teeth where plaque can accumulate.

If use of the arms or hands is limited because of disorders such as arthritis, stroke, or Parkinson's disease, people may have difficulty brushing. Several gadgets can help. Toothpaste squeezers can be used to get toothpaste out of a tube. Extenders or holders can help people hold and manipulate a toothbrush. Electric and ultrasonic toothbrushes can be especially helpful. If holding onto a piece of dental floss is awkward, a floss holder can help. Or people can tie the ends of a piece of floss together to make a loop, which is easier to hold onto. If flossing is impossible, a device that uses water pressure to help remove debris from between teeth and from pockets around teeth is available.

If people cannot open their mouth very wide, brushing is harder. Such people should not force their mouth to open completely. Instead, they can use a toothbrush with a long, flexible handle and a small head (even a children's toothbrush) to brush the teeth as well as possible.

People with dementia often need to be reminded to brush or use a rinse. Some people with dementia need to have their teeth brushed by a caregiver. Most people with dementia need a caregiver to make sure that they see a dentist regularly.

Treatment

When cavities develop, a dentist removes decayed areas of the tooth, usually with a drill. If the decay is limited to the enamel, the tooth can sometimes repair itself. Then all that is needed are prescription fluoride rinses, which help with repair. Fluoride makes the teeth more resistant to the acid produced by bacteria.

If decay is more extensive, the dentist prepares the surface of the tooth and fills the space left after removing decayed areas. New tooth-colored filling materials (composite resins and bonding agents) can sometimes be used. They help prevent cavities and appear natural. If a large area of the tooth is removed, a metal or porcelain crown may be needed. A crown fits over the whole tooth above the gum line. It is cemented securely in place.

Fillings and crowns are restorations: They help protect the remaining healthy part of the tooth and restore the tooth as much as possible to its original condition. If decay has damaged the pulp, root canal treatment is done. The pulp is removed, and the remaining space is filled with a substance that helps permanently prevent bacteria from entering that space. The tooth is then reshaped and covered with a metal or porcelain crown. If the tooth has so much decay that it cannot be restored or if other dental or medical problems make saving the tooth impossible, it may be removed (extracted).

Outlook

Treatment of tooth decay can almost always preserve the function and appearance of the tooth. Restorations can last many years. They are likely to last much longer if people brush and floss regularly and thoroughly and have regular dental checkups.

PERIODONTAL DISEASE

Periodontal disease is inflammation and infection of the tissues that support and anchor teeth.

Tissues that support and anchor the teeth include the gums (gingiva), the bone around the roots of teeth (alveolar bone), and the ligament between the alveolar bone and the root of each tooth (periodontal ligament). Most older people have periodontal disease to some degree.

Periodontal disease usually develops after plaque has been accumulating between the gum and teeth for a long time. Bacteria thrive in plaque. They produce acids and other substances that penetrate the gums and may trigger inflammation. The gums may become inflamed, infected, and swollen—a disorder called gingivitis. A deep space (pocket) may form between the gum and the root of an affected tooth. Bacteria may accumulate there and damage the tooth further. The inflammation and infection can spread to the periodontal ligaments and alveolar bone, weakening and destroying them. Then, the teeth have less support and become loose. This disorder is called periodontitis. When periodontitis continues for a long time, all the bone supporting the affected teeth may be lost, and the affected teeth may have to be removed (extracted).

Causes

Conditions that make plaque more likely to accumulate between the gum and teeth can lead to periodontal disease. Not brushing and flossing the teeth regularly allows plaque to accumulate. Plaque tends to accumulate in older people because they are likely to have receding gums. Receding gums leave spaces between gums and teeth—a place where plaque can accumulate quickly and be trapped.

If the mouth is dry, plaque is not washed away by saliva and thus remains on tooth surfaces.

Certain drugs, such as phenytoin (used to treat seizures) and calcium channel blockers (used to treat coronary artery disease), cause the gums to grow excessively (hypertrophy). Then, bacteria can invade the gums more easily. The gums may bleed and become painful. As a result, people are less likely to brush their teeth and floss in the affected areas, making gingivitis more likely to develop or worsen. Disorders and treatments that interfere with the way the body heals itself, such as undernutrition, diabetes, leukemia, or chemotherapy, increase the risk of developing periodontal disease.

Symptoms and Diagnosis

Gingivitis produces swelling that a person can feel and see. The gums are sometimes tender and may bleed during brushing or flossing. Periodontitis causes teeth to loosen. The loose teeth are usually noticed when a person chews.

A doctor or dentist can detect gingivitis during an examination of the mouth. A dentist checks for periodontitis by inserting a probe between the gum and teeth to look for spaces (pockets) and to measure how deep pockets, if present, are. Periodontitis is diagnosed when very deep pockets are found and when bone loss is seen on dental x-rays.

Prevention and Treatment

Thorough, regular care of the mouth can help prevent periodontal disease. Brushing and flossing are most helpful. Using a mouth rinse that slows the growth of bacteria may help. Having regular professional cleanings at a dentist's office is important.

Treatment of gingivitis usually involves improving the care of the mouth, including brushing and flossing. Treatment of periodontitis usually involves surgery to remove the debris and pus that accumulate as a result of inflammation and infection. Antibiotic mouth rinses and antibiotics to be taken by mouth can be prescribed. If the alveolar bone is greatly damaged, surgery may be needed to repair it.

Treatment of periodontitis takes a long time. It usually requires many dental visits and often requires repeated treatments. For treatment to be effective, people must also be diligent in brushing and flossing their teeth regularly and thoroughly.

Outlook

Gingivitis usually disappears with treatment. The gums return to normal within several days to a few weeks. Periodontitis responds to treatment more slowly. Loose teeth become tighter as the inflammation and infection subside, usually within several weeks or sometimes months. However, if periodontitis has progressed, a lot of gum, ligament, and bone tissue may be permanently lost.

DRY MOUTH

Dry mouth is a lack of moisture in the mouth.

Saliva is the fluid that keeps the mouth moist. Saliva lubricates the teeth, gums, and tongue and helps wash debris from the mouth. It helps people taste, digest, and swallow foods. It also contains substances that kill microorganisms. Saliva is produced by the salivary glands. There are three main pairs of salivary glands plus many tiny glands throughout the mouth.

Many older people have a dry mouth. Although aging itself affects moisture in the mouth only slightly, it does make people more susceptible to conditions that dry the mouth.

For many people, a dry mouth is only an occasional annoyance. For others, it is a persistent problem (called xerostomia) that interferes with tasting, chewing, swallowing, speaking, and wearing dentures. Persistent dry mouth also increases the risk of tooth decay and periodontal disease. Persistent dry mouth is usually a symptom of a disorder or a side effect of a drug.

Causes

The mouth becomes dry when too little saliva is produced or when the saliva changes so that it moistens less well. When there is too little water in the body (as occurs in dehydration), less saliva is produced, and the mouth becomes drier. Breathing through the mouth can cause dryness. Low humidity in the air can make the mouth drier.

Drugs are the most common cause of dry mouth among older people. Dry mouth can be a side effect of more than 400 drugs. The drugs most likely to cause dry mouth include:

- Antihistamines
- Tricyclic antidepressants (used to treat depression)
- Certain antipsychotics (used to treat loss of touch with reality)
- Certain drugs used to treat cancer
- Many drugs used to lower blood pressure or treat heart failure (including diuretics, which cause the kidneys to excrete more water and salt)

Many disorders can cause persistent dryness of the mouth. They include Sjögren's syndrome (which also causes dry eyes), Alzheimer's disease, sarcoidosis, hypothyroidism, and diabetes. Radiation used to treat cancers of the mouth, head, or neck causes the mouth to be permanently dry.

The mouth may become dry because stones or tumors develop in the tubes that lead from the salivary glands to the mouth (salivary ducts). Stones or tumors can block the flow of saliva. Infection or inflammation of the salivary glands can cause occasional or persistent dryness.

Dentures themselves do not cause dry mouth. If dentures cover the roof of the mouth, they may cover some salivary glands. As a result, the mouth may feel dry.

Symptoms and Diagnosis

Persistent dry mouth may cause bad breath. Chewing and swallowing food may become difficult. Sometimes undernutrition results. The dry tongue may stick in the mouth, making speaking difficult. Wearing dentures may become uncomfortable. The lips and tongue can become cracked and feel as if they are burning. The gums may become tender and bleed, suggesting gingivitis. A tooth may ache if tooth decay occurs.

A doctor or dentist usually suspects xerostomia after listening to a person's description of symptoms. Occasionally, dryness is noticed during a routine examination.

A doctor or dentist tries to determine the cause of the dryness. The drugs the person is taking are reviewed to determine whether any could be the cause. The mouth is carefully inspected. The doctor or dentist feels (palpates) the inside of the mouth to check for swelling or blockage in the salivary glands. The openings of the salivary ducts are inspected for evidence of blockage. Computed tomography (CT) or magnetic resonance imaging (MRI) is sometimes done to confirm the presence of inflammation or a blockage. If Sjögren's syndrome is suspected, the eyes are examined. Blood tests are done to confirm the diagnosis. Or a dentist or doctor may remove a tissue sample from a salivary gland and examine it under a microscope (biopsy).

Prevention and Treatment

Drinking enough fluids helps prevent dehydration, one cause of dryness. People with dry mouth should not drink fluids that contain sugar to reduce the risk of developing cavities. If people breathe mainly through their mouth during sleep, they can use a humidifier by the bedside to prevent the mouth from becoming dry.

If a dry mouth is caused by dehydration, a person is usually given fluids, which can reverse the dryness.[1] If a dry mouth is a side effect of a drug, a doctor reduces or discontinues the drug if possible.

If a blockage in the salivary glands or ducts is the cause, the blockage is removed. If inflammation or infection of the salivary glands is the cause, taking a prescription drug may lessen or relieve dryness. Inflammation can be treated with drugs such as ibuprofen. An infection is usually treated with antibiotics such as amoxicillin.

Dry mouth caused by certain disorders is not relieved by treatment. In such cases, sucking on sugarless candy (including mints) and chewing sugarless gum may slightly stimulate pro-

1. see page 250

duction and flow of saliva. Saliva substitutes, usually used as sprays, are available. They must be used frequently.

Two prescription drugs, pilocarpine and cevimeline, can stimulate the salivary glands to produce more saliva. These drugs help relieve dryness, particularly during mealtime. Occasionally, they have side effects such as sweating and diarrhea.

Measures, including drugs, that stimulate saliva flow can help improve a person's ability to chew and speak. They may improve the way the mouth feels.

Some nonprescription products are made especially for people with dry mouth. These products contain the substances that kill bacteria normally present in saliva. They also contain ingredients that help keep the mouth moist and prevent cavities. These products are available as toothpastes, mouth rinses, oral gels, and chewing gums.

People with a dry mouth have to take extra care to prevent tooth decay and gingivitis. They must brush their teeth or dentures carefully after each meal. Frequent dental examinations are needed to check for and treat tooth decay and periodontal disease.

TOOTH LOSS

Only a generation ago, most people expected to go through old age with false teeth or no teeth at all. This expectation has changed substantially during the last several decades. Although nearly half of people 85 or over have none of their natural teeth, the likelihood of losing teeth with aging is steadily decreasing. There are several reasons for this change: improved nutrition, better access to dental care, and better treatment for tooth decay and periodontal disease (common causes of tooth loss).

When teeth are lost, chewing is greatly hindered, and speaking becomes a challenge. The face looks dramatically different without the support teeth normally provide for the lips, cheeks, nose, and chin. In older people, loss of teeth can speed the loss of bone around the roots of teeth (alveolar bone). The loss of bone may make getting dentures that fit much harder.

The most common cause of tooth loss is not taking good care of the mouth—that is, not brushing and flossing each day and not having regular dental checkups. Even when tooth decay and periodontal disease can be treated, teeth can be lost if people are unwilling or unable to see a dentist. Sometimes teeth are removed when advanced periodontal disease makes chewing painful or ineffective.

People who have lost some or all of their teeth can still eat, but they tend to eat soft foods. Soft foods tend to be relatively high in carbohydrates and low in protein, vitamins, and minerals. Foods that are high in protein, vitamins, and minerals, such as meats, poultry, grains, and fresh fruits and vegetables, tend to be harder to chew. Consequently, people who eat mainly soft foods may become undernourished.

Replacing lost teeth is important for the same reasons as for preventing tooth loss. The type of replacement depends on the number of teeth lost, the location of the lost teeth, and the health of the remaining teeth, gums, and the bone around the teeth's roots. Teeth can be replaced with appliances that are fixed or cemented to existing teeth (bridges), implants, or removable appliances (partial or full dentures).

Bridges can replace one or a few teeth. They, like teeth, have to be cleaned daily. But unlike dentures, they are cemented to tooth surfaces and thus do not have to be removed for cleaning. Floss threaded between the gum and bridge with a flexible plastic "needle" or between-the-teeth brushes (proxy) can be used. Dental implants are a safe, effective replacement for one, a few, or even all of the teeth. They involve surgery to place a metal implant into the jaw bone (upper or lower) for each tooth that is being replaced. The implant extends beyond the gum line, providing a place to attach a crown. Time is allowed for the gum around the implant to heal and the bone around it to grow and hold it firmly in place. Then, a crown is attached to each implant.

Partial or full dentures are useful for people who have lost nearly all or all of their teeth. They are used when all of the teeth of the upper jaw, lower jaw, or both are lost. Dentists carefully construct dentures so that they fit well and look natural. Dentures are also constructed to help a person chew as well as possible. Typically, constructing dentures takes several months and involves a sequence of carefully planned steps.

Dentures require a lot of care. They must be kept clean. They should be removed after each meal and cleaned with toothpaste or baking soda on a toothbrush or denture brush. Also, the mouth should be cleaned with toothpaste and a toothbrush to remove food debris. The toothbrush should also be used to massage the interior of the mouth. Dentures should be removed before going to sleep, cleaned carefully, and kept in a safe place. Soaking dentures overnight in a cleaning solution can be helpful but is not necessary if dentures are cleaned well with a toothbrush.

Just because people lose their teeth does not mean that they lose their need to see a dentist. They still need to see the dentist at least once a year. The dentist checks for cancer or other problems in the mouth and evaluates the dentures' fit. The shape of the mouth can change over time or because of weight loss or gain. Then dentures have to be refitted.

Dentures can improve appearance and speech. But they are far from a perfect solution. They restore less than 20% of the chewing ability provided by natural teeth. Dentures can also cause discomfort and interfere with tasting. Some people find dentures embarrassing. If dentures do not fit well, they can interfere with chewing and swallowing. They may also cause burning sensations and sores in the mouth.

BURNING MOUTH SYNDROME

Burning mouth syndrome is a poorly understood condition that involves a sensation of burning and pain in the tongue, gums, roof of the mouth, and cheeks. Occasionally, it also involves the lips.

Burning mouth syndrome is most common among postmenopausal women. The cause is unknown. Some people may have dryness, but burning mouth syndrome is not caused by a dry mouth. The burning may be steady and persistent, or it may worsen through the day and lessen at night. Low doses of antidepressants such as nortriptyline or antianxiety drugs such as clonazepam may help relieve the burning and pain.

MOUTH SORES

Sores commonly develop on the lips and inside the mouth. These sores may be painful or bothersome, but most are harmless. Occasionally, they result from a serious disorder. Any sore that is present for more than 3 to 4 weeks should be evaluated by a dentist or doctor.

Cold sores: The most common sore on the lips is a cold sore (herpes labialis). Cold sores are caused by a viral infection. Exposure to sunlight or cold can trigger a cold sore. Cold sores are small and filled with fluid. Often, they occur in clusters. Typically, cold sores appear on the lips and reappear in the same place. Often, an area of the lips tingles or burns before the sore develops. The sore forms a crust, then disappears after 5 to 7 days. A prescription drug used immediately after the tingling is felt can make the sore disappear more quickly. Some of these drugs, such as penciclovir, are applied to the lips. Some, such as valacyclovir or acyclovir, are taken by mouth.

Canker sores: The most common sore inside the mouth is a canker sore (aphthous stomatitis). Canker sores are more likely to develop during stress or illness. They are white, flat, and surrounded by a red area. They can be painful. Many are round, but sores may be irregularly shaped. They usually last 7 to 10 days and heal without a scar. They often recur. Prescription drugs that resemble corticosteroids, such as triamcinolone, or anesthetics, such as lidocaine or benzocaine, can be applied to the sores to help them heal.

Thrush: Thrush (candidiasis) is a fungal infection. It tends to develop in the mouth in people who take antibiotics or have a dry mouth. Thrush often appears as a white, curdlike film coating the gums, including the gums under dentures, and the inside of the mouth. Thrush is usually painless, although the affected areas sometimes appear red and burn. Thrush may also affect the corners of the mouth, which become cracked, red, and dry. Antifungal creams and rinses are effective in most cases. When thrush is severe, antifungal drugs may be taken by mouth.

Oral cancer: Oral cancer starts as a red or white sore on the lips or mouth.[1] The sores may or may not be painful. They do not heal and gradually get larger. Any red or white sore that does not heal after 3 to 4 weeks should be checked by a dentist or doctor because it may be an early sign of cancer. A biopsy, culture, x-ray, or blood test may be done to check for oral cancer or another disorder.

1. see page 785

Other sores: Other disorders can cause sores that resemble those due to oral cancer. Lupus (systemic lupus erythematosus), a disorder in which the immune system malfunctions, causes mouth sores that are usually painless. They are a mixture of red and white sores that can occur on the tongue, inside of the cheeks, roof of the mouth, and gums. Lichen planus, a skin disorder that causes itching and a rash, causes mouth sores that are usually painless. They are bluish white and flat with an irregular shape that can resemble a spider's web. If lupus, lichen planus, or another disorder causes sores near the back of the mouth, eating and swallowing become difficult. Because these sores are difficult to distinguish from oral cancer, they should be checked by a dentist or doctor.

In 1936, I graduated from high school in Cove, Oregon. In 1938, I received a teacher's certificate from Eastern Oregon Normal School, which later became Eastern Oregon University. After teaching the next year, I met and married the man who was to be my husband for 62 years. Like most families we worked, we played, we struggled, and we raised our children. Money wasn't always plentiful, but ultimately we retired.

I had always wished that I might have continued with my schooling and received a bachelor's degree. It was one of those dreams of what might have been. However, when my husband's health began to fail, it was necessary for me to stay at home almost all of the time, and I looked around for something I could do to occupy my mind. It was then that I read about the Distance Education Program offered by Eastern Oregon University and contacted the local counselor.

It was a wonderful experience. She found that I was interested in obtaining a degree, and she helped me outline a program that would allow me to obtain a degree with a dual minor in history and writing. After the first class I was hooked. It was such fun. The instructors were extremely helpful. The classes were given over the Internet, and did require a lot of study at home. This was probably the hardest part. It had been a long time since I had been in a situation that needed self-discipline, and frankly, I really enjoyed the latest novel more than I did the textbooks, even though the texts have improved considerably since I was in school.

After my husband's death, my own health deteriorated and it was necessary to limit myself to one class a term. Consequently, it took a year longer than first planned. However, this spring I had the privilege, at 84, of taking part in the June graduation ceremonies at Eastern Oregon University, a dream come true!

Lona P. Downing

40

Foot Disorders

People ask much from the bones, skin, muscles, tendons (which connect muscles to bones), ligaments (which connect bones to each other), blood vessels, and nerves that make up the foot. After receiving years of trouble-free transportation from their feet, some older people expect such uncompromising service to continue indefinitely. However, although the feet are well designed and are built for high mileage, time and a variety of conditions that become more common with aging do take their toll.

CORNS AND CALLUSES

Corns and calluses are areas of thickened skin.

Corns usually develop between the toes or on the tops of the toes. Calluses usually develop on the bottoms (soles) of the feet, although they can form on the sides or on the toes. Corns and calluses are very common among older people. These conditions can be merely annoying at first but can become very painful. Some corns and calluses become inflamed and infected, especially in people with poor blood flow to the feet. Corns and calluses are often preventable. When they do form, however, they respond well to treatment.

Causes

Corns and calluses develop in response to friction or pressure. Friction occurs when skin rubs against skin (as often happens between adjacent toes) or when a sock or shoe rubs against a toe or another part of the foot. Pressure may occur when an ill-fitting shoe presses on the skin. Tight shoes and shoes that have a flat, hard toe box (the portion of the shoe where the toes fit) are especially likely to increase pressure on the skin. Also, fat and muscle tissue on the bottom of the feet thin with aging; thus pointy outgrowths of bone (spurs) and bumpy outgrowths of bone are more likely to press against the skin. When friction or pressure occurs regularly in the same area, a corn or callus forms gradually.

Symptoms and Diagnosis

A corn may be soft or hard. It is thickest at its center, or core. A callus is hard and is usually of equal thickness throughout. Some corns and calluses do not cause symptoms and can be merely annoying. However, most cause at least mild discomfort. Some cause enough pain to make walking difficult. Pain may

---

FOOT CARE GUIDELINES

Many diseases that are common in older people, such as diabetes mellitus, can increase the risk of serious foot problems by damaging blood vessels and nerves. Good foot care is a critical part of decreasing the risk of serious problems.

• The feet should be washed daily with mild soap and warm (not hot or cold) water. All soap should be rinsed off. A soft towel can be used to dry the feet thoroughly, especially between the toes.

• Toenails should be trimmed straight across and not too short. Toenails that have sharp edges may cut into the adjacent toes. People with diabetes, or other diseases that damage blood vessels and nerves, should have a podiatrist cut their toenails.

• Shoes should be comfortable and need to have wide toe boxes. Shoes should be worn daily—people should never go barefoot.

• Clean socks or stockings should be worn daily. Appropriate fit is necessary (that is, not too short, not too tight).

• If the feet are cold, thick warm socks should be worn. Heating pads and hot water bottles should be avoided.

• Daily inspection of the feet for cracks, cuts, sores, corns and calluses, and color changes is recommended. People who cannot see the bottom of their feet need another person to do that part of the inspection or must use a mirror so that the bottom of each foot can be seen.

• Lanolin should be gently massaged into dry scaly areas of the feet.

• Corns or calluses should be treated by a podiatrist—people should not attempt to treat themselves by cutting or shaving corns or calluses, nor should they apply nonprescription drugs (for example, wart removers), which can burn the skin.

worsen, and redness and warmth may develop if a corn or callus becomes inflamed and infected. Warts may resemble corns and calluses and may cause similar symptoms.

A doctor diagnoses a corn or callus by recognizing its typical appearance during a physical examination of the foot.

Prevention

Wearing properly fitting footwear is the best way to prevent corns and calluses. Shoes should be long enough and have enough space in the toe box so that there is no pressure on the tops of the toes. Finding footwear that fits properly is sometimes easier said than done. Spurs or bumpy outgrowths of bone can interfere with the fit and comfort of shoes. This discomfort can sometimes be lessened by affixing into the shoe a soft material, such as moleskin, lamb's wool, felt, or foam padding. If these measures are unsuccessful, an orthotist (a person skilled in the fitting of devices such as braces, splints, and inserts) can sometimes modify a shoe to reduce friction and pressure at certain points.

Treatment and Outlook

A doctor treats a corn or callus by using a scalpel to shave or pare away the thickened skin. Soft padding over the area is usually recommended to reduce pressure and protect the area where the corn or callus has been removed as well as to protect the surrounding healthy skin. The doctor may suggest adding a cream that softens thickened and hardened skin (emollient cream) to the padding. The doctor may also help the person modify his shoes to reduce pressure on the area where the corn or callus has been removed, refer the person to an orthotist, or recommend alternative footwear.

After a corn or callus has been removed, it will not likely recur if the person can find and continue to wear footwear that fits properly.

Self-treatment with the use of razor blades, knife blades, or nonprescription preparations of salicylic acid should not be attempted because of the risk of injury and infection. In addition, self-treatment rarely succeeds.

BUNION

A bunion is a bumpy outgrowth of the joint between the big toe and the foot (the first metatarsophalangeal joint).

A bunion is almost always accompanied by deviation of the big toe toward the second toe. Bunions are common in older people. Treatment often helps control symptoms, or bunions can be removed surgically.

A bunion usually develops over many years. However, as a bunion becomes more noticeable and the big toe deviates, troublesome changes may occur in and around the joint. Calluses may form around the joint. Osteoarthritis may develop. Pointy protrusions (spurs) may form at the ends of the two bones that come together in the joint. Sacs around the joint (bursa) can become inflamed. Wearing proper footwear can reduce symptoms. Surgical removal of a bunion is sometimes necessary.

WHAT IS A BUNION?

Sometimes the joint at the base of the big toe (first metatarsophalangeal joint) bulges sideways and away from the foot. This bulge, called a bunion, is caused by extra bone that forms at the joint. Usually, the tip of the big toe tilts toward the second toe and may push over or under it. The fluid-filled sac (bursa) at the base of the big toe may swell, causing pain.

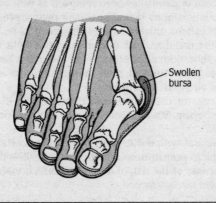

Swollen bursa

Causes

Heredity may play a role, because bunions seem to run in families. Ill-fitting footwear may also contribute to the development of bunions. Wearing footwear with a narrow toe box (the portion of the shoe where the toes fit) puts pressure on the base of the big toe, where the first metatarsophalangeal joint is located.

Symptoms and Diagnosis

For many people, bunions prove to be nothing more than cosmetically unappealing. Any callus that forms, however, may cause discomfort. Because footwear puts increasing pressure on the joint as the prominence grows, the bunion often becomes painful. Pain may worsen if osteoarthritis develops. Pain may also worsen if spurs form or if sacs (bursas) form and become inflamed. Walking may become difficult because of pain and deviation of the big toe, which may push over or under the other toes.

A doctor diagnoses a bunion during a physical examination. An x-ray can show changes in the bone, including osteoarthritis and bumpy outgrowth of bone, but in most cases, an x-ray is done only if surgery is being considered.

Treatment and Outlook

Wearing proper footwear can reduce symptoms. People with a bunion benefit from wearing shoes with more room and flexibility in the toe box, so that pressure on the first metatarsophalangeal joint is lessened. The doctor may recommend an insert (orthotic) for the shoe to reduce friction and pressure. Wearing footwear that fits properly may help reduce pain and inflammation. The bunion may even shrink, although it will not disappear completely.

Surgery is sometimes performed as a last resort when pain cannot be relieved by adjusting the shoe. Surgery consists of shaving away the bumpy areas of bone that have formed at the ends of the two bones that join in the metatarsophalangeal joint. Surgery can also remove any spurs that have formed. During surgery, a wire or rod may be inserted temporarily into the big toe, so that the toe can be realigned to its normal position. After surgery, bunions rarely recur.

HAMMER TOE

A hammer toe is a toe that becomes permanently bent in the middle so that the end of the toe points downward. The portion of the toe before the joint where the bend occurs tends to arch upward.

A hammer toe takes years to develop. Once the toe becomes permanently bent, corns or calluses may form. Treatment helps control symptoms in many people, but surgery is sometimes needed to straighten the toe.

Causes

Wearing ill-fitting shoes is probably the main cause of hammer toe. As the toe bends, tendons add to the problem by contracting in such a way that the bending is reinforced to the point of becoming permanent. In some cases, tendons that are abnormal to begin with may start the bending process.

Symptoms and Diagnosis

For some people, a hammer toe is nothing more than an unsightly deformity that detracts from the appearance of the foot. However, discomfort may develop if a corn or callus develops on the end or top of the toe. If pressure and friction continue on the end or top of the toe, a painful ulcer may develop. Discomfort or pain can lead to difficulty walking.

Treatment

People with a hammer toe benefit from wearing shoes in which the toe box is made of a flexible material and is wide enough and high enough to provide adequate room for the toes. High-heeled shoes should be avoided, because they tend to force the toes into a narrow, flat toe box. A doctor may recommend an insert (orthotic) for the shoe to help reduce friction and pressure on the hammer toe. Wearing properly fitted shoes may reduce pain and inflammation. It may also prevent ulcers from developing and help existing ulcers heal. However, the hammer toe does not disappear.

Surgery to straighten the toe may be needed if an ulcer has formed on either the end or the top surface of the toe. Surgery sometimes involves cutting the tendons that support movement in the toe so that the toe can be straightened. Cutting the tendons, however, takes away the ability to bend the very end of the toe. Another type of surgery combines temporary insertion of a pin or rod into the toe and alteration or repair of the tendons, so that the toe is straightened. After surgery, the deformity rarely recurs.

HEEL OR ARCH PAIN

Heel or arch pain may occur in an older person simply because the fat padding that lies between the bones and the skin becomes thinner with aging. Pain also may be due to repetitive activity, such as going down stairs often; this increases pressure on the arch and in the heel. Heel or arch pain may also be a symptom of a larger problem.

The most common cause of heel pain is a pointy outgrowth of bone (spur). Pain results when the foot presses against something at the site of the spur. A spur can also cause pain if a person alters the way in which he walks to keep pressure off the foot. Doing so stretches the Achilles tendon and the flat sheet of connective tissue on the bottom of the foot (plantar fascia) where they attach to the heel. Inflammation of the Achilles tendon (Achilles tendinitis) and of the plantar fascia (plantar fasciitis) adds to the pain.

Heel pain can also result from inflammation of the sac situated between the large bone in the heel and the Achilles tendon (Achilles bursitis). Diseases such as rheumatoid arthritis[1] and gout[2] sometimes cause heel pain as well.

Diagnosis and Treatment

A doctor determines the cause of heel pain by reviewing the person's symptoms and examining the foot. X-rays may be performed to look for abnormalities such as spurs.

Treatment depends on the cause. Pain due to thinning of the fat pad on the bottom of the foot may be relieved simply by using inserts (orthotics) in footwear. Inserts provide more padding and support for the heel or arch. Some inserts are sold without a prescription, but others are prescribed by a doctor or

1. see page 591
2. see page 598

WHAT IS A HEEL SPUR?

Growths of extra bone, called heel spurs, sometimes form on the heel bone. A spur may form when the plantar fascia, the sheet of connective tissue that extends from the bottom of the heel bone to the base of the toes, pulls on the heel too much.

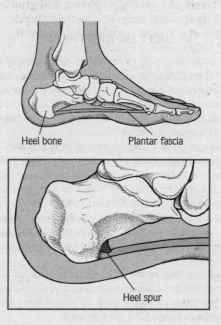

Heel bone   Plantar fascia

Heel spur

a foot doctor (podiatrist) and are fitted by a doctor, foot doctor, or orthotist (a person skilled in the fitting of devices such as braces, splints, and inserts).

Nonsteroidal anti-inflammatory drugs (NSAIDs) are sometimes taken by mouth to relieve the pain caused by bursitis and fasciitis. Injections of a corticosteroid and a numbing drug (anesthetic) are sometimes given for severe pain.

Shock wave therapy may help relieve pain if drug therapy is ineffective or may be used instead of drug therapy. A dome-shaped device, placed on the skin over the painful area in the heel, is used to generate the shock waves.

Surgery is sometimes needed to remove a bone spur that is causing pain. However, spurs sometimes recur.

ONYCHAUXIS AND ONYCHOGRYPHOSIS

In onychauxis and onychogryphosis, nail growth goes awry. Onychauxis is thickening of a toenail. Onychogryphosis is thickening of a toenail to the point where the nail curves, giving it a clawlike appearance.

Affected nails tend to grow very long, because the thickening and curving make cutting or trimming very difficult. Affected nails may also become infected by fungi.

Ill-fitting shoes, injury, poor blood flow to the feet, diabetes, or a nutritional deficiency may cause either onychauxis or onychogryphosis. At any point in time, one or more nails on a foot may be affected by either onychauxis or onychogryphosis.

Symptoms

Discomfort can result when footwear or even bed sheets press on thickened nails, because the surface beneath the nails (the nail plate) is also thickened and tender. Therefore, whatever presses on the nail indirectly presses on the nail plate. Nails can become so long and deformed that they impair walking. Long curved nails can also penetrate adjacent toes, resulting in pain and infection of the skin.

Treatment

Treatment involves frequent nail cutting or trimming. This cutting and trimming almost always requires the expertise of a nurse, doctor, or foot doctor (podiatrist) and the use of special clippers or other tools. Occasionally, if conditions that are causing or contributing to the abnormal nail growth can be remedied or treated more effectively, nail care may become more routine, without the need for special expertise or equipment.

ONYCHOMYCOSIS

Onychomycosis is a fungal infection of the toenails.

Onychomycosis usually occurs in people with a fungal infection of the skin between the toes. Injury to nails or to the surface beneath nails (the nail plate) and moisture around the toes makes the development of onychomycosis more likely. Onychomycosis is common among older people, especially among those with diabetes.

Symptoms and Diagnosis

A nail affected by onychomycosis becomes white or yellow. It can thicken and develop a coarse, irregular surface. The nail can partly crumble or partly separate from the underlying nailbed. The nail may curl up or down (gryphosis).

Onychomycosis can usually be diagnosed on the basis of the nail's appearance. However, laboratory testing of material scraped or swabbed from the surface underneath the toenail may be done to confirm the diagnosis.

Prevention and Treatment

Keeping feet dry and treating athlete's foot may help prevent onychomycosis.

Although it rarely causes serious health problems, onychomycosis can trouble older people or their caretakers. The nails can become difficult or nearly impossible to trim. Using special clippers or other tools, a nurse, doctor, or foot doctor (podiatrist) can provide nail care. Onychomycosis is a special problem for people with diabetes or poor blood flow to the foot, for whom infections of the toes or feet can have serious consequences.

Most people do not need antifungal treatment. Antifungal drugs often fail to cure the infection, but the drugs may help to suppress the infection and improve the appearance of the affected nails. The two drugs that are used, itraconazole and terbinafine, are taken by mouth. Sometimes drug therapy helps in as little as 3 months, but for most people, especially people with poor blood flow to the foot, treatment must be continued until the nails grow out, which can take up to a year in older people. Because itraconazole and terbinafine may interact with other drugs and may cause side effects, treatment is worthwhile only if onychomycosis causes health risks or bothersome symptoms. Both itraconazole and terbinafine are available as less expensive creams, but they do not help when they are applied to the surface of infected nails.

A compromise approach, which is far safer but much less likely to cure the infection, is painting the nails daily with an antifungal (ciclopirox) solution. Most often, this treatment has little or no effect. When this solution does help, there is a very good chance that the infection will return soon after treatment is stopped. The spaces between the toes and the bottoms of the feet can be treated with an antifungal cream or powder to reduce the likelihood of reinfection of the nails.

41

Arthritis

Arthritis means "inflammation of joints." Yet when older people are afflicted with arthritis, they tend to be bothered less by the inflammation and more by the pain and stiffness that accompany arthritis.

Many people assume arthritis to be an unavoidable part of growing old. Although aging itself does not cause arthritis, arthritis does become more common as people age, for various reasons. The development of arthritis brings many older people much distress. Jack Benny may have captured a sense of that distress when, as he was being honored, he remarked about his arthritis, "I don't deserve this award, but I have arthritis and I don't deserve that either."

Among the different types of arthritis, several affect mostly older people. The most common of these is osteoarthritis. Others include rheumatoid arthritis, gout, pseudogout, and infectious arthritis.

OSTEOARTHRITIS

Osteoarthritis is a chronic disorder of cartilage (the connective tissue that cushions and protects the surface of bones

where they meet to form joints), bones, and some of the tissues that surround joints. Osteoarthritis is sometimes called degenerative arthritis. Osteoarthritis results in pain, stiffness, deformity, and loss of function.

Osteoarthritis is the most common type of arthritis and is very common in old age. Indeed, osteoarthritis affects most people to some degree by age 70. Whereas some people with osteoarthritis experience only annoying aches and pains, others are significantly disabled by it. A number of therapies can help relieve pain and improve joint function. For those with the most vexing problems, surgical replacement of joints relieves symptoms but poses risks.

Causes

Osteoarthritis is caused in part by wear and tear on the joints. However, use alone does not lead to arthritis. Joints that have been injured or that bear the stress of an inordinate amount of weight (as occurs in obesity) are especially susceptible to the effects of wear and tear. After arthritis begins to develop, the joints sustain further damage as the person continues to use them, particularly the joints in the shoulders, hips, knees, and lower back.

Osteoarthritis may also be caused in part by an abnormality in the way joint cartilage is formed, which causes it to swell and crack. Ultimately, the surface of the cartilage becomes pitted, and tiny cavities develop in the bone beneath the cartilage. In addition, bony outgrowths or protrusions (spurs) may form. Alternatively, the entire end of the bone may enlarge irregularly. Sometimes, outgrowths and bony enlargement occur together in the same joint.

Symptoms

Symptoms usually develop gradually. At first, only one or a few joints are affected, such as those of the fingers, base of the thumbs, neck, lower back, big toes, hips, or knees. Pain often increases when the joint is used to perform work, such as lifting or bearing weight. The joint may become stiff from lack of use but usually loosens up within 30 minutes of use. Thus, many people experience more pain when they start to move; once they are in motion, the pain decreases.

Nonetheless, affected joints tend to become increasingly damaged and painful over months and years. In addition, the supporting ligaments (tough fibrous cords that connect bones) may stretch, making the joint increasingly unsteady. Alternatively, a joint's degree of movement (range of motion) may be reduced.

Bony outgrowths may press on nerves or on blood vessels, resulting in further pain or in impaired blood flow to tissues supplied by the blood vessels.

ACHES AND PAINS AFFECTING SOFT TISSUE NEAR JOINTS

Aches and pains of soft tissue that are not due to joint abnormalities are sometimes referred to as nonarticular rheumatism. Tissues affected may include ligaments, tendons, bursae, and muscles. The following discussion focuses only on problems affecting tendons and bursae.

Tendons

Tendons are cords consisting largely of fibrous tissue that connect muscles to bone. Therefore, tendons allow muscles to move joints. Tendons typically run inside tendon sheaths, which provide lubrication to the tendons, allowing them to move easily and with low friction.

A number of disorders can affect tendons (including tendon rupture). However, the typical rheumatic disorder that affects tendons is inflammation (tendinitis). The inflammation generally affects the tendon and its sheath. The result is pain and difficulty in moving the tendon—or even complete immobilization of the tendon. The cause is often unknown. However, the aches and pain are often caused by overuse. Other, less common, causes include a variety of body-wide disorders such as gout and diabetes. Treatment involves treating the underlying cause, such as trying to avoid further overuse, and resting the affected joint—using temporary splinting if necessary. Drugs that reduce inflammation, such as nonsteroidal anti-inflammatory drugs (NSAIDs), are often given. Sometimes, a corticosteroid is injected into the tendon sheath.

Bursae

Bursae are fluid-filled sacs that lie between a tendon (and its sheath) and the underlying bone. Thus, bursae cushion movements between tendons, muscles, skin, and bones, allowing tendons to move easily in the vicinity of a joint.

Inflammation of a bursa (bursitis) results in pain and interferes with such movement. Bursitis is most often caused by overuse (like tendinitis). It may also be caused by injury, by disorders such as rheumatoid arthritis, or by infection of the bursa. Treatment depends on the underlying cause (such as antibiotics for infection). Treatment of the symptoms is virtually identical to that for tendinitis.

A grating or creaking sound (crepitus) may be heard when large joints (for example, the knees) are moved. Also, joints can become enlarged and deformed (giving rise, for example, to the knotty, gnarled appearance of the finger joints often referred to as Bouchard's and Heberden's nodes). In addition, fluid accumulation (effusion) in large joints may cause swelling.

Diagnosis

A doctor diagnoses osteoarthritis on the basis of the typical symptoms, a physical examination, and x-rays of the joints. X-rays may show bone enlargement and narrowing of the space between the bone surfaces at the joint. However, x-rays are of limited usefulness in the early stages of osteoarthritis because they can show damage to the bone but are unable to show damage to the cartilage, where much of the problem exists. Magnetic resonance imaging (MRI) can detect even early changes in cartilage but is too expensive for routine use. Blood tests and analysis of the synovial fluid (the normal fluid within the joints) aid in excluding other types of arthritis, such as that in gout and pseudogout.

Prevention

Little can be done to prevent osteoarthritis, but people with early-stage osteoarthritis can try to minimize further damage. Limiting the use of affected joints is advised. People who are overweight should lose weight, which reduces the pressure on weight-bearing joints (such as knee joints). Exercises that strengthen the muscles and ligaments surrounding affected joints are also recommended.[1]

Treatment

Osteoarthritis that neither causes symptoms nor interferes with function does not require treatment. Treatment, when necessary, aims to relieve pain, improve joint function, and enable a person to perform daily activities. To meet these treatment goals, the person should inform the doctor and other health care practitioners of the precise problems that affected joints are causing. During these discussions, both short- and long-term goals of treatment should be established.

1. see page 589

Short-term goals may include sufficient relief of pain and stiffness so as to permit increased use of the joints. Achieving such goals allows the person to gain confidence. This confidence, in turn, increases the likelihood of achieving long-term goals, such as preserving the ability to perform daily activities. Unrealistic short-term goals and expectations of treatment (for example, complete relief of pain and resumption of all activities), however, can lead to frustration and depression.

Exercise: Regular exercise, including range-of-motion, strengthening, and endurance exercises, can help reduce joint stiffness and pain, increase flexibility and strength, and prevent further damage.[1] However, excessive exercise should be avoided. The types of exercise that can be helpful include aerobic exercise (such as walking) combined with resistance training (such as weight training) and stretching.

Exercises performed in warm water are particularly helpful, because the buoyancy of the water provides support and reduces weight on the joints. The warmth helps reduce stiffness and discomfort during movement. Certain precautions must be taken, however, when exercising in warm water. Keeping the water temperature between about 83° and 88° F prevents overheating. In very warm water (between 98° and 104° F), time spent exercising should not exceed 15 minutes. Someone should be available to help the person get into and out of the water. Using alcohol or certain drugs can make use of a pool or spa dangerous.

Physical therapy: Physical therapy,[2] including heat therapy and cold therapy, can be helpful. Heat therapy may involve deep heat treatment with ultrasound or with diathermy—a technique of heating parts of the body with the use of high-frequency alternating electric current applied by electrodes. Cold therapy may involve the use of ice packs.

Physical therapy may include the use of other devices and procedures as well. Splints or supports (such as soft or rigid braces) can protect joints during exercise by reducing unwanted joint movement. Shoe inserts (orthotics) often reduce pain caused by walking. Although not well studied, massage therapy may relieve pain and improve joint function when performed by

1. see page 907
2. see page 171

a trained therapist. Sitting or lying on chairs or beds that provide firm support is also advised. Adaptive aids, such as braces and canes (which assist with walking) and grippers (which assist with opening jars) may be used. Weight loss is important for people who are overweight, because too much weight places additional strain on affected joints.

Drug therapy: Drugs may be used in addition to exercise and physical therapy to relieve symptoms.[1] Pain relievers (analgesics), such as acetaminophen, may be useful. Nonsteroidal anti-inflammatory drugs (NSAIDs) may reduce inflammation and relieve pain. NSAIDs must be used with caution in older people, however, because these drugs pose a higher risk of side effects, such as bleeding in the digestive tract. New NSAIDs called cyclooxygenase-2 (COX-2) inhibitors (coxibs) reduce pain much like other NSAIDs but are less likely to irritate the stomach and cause bleeding. All NSAIDs, including coxibs, can cause kidney damage and impair kidney function.

Glucosamine[2] and chondroitin[3] are nutritional supplements that can be used to treat osteoarthritis. Many preparations combine the two substances. Glucosamine and chondroitin may help the body prevent further damage to cartilage and repair existing damage to cartilage. In addition, glucosamine and chondroitin help relieve the pain of osteoarthritis.

Some drugs are applied to the skin (topically) to relieve pain in underlying joints. For example, capsaicin (derived from cayenne pepper) applied directly over the affected joint may offer relief. Capsaicin is available as a cream, gel, or lotion.

When joints are swollen, joint fluid is removed to relieve pain. A corticosteroid can be injected into the joint to further reduce inflammation. However overuse of corticosteroid injections may result in damage. Hyaluronate (a component of synovial fluid) may also be injected into the joint to relieve pain; its effects may last up to several months.

Surgery: Surgery may be performed when other treatments do not relieve pain or improve joint function.

In joint replacement, the most common surgery performed for osteoarthritis, an abnormal joint is replaced with an artificial

1. see page 335
2. see page 80
3. see page 73

joint. Joint replacement is most commonly performed on the hip[1] and knee.[2] Replacement almost always improves range of motion and function and dramatically decreases pain. A variety of techniques and types of artificial joints are used, depending on the affected joint.

Outlook

Osteoarthritis tends to worsen steadily with time. When drug therapy is no longer effective, patients may benefit from joint replacement.

RHEUMATOID ARTHRITIS

Rheumatoid arthritis (RA) is a disorder in which affected joints, usually including those of the hands and feet, are inflamed, resulting in swelling, pain, and, often, significant damage.

Typically, RA first appears between ages 25 and 50, although it may begin at any age. RA affects about 1% of the population worldwide and affects about two to three times more women than men.

In RA, damage to joints is usually gradual but may be relentless and can result in significant disability. Sometimes, however, RA is limited and becomes dormant (goes into remission) before significant damage occurs. The progression of RA depends on many factors, including a person's family history.

Most people with RA have mild anemia (an insufficient number of red blood cells). Rarely, the white blood cell count becomes abnormally low. When a person with RA has a low white blood cell count and an enlarged spleen, the disorder is called Felty's syndrome.

Causes

The cause of RA is unknown, although it is thought to be an autoimmune disease. The body's immune system attacks the connective tissue that lines joints (synovium) and can also at-

1. see art on page 324
2. see art on page 592

REPLACING A KNEE

A knee joint damaged by arthritis may be replaced with an artificial joint (prosthesis). After a general anesthetic is given, the surgeon makes an incision over the damaged knee. The knee cap is removed. Then, the ends of the thigh bone and shinbone are smoothed so that the artificial joint can be attached more easily. One part of the artificial joint is inserted into the thigh bone, and the other part into the shinbone. The parts are cemented in place.

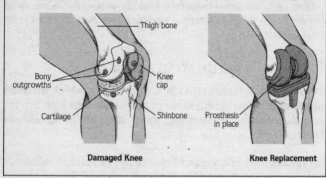

Damaged Knee   **Knee Replacement**

tack connective tissue in many other parts of the body, such as the blood vessels and lungs. Eventually, the joints are damaged.

Symptoms

RA may be mild, with occasional flare-ups followed by long periods of remission, or may progress steadily, either slowly or rapidly. Rheumatoid arthritis may start suddenly, affecting many joints of the lower and upper extremities but especially the hands. More often, it starts gradually, affecting different joints at different times. Usually, the inflammation is symmetric, affecting the same joint on both sides of the body. Typically, toes, feet, wrists, elbows, ankles, and the small joints in the fingers become inflamed first.

Affected joints are usually painful and often stiff, especially just after awakening. Stiffness often lasts for at least several hours after awakening but may diminish with use of the joints. Some people feel tired and weak, especially in the early afternoon. A low-grade fever (around 100.4° F) may occur intermittently.

℞ SOME DRUGS USED FOR RHEUMATOID ARTHRITIS

Type	Drug	Selected Side Effects	Benefits
Nonsteroidal anti-inflammatory drugs (NSAIDs)	Aspirin Ibuprofen Naproxen Diclofenac	Upset stomach, stomach ulcers, bleeding in the digestive tract, increased blood pressure, kidney toxicity	Effective in treating symptoms by decreasing inflammation
fewer	Cyclooxy-genase-2 (COX-2) inhibitors (coxibs)	Stomach ulcers (but less risk than with other NSAIDs) increased blood pressure, kidney toxicity	As effective as other NSAIDs but with side effects
Corticosteroids	Prednisone	Numerous side effects throughout the body with long-term use, including moonlike face; buffalo hump on back; thin, fragile skin; stretch marks; muscle weakness; bone thinning; stomach ulcer; swelling of the abdomen, with thin arms and legs	Can reduce inflammation much more quickly than alternative treatments
Disease-modifying anti-rheumatic drugs (DMARDs)	Gold com-pounds	Kidney damage, rashes, itchy skin,decreased numbers of blood cells	Can slow progression of joint damage

Table continues on the following page.

Type	Drug	Selected Side Effects	Benefits
	Methotrexate Leflunomide Azathioprine Cyclophosphamide Cyclosporine	Liver disease, lung inflammation, an increased susceptibility to infection, the suppression of blood cell production in the bone marrow	Methotrexate or leflunomide can be used early for severe rheumatoid arthritis; can slow progression of joint damage
	Penicillamine	Suppression of blood cell production in the bone marrow, kidney problems, muscle disease, rash, bad taste in the mouth	Can slow progression of joint damage
	Hydroxychloroquine	Rashes, muscle aches, eye problems	Can slow progression of joint damage
	Sulfasalazine	Stomach upset, liver problems, blood cell disorders, rashes	Can slow progression of joint damage
Anti-cytokines	Tumor necrosis factor inhibitors (adalimumab, etanercept, infliximab)	Potential risk of infection, cancer (especially lymphoma), nerve damage, reactivation of latent (dormant) tuberculosis	Dramatic, prompt response in most people; can slow progression of joint damage
	Anti-interleukin-1 receptor	A decreased number of white blood	Dramatic, prompt response in

Type	Drug	Selected Side Effects	Benefits
	antagonists (anakinra)	cells (neutropenia), possibly increased risk of infection and cancer	most people; can slow progression of joint damage

Affected joints are painful and red and tend to swell. They may become dislocated. Unless exercised, affected joints may freeze in one position. Swollen wrists can pinch a nerve and result in numbness or tingling due to carpal tunnel syndrome.[1] Fluid-filled swellings called cysts may develop behind affected knees and rupture, causing pain and swelling in the lower legs. Hard bumps may develop under the skin, usually near pressure points, such as the back of the forearm near the elbow.

Rarely, RA affects parts of the body other than the joints. For example, blood vessels may become inflamed (vasculitis). Inflamed blood vessels lead to reduced blood supply to tissues and may result in nerve damage or leg sores (ulcers). The membranes that cover the lungs may become inflamed (pleuritis), as may the sac that surrounds the heart (pericarditis). Inflammation and scarring of the lungs can lead to chest pain or shortness of breath. Excessive dryness of the eyes or mouth (Sjögren's syndrome) or swollen lymph nodes may develop.

Diagnosis

A doctor diagnoses RA on the basis of the typical symptoms. Tests to support the diagnosis may include blood tests, an examination of a sample of joint fluid obtained with a needle (aspiration), and a biopsy (in which a tissue sample from a rheumatoid nodule is removed and examined under a microscope). Characteristic changes in the joints may be seen on x-rays.

In most affected people, the erythrocyte sedimentation rate (ESR) is increased. ESR is a test that measures the rate at which red blood cells settle to the bottom of a test tube containing blood. An increased ESR indicates active inflammation. A doc-

1. see box on page 398

tor may monitor the ESR when symptoms are mild to help determine whether RA is still active.

Many people with RA have distinctive antibodies in their blood. Antibodies are substances formed in the body to fight disease, but in the case of RA, they attack the body's own joint tissues. For instance, an antibody called rheumatoid factor is present in most people with RA. Usually, as the level of rheumatoid factor increases, the RA is more severe and the outlook is poorer. The level of rheumatoid factor may decrease when joints are less inflamed.

Treatment

Treatment of RA ranges from simple life-style modifications to specific drug and nondrug therapies.

Diet: Rarely, people experience symptom flare-ups after eating certain foods. If so, these foods should be avoided. A diet rich in fish and plant oils but low in red meat may slightly reduce inflammation.

Rest: Regular rest periods often help relieve pain in affected joints. Sometimes a short period of bed rest helps relieve a severe flare-up in its most active, painful stage. Rest is especially important when symptoms are severe. However, prolonged bed rest weakens muscles and reduces the ability to exercise and may lead to permanent loss of independence. Splints can be used to immobilize and rest one or several joints, but some systematic exercise of the joints is needed to prevent muscles from weakening and joints from freezing in place.

Drug therapy: Drugs used to treat RA fall into four categories: Nonsteroidal anti-inflammatory drugs (NSAIDs),[1] such as ibuprofen; corticosteroids, such as prednisone; disease-modifying anti-rheumatic drugs (DMARDs), such as methotrexate; and anti-cytokines, such as infliximab. Corticosteroids, DMARDs, and anti-cytokines are sometimes referred to as immunosuppressive drugs because they suppress certain functions of the immune system involved in the progression of RA.

Corticosteroids, DMARDs, and anti-cytokines not only relieve symptoms but also may slow the progression of RA.

Nondrug therapies: Nondrug therapies are used in addition to drugs to reduce joint inflammation. These therapies include

1. see page 335

exercise, physical or occupational therapy, and, sometimes, surgery.

Gentle exercise helps maintain motion in inflamed joints so that they do not freeze in one position.[1] As the inflammation subsides, regular aerobic exercise can help improve function, although a person should not exercise to the point of fatigue. For many people, exercise in water may be easier.[2]

Physical therapy can be especially useful when degree of movement (range of motion) in the joints has been severely reduced by pain and inflammation. Physical therapists sometimes use heat therapy, which may involve applying hot packs or infrared heat to joints. Heat therapy may also involve immersing small joints (such as those in the hands) in a paraffin bath and immersing specific body parts or the whole body from the neck down in warm water (usually about 85° F). Cold therapy (for example, with ice packs) is an alternative. Intensive exercises and, occasionally, splints may also be used to gradually extend the joint and help prevent deformities. Instruction may be given for performing exercises at home.

Occupational therapy for people who are disabled by RA can involve training in the use of several aids or devices that make it possible to accomplish daily tasks. For example, a device called a gripper enables a person to grasp an object without having to squeeze the hand forcefully. Walking can be made less painful by wearing specially modified shoes, which can be fitted by an orthotist.

Surgically replacing knee[3] or hip[4] joints is the most effective way of restoring mobility and function when RA is in an advanced stage and drug therapy has not helped sufficiently. Joints can also be removed or fused together, especially in the foot, to make walking less painful. The thumb can be fused to enable a person to grasp. Unstable vertebrae at the top of the neck can be fused to prevent them from compressing the spinal cord.

Outlook

In general, the long-term outlook is poor for people with long-standing, severe RA. Although treatment usually relieves

1. see page 907
2. see page 589
3. see art on page 592
4. see art on page 324

symptoms, joint damage often continues, and at least 1 out of 10 people with RA eventually becomes severely disabled. In addition, people with active RA have higher rates of serious infections and cardiovascular disease compared with the general population. In rare cases, RA resolves without aggressive treatment.

GOUT

Gout is a disorder that results when a type of urate crystal accumulates in the joints because of high levels of uric acid in the blood (hyperuricemia), leading to painful attacks of joint inflammation.

Gout is more common in men than in women. It usually develops during middle age in men and any time after menopause in women. Drug treatment is generally effective. However, despite treatment, over time and after repeated attacks, joint motion may become progressively restricted by damage caused by deposits of urate crystals in the joints and tendons. Significant disability may result.

Kidney stones, primarily uric acid stones, develop in one fifth of the people who have gout. If left untreated, kidney stones may lead to infection and kidney damage.

Causes

Normally, uric acid is present in small amounts in the blood because of the breakdown of cells. Also, the body transforms substances in foods called purines into uric acid. Uric acid is usually excreted in the urine, keeping blood levels of uric acid normal.

Levels of uric acid may become abnormally high when the kidneys cannot eliminate enough uric acid in the urine. In most people, the cause is unknown. However, levels are especially likely to increase in people with kidney damage due to diseases such as diabetes and high blood pressure. Certain drugs (e.g., thiazide diuretics) directly impair the kidneys' ability to eliminate uric acid, also causing levels of uric acid to rise. In some people, a disease such as leukemia causes excessive uric acid to be produced. The kidneys are overwhelmed by the large amount of uric acid and are unable to excrete it sufficiently.

When the levels of uric acid in the blood are high, urate crystals may form and accumulate in joints. Hard lumps of urate crystals (tophi) are first deposited in the joint lining (synovium) or cartilage or in bone near the joints and then under the skin around joints. Tophi can also develop in the kidneys, under the skin on the ears, in the tough band extending from the calf muscles to the heel (Achilles tendon), or around the elbows. If untreated, tophi can burst and discharge chalky masses of urate crystals through the skin.

Regardless of the underlying cause of gout, a high-purine diet (which includes such foods as anchovies, asparagus, consommé, herring, meat gravies and broths, mushrooms, mussels, all organ meats, sardines, and sweetbreads) worsens matters. Alcohol ingestion makes things worse because alcohol both increases the production of uric acid and interferes with its elimination by the kidneys.

Symptoms

Painful gout attacks (acute gouty arthritis) can occur without warning. These attacks may be triggered by an injury, surgery, consumption of large quantities of alcohol or purine-rich food, fatigue, emotional stress, or illness. Typically, severe pain occurs suddenly in one or more joints, often at night. The pain becomes progressively worse and is often excruciating, particularly when the joint is moved or touched. Even a sheet or blanket touching a toe affected by gout can hurt. The joint becomes inflamed—it swells and feels warm, and the skin over the joint appears red or purplish, tight, and shiny. The joints most likely to be affected are those in the feet, particularly at the base of the big toe. Other joints commonly affected include those in the ankles, knees, wrists, and elbows. The joints of the spine, hips, and shoulders are rarely affected.

Other symptoms of an attack can include fever (which may reach 102° F), chills, a general feeling of illness, and a rapid heartbeat. The first few attacks usually affect only one joint and last for a few days. The symptoms gradually disappear, joint function returns, and no symptoms appear until the next attack. However, if the disorder progresses, untreated attacks last longer, occur more frequently, and affect several joints.

If kidney stones develop in the urinary tract (urolithiasis), excruciating pain may result.

Diagnosis

Doctors often diagnose gout on the basis of its distinctive symptoms and an examination of the affected joints. The diagnosis is confirmed when urate crystals are identified in a sample of a tophus or in joint fluid that has been removed with a needle (joint aspiration) and viewed under a microscope.

Other tests are sometimes performed to support the diagnosis and to provide additional information. They also help exclude other possible causes. A blood test may show a high level of uric acid in the blood, which supports the diagnosis. A blood test may also show a high white blood cell count due to the inflammation caused by the urate crystals. X-rays may show joint damage and the presence of tophi.

Treatment

The first step is to relieve the painful joint by controlling the inflammation with drugs.

Nonsteroidal anti-inflammatory drugs (NSAIDs),[1] including the cyclooxygenase-2 (COX-2) inhibitors (coxibs), are often effective. NSAIDs must be used with caution in older people, however, because these drugs pose a higher risk of side effects, primarily bleeding in the digestive tract and kidney damage. Rarely, opioid analgesics, such as codeine, are needed. Colchicine, the traditional but no longer the most common first-step treatment, begins to ease joint pain after 12 hours. The pain is relieved within 36 to 48 hours. However, it tends to cause diarrhea. Corticosteroids, such as prednisone, are sometimes used to reduce joint inflammation in people who cannot tolerate the other drugs. Corticosteroids may also be injected into an inflamed joint to relieve pain.

In addition to drug therapy, the inflamed joint may be immobilized with a splint to help further reduce pain.

The second step is to avoid recurrences of gout attacks. Avoiding alcoholic beverages, losing weight, discontinuing drugs that cause elevated blood levels of uric acid, and eating smaller amounts of purine-rich foods may be all that is needed. Many people who have gout are overweight. As they gradually lose weight, their blood levels of uric acid often return to normal or near normal, and gout attacks cease. Most tophi on the

℞ DRUGS USED FOR GOUT

Drug	Selected Side Effects	Comments
Nonsteroidal anti-inflammatory drugs, including cyclooxygenase-2 (COX-2) inhibitors (coxibs)	Upset stomach, bleeding, kidney damage, high potassium levels, retention of sodium and potassium	Taken by mouth; effective in preventing and treating attacks
Colchicine	Diarrhea (occurs often), abdominal pain, damage to the bone marrow (rare)	Taken by mouth; effective in preventing and treating attacks
Prednisone	Retention of sodium, causing swelling or high blood pressure	Taken by mouth; dramatic benefit, but used only if other treatments cannot be used
Prednisolone Triamcinolone	Pain, discomfort, joint damage with overuse, inflammation (occasionally), infection (rarely)	Given by injection; very effective if injected into the joint—used if only one or two joints are affected
Probenecid Sulfinpyrazone	Headache, nausea, vomiting, kidney stones	Taken by mouth; can be used long term to lower blood levels of uric acid for preventing attacks (aspirin should not be used at the same time)
Allopurinol	Upset stomach, skin rash, decrease in the number of white blood cells, liver or kidney damage, inflammation of blood vessels (vasculitis)	Taken by mouth; can be used long term to lower blood levels of uric acid for preventing attacks; may also remove crystals or stones already in the kidney

ears, hands, elbows, or feet shrink slowly when the uric acid level falls sufficiently. However, extremely large tophi may have to be removed surgically. Uric acid stones in the urinary tract can be broken up and thereby washed out in the urine, with ultrasound directed at the stones from outside the body (extracorporeal shock wave lithotripsy).

Preventive daily drug treatment may be needed for people who experience repeated, severe attacks. Colchicine may be taken daily to prevent attacks or to greatly reduce their frequency. NSAIDs may also be taken daily, but continued use is not encouraged because of potential side effects. NSAIDs pose some risks for people who have kidney or liver disease. Preventing attacks does not prevent or heal existing joint damage caused by urate crystals, because the crystals remain in the joints.

Drugs that cause excretion of uric acid in the urine (uricosuric drugs), such as probenecid and sulfinpyrazone, can be used to lower the uric acid level in the blood (in people who have normal kidney function) by increasing the kidney's excretion of uric acid. Aspirin, even in low doses, blocks the effects of probenecid and sulfinpyrazone and thus should be avoided when a person is taking either of these drugs.

Although uricosuric drugs lower the level of uric acid in the blood, they can increase the concentration of uric acid in the urine; drinking plenty of fluids—at least 3 quarts a day—may help reduce the risk of uric acid stones developing in the urinary tract. Uricosuric drugs can cause a gout attack when they are first taken. Because low doses of colchicine or an NSAID can decrease this risk, one of these drugs is usually taken for a few months as well.

Allopurinol is another drug that is used to lower the level of uric acid in the blood. This drug blocks the production of uric acid in the body and is especially helpful for people who have a high level of uric acid in the blood as well as urate stones or impaired kidney function. However, allopurinol can cause stomach upset, a skin rash, a decreased white blood cell count, or liver damage. In addition, as with uricosuric drugs, allopurinol can cause a gout attack when it is first taken. To decrease this risk, a doctor may prescribe low-dose colchicine or an NSAID to be taken as well for a few months.

PSEUDOGOUT

Pseudogout, sometimes called calcium pyrophosphate dihydrate crystal deposition disease, is caused by deposits of these crystals in the cartilage and then in the fluid of the joints. These crystal deposits lead to intermittent attacks of painful joint inflammation.

Pseudogout usually occurs in older people and affects men and women equally. In most cases, joints heal without problems, but permanent joint damage can occur. Drug therapy is generally able to control symptoms.

Causes
The cause of pseudogout is unknown. It may occur in people who have other diseases, such as an abnormally high calcium level in the blood due to a high level of parathyroid hormone (hyperparathyroidism), an abnormally high iron level in the tissues (hemochromatosis), or an abnormally low magnesium level in the blood (hypomagnesemia). However, most people with pseudogout have none of these diseases. Pseudogout may be hereditary.

Symptoms
Symptoms vary widely but tend to resemble those of gout. Some people have attacks of painful joint inflammation, usually in the knees or wrists. Attacks may resemble those of gout but are usually less severe. Attacks of pseudogout, like those of gout, can cause fever. Some people have lingering, chronic pain and stiffness in joints of the arms and legs, including the shoulders, elbows, and hips. Other people have no pain between attacks, and some have no pain at any time, despite large deposits of crystals.

Diagnosis
A doctor diagnoses pseudogout by taking fluid from an inflamed joint through a needle (joint aspiration). The diagnosis is confirmed when calcium pyrophosphate crystals are identified in the joint fluid and viewed under a microscope. Calcium from calcium pyrophosphate crystals may be deposited in cartilage, joints, bursae (fluid-filled sacs near joints that help cushion

COMPARING GOUT AND PSEUDOGOUT

Feature	Gout	Pseudogout
Cause	Crystals of urate in the joint	Crystals of calcium pyrophosphate dihydrate in the joint
People most commonly affected	Older people, mostly men	Older people, men and women affected equally
Joints most commonly affected	Joints of the foot, especially the big toe, and the wrists and hands; also, ankles, knees, and elbows	Large joints, such as the knees, shoulders, and hips
Symptoms	Very painful joints. Pain occurs in attacks. Fever may occur during attacks	Joints may or may not be painful, and intensity of pain varies. Pain may occur in attacks or as persistent pain. Fever may occur when symptoms are present
	Hard lumps of crystals (tophi) seen or felt	No lumps of crystals can be seen or felt
	Kidney stones in some cases	No kidney stones
Diagnosis	Tophi and joint erosion may be seen on x-ray	Calcification may be seen on x-ray
	High or normal uric acid levels	High or normal calcium levels

movements), ligaments, and tendons. Deposition of calcium is called calcification, which can be seen on x-ray.

Prognosis and Treatment

Often, the inflamed joints heal without any residual problems, but many people experience permanent joint damage.

Usually, treatment can stop attacks and prevent new attacks

but cannot prevent damage to the affected joints. Most often, nonsteroidal anti-inflammatory drugs (NSAIDs),[1] including the cyclooxygenase-2 (COX-2) inhibitors (coxibs), are used to reduce the pain and inflammation. NSAIDs must be used with caution in older people, because these drugs pose a higher risk of side effects, such as bleeding in the digestive tract and kidney damage. Colchicine in low doses can be taken daily by mouth to prevent attacks. Sometimes, excess joint fluid is drained and a corticosteroid is injected into the joint to reduce the inflammation. No effective long-term treatment is available; however, physical therapy (such as muscle strengthening and range-of-motion exercises) may be helpful.

INFECTIOUS ARTHRITIS

Infectious arthritis (septic arthritis) is a serious disorder in which affected joints are inflamed because of infection. Fluid then accumulates in the inflamed joint.

The risk of developing infectious arthritis increases with age. Risk is also greater for people whose immune system is impaired because of cancer, diabetes, or treatment with drugs such as corticosteroids.

Causes

Among older people, bacteria are almost always the cause of the infection. Bacteria usually get directly into the joint as a result of injury or surgery. Alternatively, bacteria travel from a nearby infection in the body or through the bloodstream from a more distant site. Sometimes the source of the bacteria is unknown. Infectious arthritis most often affects joints already damaged by disease, usually osteoarthritis or RA.

Symptoms and Diagnosis

Infectious arthritis usually begins with the sudden onset of fever, a general sick feeling, and pain in one or more joints. Primarily the large joints are affected, most commonly the shoulders, elbows, wrists, hips, and knees. The affected joint is often

1. see page 335

red, warm, and swollen. However, some people with infectious arthritis look and feel as they normally do, except that they may have a slight fever.

A doctor diagnoses infectious arthritis by examining the affected joint and removing fluid from it. Analysis of the fluid may show a high white blood cell count, which indicates infection. The bacteria causing the infection may also be identified in the sample. Blood samples are also obtained to determine whether the bacteria traveled from the bloodstream.

Treatment

Immediate treatment with antibiotics given intravenously and removal of joint fluid (aspiration) is needed to avoid permanent damage to the joint and to the cartilage inside the joint. Joint fluid is drawn out as completely as possible to help speed the body's ability to clear the infection. This procedure is repeated daily until the white blood cell count in the joint fluid decreases. Antibiotics given intravenously are later switched to antibiotics taken by mouth. If fever and joint pain are not substantially reduced in 48 to 72 hours, joint fluid may be surgically removed (surgical drainage).

42

Temporal Arteritis and Polymyalgia Rheumatica

In temporal arteritis (sometimes called giant cell arteritis), certain arteries in the head and elsewhere become inflamed. The temporal arteries (located on the temple, beside the eye) are most commonly affected, often causing a throbbing headache. In polymyalgia rheumatica, the lining of some joints (such as those in the neck, shoulders, and hips) becomes inflamed, causing muscle pain and stiffness. Temporal arteritis and polymyalgia rheumatica are separate disorders but closely related. They occur together so often that they may be thought of as Frick and Frack disorders. At least half of people who have temporal arteritis also have polymyalgia rheumatica. And about one fourth of people who have polymyalgia rheumatica develop temporal arteritis.

Temporal arteritis and polymyalgia rheumatica develop only in people over 50, and they become more common as people age. Polymyalgia rheumatica, which affects 7 out of 1,000 people over 50, is more common than temporal arteritis, which affects about 2 out of 1,000 people over 50. Both disorders affect more women than men.

People rarely die of temporal arteritis or polymyalgia rheumatica. But without treatment, the pain these disorders cause, whether they occur together or separately, can make everyday living miserably difficult. If not treated promptly, temporal arteritis can cause blindness.

Causes

No one knows what causes temporal arteritis or polymyalgia rheumatica. However, what happens in the body when the two disorders develop is known. In both disorders, cells that are part of the body's immune system malfunction.

In temporal arteritis, cells of the immune system (mainly certain white blood cells) invade the wall of the arteries that carry blood to the head. These cells cause inflammation in segments of the arteries (arteritis). These segments may become partially or completely blocked. Most often, the temporal arteries are affected. Sometimes other arteries in the head, including those that carry blood to the eyes (ophthalmic arteries) or to the chin, mouth, and nose (facial arteries), are affected, as are arteries in the neck (carotid arteries) and arteries elsewhere in the body. Rarely, a bulge (aneurysm) develops in the body's largest artery, the aorta.

In polymyalgia rheumatica, cells of the immune system enter joints such as those in the neck, shoulders, and hips. These cells cause inflammation of the lining of joints (synovitis). The cells do not invade the muscles, even though polymyalgia rheumatica causes muscle pain more than joint pain.

Symptoms

Temporal arteritis and polymyalgia rheumatica cause the same general symptoms, such as fatigue, slight fever, loss of appetite, and weight loss. People with either of the disorders may have one or more of these symptoms. People may have additional symptoms that are caused only by temporal arteritis. These symptoms vary depending on which arteries are affected. People may also have symptoms caused only by polymyalgia rheumatica.

Temporal arteritis can cause double vision (diplopia) and blurred vision. A person may also be unable to see when looking in one direction. Or a person may completely lose vision in one eye. Loss of vision may be temporary. However, unless temporal arteritis is treated promptly, vision may be lost permanently, sometimes in both eyes.

Many people with temporal arteritis have headaches. Often described as continuous and throbbing, the headaches are usually felt at the temple. The temple may be tender when touched. The temporal artery may bulge because it is inflamed and swollen. It may feel bumpy. Temporal arteritis may cause aching pain in the jaw during chewing or talking (jaw claudication). Some people experience dizziness that feels like spinning (vertigo).

An aneurysm in the aorta[1] due to temporal arteritis often causes no symptoms. But occasionally, an aneurysm leaks or ruptures, causing sudden chest or back pain, weakness, lightheadedness, confusion, and even death.

Polymyalgia rheumatica causes muscle pain and stiffness, most often in the neck, shoulders, and hips. The pain tends to be worse in the morning. But pain may awaken a person during the night. Usually, stiffness is more noticeable in the morning and after periods of inactivity. A person may be unable to move the shoulders and hips freely because they are too stiff. Pain may make getting out of bed difficult. Affected muscles may be slightly tender when touched. Less often, mild pain and swelling occur in the wrists, fingers, and knees.

1. see page 640

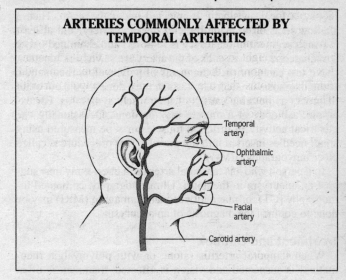

ARTERIES COMMONLY AFFECTED BY TEMPORAL ARTERITIS

Temporal artery

Ophthalmic artery

Facial artery

Carotid artery

Diagnosis

Doctors may suspect temporal arteritis, polymyalgia rheumatica, or both in a person who has fatigue, fever, loss of appetite, and weight loss. If headaches or sudden changes in vision are also present, temporal arteritis is suspected. Doctors check the temporal artery on each side of the head to see if it is swollen, bulges more than usual, or feels bumpy. If the neck, shoulders, and hips are painful and stiff, polymyalgia rheumatica is suspected.

Blood tests help doctors diagnose both disorders. The most common blood test is measurement of the erythrocyte sedimentation rate (ESR). This test helps determine how much inflammation is present. In most people with either or both disorders, the ESR is much higher than normal. But in a few people, it is normal. If the ESR is normal but symptoms suggest one of these disorders, another blood test—measuring the level of C-reactive protein—may help. The presence of this protein indicates inflammation.

A biopsy of the affected temporal artery is always recommended to confirm a diagnosis of temporal arteritis. For the biopsy, a local anesthetic is injected under the scalp. Then a shallow incision is made directly over the artery, and at least a 1-inch segment of the artery is removed and examined under a microscope. The cut ends of the artery are sewn back together.

No test can confirm a diagnosis of polymyalgia rheumatica. If the diagnosis is uncertain, tests may be done to rule out other disorders as possible causes of the muscle symptoms. For example, a biopsy of a muscle may be done. Occasionally, the electrical activity of different muscles may be measured using small needles inserted into the muscle. This procedure is called electromyography (EMG).[1]

In a person who has temporal arteritis, a chest x-ray may suggest an aneurysm in the aorta. Ultrasonography, computed tomography (CT), or magnetic resonance imaging (MRI) may be done to confirm the diagnosis of an aneurysm.

Treatment and Outlook

When temporal arteritis (alone or with polymyalgia rheumatica) is suspected and vision is affected, treatment is often begun immediately. It is usually begun even before a biopsy is done to confirm the diagnosis. Any delay in the treatment of temporal arteritis increases the risk that blindness may occur and that blindness, if present, may become permanent. However, when vision is not affected and biopsy results can be obtained in a few days, many doctors wait for biopsy results before starting treatment. Treatment may be given when biopsy results are negative but the results of the physical examination and blood tests strongly suggest temporal arteritis. A biopsy does not always detect temporal arteritis.

Treatment usually consists of a corticosteroid, such as prednisone. Prednisone is taken as a tablet. The starting dose of prednisone for temporal arteritis is much higher than that for polymyalgia rheumatica. If prednisone relieves symptoms in people who are thought to have polymyalgia rheumatica (but do not have temporal arteritis), the diagnosis is supported.

If the biopsy does not show any evidence of temporal arteritis or if prednisone has been tried but has not been effective, doctors look for other causes of the symptoms.

Many people with temporal arteritis (alone or with polymyal-

1. see page 139

gia rheumatica) begin to improve dramatically during the first week of treatment with prednisone. Some improve within 1 day. After only a few days of treatment, headaches from temporal arteritis may subside. After having been barely able to get out of bed because of polymyalgia rheumatica, people may be walking and doing light household chores.

Prednisone is often continued at the starting dose for several weeks to make sure that symptoms are under control. Then, doctors usually slowly and cautiously reduce the dose. They monitor the person's response to the reductions in dose by periodically asking how well prednisone is controlling the symptoms and by measuring the ESR to check for evidence of inflammation. If symptoms worsen or if the ESR increases, doctors usually delay the next reduction in dose or even increase the dose.

The goal is to keep reducing the dose until the person no longer needs to take the drug. This approach is important because prednisone is more likely to cause problems when it is given at a high dose or for a long time. These problems include high blood pressure, thinning of the skin, poor wound healing, osteoporosis, diabetes, and cataracts. Nonetheless, treatment usually must be continued for at least 1 to 2 years and sometimes longer.

If an aneurysm develops in the aorta because of temporal arteritis, the aneurysm may be surgically repaired. Whether an aneurysm is repaired depends on its size and location.[1]

Temporal arteritis and polymyalgia rheumatica rarely cause death. For the most part, problems caused by these disorders can be prevented or effectively treated. Treatment also enables most people who have one or both disorders to regain their ability to function. A complete recovery is the reward for many of the people who faithfully continue treatment as instructed.

1. see page 640

43

High Blood Pressure

High blood pressure (hypertension) is blood pressure that is consistently higher than normal. Blood pressure is the force exerted by blood against the walls of arteries (the blood vessels that carry blood from the heart to the rest of the body).

The "tension" part of "hypertension" does not imply being tense or anxious. Many people who are calm and relaxed have hypertension, and some people who are tense and anxious have normal blood pressure. Also, the "hyper" part of "hypertension" does not imply being hyperactive.

In the United States, high blood pressure becomes more common as people age. More than half of people aged 65 or over have high blood pressure.

Persistently high blood pressure damages arteries. It speeds up the deposit of cholesterol and other fatty materials in arteries (atherosclerosis). It may make arteries weaken and sometimes even bulge and rupture. It may cause the heart to enlarge. As a result, tissues (particularly in the brain, heart, and kidneys) are damaged, sometimes resulting in an early death. As blood pressure increases, the risk of stroke, heart attack, heart failure, and kidney failure also increases. Rarely, very high blood pressure impairs vision. Treatment can effectively control high blood pressure and help prevent the problems it causes.

When a person's blood pressure is measured, the result consists of two numbers. The higher number (systolic pressure) represents the pressure when the heart beats. The lower number (diastolic pressure) represents the pressure when the heart relaxes between beats. Ideally, blood pressure is about 120/80 mm Hg (millimeters of mercury). This reading is referred to as "120 over 80." Blood pressure (often abbreviated BP) is considered high when the systolic pressure is 140 mm Hg or higher or when the diastolic pressure is 90 mm Hg or higher. In younger people with high blood pressure, both systolic pressure and diastolic pressure are usually high. In older people with high blood pressure, systolic pressure is often high (more than 140 mm Hg) while diastolic pressure remains in the normal range (less than 90 mm Hg). This disorder, called isolated systolic hypertension, may have even greater risks than when both systolic pressure and diastolic pressure are high.

A person's blood pressure is determined partly by how well the heart, arteries, and kidneys are working together. The drugs used to treat high blood pressure (antihypertensive drugs) lower blood pressure by affecting how these organs function.

ADDITIONAL DETAIL

The way the body determines and controls blood pressure is complex. It involves the heart, arteries, and kidneys working together. Blood pressure is affected by the following:

• How fast the heart is beating (heart rate) and how forcefully it contracts. An increase in rate or force tends to increase blood pressure.

• Whether the small arteries that carry blood to the tissues can expand (dilate) and contract (constrict). If the vessels do not readily dilate, are blocked, or are stiff, the heart must work harder to pump blood into them. And blood pressure increases.

• Whether the kidneys can remove (excrete) enough salt and water from the body. If salt and water are not excreted effectively, the amount of blood in the body (blood volume) increases. When blood volume increases, the heart has to work harder, causing blood pressure to increase.

The nervous system and certain hormones also affect blood pressure. They help regulate the heart rate, the force of the heart's contractions, and the diameter of arteries (by causing them to dilate or constrict). Some hormones affect the amount of salt and water that the kidneys excrete.

Causes

The two main types of high blood pressure are essential (or primary) hypertension and secondary hypertension.

Essential hypertension—when the cause is unknown—is by far the most common type. Changes due to aging may contribute. As people age, large arteries gradually stiffen and small arteries may become partially blocked. Also, blood pressure tends to increase. Putting two and two together, some experts conclude that the stiffening of larger arteries and blockages in small arteries partly explain why blood pressure tends to increase as people age. An unhealthy diet (for example, too much salt or alcohol) and chronic stress may also contribute to high blood pressure. Obesity and changes in the way the kidneys function play an important role in the development of high blood pressure. In many nonindustrialized countries, blood pressure is less likely to increase as people age. This difference may be explained by differences in diet and stress, among other things.

Secondary hypertension, which is relatively rare, results from several disorders. Examples are disorders that partially block the arteries to the kidneys (such as atherosclerosis) and disorders that damage the kidneys (such as infections or diabetes). A tumor in the adrenal glands (located on top of the kidneys) or sleep apnea may cause secondary hypertension.

Secondary hypertension can result from using certain drugs. They include nonsteroidal anti-inflammatory drugs (NSAIDs), corticosteroids, and nonprescription allergy drugs and cold remedies that contain phenylephrine or pseudoephedrine.

Symptoms

People with high blood pressure may have no symptoms. They may blame high blood pressure for headaches, nosebleeds, or ringing in the ears. But these symptoms may occur whether blood pressure is high or not. Some people with high blood pressure sometimes feel flushed or just do not feel right.

Occasionally, the first symptoms develop because high blood pressure has damaged one or more organs (particularly the brain, heart, or kidneys). Organ damage and symptoms are more likely if high blood pressure is not treated or not adequately treated.

Very high blood pressure sometimes causes sudden headache with loss of sensation in and paralysis of one half of the body. These symptoms result from rupture of an artery in the brain (hemorrhagic stroke).

Chest pain due to coronary artery disease may occur. If heart failure develops, the legs and feet may swell and people may become short of breath during physical activity and eventually during rest. If the kidneys are damaged, people may urinate frequently. If damage is severe, they may feel nauseated and tired.

Vision may become blurred when blood pressure is very high. Arteries in the eyes can be damaged. If one of these arteries ruptures, a blind spot in vision may develop.

Diagnosis

In most people, the only way to diagnose high blood pressure is to measure blood pressure—a simple, painless procedure. To measure blood pressure, a health care practitioner places an inflatable cuff around the person's arm just above the elbow. The person's arm is supported (for example, by a table or desk) and kept at about the same level as the heart. The cuff is connected to a device that measures pressure (called a sphygmomanometer). The practitioner tucks a stethoscope just under the edge of the cuff to be ready to listen. The cuff is inflated until it squeezes (compresses) the main artery in the upper arm (brachial artery) so that blood flow is temporarily stopped. Then the air in the cuff is slowly and steadily released. The practitioner notes pressure on the sphygmomanometer twice: (1) when blood first begins to flow through the artery and the sounds of the heartbeat can be heard (systolic pressure) and (2) when blood flow becomes continuous and heartbeat sounds cannot be heard (diastolic pressure).

Typically, measurements are taken on at least two or three occasions to confirm that blood pressure is consistently high. Ideally, blood pressure is measured in both arms at least the first time, because there may be a difference. The measurement from the arm with the higher reading is usually used to determine whether treatment is necessary. Measurements are made while the person is sitting, usually after several minutes of rest.

A device that can be used to measure blood pressure at home may be recommended. It enables people to check their blood pressure at different times of the day or night. However, taking blood pressure measurements at home is meant to supplement, not replace, having measurements taken by a health care practitioner. Measurements taken at home show what happens to a person's blood pressure under a variety of conditions. Thus, they provide information that may help the doctor determine how to best treat the person.

Some home blood pressure–measuring devices are digital and do not require use of a stethoscope. They measure blood pressure automatically, and the results are displayed on a screen. Digital devices can be especially helpful for people who live alone or who have hearing problems.

Most devices used to monitor blood pressure at home are accurate. However, measurements made at a finger or wrist may not be reliable.

Sometimes blood pressure is high when measured by a doctor or other health care practitioner but is normal when measured at home or somewhere other than a doctor's office. This phenomenon is called white-coat hypertension: The person is reacting to the doctor's white coat. The stress of being in a doctor's office causes blood pressure to be high temporarily. White-coat hypertension, once considered to be of little medical significance, should not be ignored. Higher blood pressure during a visit with a doctor may mean that blood pressure also increases during other stressful situations. If blood pressure is consistently higher than 140/90 mm Hg in a doctor's office despite being lower at home, the doctor occasionally recommends blood pressure monitoring during the person's normal daily activities (home blood pressure measuring).

Ambulatory monitoring involves wearing a cuff that automatically inflates and deflates every 15 to 20 minutes and a small device that records the readings. Ambulatory monitoring is usually done for 24 or 48 hours. It provides measurements that may be more reliable and accurate than isolated measurements taken in a doctor's office. Undergoing ambulatory monitoring is more expensive than using home blood pressure–measuring devices.

In people who have unusually stiff arteries, the inflated blood pressure cuff may not adequately compress the artery. Thus, measurements are sometimes higher than actual blood pressure (a condition called pseudohypertension). In such cases, blood pressure may be normal, or it may be high but not as high as the measurement indicates. In a few people with pseudohypertension, taking drugs to lower blood pressure (antihypertensive drugs) makes blood pressure fall too low. As a result, they may feel light-headed.

To determine whether another disorder is causing high blood pressure, doctors ask questions about symptoms. For example, doctors may ask about snoring and daytime sleepiness to determine whether sleep apnea could be the cause. A physical examination and simple laboratory tests can also help identify a cause. Typically, tests include analysis of urine (urinalysis) and some blood tests. Other tests, most commonly electrocardiography, may be done to determine whether the heart has been damaged by high blood pressure. Occasionally, more tests, such as echocardiography[1] or exercise stress testing, are necessary.

Treatment

Changes in lifestyle may help lower blood pressure. For example, people should maintain a desirable body weight and exercise regularly. Drinking no more than two alcoholic beverages (10 ounces of wine, 24 ounces of beer, or 2 ounces of whiskey) a day and limiting intake of salt may help. People can learn to manage stress better. Changes in lifestyle also help when antihypertensive drugs are needed, because lower doses may be used.

If high blood pressure is caused by another disorder, treating that disorder may lower blood pressure. If a drug is causing high blood pressure, discontinuing the drug may help.

If these measures do not lower blood pressure enough, antihypertensive drugs are needed. More than three fourths of people with high blood pressure have to take antihypertensive drugs.

Several types of antihypertensive drugs are available. When selecting the most appropriate drug, doctors consider how severe the high blood pressure is, whether other risk factors for heart attacks (such as diabetes or abnormal cholesterol levels) are present, and whether the heart is damaged. They also consider side effects that may occur. For older people, taking anti-

1. see page 130

℞ DRUGS USED FOR HIGH BLOOD PRESSURE

Type	Examples	Possible Side Effects	People Who May Benefit from the Drug
Alpha-beta-blockers	Carvedilol Labetalol	Low blood pressure when a person stands (orthostatic hypotension)	People with angina pectoris People who have recently had a heart attack People with heart failure
Alpha-blockers	Doxazosin Prazosin Terazosin	Awareness of rapid heartbeats (palpitations), dizziness, and fluid retention (edema)	Men with an enlarged prostate People with abnormal cholesterol levels
Angiotensin-converting enzyme (ACE) inhibitors	Benazepril Captopril Enalapril Fosinopril Lisinopril Quinapril Ramipril Trandolapril	Dry cough, low blood pressure, impairment of kidney function, an increased potassium level, and an allergic reaction called angioedema (swelling that affects the face, lips, and windpipe and may interfere with breathing)	People with heart failure People with diabetes (especially if they have a kidney disorder)
Angiotensin II receptor blockers	Candesartan Eprosartan Irbesartan Losartan Valsartan	Dizziness, low blood pressure, impairment of kidney function, and an increased potassium level	People with heart failure People with diabetes
Beta-blockers	Acebutolol Atenolol Bisoprolol Metoprolol Nadolol Penbutolol Propranolol	Spasm of the airways, an abnormally slow heart rate (bradycardia), insomnia, fatigue, shortness of breath, Raynaud's	People with angina pectoris People who have recently had a heart attack People with migraine headaches

Type	Examples	Possible Side Effects	People Who May Benefit from the Drug
		phenomenon, vivid dreams, and sexual dysfunction	People with essential tremor People with an abnormal heart rhythm People with heart failure
Calcium channel blockers	Amlodipine Diltiazem Felodipine Isradipine Nicardipine Nisoldipine Verapamil	Dizziness, heart failure, fluid retention (edema) in the ankles, flushing, head-ache, heartburn, enlarged gums, and an abnormally fast heart rate With verapamil and diltiazem, an abnormally slow heart rate With verapamil and, less frequently, with diltiazem, constipation	People with angina People with migraine headaches People with isolated systolic hypertension People with an abnormal heart rhythm
Diuretics	Chlorothia-zide Chlorthali-done Hydrochlor-othiazide Indapamide Methyclothi-azide Metolazone	Decreased levels of potassium and magnesium, increased levels of calcium and uric acid, and, in men, sexual dysfunction	Most older people Obese people People with heart failure People with isolated systolic hypertension

hypertensive drugs can make blood pressure fall too low in certain situations—for example, when they stand up (a disorder called orthostatic hypotension). As a result, they may feel light-headed. Many antihypertensive drugs are effective and relatively free of side effects. Many people need to take more than one type.

Thiazide diuretics (such as hydrochlorothiazide) are often given first. Diuretics increase the amount of salt and water excreted by the kidneys and may expand (dilate) blood vessels. Beta-blockers are sometimes given first. They slow the heart rate and reduce the force of the heart's contractions. Diuretics and beta-blockers reduce the risk of heart attacks, heart failure, strokes, and kidney failure.

Other types of antihypertensive drugs may be used. Each type dilates arteries but may do so in different ways. Alpha-blockers interfere with the action of a hormone called norepinephrine, which causes arteries to contract (constrict). Alpha-beta-blockers combine the actions of beta-blockers and alpha-blockers. Angiotensin-converting enzyme (ACE) inhibitors interfere with the formation of a hormone called angiotensin, which causes arteries to constrict. Angiotensin II receptor blockers interfere with the action of angiotensin. Calcium channel blockers block calcium from entering cells. As a result, arteries dilate and blood pressure is reduced. Some of these drugs also reduce the force of the heart's contractions.

Some people have conditions that make a certain type of antihypertensive drug particularly well suited for them. For example, obese people may respond particularly well to a diuretic or calcium channel blocker. For people with high blood pressure plus diabetes or heart failure, an angiotensin-converting enzyme (ACE) inhibitor or an angiotensin II receptor blocker is recommended because these drugs help protect the kidneys. For people who have had a heart attack or who have angina, migraine headaches, or glaucoma, a beta-blocker is recommended. For men with an enlarged prostate (benign prostatic hyperplasia), an alpha-blocker or alpha-beta-blocker is particularly useful. Alpha-blockers and alpha-beta-blockers relax muscles in the bladder and urethra. Then urine can flow more easily. However, in older people, taking an alpha-blocker or alpha-beta-blocker may cause light-headedness and urinary incontinence.

In general, the goal of treatment is to lower blood pressure below 140/90 mm Hg or even lower in people with diabetes or a kidney disorder. However, in older people, meeting this goal is not always possible. For example, the number of drugs or the dose of drugs needed to decrease blood pressure below 140/90 mm Hg may cause annoying side effects. But any decrease in blood pressure is better than none.

Outlook

Most people with high blood pressure have to take antihypertensive drugs for the rest of their life. If treatment is discontinued, blood pressure is likely to go back up, although it may stay down for the first several months. Sometimes doctors try reducing the dose. If blood pressure increases, the dose is increased again.

If people are concerned about side effects or if they are taking several drugs, they can ask their doctor about reducing the dose or changing the drug. As long as treatment is adequate, people can expect to lead a long life with few restrictions.

44

Blood Vessel Disorders

In blood vessel disorders, blood vessels may become blocked, bulge abnormally, or tear. Or they may become stretched out or inflamed. As a result, blood does not circulate through the body as it normally does.

Essentially, blood vessels are the body's plumbing system. Blood vessels (arteries, capillaries, and veins) carry blood throughout the body, delivering oxygen and nutrients to tissues and carrying waste products away from tissues. The body's tissues need a constant supply of oxygen and nutrients to survive.

Arteries carry blood from the heart to the body's tissues. The heart pumps blood into the body's main artery, the aorta. The aorta divides into smaller and smaller arteries and finally into capillaries—tiny blood vessels that connect arteries and veins. In capillaries, oxygen and nutrients leave the blood and enter the tissues, and waste products leave the tissues and enter the blood. Capillaries lead to veins, which become larger and larger as they approach the heart. Veins carry blood back to the heart.

The heart pumps the blood that has returned from the veins to the lungs (through the pulmonary arteries). In the lungs, oxygen is added to blood (the blood becomes oxygenated). Oxygenated blood flows from the lungs to the heart (through the pulmonary veins). The heart then pumps this blood into the arteries and to the tissues.

Both arteries and veins are elastic. Arteries can change size: They expand (dilate) and contract (constrict). Thus, they help control blood pressure and can deliver enough blood to tissues. For example, when arteries dilate, they provide more space for blood to flow through, so blood pressure decreases. Veins dilate when blood flow through them increases and constrict when blood flow decreases. Thus, they help adjust how much blood the bloodstream can hold.

The heart pumps blood through the arteries, so blood travels through arteries under high pressure. In contrast, the heart does not pump blood through the veins, so blood travels through veins under low pressure. Blood in some veins (such as the veins in the legs) has to travel against gravity to reach the heart. These veins have one-way valves with two flaps (cusps) that prevent blood from flowing backward. The flaps open to allow blood to flow toward the heart and close if blood starts to flow backward. Blood in the leg veins is propelled toward the heart by contractions of the leg muscles, which squeeze the veins in the legs.

Blood vessels hold up quite well to a lifetime of use, considering that blood makes more than 1,000 trips around the body each day. To some degree, the body can repair damaged blood vessels and create new vessels when needed. Nevertheless, aging itself and disorders that may develop as people age take a toll on blood vessels.

If a disorder affects arteries, severe symptoms can occur within seconds because lack of oxygen affects tissues immediately. If a disorder affects veins, symptoms usually are less severe or develop more slowly. Many blood vessel disorders can be effectively prevented or treated.

ARTERIES AND VEINS: CIRCULATING THE BLOOD

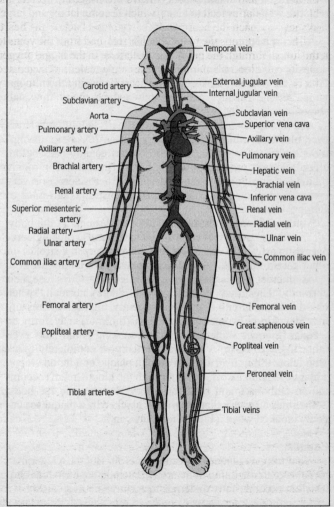

Temporal vein

Carotid artery
Subclavian artery
Aorta
Pulmonary artery
Axillary artery
Brachial artery
Renal artery
Superior mesenteric artery
Radial artery
Ulnar artery
Common iliac artery

External jugular vein
Internal jugular vein
Subclavian vein
Superior vena cava
Axillary vein
Pulmonary vein
Hepatic vein
Brachial vein
Inferior vena cava
Renal vein
Radial vein
Ulnar vein
Common iliac vein

Femoral artery
Popliteal artery
Tibial arteries

Femoral vein
Great saphenous vein
Popliteal vein
Peroneal vein
Tibial veins

ATHEROSCLEROSIS

In atherosclerosis (sometimes called hardening of the arteries), the walls of arteries thicken as well as harden.

Atherosclerosis begins when cholesterol and other fatty materials in the blood gradually accumulate in arteries and form deposits (plaques or atheromas). Over time, calcium accumulates in the plaques, making them stiff and causing them to enlarge. As the plaques enlarge, they reduce blood flow and sometimes block the arteries.

Atherosclerosis often begins during early adulthood. However, blood flow must be reduced by at least 70% before symptoms are likely to occur. Several decades usually pass before atherosclerosis progresses to this point. Thus, it is commonly thought of as an older person's disease. Atherosclerosis is very common in the United States, Canada, Australia, and most of Europe.

Atherosclerosis tends to affect arteries throughout the body. It can affect arteries that carry blood to the heart (causing coronary artery disease), brain (sometimes resulting in a stroke), or other parts of the body (causing peripheral arterial disease).

As atherosclerosis progresses, the affected arteries lose their elasticity. Then they cannot expand (dilate) normally when blood is pumped into them. Consequently, high blood pressure may develop or worsen. Blood clots (thrombi) may form on plaques. Plaques sometimes rupture, making blood clots even more likely to form. A clot can partially or completely block blood flow through an artery. Part of a plaque or a blood clot on a plaque may break off, travel through the bloodstream (becoming an embolus), and block an artery elsewhere in the body. Sometimes an artery that is partially blocked by a plaque is suddenly blocked when a blood clot lodges in it.

Causes

What triggers plaques to form is unclear. But the trigger may be damage to the lining of an artery. Such damage enables cholesterol and other fatty materials to accumulate in an artery.

ATHEROSCLEROSIS: BLOCKING AN ARTERY

The wall of an artery consists of several layers. The lining or inner layer (endothelium) is usually smooth and unbroken. Atherosclerosis begins when the lining is damaged. Then fatty materials, mainly cholesterol, may accumulate there, forming a deposit (plaque, or atheroma). Other materials, such as connective and elastic tissue, cell debris, and calcium, may also accumulate. As more materials accumulate, the plaque bulges into the channel of the artery. A plaque may partially or completely block an artery, thus reducing or stopping blood flow.

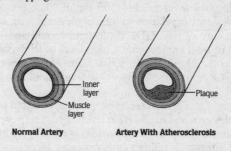

Normal Artery   Artery With Atherosclerosis

Certain conditions (called risk factors) make atherosclerosis more likely to develop or worsen. Some risk factors cannot be changed. They include a family history of early atherosclerosis (having a close relative who developed the disease at a young age), older age, and male sex. Other risk factors can usually be corrected or treated. They include abnormal levels of cholesterol and other fats (lipids) in the blood, high blood pressure, diabetes, smoking and exposure to tobacco smoke, excess body weight, and physical inactivity.

LEVELS OF FATS IN THE BLOOD

Type of Fat	Desirable Level
Total cholesterol	Less than 200 mg/dL
Low-density lipoprotein (LDL)	Less than 100 mg/dL cholesterol
High-density lipoprotein (HDL)	More than 40 mg/dL cholesterol
Triglycerides	Less than 150 mg/dL after a person fasts at least 8 hours

Having a high level of low-density lipoprotein (LDL, the "bad" cholesterol) or a low level of high-density lipoprotein (HDL, the "good" cholesterol) increases the risk of atherosclerosis. Generally, experts recommend that the LDL cholesterol level be less than 100 mg/dL (milligrams per deciliter of blood) and that the HDL cholesterol level be more than 40 mg/dL. The total cholesterol level includes LDL and HDL cholesterol. For most people, the total cholesterol level should be less than 200 mg/dL. The risk of a heart attack more than doubles when the total cholesterol level reaches 300 mg/dL. The percentage of HDL cholesterol in relation to total cholesterol is an especially useful measure of risk. HDL cholesterol should account for at least 25% of total cholesterol. A high level of triglycerides, another fat in the blood, is also a risk factor. After a person fasts for at least 8 hours, the triglyceride level should be less than 150 mg/dL.

Cholesterol levels increase as people age. Diet and genes also affect cholesterol and triglyceride levels. For most people, a diet high in saturated fats, trans fatty acids (artificially hydrogenated fats), and simple or refined carbohydrates increases the total cholesterol level. Eating excess calories can result in a high triglyceride level, as can drinking large amounts of alcohol. However, for some people, diet has little effect. Some people can eat large amounts of saturated fat and trans fatty acids, and their total cholesterol level stays at an acceptable level. Others can follow a strict low-fat diet, and their total cholesterol level remains well above the highest acceptable level. Such differences seem to be mostly determined by genes. A person's genetic makeup influences the rate at which the body makes, uses, and eliminates fats.

Abnormal cholesterol or triglyceride levels can be due to certain disorders. They include diabetes that is poorly controlled, kidney failure, some liver disorders, and an underactive thyroid gland (hypothyroidism).

Smoking increases the risk of atherosclerosis in several ways. It decreases the HDL cholesterol level and increases the triglyceride level. Smoking also increases the level of carbon monoxide in the blood. Excess carbon monoxide may make damage to the lining of arteries more likely. Smoking causes the muscle layer of the artery's wall to contract (constrict). If an artery is already partially blocked, constriction of the artery's wall decreases the amount of blood reaching the tissues even more. Also, smoking makes blood more likely to clot. Secondhand smoke—smoke breathed in from someone else's smoking—should also be avoided.

Being overweight increases the risk of atherosclerosis.[1] It also increases the risk of high blood pressure, diabetes, and abnormal cholesterol levels—all risk factors for atherosclerosis.

Physical inactivity appears to increase the risk of atherosclerosis and several of its risk factors: high blood pressure, abnormal cholesterol levels, and being overweight.

A high level of homocysteine (an amino acid, one of the building blocks that make up protein) in the blood can directly damage the lining of arteries. As a result, plaques are more likely to develop. A high homocysteine level may also make blood clots more likely to form. The homocysteine level increases as people age. Kidney failure, some cancers (such as breast cancer), heavy smoking, or a deficiency of certain vitamins (folic acid or vitamin B_6 or B_{12}) can cause the homocysteine level to increase.

Infection can damage the lining of arteries, making atherosclerosis more likely to develop.

Symptoms and Diagnosis

Symptoms may first occur during physical activity, when tissues need more oxygen. Pain or muscle cramping may be felt, often in the legs. These symptoms occur because the artery supplying the affected area is partially blocked and is not receiving enough blood and oxygen.

Typically, symptoms such as pain, cramping or tightness in muscles, and weakness develop gradually as a plaque slowly enlarges and reduces blood flow through an artery. However, the first symptoms sometimes occur suddenly because an artery is suddenly blocked.

Other symptoms depend on where the blockage is:

• If one or more arteries supplying the heart (coronary arteries) are partially blocked, chest pain (angina) can result.[2] If an artery is completely blocked, a heart attack can result.

1. see page 244
2. see page 659

• If an artery supplying the brain (a carotid or vertebral artery) is completely blocked, a stroke can result.[1]

• If arteries in the legs are partially blocked, leg cramps (intermittent claudication)[2] can result.

• If arteries supplying one or both kidneys become blocked, kidney failure or dangerously high blood pressure (malignant hypertension) can result.

Often, atherosclerosis is diagnosed only after it causes symptoms or other problems. Atherosclerosis is sometimes diagnosed when arteries appear outlined or highlighted on an x-ray taken for other reasons. Arteries may appear outlined because of calcium deposits in plaques. Other tests, depending on symptoms, may be done.

Prevention and Treatment

Correcting or treating risk factors can prevent atherosclerosis from worsening and may even cause some of the plaques to shrink. The sooner risk factors are changed, the greater the potential benefit. Because abnormal cholesterol levels are an important risk factor, older people should have their cholesterol levels measured even if they do not have symptoms of atherosclerosis.

FATS IN FOOD

Type	Sources
Saturated fats	Meat, eggs, and dairy products
Trans fatty acids	Margarine, shortening, and many processed foods such as cookies, crackers, doughnuts, and chips
Monounsaturated fats	Olive oil, canola oil, peanut oil, avocados, and nuts
Omega-3 fats	Deep-sea fish such as mackerel, salmon, and tuna

---

1. see page 374
2. see page 632

Limiting the amount of saturated fats, trans fatty acids, and simple or refined carbohydrates in the diet can help control cholesterol levels. When possible, people should substitute monounsaturated fats and omega-3 fats for saturated fats and trans fatty acids.

Eating plenty of fruits, vegetables, and whole-grain foods also helps control cholesterol levels. These foods are naturally low in fat and contain no cholesterol. Many of the same foods are also rich in soluble fiber, which helps lower cholesterol levels. Examples are oat bran, oatmeal, beans, peas, rice bran, barley, citrus fruits, strawberries, and apple pulp.

If needed, drugs can be taken to control abnormal cholesterol levels. Many types of cholesterol-lowering drugs are available. For some people, taking one cholesterol-lowering drug is effective. Other people need to take two or, rarely, three drugs. Statins, such as atorvastatin, fluvastatin, pravastatin, and simvastatin, are commonly used. Bile acid binders and fibric acid derivatives are sometimes helpful. Lowering high cholesterol levels using drugs can reduce the risk of heart attacks, strokes, and death.

People should stop smoking if they smoke. Stopping smoking reduces the risk of atherosclerosis by half. The benefits of stopping smoking begin immediately and increase with time.

People with atherosclerosis should lose weight if they are overweight. Losing weight reduces the risk of several risk factors for atherosclerosis: high blood pressure, diabetes, and abnormal cholesterol levels.

Regular physical activity reduces the risk of atherosclerosis. Exercise can help change other risk factors for atherosclerosis—by lowering blood pressure and cholesterol levels and by helping with weight loss.

Eating foods rich in folic acid and vitamin B_6 and B_{12} may help lower homocysteine levels and thus decrease the risk of atherosclerosis. Such foods include raw leafy green vegetables, citrus fruits, mushrooms, nuts, and enriched breads, pastas, and cereals. Even with changes in diet, some older people may still have low levels of folic acid and vitamins B_6 and B_{12}. Therefore, many experts recommend taking a daily multivitamin supplement containing these vitamins.

℞ CHOLESTEROL-LOWERING DRUGS

Type	Examples	Side Effects	Comments
Bile acid binders	Cholestyramine Colesevelam Colestipol	Constipation, abdominal pain, nausea, bloating, and an increased triglyceride level	These drugs lower the LDL cholesterol level. However, they can bind with other drugs and reduce their effectiveness
Cholesterol absorption inhibitor	Ezetimibe	Abdominal pain, diarrhea, and fatigue	Ezetimibe lowers LDL and total cholesterol levels. Often, ezetimibe is used with a statin to further lower these levels
Fibric acid derivatives	Fenofibrate Gemfibrozil	Diarrhea, nausea, bloating, abdominal pain, rash, abnormal levels of liver enzymes, muscle inflammation, and gallstones	These drugs may slightly increase the HDL cholesterol level and decrease the triglyceride level
Lipoprotein synthesis inhibitor	Niacin	Flushing, itching, digestive upset, ulcers, increased levels of liver enzymes, gout, and a high blood sugar level (hyperglycemia)	Niacin lowers the LDL cholesterol level and increases the HDL cholesterol level
Statins (HMG-CoA	Atorvastatin Fluvastatin	Mild constipation,	These drugs lower the LDL

Type	Examples	Side Effects	Comments
reductase inhibitors)	Lovastatin Pravastatin Rosuvastatin Simvastatin	loose stools, bloating, headaches, rashes, fatigue, muscle soreness (due to inflammation and degeneration), and inflammation of the liver	cholesterol level. They slightly lower the triglyceride level and moderately increase the HDL cholesterol level.

HMG-CoA = 3-hydroxy-3-methylglutaryl coenzyme A.

Symptoms and other problems due to atherosclerosis are treated. Specific treatment is needed for angina, heart attacks,[1] strokes,[2] and peripheral arterial disease (below).

PERIPHERAL ARTERIAL DISEASE

In peripheral arterial disease (also called peripheral vascular disease), blockages in peripheral arteries reduce or stop blood flow.

Peripheral arteries carry blood to tissues other than those of the brain, heart, and lungs. Most commonly, peripheral arterial disease develops in the legs. Having this disease is a bit like having clogged plumbing.

Peripheral arterial disease is very common among older people. The most common cause is atherosclerosis, which becomes increasingly common as people age. Atherosclerosis usually causes gradual blockage of arteries. Peripheral arterial disease may also result from sudden, complete blockage by part of a blood clot that formed in the heart, aorta, or another artery. Part of the clot can break off and travel through the bloodstream (becoming an embolus) until it reaches an artery that is too small for it to pass through. Some disorders (such as atrial fibrillation, aneurysms, and clotting disorders) increase the risk of blood clots.

1. see page 666
2. see page 374

Peripheral arterial disease damages tissues by depriving them of blood and thus oxygen and nutrients. The damaged tissues may die if blood flow is not improved.

Peripheral arterial disease usually causes problems in the legs first. Problems may be first noticed during walking because muscles need more oxygen during physical activity. As the disease progresses, it may affect more peripheral arteries. Sometimes arteries that carry blood to internal organs such as the stomach or intestines are affected. If peripheral arterial disease is caused by atherosclerosis, the arteries that carry blood to the heart, brain, or lungs may also be affected. Then, the risk of heart attacks, heart failure, and strokes is increased.

Peripheral arterial disease can be prevented in many people. Treatment can help control symptoms and make problems less likely to develop.

Symptoms

At first, peripheral arterial disease usually causes no symptoms. When symptoms occur, they usually involve the legs.

Most commonly, pain, tightness, or weakness is felt in the legs or buttocks during walking. This symptom is called intermittent claudication. Claudication results from a gradual blockage of leg arteries. Often, both legs are affected, but one leg can be affected more than the other. The pain, usually felt in the calves, is typically dull and achy. The legs may feel as if they are being squeezed. The pain often begins predictably. For example, it may develop after a person walks a certain number of blocks. Resting for a few minutes relieves the pain. If the blockage enlarges, the pain may begin after less activity or last longer.

At first, the leg may look almost normal. But as the blockage enlarges, muscles may shrink (atrophy). The skin may become shiny, thin, and cracked. Sores may develop on the toes or foot. Sores and wounds, including scratches and cuts, tend to heal slowly and incompletely and can easily become infected. Redness, warmth, pain, or pus around a sore or wound or a fever may indicate an infection.

If an artery is almost completely blocked, pain may occur even when a person is resting. The pain may feel like pins and needles or severe burning. It is often worse at night. The foot may become cool, pale, or turn blue. Toes or parts of the foot may die, becoming black and numb (a condition called dry gangrene). Dry gangrene sometimes leads to an infection called wet gangrene. The infection can spread up the leg within hours, destroying large amounts of tissue. The infection can also spread within the bloodstream. In either case, the person can become gravely ill very quickly, sometimes within a few hours. When the infection spreads, fever and low blood pressure usually develop, and some people die.

Excruciating pain can occur suddenly when an artery is blocked by an embolus. The pain can become unbearable within seconds. The affected foot or leg may become cool, pale, or blue within seconds and numb within minutes or hours.

Other symptoms may occur, depending on which arteries are blocked, which organ is deprived of blood, and how quickly the blockage developed. For example, gradual blockage of arteries to the intestines may cause abdominal pain that is worse after eating (bowel ischemia). Sudden blockage of arteries to the stomach or intestines can cause sudden, severe abdominal pain. In men, blood flow to the penis may be reduced, causing erectile dysfunction.

Diagnosis

To assess the blood supply to the legs, a doctor usually checks the pulse in the feet and legs. If arteries are extensively blocked, the pulse is decreased or absent. Using a blood pressure cuff, the doctor may measure blood pressure in the arms and legs. Normally, blood pressure in the thighs is as high as or a bit higher than that in the arms. If arteries in the legs are blocked, blood pressure in the part of the legs above the blockage is likely to be much higher than blood pressure in the arms. But blood pressure below the blockage is usually much lower than that in the arms. Several blood pressure cuffs may be used to check for differences in blood pressure in various parts of the leg. Blood pressure is measured on both sides of the body. Normally, the pressures are about equal. But blood pressure may be much lower on one side if arteries are blocked.

Doppler ultrasonography can be used to measure blood flow

and thus can help determine the extent of the blockage.[1] This test is simple and painless. It uses sound waves rather than radiation to produce an image. Slight blockage may not be detected if the test is done when the person is resting. So sometimes the test is done while the person is exercising the leg.

Angiography done with a long, thin tube (catheter) is the most accurate test for determining the location and extent of a blockage. In this test, dye is injected through the catheter inserted in an artery and positioned as close as possible to the affected area. Then x-rays are taken. Magnetic resonance angiography (MRA) is almost as accurate as angiography with a catheter but is safer and more comfortable. No radiation is involved. A contrast agent may be injected, but a needle (not a catheter) is used, and the needle is inserted into a vein (not an artery) and is removed as soon as the injection is complete.

Once a blockage is detected, other tests may help determine the cause. Blood tests are usually done to look for disorders that can cause atherosclerosis or blood clots. Tests are also done to determine whether atherosclerosis has affected arteries that carry blood to the heart or brain. Tests to check for coronary artery disease, such as electrocardiography or exercise echocardiography (ultrasonography of the heart during exercise stress testing), are commonly done, especially if surgery is planned. Ultrasonography may be used to check the arteries in the neck, because they carry blood to the brain.

Treatment

The goals of treatment include preventing blockages from worsening and relieving symptoms (usually claudication). Treatment may also improve the condition of the skin and help sores and wounds heal. Treatment may even prevent death due to a heart attack or stroke.

Treatment differs depending on whether the blockage occurred suddenly or developed gradually. A sudden blockage requires emergency treatment. The goal is to open the artery as quickly as possible so that tissues receive oxygen and do not die. The effects of sudden blockage may be reversed if treatment is given within hours. To open the artery, doctors try to dissolve or remove the blockage. If a blood clot is causing the

1. see page 130

blockage, a drug that dissolves clots (thrombolytic drug), such as tissue plasminogen activator or streptokinase, may be given. Sometimes these drugs can be applied directly to the clot through a catheter during angiography. If drugs do not work, surgery may be needed to remove the clot. If the clot is in a large artery, surgery may be the treatment of choice.

For blockages that developed gradually, treatment usually involves correcting or treating the risk factors for atherosclerosis.[1] These measures may prevent atherosclerosis from worsening and may even make some of the blockages in arteries shrink.

Gradually exercising the legs more can help relieve symptoms. For example, a person should walk until symptoms occur, stop and rest until symptoms resolve, then walk further. This strategy, done repeatedly, gradually increases the distance the person can walk.[2]

Drugs that prevent platelets from sticking together (antiplatelet drugs), such as aspirin, ticlopidine, and clopidogrel, may be prescribed. Platelets are small cell-like particles in the blood. They stick together to help blood clot and plug breaks in blood vessels. Thus, antiplatelet drugs can prevent clots from forming and causing more blockages. These drugs relieve symptoms. They may also prolong life because they help prevent heart attacks and strokes.

Drugs such as cilostazol and pentoxifylline, taken by mouth, are used to treat claudication, but the effectiveness of pentoxifylline has not been proved. Acetyl-L carnitine, ginkgo biloba, and vitamin E supplements are used less often. Their effectiveness is uncertain. Many other treatments, including drugs that may stimulate the growth of new blood vessels, are being studied.

Somewhat like a plumber trying to clear a clogged drain, doctors may try to mechanically open blocked arteries. For example, if an artery is blocked in only one place, a catheter with a small balloon can be inserted through the skin and into the blocked artery. Once in place, the balloon is inflated and used to clear the blockage. This procedure is called percutaneous transluminal angioplasty (PTA). It can often be done at the same

1. see page 625
2. see page 913

COLLATERAL CIRCULATION: A WAY AROUND A BLOCKAGE

Sometimes when an artery is blocked, the body forms new blood vessels—very small arteries and capillaries—to carry blood around the blockage. These blood vessels are called collateral circulation. As the blockage enlarges, more and more collateral vessels may form, depending on where the blockage is. The ability to form collateral circulation varies from person to person. The reasons for this variation are unknown. But aging itself does not appear to affect it.

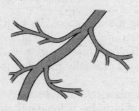

Normal Artery

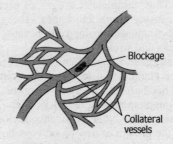

Blockage

Collateral vessels

Collateral Circulation

time as angiography. During angioplasty, a small tube of wire mesh (stent) can be inserted into the artery to keep it open.

If gradual blockage causes severe symptoms, such as pain during rest, surgery to open the blocked arteries may be necessary. Many types of surgery can be effective. For example, if the blockage is caused by atherosclerosis, the blocked portion of the artery can often be replaced with an artificial tube (graft) that bypasses the blockage.

Good foot care helps prevent infection or gangrene.[1] Each day, the feet, legs, and sores (if present) should be washed with a gentle soap. Sores should be covered with clean, dry bandages. Keeping the legs below the level of the heart helps improve blood flow and thus may speed healing. Tight shoes should not be worn. A doctor should check any sore on the foot that has not begun to heal after several days. If the sore is infected, doctors usually prescribe antibiotics. People with an infected sore may need to be hospitalized.

If people have persistent pain, severe infection, or gangrene, the leg may have to be surgically removed (amputated). A leg may be amputated below the knee, above the knee, or at the hip. Sometimes only a toe or part of the foot is amputated. Doctors usually recommend an artificial leg (prosthesis). Taking care of the remaining part of the leg (stump) is crucial. It should be kept clean and dry and checked daily for irritation, redness, and sores. Rehabilitation after amputation is intensive.[2] After surgery, physical therapy is started as soon as the person is able.

Outlook

In many people with claudication, blockage of leg arteries continues to progress. However, symptoms often do not worsen as much as blockage does because the body can form new vessels to aid blood flow. Formation of new blood vessels is called collateral circulation.

If peripheral arterial disease is part of widespread atherosclerosis, blood flow to a vital organ such as the heart or brain may be blocked. Then, serious consequences such as a heart attack or stroke may occur. Death may occur within months or years. It is often due to a heart attack or stroke.

AORTIC DISSECTION

Aortic dissection is a tear in the inner layer of the aorta's wall. Blood can surge through the tear, separating (dissecting) the inner layer from the middle and outer layers.

1. see box on page 576
2. see page 184

UNDERSTANDING AORTIC DISSECTION

In an aortic dissection, the inner layer of the aorta's wall tears. Blood can surge through the tear, separating (dissecting) the inner layer from the other layers of the wall. As a result, blood can flow between the layers, distorting that part of the aorta.

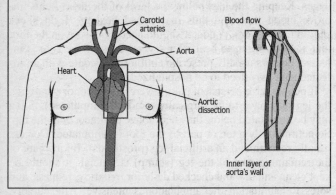

Most aortic dissections occur in people with high blood pressure, particularly men. About half occur in people over 60. Aortic dissection becomes more likely as people age.

When blood surges through the layers of the aorta's wall, it may accumulate. Then the wall may swell and become distorted. The swelling can completely block the opening of arteries that branch off the aorta. If the arteries that supply blood to the heart (coronary arteries) are blocked, the aortic valve (which controls blood flow between the left ventricle and aorta) may be damaged. Thus, blood cannot flow to vital organs, depriving them of oxygen. Blood sometimes accumulates in the sac around the heart (pericardium), causing a disorder called pericardial effusion. The accumulation of blood prevents the heart from pumping enough blood. The dissection can also cause rupture of the aorta.

Treatment involves controlling blood pressure. Surgery is often needed. Aortic dissection is often fatal. However, for some types of dissections, surgery can prolong life for many years.

Causes and Symptoms

In older people, aortic dissection often results from high blood pressure. The high pressure can cause part of the aorta's wall to deteriorate. Aging itself can cause similar deterioration. Birth defects and connective tissue disorders can cause aortic dissection but usually do so before people reach old age.

Aortic dissection typically causes pain. Usually, the pain is sudden and severe and feels like ripping or tearing. It can be felt in the back, often between the shoulder blades, or in the chest. Sometimes dissection causes only mild back pain, similar to other backaches.

When arteries are blocked, organs may not get enough blood. The consequences depend on which organs are affected and can include the following:

- Stroke if the brain is affected
- Heart attack if the heart is affected
- Sudden abdominal pain if the intestine is affected
- Lower back pain if the kidneys are affected
- Nerve damage that causes numbness, tingling, paralysis, or incontinence if the spinal cord is affected
- Pain in the feet if the leg arteries are affected

Other symptoms may include shortness of breath, loss of consciousness, low blood pressure, or shock. These symptoms can develop if blood accumulates in the sac around the heart, preventing the heart from pumping enough blood. Heart failure may develop if the aortic valve is damaged. The dissected aorta may rupture, causing a person to go into shock and die quickly.

Diagnosis

Doctors may suspect aortic dissection when the pulse or blood pressure is decreased in one or more limbs. With a stethoscope, they may hear a heart murmur.

A chest x-ray sometimes shows signs of dissection but is not conclusive. The diagnosis must be confirmed by another test. The preferred tests are computed tomography (CT) done after dye is injected into a vein, magnetic resonance imaging (MRI), and transesophageal echocardiography. For transesophageal echocardiography, an imaging device is passed down the throat into the esophagus. Occasionally, angiography is necessary. For this test, x-rays are taken while dye is injected through a long, thin tube (catheter) into the aorta.

Treatment and Outlook

People with aortic dissection are admitted to an intensive care unit. Drugs are given intravenously to lower blood pressure and reduce the force of the heart's contractions. Thus, pressure on the aorta's wall is reduced. If the dissection occurs in the part of the aorta close to the heart, surgery is done. The affected part of the aorta is usually replaced with an artificial tube (graft). If the dissection occurs in a part of the aorta farther from the heart, surgery may not be necessary. In these cases, lowering blood pressure may be sufficient.

Without treatment, most people with aortic dissection die within 2 weeks. Dissections that occur in the part of the aorta close to the heart are the most deadly. With treatment, most people who survive the first 2 weeks live for at least another 5 years.

ANEURYSMS

An aneurysm is a bulge that develops in the wall of an artery. Aneurysms usually develop in large arteries (such as the aorta), but they can develop in any artery.

Aneurysms are common. Most develop in older people, particularly in men and in people who have atherosclerosis and high blood pressure.

Most aneurysms are small and do not cause serious problems. Large aneurysms may rupture, causing bleeding. If an aneurysm in the aorta ruptures, the bleeding can be massive or fatal. When aneurysms rupture, the tissues supplied by the artery are deprived of blood and thus oxygen and nutrients. Occasionally, aneurysms of the aorta result in dissection of the aorta's wall.

Because blood does not flow normally through aneurysms, blood clots (thrombi) can develop and block blood flow through them. Part of a clot may break off, travel through the bloodstream (becoming an embolus), and eventually block a small artery in another part of the body. Occasionally, an aneurysm presses on adjacent body structures, producing pain or causing tissues to break down (deteriorate).

Most aneurysms, if detected early, can be treated. Treatment is more likely to be effective if it is given before an aneurysm ruptures.

In older people, aneurysms most commonly develop in the part of the aorta that is in the abdomen. They are called abdominal aortic aneurysms. The second most common site is the popliteal artery, located at the back of the knee. Aneurysms may also develop in the part of aorta that is in the chest. They are called thoracic aortic aneurysms. Aneurysms can develop in the arteries that lead from the aorta to the leg arteries (iliac arteries), the main arteries of the thighs (femoral arteries), arteries in the neck (carotid arteries—which carry blood to the brain), and the heart's arteries (coronary arteries). Aneurysms can develop in the arteries within the brain,[1] but these aneurysms usually cause symptoms and are diagnosed and treated before age 65.

Causes

In older people, most aneurysms develop because the arteries have been weakened by years of atherosclerosis.[2] High blood pressure (which puts added pressure on arteries) and cigarette smoking (which can damage arteries) make aneurysms more likely to develop. High blood pressure also tends to make existing aneurysms enlarge and sometimes rupture.

Symptoms

Often, aneurysms do not produce symptoms until just before they rupture.

Before an abdominal aortic aneurysm ruptures, a pulsing sensation may be felt in the abdomen. Typically, when the aneurysm begins to rupture, pain is first felt as a deep, penetrating pain in the back or abdomen. The area over the aneurysm may become tender. As the rupture progresses, it often causes sudden, excruciating pain in the lower abdomen and back. If the resulting internal bleeding is severe, the person rapidly goes into shock, often losing consciousness and collapsing. Sometimes an aneurysm causes mild pain in the back or abdomen

1. see page 378
2. see page 624

that comes and goes. The pain is usually caused by a series of small ruptures that become covered with blood clots.

Thoracic aortic aneurysms may become very large without causing symptoms. Symptoms vary but can include pain (usually high in the back), coughing, and wheezing. Rarely, a person coughs up blood if an aneurysm presses on an airway wall, causing it to break down. Swallowing may be difficult and hoarseness may develop if an aneurysm presses on the lower part of the throat.

Rupture of a thoracic aortic aneurysm usually causes excruciating pain high in the back. The pain may radiate down the back and into the abdomen as the rupture progresses. Pain may also be felt in the chest and arms. Internal bleeding may cause the person to rapidly go into shock.

Usually, aneurysms in arteries in the limbs do not cause pain unless they rupture, and they rupture much less often. But if blood clots develop and part of the clot breaks off and blocks a small artery, the skin over areas beyond the blockage may become pale and cool. If the blockage persists, gangrene may develop in the limb, which sometimes must be amputated.

Diagnosis

Aneurysms, particularly abdominal aortic aneurysms, may be found unexpectedly when a doctor performs a physical examination or a test for another reason. A doctor checks the aorta by pressing deeply on the abdomen. If the aorta feels unusually large or is pulsing too forcefully, the doctor suspects an abdominal aortic aneurysm. With a stethoscope placed over the aneurysm, the doctor can sometimes hear a whooshing sound (bruit).

Abdominal aortic aneurysms are usually diagnosed and measured using ultrasonography. Computed tomography (CT) and magnetic resonance imaging (MRI) are sometimes used. A thoracic aortic aneurysm can be diagnosed using CT, MRI, or transesophageal echocardiography (in which an imaging device is passed down the throat into the esophagus). Angiography of the aorta may be needed. For this test, dye is injected through a long, thin tube (catheter) that is inserted into a vein and threaded to the aorta. Then x-rays are taken. The dye outlines the aneurysm.

ANEURYSMS IN THE AORTA

Most commonly, aneurysms develop in the part of the aorta that is in the abdomen. These aneurysms are called abdominal aortic aneurysms. Other aneurysms, called thoracic aortic aneurysms, may develop in the part of the aorta in the chest. However, aneurysms can develop in any artery.

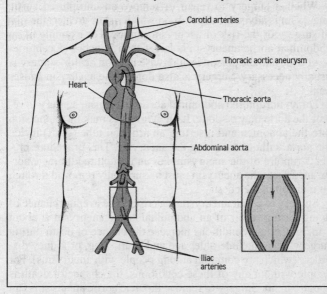

Aneurysms of leg arteries can be accurately diagnosed using ultrasonography or CT. Angiography is accurate and provides even more details about the aneurysm. But usually, angiography is done only when surgery to repair the aneurysm is being planned.

Because the chance of an aneurysm rupturing without warning often depends on its size, tests may have to be repeated periodically to see whether the aneurysm is enlarging. For example, if an abdominal aortic aneurysm is more than 1½ inches (4 centimeters) wide, ultrasonography or CT should be done every 6 months.

Treatment

Controlling blood pressure as closely as possible with drugs[1] can help prevent an aneurysm from enlarging. Beta-blockers, which decrease the force of the heart's contraction, are particularly useful.

Whether surgery to repair or remove an unruptured aortic aneurysm is advisable depends on which risk is greater: the risk of surgery or the risk of aneurysm rupture. For example, if an abdominal aortic aneurysm is larger than 2 inches (5 centimeters) wide and the person is otherwise in good health, surgery is usually necessary. Surgery is also done if the aneurysm causes pain.

For an unruptured abdominal aortic aneurysm, surgery to repair the aorta may be done. It often involves making an incision into the abdomen and inserting an artificial tube (graft) inside the aorta without removing the aneurysm. This procedure prevents rupture of the aneurysm. For an unruptured thoracic aortic aneurysm, the aneurysm must be surgically removed through an incision in the chest.

Surgery to repair aneurysms has risks. The average chance of dying during repair of an abdominal aortic aneurysm is about 1 in 20. Certain conditions increase the chance of death during surgery. They include older age and heart, lung, or kidney disorders (which are common among people with aneurysms). For people without any of these conditions, the chance of death is about 1 in 50. Surgery to remove thoracic aortic aneurysms can be comparably risky.

A new, nonsurgical technique (called endovascular repair) can be used to repair unruptured abdominal aortic aneurysms. After numbing the insertion site with a local anesthetic, the doctor inserts an artificial tube into an artery near the top of the leg and guides it into the aneurysm. The tube is similar to the one inserted during surgery, but it is collapsed, so that it can fit into a blood vessel. Once inside the aneurysm, the tube expands, forming a new channel for blood flow. This technique appears to be effective.

If an aneurysm causes pain, surgery is usually necessary because rupture is very likely. If an abdominal or thoracic aortic aneurysm ruptures, the only chance for survival is emergency

1. see page 617

surgery. The goal of emergency surgery is to replace the ruptured part of the aorta with a graft. Even with surgery, rupture
of an abdominal or a thoracic aortic aneurysm is fatal more than
half of the time. Death often results from loss of blood.

Leg artery aneurysms, whether ruptured or not, are usually
repaired surgically. The risk of death during surgery is slight,
and if surgery is not done, the risk of losing the leg is high because clots can form and block blood flow.

Outlook

Aneurysms tend to enlarge, particularly if subjected to the
wear and tear caused by high blood pressure. However, they
tend to enlarge slowly. The larger the aneurysm, the greater the
chance of rupture. Rupture is unlikely for abdominal aortic
aneurysms smaller than 2 inches (5 centimeters) wide, for thoracic aortic aneurysms smaller than $2^{1}/_{2}$ inches (6 centimeters)
wide, and for most leg artery aneurysms. Abdominal aortic
aneurysms larger than 3 inches ($7^{1}/_{2}$ centimeters) are likely to
rupture eventually and without warning.

VARICOSE VEINS

**Varicose veins are swollen, stretched, or twisted veins lo-
cated just under the skin (superficial veins). Varicose veins
usually develop in the legs and are often visible.**

Varicose veins are very common. They affect more women
than men. Varicose veins frequently develop after age 40 and
worsen as people age. Sometimes they are a symptom of another disorder.

Varicose veins can cause bothersome symptoms and minor
blood clots, and they can mar the appearance of the legs. However, they usually do not cause serious problems.

Individual varicose veins can be treated. However, unless the
cause is a curable disorder, no treatment can cure all of a person's varicose veins.

Causes

Aging itself can contribute to varicose veins because veins
become less elastic. Then, veins widen when blood flow increases but may not return to their original size when blood flow

VALVES IN VARICOSE VEINS

In a normal vein, the valves close to prevent the backward flow of blood.
In a varicose vein, the valves cannot close because the vein is abnormally
widened. Consequently, blood can flow backward.

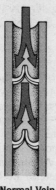

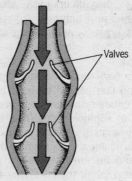

Valves

Normal Vein   **Varicose Vein**

decreases. They may become permanently widened. As a result,
the flaps of the vein's valves are too far apart and cannot close
to keep blood from flowing backward. The backward flow of
blood can widen the veins even more.

Varicose veins often develop in people who are overweight,
in women who have been pregnant several times, and in people
who repeatedly stand for long periods of time. Varicose veins
also tend to run in families.

Varicose veins can develop when veins deeper in the legs are
blocked by clots or are damaged and cannot carry enough
blood. As a result, blood from these veins backs up in the superficial leg veins and increases pressure in them.

Varicose veins sometimes develop when large veins in the
abdomen are blocked and pressure in them increases. Blood
then backs up in the veins of the legs, increasing pressure in
them. Cirrhosis and some pelvic or abdominal tumors can cause
varicose veins in this way.

Symptoms and Diagnosis

Varicose veins bulge visibly, particularly when a person is standing. They may be twisted, coiled, or blue. Usually, there are no other symptoms. Itching or a rash may develop. If the veins are very large, the affected leg may tire more easily. Occasionally, pain occurs in the affected leg. If cut, a varicose vein can bleed profusely.

Many people with varicose veins also have spider veins, which are, despite the name, enlarged capillaries, not veins. Capillaries are tiny blood vessels that connect the arteries and veins. Spider veins appear as purple or red branches, resembling a spider web.

If varicose veins result from problems with deep leg veins, the area just above the ankle may become chronically swollen, and brown areas may develop on the skin. Sometimes deep sores (venous ulcers)[1] also develop.

Occasionally, a varicose vein becomes inflamed and painful because a clot forms in it. This disorder is called superficial thrombophlebitis.

Varicose veins are usually diagnosed based on symptoms and results of the physical examination.

Treatment and Outlook

Wearing elastic stockings to compress the legs is usually the only treatment recommended for older people. The stockings squeeze the legs and help prevent excess blood from accumulating, stretching the veins, and causing pain. Elevating the legs and avoiding standing for long periods of time may also help.

Treatments designed to remove or hide individual varicose veins can make the veins less obvious, but such treatments do not improve a person's health. One of these treatments, called sclerotherapy, involves injecting an irritating solution into the veins. The solution makes the veins scar and shrink. Varicose veins can also be removed surgically. This procedure is called vein stripping. Laser treatment is being tried, but whether it is effective and safe is unclear.

For most people, the most troubling aspect of varicose veins is their appearance. Serious problems are rare.

1. see page 509

SUPERFICIAL THROMBOPHLEBITIS

Superficial thrombophlebitis is pain and inflammation in a vein just under the skin (superficial vein).

Superficial thrombophlebitis is common. The cause is a blood clot (thrombus) in the vein. Veins in a leg are most often affected. Superficial thrombophlebitis usually develops in a varicose vein, but most varicose veins are not affected.

Superficial thrombophlebitis does not usually cause serious problems. Some people with superficial thrombophlebitis in the leg also have deep vein thrombosis, which is more serious.

Causes

Any condition that causes blood to pool and clot, such as varicose veins or a minor injury that causes swelling in a vein, can lead to superficial thrombophlebitis. Occasionally, superficial thrombophlebitis develops after a long, thin tube (catheter) is inserted into a vein as part of treatment, especially if the vein is irritated or an infection develops.

Rarely, thrombophlebitis occurs repeatedly in normal veins. This disorder is called migratory phlebitis or migratory thrombophlebitis. It may be a sign of a serious underlying disorder, such as cancer or excessive blood clotting.

Symptoms and Diagnosis

The skin over the affected vein becomes red, swollen, warm, and tender. This area is sometimes very painful. Because blood in the vein is clotted, the vein feels like a hard cord under the skin. The vein may feel hard along its entire length.

The diagnosis is based on symptoms and results of a physical examination. If superficial thrombophlebitis develops in a leg—particularly if the person is at risk of having deep vein thrombosis or if the leg is swollen—tests such as Doppler ultrasonography may be done to check for blood clots in deep leg veins.

Treatment and Outlook

Usually, superficial thrombophlebitis resolves within several days. Occasionally, swelling and hardness persist for weeks. If the cause is a serious disorder or if the person has deep vein thrombosis, superficial thrombophlebitis may last longer or may recur.

The goal of treatment is to relieve symptoms. Usually, a non-steroidal anti-inflammatory drug (NSAID) is recommended. Soaking the leg in warm water or placing warm compresses on the affected area and elevating the leg may help.

Superficial thrombophlebitis rarely causes serious problems. In superficial thrombophlebitis, blood clots are unlikely to break off, travel through the bloodstream, and block an artery elsewhere in the body. The clots usually adhere to the vein. Drugs that make blood less likely to clot (anticoagulants) are not needed, unless the clot extends into the femoral vein, the largest vein in the leg.

DEEP VEIN THROMBOSIS

Deep vein thrombosis (also called deep vein thrombophlebitis, or DVT) is the formation of blood clots (thrombi) in the deep veins. Deep veins are located in the muscles or deeper.

Deep vein thrombosis is common. Inactivity increases the chance of developing deep vein thrombosis. This disorder usually affects veins in the calves or thighs.

Occasionally in deep vein thrombosis, part of one or more blood clots breaks off, travels through the veins and heart (becoming an embolus), and blocks the arteries that carry blood to the lungs. This blockage is called pulmonary embolism, which can have serious consequences.

If deep vein thrombosis persists or recurs, leg veins and the valves in them can be permanently damaged. Then blood flow back to the heart is reduced. Blood pools in veins, causing fluid to leak from the veins into tissues. This disorder is called chronic venous insufficiency.

If diagnosed before much damage has occurred, deep vein thrombosis can usually be treated effectively.

Causes

Usually, deep vein thrombosis develops in the leg veins. When a person is inactive, the leg muscles do not contract and squeeze blood vessels forcefully enough to propel blood to the heart. Blood then pools in the leg veins, where it can clot easily. Any long period of inactivity can cause deep vein thrombosis. For example, paralysis of the legs, bed rest (as required for treatment of heart failure or after hip surgery), and even long airplane flights or car trips can cause deep vein thrombosis.

Deep vein thrombosis usually develops in people whose blood is otherwise normal. However, abnormalities that make blood more likely to clot (such as some cancers, clotting disorders, and dehydration) can result in deep vein thrombosis. It can also result from damage to veins, such as that due to an injury or surgery.

Symptoms

Many people with deep vein thrombosis have no symptoms or only mild symptoms. Symptoms can include deep aching pain. The calf or thigh often swells. Swelling worsens after the leg has been lower than the body (often during the day, after walking and sitting) and lessens after the leg is elevated (often at night, after lying in bed). Sometimes the skin over the affected vein (often in the calf) appears red and feels warm or tender. Deep vein thrombosis can cause varicose veins.[1]

If pulmonary embolism occurs, people can become short of breath, develop a rapid heart rate or low blood pressure, or lose consciousness. The severity of the symptoms depends on the size and number of pulmonary emboli. Rarely, death occurs without warning.

If chronic venous insufficiency develops, the legs may become chronically swollen.

Diagnosis

Because deep vein thrombosis can lead to serious problems, tests are often done to detect the disorder even when symptoms are mild. Deep vein thrombosis can usually be diagnosed using Doppler ultrasonography.[2]

Doctors may use a specific blood test to help them diagnose deep vein thrombosis or pulmonary embolism. This test can detect blood clots by measuring a protein called D-dimer. D-dimer is released into the bloodstream when blood clots are being

1. see page 645
2. see page 130

formed and broken down. However, the test is not always helpful, because the level of D-dimer in the blood can be high in other disorders.

If a person is short of breath, doctors may measure the level of oxygen in the blood (oxygen saturation). Doctors may use a device called a pulse oximeter, which is attached to a finger, toe, or ear lobe for several seconds. Or the oxygen level may be measured in a sample of blood. A low oxygen level suggests pulmonary embolism. However, an imaging study is needed to confirm the diagnosis. Usually, nuclear scanning of the lungs is done. For this test, a small amount of a radioactive material is injected into a vein, and a scanner produces a picture of how the material flows through the lungs' blood vessels. Sometimes angiography is necessary. For this test, x-rays are taken while dye is injected into the pulmonary artery. Sometimes a type of computed tomography (CT) called helical (spiral) CT may be used for diagnosis.

Prevention

Preventing deep vein thrombosis is important because serious problems can develop without warning. Many preventive measures can be effective. During any period of inactivity (such as sitting or having to stay in bed for a long time), the legs should be stretched frequently. During long flights or car trips, a person should walk every 2 hours.

If a person is temporarily confined to bed, pneumatic stockings effectively prevent deep vein thrombosis. These stockings are repeatedly inflated then deflated by an electric pump. Inflating them helps squeeze the calves and empty the veins. The stockings can be applied before surgery and kept on until the person can walk. Pneumatic stockings are also helpful for people permanently confined to bed.

Drugs that make blood less likely to clot (anticoagulants, sometimes called blood thinners) can be given to people who are hospitalized and who are at high risk of deep vein thrombosis. For example, these drugs may be given to people confined to bed after certain types of surgery. Usually, the anticoagulant heparin or a related drug is injected under the skin daily.

When not in bed, people with chronic venous insufficiency can wear elastic stockings. These stockings help prevent deep vein thrombosis and leg sores and reduce swelling.

UMBRELLAS:
PREVENTING PULMONARY EMBOLISM

In people who have deep vein thrombosis, part of a blood clot in an affected leg vein may break off and travel through the bloodstream (becoming an embolus). After traveling through veins and the heart, the embolus can become lodged in one of the arteries that carry blood to the lungs (pulmonary arteries). It may block blood flow, causing pulmonary embolism. To prevent pulmonary embolism, doctors may recommend that a filter, called an umbrella, be permanently placed in the vein that carries blood from the legs to the heart (inferior vena cava). The filter traps emboli before they reach the heart but allows blood to flow through freely.

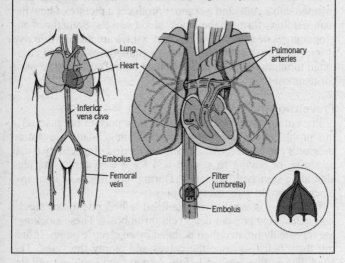

Treatment and Outlook

The goal of treatment is to dissolve the clot and prevent pulmonary embolism. Hospitalization is often necessary. Usually, an anticoagulant, such as heparin or a related drug, is injected into a vein. After a few days, another anticoagulant, warfarin, taken by mouth, is started. The heparin injections are discontinued within the next several days. People may need to take an anticoagulant for several months. Because taking an anticoagulant increases the risk of excessive bleeding, blood tests must be done periodically to check whether the blood is taking too long to clot. The doctor can then increase or decrease the dose of the anticoagulant if needed.

A drug that dissolves blood clots (thrombolytic drug), such as tissue plasminogen activator, urokinase, or streptokinase, is sometimes given, particularly if symptoms are severe.

If pulmonary embolism develops, anticoagulants are given to prevent more pulmonary emboli. A thrombolytic drug may be given to dissolve a pulmonary embolus.

Sometimes doctors insert a filter (umbrella) into the vein that carries blood from the legs to the heart (inferior vena cava). The filter traps blood clots, preventing them from traveling from the legs to the lungs. The filter can be used if anticoagulants are ineffective or if a person has a condition (such as a bleeding ulcer) that makes anticoagulants particularly risky.

Unless chronic venous insufficiency or pulmonary embolism develops, the outlook for people with deep vein thrombosis is good. For people with pulmonary embolism, death is more likely if the level of oxygen in the blood has decreased, if they have lost consciousness, or if low blood pressure develops.

People often ask me how I still have the stamina to ice skate often at age 95. The answer is simple . . . I exercise and eat correctly and have a positive attitude.

For one thing, to grow old gracefully you have to keep moving. We move before we are born, and that movement must be continued throughout life. Clearly you will live longer if you exercise. Even laughing is an excellent exercise. There are special exercises for the elderly and the handicapped that can be done right in bed. Currently I am teaching an exercise class for the elderly and a separate class for those in wheelchairs.

It is best to start exercising early in life, the earlier the better. Take ice skating for example. Anyone can skate whether they are 9 or 90. Skating is easier than walking, because when you glide, you don't even have to lift your feet.

Basically you can tighten flabby muscles with contractions and stretching; you can enhance the cardiovascular system; you can correct maladjusted posture and maintain a more youthful figure and appearance . . . all through exercise.

People eat much too fast, without thought as to what they are eating and without enjoyment and without regard to their health. For example, white bread contains bleached flour. The bleach is a chemical and is not good for you. Whole wheat bread is the bread you should eat. Eating things that contain natural substances (the natural sugar in fruit for example, as opposed to artificial or refined sugar) makes sense for good health. I am living proof.

There are people who seem to be born to be lethargic. When they get sick, they don't understand why. People must be active mentally and physically and must project their mind into their energy expenditure (doing things by rote just isn't enough). Naturally, one's attitude plays an important part in the quality of life as you grow older. Positiveness is critical.

Don't think about getting older. Don't say you can't meet your goals; have faith in yourself. Think young to stay young, eat right, and exercise your mind and body every day. Remember to laugh. An old Japanese "Laughing Ritual" says to laugh heartily 3 times: Once to give thanks for yesterday, once to pray for tomorrow, and once to cleanse the mind and heart.

Melitta Brunner

45

Coronary Artery Disease

In coronary artery disease (CAD), the arteries that supply the heart with blood (coronary arteries) are partially or completely blocked.

CAD can limit activities and prevent people from living as they would like. It can also result in death, usually due to a heart attack, a disorder involving an abnormal heart rhythm (arrhythmia), or heart failure. However, much can be done to prevent and treat CAD.

In the United States, about 1 out of 6 people 65 and over has CAD. After age 65, the likelihood that a person will develop CAD increases with each passing year. In older men and women, CAD is the most common cause of death.

The heart, like other organs, needs a constant supply of blood to bring oxygen and nutrients to it and to remove waste products. The amount of oxygen the heart needs depends on how hard it is working. During physical activity, the heart has to work harder and so needs more oxygen. The right and left coronary arteries supply heart tissue with blood. They branch off the aorta just after it leaves the heart, then divide into smaller arteries.

When one or more of the arteries supplying the heart is partially blocked, the heart may not get enough oxygen. This inadequate supply of oxygen, called ischemia, often causes chest pain (angina). If an artery is completely blocked, some heart tissue may die. Death of heart tissue is called a heart attack. If a lot of heart tissue dies, the heart's ability to pump blood to the rest of the body is impaired, causing heart failure.[1] If ischemia or a

---

1. see page 680

heart attack affects certain areas of the heart, the heart's electrical system may malfunction, leading to an abnormal heart rhythm.[1]

Causes

CAD is almost always caused by atherosclerosis.[2] In atherosclerosis, cholesterol and other materials are deposited in the wall of an artery, forming plaques (atheromas). As these plaques enlarge, they partially or completely block the artery. With time, calcium accumulates in the plaques. This process usually takes many years or even decades. For this reason, CAD is more common among older people. Occasionally, a blood clot forms on a plaque, making the degree of blockage greater and sometimes blocking the artery completely.

Certain circumstances and disorders (called risk factors) can make atherosclerosis and thus CAD more likely to develop. They include the following:

- Smoking
- Physical inactivity
- Excess body weight
- Parents or siblings who developed CAD before age 50 to 55 (family history)
- Older age
- Male sex
- High blood pressure
- Abnormal levels of cholesterol and triglycerides in the blood
- Diabetes
- A high level of C-reactive protein (CRP) in the blood

If CAD is present, these risk factors can make it worse.

Smoking greatly increases the risk of developing CAD and of making it worse. The more cigarettes smoked, the greater the risk. Also, older people who continue to smoke after having a heart attack are two to three times more likely to have another heart attack or to die within 5 years than those who stop.

1. see page 694
2. see page 624

BLOOD FLOW THROUGH THE HEART

Blood follows a particular path from the heart to the body and back. As blood follows this path, it takes oxygen to the body's tissues and removes waste products from them.

Blood from the body enters the upper right heart chamber (right atrium), then moves through the tricuspid valve into the lower right chamber (right ventricle). This blood contains a little oxygen and a lot of carbon dioxide (a waste product of cell activity). Blood is pumped through the pulmonary valve into the pulmonary arteries and to the lungs. There, oxygen is added and carbon dioxide is removed from the blood.

This oxygen-rich blood travels back to the heart through the pulmonary veins. It enters the left atrium, then moves through the mitral valve into the left ventricle. The left ventricle pumps blood through the aortic valve into the aorta and to all of the body.

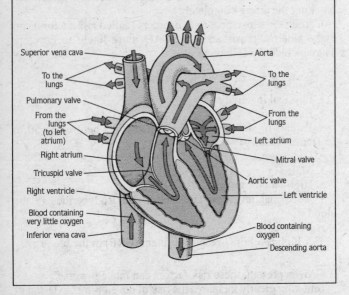

Labels (left side, top to bottom): Superior vena cava; To the lungs; Pulmonary valve; From the lungs (to left atrium); Right atrium; Tricuspid valve; Right ventricle; Blood containing very little oxygen; Inferior vena cava

Labels (right side, top to bottom): Aorta; To the lungs; From the lungs; Left atrium; Mitral valve; Aortic valve; Left ventricle; Blood containing oxygen; Descending aorta

Men tend to develop CAD about 10 years earlier than women, because until menopause, women seem to be protected by female hormones such as estrogen. After menopause, blood pressure and cholesterol levels tend to increase, and the risk of CAD increases.

High blood pressure is the most common risk factor for CAD

in older people. For most older people, blood pressure should be lower than 140/90 mm Hg (millimeters of mercury).

Diabetes is a risk factor for CAD regardless of what the levels of sugar in the blood are. If blood sugar levels are poorly controlled, the risk is even greater.

Abnormal cholesterol levels include a high level of total cholesterol, a high level of low-density lipoprotein cholesterol (LDL, the "bad" cholesterol), and a low level of high-density lipoprotein cholesterol (HDL, the "good" cholesterol).[1] High levels of triglycerides (another fat in the blood) may also increase the risk of CAD. Diet, exercise, weight, and genes affect cholesterol and triglyceride levels.

A high level of C-reactive protein in the blood indicates persistent inflammation (as occurs in rheumatoid arthritis). Inflammation, regardless of where it occurs in the body, may damage arteries, enabling plaques to form.[2]

A high level of homocysteine (an amino acid) in the blood may increase the risk of CAD. But the importance of a high homocysteine level is not yet known. Depression and significant stress (such as the death of a spouse) may increase risk.

Rarely, the muscle layer of a coronary artery's wall suddenly and temporarily contracts (constricts), causing a spasm. A spasm can temporarily reduce or cut off blood flow to the heart.

Symptoms

Symptoms of CAD may occur when part of the heart does not get enough oxygen, causing ischemia in heart tissue (myocardial ischemia). Or symptoms may occur when part of the heart dies—that is, when a heart attack (myocardial infarction) occurs.

The most common symptom of myocardial ischemia is discomfort in the center of the chest, behind the breastbone. This discomfort, known as angina, is often described as pressure, tightness, squeezing, or heaviness (like a weight on the chest). Angina may or may not be painful. It may be felt only in the chest, or it may move. Most commonly, it moves down the left arm. It may move to the back, throat, neck, jaw, teeth, or right arm. Angina is usually triggered by situations in which the heart

1. see box on page 625
2. see page 624

is working harder and needs more oxygen than usual. Examples are physical activity or emotional stress. The discomfort usually develops gradually (without a sudden, sharp pain) and subsides gradually after a few minutes (up to about 20 minutes). Angina may occur several times a day or only once in a while. Angina is usually relieved by resting or by taking nitroglycerin (placed or sprayed under the tongue).[1]

Occasionally, angina is accompanied by shortness of breath, nausea, dizziness, or fatigue. People may also break out in a cold sweat or feel their heart pounding (as palpitations). In older people, the only symptom may be shortness of breath that is triggered by physical activity or stress. Some people have only a sensation that resembles indigestion but is unrelated to eating. This sensation is more likely to occur during physical activity. Sometimes the only symptom is a feeling of impending doom. Any combination of these symptoms may occur. Occasionally, ischemia may cause an older person to faint.

In many people with CAD, the pattern of symptoms remains about the same for months to years. That is, symptoms are produced by the same level of physical activity, and they do not change much in severity or frequency. In other people, symptoms gradually worsen over time. In contrast, symptoms sometimes suddenly worsen: They may become more severe, occur more often, or occur during less strenuous activity. Such sudden worsening of symptoms, called unstable angina, may mean that CAD has suddenly become worse. Immediate evaluation and treatment by a doctor are essential.

Sometimes myocardial ischemia causes no symptoms. In such cases, it is called silent ischemia.

Symptoms of a heart attack are similar to those of myocardial ischemia, but they usually last longer and are more severe. As with angina, pain due to a heart attack may be felt in the chest, neck, throat, jaw, teeth, or arms. However, in older people, a heart attack may cause little or no chest pain or discomfort. Instead, a heart attack may cause shortness of breath, a smothering feeling, nausea, vomiting, sweating, dizziness, indigestion, palpitations, overwhelming fatigue, fainting, a feeling of impending doom, or any combination of these symptoms. Less commonly, older people who are having a heart attack become

1. see page 671

confused, disoriented, or restless. About one fourth of heart attacks occur without symptoms, as silent heart attacks. Silent heart attacks are more common among people with diabetes.

As people age, the heart becomes less able to handle the stress of a heart attack. Heart failure may cause accumulation of fluid in the lungs (pulmonary edema). Other common problems include low blood pressure (hypotension) and abnormal heart rhythms (arrhythmias), such as atrial fibrillation and ventricular tachycardia. Less commonly, the heart muscle may tear (rupture), or a blood clot may form in the heart. Heart attacks can also lead to cardiogenic shock, which, if untreated, results in death. In cardiogenic shock, the heart cannot pump enough blood to the brain, kidneys, and other organs. As a result, these organs cannot function. Sometimes a heart attack causes death immediately because of a very fast irregular heart rhythm (venticular fibrillation).

After a heart attack, many people feel depressed, nervous, or anxious. To some degree, these feelings are a normal reaction to having had a heart attack. However, if these feelings are too intense or if they persist for more than a few weeks, they may interfere with normal recovery, and treatment may be needed.

Diagnosis

If older people develop any of the symptoms that might be caused by CAD, they should immediately contact their doctor.

If a person has typical symptoms and risk factors for CAD, the diagnosis is usually made easily. One or more tests may be done to confirm the diagnosis and to determine how extensive CAD is.

Electrocardiography (ECG), a safe, quick, and painless test, is often done first. Small sensors (electrodes) are attached to the person's arms, legs, and chest. Electrodes detect the electrical currents produced in the heart during each heartbeat. The electrical currents are recorded as lines on a strip of graph paper (the electrocardiogram). Electrocardiography can often detect whether a heart attack is occurring or has already occurred. It may detect ischemia. However, this test does not always detect CAD, especially in people who are not having symptoms when the test is done. For this reason, a stress test is often recommended.

RECOGNIZING A HEART ATTACK

Some heart attacks are severe and sudden, and there is no doubt about what is happening. But many heart attacks begin more subtly and gradually. People may not recognize what is happening to them. However, certain symptoms may indicate that a heart attack is happening. People who have one or more of these symptoms, even if the symptom goes away, should immediately call an emergency telephone number (usually 911) or go to the hospital.

Getting treatment as soon as possible can reduce the amount of damage done to the heart and increase the chances of a good recovery. Symptoms of a heart attack include the following:

• Discomfort—pressure, tightness, squeezing, heaviness, or pain—in the center of the chest that lasts more than a few minutes
• Discomfort or pain in other areas of the upper body, especially the left arm, that lasts more than a few minutes
• Shortness of breath that lasts more than a few minutes, especially if it is not caused by a person's activities (such as vigorous exercise) or another disorder (such as chronic obstructive pulmonary disease, or COPD)
• Indigestion that lasts more than a few minutes and that is unrelated to eating
• Fainting
• A cold sweat

In a stress test, the heart has to work harder. Then, heart problems are more likely to be detected. This test is safe and can detect most cases of CAD. Stress tests often involve exercise, usually walking on a treadmill or pedaling a stationary bicycle. For people who cannot exercise, a drug such as dobutamine or adenosine can be given intravenously to stress the heart. Throughout a stress test, heart rate, blood pressure, and the electrocardiogram are recorded and closely monitored.

Echocardiography or nuclear (radionuclide) scanning may be done during a stress test. These tests are used to detect ischemia. They can also detect damage to the heart (such as that due to a heart attack) and determine how well the heart is pumping. In echocardiography, a hand-held device that sends and receives high-frequency sound (ultrasound) waves is placed on the person's chest. The ultrasound waves are used to produce a moving image of the heart. In nuclear scanning, pictures of the heart are taken after a tiny amount of a radioactive substance (radionuclide) is injected into a vein.

Sometimes computed tomography (CT) is used to detect

CAD.[1] It is done to check for calcium that can accumulate in plaques in coronary arteries. This test is simple, safe, quick, and painless. But its value in diagnosing CAD in older people is unclear. In this test, several x-rays are taken, and a computer is used to produce images of the coronary arteries.

Coronary angiography (cardiac catheterization) is the most accurate way to detect CAD and to determine the extent and location of blockages.[2] This information helps doctors decide which treatments are best—for example, whether angioplasty or bypass surgery is needed. Cardiac catheterization can usually be done safely in people of all ages. However, it involves more risks than other tests, because it is invasive. (Invasive tests involve an incision or insertion of an instrument into the body.) The risk of serious problems is small, although the risk is somewhat higher for older people. The value of the information it provides greatly outweighs its small potential risk.

Cardiac catheterization is often recommended if symptoms and the results of other tests suggest that blockage of the coronary arteries could have serious consequences. Cardiac catheterization may also be done if other tests cannot confirm the diagnosis.

In cardiac catheterization, a long thin tube (catheter) is inserted into an artery near the hip (usually) or elbow and threaded to the heart. A dye is injected through the catheter to outline the coronary arteries and heart's chambers. Many x-rays are taken to look for blockages and to determine how well the heart is functioning.

After cardiac catheterization, the most common problem is bleeding at the site where the catheter was inserted. Usually, bleeding is mild, resulting in a bruise. Occasionally, bleeding is severe enough that a blood transfusion is needed. The risk of bleeding can be reduced by not moving the leg or arm into which the catheter had been inserted for several hours. Rarely, an artery is damaged, and surgery is needed to repair it. Other serious problems that can occur during or after cardiac catheterization include an allergic reaction to the dye, a heart attack, a stroke, an abnormal heart rhythm, and kidney failure.

If doctors suspect unstable angina or a heart attack, blood

1. see page 124
2. see page 132

tests are done. A small amount of blood is drawn every 6 to 12 hours for 1 or 2 days. The blood is tested for proteins that are released into the bloodstream when the heart is damaged. These proteins include CK-MB, troponin I, and troponin T. If the level of any of these proteins is increased, heart tissue has been damaged or has died, probably because of a heart attack.

Prevention

Eating a healthy, well-balanced diet can help prevent CAD.[1] Such a diet should be high in fiber and low in saturated fats, artificially hydrogenated fats (trans fatty acids), cholesterol, and foods containing simple or refined carbohydrates. It should include plenty of fruits, vegetables, and whole-grain foods.

Eliminating or controlling risk factors for CAD may help prevent the disease.

Stopping smoking is the single most important thing a person can do to prevent a heart attack. For people who smoke cigarettes, stopping smoking cuts the risk of having a heart attack in half. The benefit of stopping smoking is at least as great for older people as for younger people.

Exercising regularly can help reduce the risk of CAD.[2] Any regular exercise is better than no exercise. A good goal is 30 minutes of exercise at least 4 days a week. For most older people, walking is best. But jogging, swimming, and stationary cycling are good alternatives. These activities are aerobic exercise. That is, they require getting a continuous supply of oxygen from the air to the muscles being exercised. Aerobic exercise improves endurance and is particularly helpful in preventing CAD. But other types of exercise—flexibility (stretching) and strengthening exercises (such as weight training)—also help by maintaining general health and fitness. Exercising regularly, even in small amounts, is particularly beneficial for people who have been doing very little or no exercise.

Before starting an exercise program, older people should check with their doctor. If chest pain, shortness of breath, dizziness, or other symptoms occur, people should stop exercising and contact their doctor.

In addition to regular exercise, developing and maintaining a

1. see page 41
2. see page 909

more active lifestyle can also help prevent CAD. For example, daily activities, such as gardening or housecleaning, can be done more vigorously or more often. Other ways to become more active are to walk instead of drive and to take the stairs instead of the elevator whenever possible.

The risk of developing high blood pressure can be reduced. Ways to help reduce the risk include exercising regularly, maintaining a healthy weight, eating a healthy diet, and limiting the amount of salt and alcohol consumed. People who already have high blood pressure may need to take antihypertensive drugs[1] in addition to exercising and changing their diet. Losing weight if overweight and stopping smoking are also recommended.

If cholesterol levels are abnormal, stopping smoking, exercising regularly, and eating a healthy diet can help. People should reduce the amount of saturated fat and trans fatty acids they consume. When possible, monounsaturated fats and poly-unsaturated fats, particularly omega-3 fats,[2] should be substituted for saturated fats and trans fatty acids. Eating plenty of fruits, vegetables, and whole-grain foods also helps control cholesterol levels. However, most older people with high cholesterol levels need to take drugs. Statins, such as atorvastatin, fluvastatin, lovastatin, pravastatin, rosuvastatin, and simvastatin, are commonly used. Statins are especially helpful for older people with diabetes, regardless of what their cholesterol levels are. Other cholesterol-lowering drugs, such as cholestyramine, ezetimibe, gemfibrozil, and niacin, are also used.[3]

Low levels of vitamins B_6 and B_{12} and folic acid may contribute to the risk of CAD. Many older people have low levels of these vitamins. Therefore, many experts recommend a daily multivitamin supplement containing these vitamins. Other dietary supplements do not appear to help prevent CAD.

Reaching and maintaining a healthy weight can help control several risk factors for CAD: diabetes, high blood pressure, and abnormal cholesterol and triglyceride levels. Eating a healthy diet and exercising regularly can help people reach and maintain a healthy weight.

For people with diabetes, controlling the levels of sugar in

1. see table on page 618
2. see table on page 628
3. see table on page 630

the blood can help reduce the risk of CAD. Blood sugar levels can be controlled effectively with drugs combined with diet and exercise.[1]

Treatment

Treatment of CAD varies depending on how severe the symptoms are and how extensive the blockages are. Most older people who have stable angina can be treated with drugs without being hospitalized. However, people who have unstable angina or who are having a heart attack must be hospitalized and treated immediately.

The main goals of treatment are to improve blood flow through the coronary arteries, relieve symptoms, and prevent additional problems.

Several different types of drugs may be prescribed to treat stable angina. If drugs are not effective or if the blockage is substantial, angioplasty or coronary artery bypass graft surgery may be necessary. Both procedures are good options for older people. Both relieve symptoms and may prolong life. Which procedure is done depends largely on the location and degree of blockage.

Drugs: Most people with CAD take several types of drugs: aspirin (or a similar drug), beta-blockers, and nitrates. Some people also take calcium channel blockers, angiotensin-converting enzyme (ACE) inhibitors, and statins.

℞ DRUGS USED FOR CORONARY ARTERY DISEASE

Type	Examples	Possible Side Effects	Comments
Angiotensin-converting enzyme (ACE) inhibitors	Benazepril Captopril Enalapril Fosinopril Lisinopril Moexipril Perindopril Quinapril Ramipril Trandolapril	Dry cough (most common), low blood pressure, impairment of kidney function, an increased potassium level, and allergic reactions	These drugs lower blood pressure and reduce the amount of work the heart has to do. They reduce the risk of heart attacks, heart failure, and death

Type	Examples	Possible Side Effects	Comments
Angiotensin II receptor blockers	Candesartan Eprosartan Irbesartan Losartan Olmesartan Telmisartan Valsartan	Dizziness, low blood pressure, impairment of kidney function, and an increased potassium level	The effects of these drugs are similar to those of ACE inhibitors. They are used to treat people with high blood pressure. They are sometimes used instead of an ACE inhibitor to treat people with a heart disorder
Anticoagulants	Dalteparin Enoxaparin Heparin Lepirudin Tinzaparin Warfarin	Bleeding, especially when used with other drugs that have a similar effect (such as aspirin, many other nonsteroidal anti-inflammatory drugs, and other antiplatelet drugs)	These drugs make blood less likely to clot. They are used to treat people who have unstable angina or who have had a heart attack
Antiplatelet drugs	Aspirin Clopidogrel Ticlopidine	Bleeding, especially when used with other drugs that have a similar effect (such as anticoagulants) With aspirin, stomach irritation With ticlopidine and less so with clopidogrel, a small risk of reducing the number of platelets or white blood cells	These drugs prevent platelets from clumping and blood clots from forming. They also reduce the risk of heart attacks. They are used to treat people who have stable or unstable angina or who have had a heart attack. Aspirin is taken as soon as a heart attack is suspected. People with an allergy to

Table continues on the following page.

Type	Examples	Possible Side Effects	Comments
			aspirin may take clopidogrel or ticlopidine as an alternative
Glycoprotein IIb/IIIa inhibitors (a type of antiplatelet drug)	Abciximab Eptifibatide Tirofiban	Bleeding, especially when used with drugs that have a similar effect (such as anticoagulants or thrombolytic drugs), and reduction of the number of platelets	These drugs prevent other platelets from clumping and blood clots from forming. They are used to treat people who have unstable angina or who have had a heart attack
Beta-blockers	Acebutolol Atenolol Betaxolol Bisoprolol Carteolol Carvedilol Metoprolol Nadolol Penbutolol Propranolol Timolol	Spasm of the airways (bronchospasm), an abnormally slow heart rate (bradycardia), heart failure, cold hands and feet, insomnia, fatigue, shortness of breath, Raynaud's phenomenon, vivid dreams, hallucinations, and sexual dysfunction. With some beta-blockers, an increased triglyceride level	These drugs slow the heart rate and reduce the heart's need for oxygen. They also reduce the risk of heart attacks and sudden death. They are used to treat people who have stable or unstable angina or who are having or have had a heart attack
Calcium channel blockers	Amlodipine Diltiazem Felodipine Isradipine	Dizziness, heart failure, fluid accumulation (edema) in the	These drugs dilate blood vessels, improve blood flow to the heart,

Type	Examples	Possible Side Effects	Comments
	Nicardipine Nifedipine Nisoldipine Verapamil	ankles, flushing, headache, heartburn, enlarged gums, and an abnormally fast or slow heart rate. With verapamil and, less frequently, with diltiazem, constipation	and lower blood pressure. Diltiazem and verapamil slow the heart rate. Calcium channel blockers are used to treat people who have stable angina
Nitrates	Isosorbide dinitrate Isosorbide mononitrate Nitroglycerin	Flushing, headache, dizziness, fainting, and a temporarily fast heart rate (tachycardia)	These drugs dilate blood vessels. They relieve angina and prevent episodes of angina. They are used to treat people who have stable or unstable angina. People with angina should keep nitroglycerin with them at all times
Opioids	Morphine	Drowsiness, slowed breathing low blood pressure when standing up, constipation, nausea, vomiting, and confusion (especially in older people)	In people who are having a heart attack, these drugs are used to relieve anxiety and pain
Statins	Atorvastatin Fluvastatin Lovastatin	Mild constipation, loose stools, bloating,	These drugs are used primarily to control abnormal

Table continues on the following page.

Type	Examples	Possible Side Effects	Comments
	Pravastatin Rosuvastatin Simvastatin	headaches, rashes, fatigue, muscle sore-ness, and inflammation of the liver	cholesterol levels. They also reduce the risk of heart attack, stroke, and death in older people with coronary artery disease
Thrombo-lytic drugs	Anistreplase Recombinant tissue plasmino-gen activator (alteplase) Reteplase Streptokinase Tenecteplase Urokinase	Bleeding from the skin, gums, nose, or digestive tract and, rarely, bleeding within the brain (intracerebral hemorrhage)	These drugs dissolve blood clots. They are used to treat people who are having a major heart attack

Aspirin, an antiplatelet drug, reduces the risk of heart attacks and death. Antiplatelet drugs make blood clots less likely to form by preventing platelets from sticking together. The normal function of platelets is to stick together and help form blood clots that plug tears in the lining of blood vessels. However, if platelets form a clot on fatty deposits in a coronary artery, the clot may partially or completely block the artery. A heart attack may result. Doctors recommend that most people who have CAD take a small dose of aspirin (such as one children's as-pirin) daily. People with an allergy to aspirin may take another antiplatelet drug, such as ticlopidine or clopidogrel. Because aspirin and other antiplatelet drugs prevent blood from clotting normally, bleeding problems occasionally occur. Doctors may advise older people with chronic bleeding (such as that due to a bleeding ulcer) not to take antiplatelet drugs.

Beta-blockers slow the heart rate and reduce the heart's need for oxygen. They also lower blood pressure. As a result, myo-cardial ischemia is less likely to develop, and angina occurs less often. Beta-blockers also reduce the risk of heart attacks and sudden death and prolong life in people with CAD.

Nitrates, such as nitroglycerin, expand (dilate) blood vessels. Thus, they improve blood flow to the heart. Also, the heart does not have to work as hard to pump blood. Nitrates reduce the heart's need for oxygen. As a result, they relieve angina. Nitroglycerin can relieve angina in a few minutes. It is usually taken as a tablet or spray under the tongue. When the drug is taken this way, its effects last up to 30 minutes. People with angina should keep nitroglycerin with them at all times. Other nitrates, such as isosorbide, have effects that last longer. These drugs can be taken to prevent angina. They are available as tablets taken by mouth and as skin patches or ointments. When nitrates are used continuously, their effects wear off after a few hours. Consequently, people should not take nitrates for more than about 16 hours each day.

The most common side effect of nitrates is headache. For most people, headaches subside after a few days and do not interfere with long-term use of the drugs. Nitrates can also lower blood pressure, resulting in dizziness and sometimes fainting, especially in older people. Therefore, when taking nitroglycerin under the tongue, older people should sit or lie down.

Calcium channel blockers dilate blood vessels, improve blood flow to the heart, and lower blood pressure. These drugs also prevent spasms of the arteries. Calcium channel blockers are often used when people cannot take beta-blockers or when beta-blockers and nitrates do not relieve symptoms.

ACE inhibitors lower blood pressure and reduce the amount of work the heart has to do. These drugs reduce the risk of heart attacks, heart failure, and death. They are not used to relieve angina. The most common side effect is a dry, hacking cough. Occasionally, the cough is severe enough that the drug must be discontinued.

Statins are used primarily to control abnormal cholesterol levels. They reduce the risk of heart attacks, strokes, and death in older people with CAD. Muscle soreness that develops while taking a statin may indicate muscle damage. So if this symptom develops, people should contact their doctor immediately.

Coronary angioplasty: Coronary angioplasty (percutaneous transluminal coronary angioplasty, or PTCA) is used to physically open a blocked coronary artery. This procedure is often preferred to bypass surgery because it is less invasive. However, angioplasty may be impossible because the affected area is too

UNBLOCKING AN ARTERY: ANGIOPLASTY

A doctor inserts a thin tube (catheter) with a balloon at its tip through a small incision in the skin and into a large artery (usually the femoral artery in the thigh). The catheter is threaded through the connecting arteries and the aorta to the partially or completely blocked coronary artery. The balloon is inflated, compressing the blockage and thus opening up the artery. Often, a tube made of wire mesh (stent) is placed over the deflated balloon at the catheter's tip and inserted with the catheter. When the balloon is inflated, the stent opens up. Then the balloon-tipped catheter is removed, and the stent is left in place to help keep the artery open.

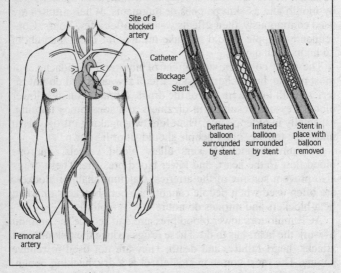

Site of a
blocked
artery

Catheter

Blockage

Stent

Femoral
artery

Deflated
balloon
surrounded
by stent

Inflated
balloon
surrounded
by stent

Stent in
place with
balloon
removed

large or there are too many blockages to be treated effectively with angioplasty.

During angioplasty, people are usually awake. The procedure is similar to angiography.[1] A thin tube (catheter) with a balloon at its tip is threaded into the blocked coronary artery. Inflating the balloon opens up the artery. Often, a small tube made of wire mesh (stent) is inserted at the same time. Angioplasty with a stent is more likely to prevent the artery from becoming blocked again than is angioplasty alone. After a stent has been

1. see pages 132 and 663

BYPASSING A CORONARY ARTERY

In coronary artery bypass surgery, a segment of an artery or a vein from another part of the body is attached (grafted) to a coronary artery. One end is attached to a coronary artery beyond the area that is blocked. The other end is attached to the aorta (which carries blood from the heart to most of the body). Blood is thus rerouted, skipping over (bypassing) the blocked area. Thus, the blood has an alternate route from the aorta to the heart, and the blocked area is bypassed. An artery near the heart (internal mammary artery) is often used. A segment of a vein, usually from a vein in the leg (saphenous vein), can also be used instead of or in addition to an artery.

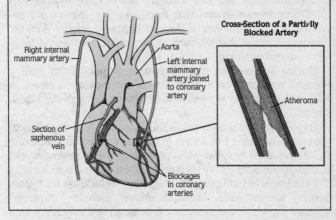

Right internal mammary artery

Aorta

Left internal mammary artery joined to coronary artery

Section of saphenous vein

Blockages in coronary arteries

Cross-Section of a Partially Blocked Artery

Atheroma

inserted, people are usually given clopidogrel or ticlopidine for up to several months. These drugs reduce the risk that a blood clot will block the artery again. Stents that are coated with a drug to further reduce the risk of blockages are available.

Sometimes angioplasty causes temporary chest pain. Other problems that can occur are the same as those for cardiac catheterization.[1] But the risk of serious problems, including heart attacks and death, is somewhat higher.

Coronary artery bypass graft surgery (CABG): In this surgery, commonly called bypass surgery, a vein or an artery from another part of the body is used to bypass the blocked coronary artery. Bypass surgery is usually recommended when there are several blockages or when the blockages occur

1. see page 663

throughout the length of a coronary artery. In such cases, angioplasty is unlikely to be effective. More than half of people who have bypass surgery are 65 or over.

For bypass surgery, a segment of an artery or a vein from another part of the body is attached (grafted) to the coronary artery. Thus, the blocked area is skipped (bypassed). Arteries are preferred to veins because they are less likely to become blocked.

Usually, more than one blockage is bypassed. A triple bypass means that three blocked coronary arteries are bypassed. A quadruple bypass means that four coronary arteries are bypassed. A higher number of blocked, bypassed arteries does not necessarily mean that the surgery was riskier or that the long-term outlook is worse.

During surgery, the heart is usually stopped from beating because operating on a heart that is not moving is easier. A heart-lung machine is used to pump blood through the bloodstream.[1]

Bypass surgery usually takes 3 to 5 hours. After surgery, people typically spend 1 to 3 days in intensive care and a total of 5 to 10 days in the hospital. Most older people need several weeks to recuperate before they can resume their normal activities.

Less invasive (and possibly less risky) techniques for bypass surgery are available. These techniques include "off-pump" surgery (in which the heart is left beating) and surgery with a smaller chest incision. The safety and effectiveness of these techniques in older people are being studied.

Bypass surgery is routine and relatively safe. However, risks are higher for older people than for younger ones, partly because older people are more likely to have other disorders that increase risk (such as diabetes, lung disorders, or kidney disorders). Problems that can occur after bypass surgery include strokes, abnormal heart rhythms, temporary confusion, difficulty breathing, pulmonary embolism, bleeding, infections, kidney failure, and death.

Emergency treatment: Anyone with angina that is worsening (unstable angina) or with symptoms that may indicate a heart attack should take one aspirin, call an emergency telephone number (such as 911), and get to a hospital immediately.

1. see box on page 721

The aspirin should be chewed so that it is absorbed more quickly.

The sooner treatment begins, the better the person's outlook. In cases of a heart attack, prompt transportation by an ambulance to an emergency department may save the person's life. Spending time trying to contact the person's doctor or waiting for family members to arrive delays treatment and is dangerous. People who have unstable angina are usually hospitalized. Those who are having a heart attack are always hospitalized.

In the emergency department, people who may have unstable angina or who have symptoms of a heart attack are given aspirin (by mouth) and oxygen (through nasal prongs or a face mask). Most people are given nitroglycerin (under the tongue, as ointment, or intravenously) and morphine (intravenously). A beta-blocker may also be given (intravenously or by mouth). Heparin, a drug that makes blood less likely to clot (anticoagulant), is often given (intravenously or by injection under the skin).

While treatment is being started, electrocardiography and blood tests are done. If these tests confirm unstable angina or a heart attack, additional treatments may be given. Glycoprotein IIb/IIIa inhibitors may be given intravenously in addition to aspirin and heparin. These drugs are powerful antiplatelet drugs that help prevent new blood clots from forming in a coronary artery.

People who have had a major heart attack may be given a drug that dissolves blood clots (thrombolytic drug). Dissolving the clot in the blocked coronary artery restores blood flow to the heart. Thus, damage to the heart is reduced, and the outlook is improved. These drugs are useful only when given within the first 6 to 12 hours of a heart attack.

Rarely, thrombolytic drugs cause serious bleeding, including bleeding into the brain. This problem occurs in fewer than 1 out of 100 people, but the risk is higher for older people. The risk is also higher for people who have very high blood pressure or who have had a stroke.

An alternative to thrombolytic drugs is cardiac catheterization, done immediately and followed by angioplasty (often with a stent). This technique opens a blocked artery more effectively than thrombolytic drugs and is less likely to result in a stroke. However, fewer than 1 out of 5 hospitals in the United States can do this procedure in an emergency situation. Rarely, cardiac catheterization done at the time of a heart attack detects extensive blockage that requires emergency bypass surgery.

Additional treatments may be needed for problems that develop after a heart attack, such as abnormal heart rhythms, heart failure, or pulmonary edema. Rarely, surgery is needed to repair a tear (rupture) in the heart caused by a heart attack.

After a heart attack, people are often given aspirin, clopidogrel or ticlopidine (especially if a stent has been inserted), a beta-blocker, an ACE inhibitor, and a statin. Some people may also be given nitrates, a calcium channel blocker, or warfarin (an anticoagulant). People who cannot tolerate an ACE inhibitor because of cough or other side effects may be given an angiotensin II receptor blocker.

Rehabilitation: After a heart attack or bypass surgery, rehabilitation is usually helpful. Rehabilitation begins in the hospital with such activities as getting out of bed, sitting in a chair, and going to the bathroom. People are encouraged to walk as soon as they are physically able. Resuming activities soon after a heart attack or bypass surgery helps prevent problems (such as blood clots in the legs)[1] and speeds recovery.

After discharge from the hospital, activities should be gradually increased over a period of 2 to 4 weeks. If possible, people should walk a little each day. People should increase their walking time gradually until they can walk 20 to 30 minutes comfortably. Most people can resume sexual activity, drive, and go back to work within 2 to 4 weeks after discharge. Lifting heavy objects or weights should be avoided for at least 4 weeks. The return to usual activities may be slower if the heart attack was extensive or if problems develop after bypass surgery.

Many older people, especially those who were not in good physical condition before the heart attack, benefit from continuing rehabilitation in a cardiac rehabilitation program.[2] These programs include exercise sessions supervised by a trained exercise specialist. People are also taught how to change to a lifestyle that can help reduce the risk of another heart attack. Typically, people attend three sessions a week for 8 to 12 weeks.

Long-term treatment: Most people who have had a heart attack must continue to take drugs for the rest of their life. These

1. see page 148
2. see page 179

drugs may include aspirin or another antiplatelet drug, a beta-blocker, an ACE inhibitor, and a statin. Some people are given an anticoagulant (usually warfarin), a nitrate, a calcium channel blocker, or several of these drugs. People who cannot tolerate an ACE inhibitor because of cough or other side effects may be given an angiotensin II receptor blocker.

Eliminating or controlling risk factors is a lifelong task, even when angioplasty or bypass surgery is done. If risk factors are not eliminated or controlled, CAD tends to worsen and cause additional problems. Blood pressure, cholesterol levels, and weight should be kept within recommended ranges if possible. Smokers should stop smoking. Eating a low-fat, healthy diet is recommended. Most people are advised to exercise regularly. Learning to manage stress, when possible, may help.

If depression lasts more than 2 weeks after discharge from the hospital, treatment is needed. If family members notice that depression is persisting, they should encourage the person to contact the doctor. Without treatment, people with depression recover more slowly and have more serious problems later. People with depression are more likely to die during the first year after a heart attack. Treatment of depression, which includes counseling and antidepressant drugs, is usually effective.[1] Regular exercise, which improves mood and strengthens the heart, may help.

Outlook

CAD tends to worsen over time. Blockages tend to worsen so that less and less blood flows through the blocked arteries, and new blockages tend to develop. Angina tends to worsen. However, eliminating or controlling risk factors can delay and even prevent development and worsening of blockages. Treatment can relieve angina for years or even decades.

For people who have had a heart attack, the outlook depends on how much of the heart has been damaged. If a heart attack is massive or causes certain abnormal heart rhythms, death may occur within seconds, minutes, or days. However, most people who survive for a few days after a heart attack recover. They may live, sometimes with few or no symptoms, for years or decades afterward. The outlook is worse for people who con-

1. see page 448

tinue to have angina or abnormal heart rhythms or who develop heart failure. Following a healthy lifestyle and taking the drugs that the doctor prescribes can help prevent a heart attack and improve the outlook.

Sometimes because of a person's condition, treatments such as bypass surgery and angioplasty are too risky or will not prolong life. For example, these treatments may not benefit older people who have very advanced CAD, extensive damage to the heart, or other serious disorders (such as severe lung disorders or advanced cancer). These people are unlikely to survive for more than a few months. Care then focuses on relieving symptoms, such as pain and shortness of breath, and on making the person's remaining days as comfortable and fulfilling as possible.[1]

In people with CAD, death often occurs without warning. Death can occur quickly, before any symptoms develop or before they become bothersome. Such a death may result from a heart attack or an abnormal heart rhythm. Or death can occur after a period of chronic illness with ups and downs. Such a death may result from heart failure. Consequently, people with CAD, even those without significant symptoms, should prepare advance directives,[2] stating what kind of care they want at the end of life.

1. see page 211
2. see page 953

When the time came to close the family business, which we operated in our community for 44 years, we hated the idea. What would we do with our lives? The 6-days-a-week job we had gave us a reason to get up each day—a purpose in life. Sure, we had a wonderful family life besides the STORE, but everything was intertwined. We worked with our parents, brother, sister-in-law, and our children. The people who worked for us became our extended family. When my brother's health forced us to sell what had been our home away from home . . . the reality hit hard. It seemed impossible to realize that we no longer had to go to the STORE. We were only 59 and 56 years old and never imagined retiring!

We had to find an outlet for our need to be useful. After working side by side for all those wonderful years, we needed a purpose for our lives. We had both been involved in volunteering in our church and synagogue, Boy and Girl Scouts, Kiwanis, League of Women Voters, our children's school but never seemed to have enough time for everything we wanted to do. Now, without anything we really had to do—what would we do???

A friend asked us to attend a meeting at our Retired Senior Volunteer Program's office. This phone call gave us a new start on the rest of our life. For four cold January mornings, we once again had to get up. We rode the bus talking to people to obtain their views on how the city bus system could be improved.

Through RSVP, wonderful and challenging opportunities opened up. During the last 10 years, we have been given a chance to mentor young people in schools and take pictures at the DMV. We have even started another generation volunteering. We take our 1-year-old grandson to volunteer at the information desk at City Hall. The list of tasks goes on and on. We feel so very fortunate that we can give back a little to our wonderful community.

Myrna and Lyle Peacock

46

Heart Failure

Heart failure develops when the heart cannot pump as much blood as the body needs. Heart failure does not mean that the heart has stopped. Rather, it means that the heart cannot keep up with the work required of it—its workload.

Heart failure is one of the most common disorders among older people. Heart failure usually worsens over a period of years, eventually leading to death. However, treatment can relieve symptoms and prolong life.

The heart is a muscular organ with four chambers designed to pump blood efficiently, reliably, and continuously over a lifetime. The right and left sides of the heart each have an upper chamber (atrium) and a lower chamber (ventricle). The right atrium receives blood from the body and pumps it into the right ventricle, which pumps blood to the lungs. The left atrium receives blood from the lungs and pumps it into the left ventricle. The left ventricle, which is the workhorse of the heart, pumps blood to the rest of the body. The four chambers contract in rhythm to pump blood efficiently.[1]

When the heart cannot pump enough blood, the tissues of the body may not get enough oxygen and nutrients. As a result, muscles may tire more quickly, and other organs may not function normally. Also, blood may back up in the veins, causing fluid to leak out and accumulate in tissues. When blood coming into the right side of the heart backs up (called right-sided heart failure), fluid may accumulate in the abdomen, legs, and feet. When blood coming into the left side of the heart backs up (called left-sided heart failure), fluid may accumulate in the lungs. The

1. see art on page 658

backup of blood, called congestion, is why heart failure is also known as congestive heart failure. Often, both sides of the heart are affected, although one side may be affected more.

As heart failure progresses, the heart works harder in an effort to pump more blood. The heart's walls may become thicker, just as arm or leg muscles do after months of weight training. The heart's chambers may also enlarge, because pressure inside the heart increases. At first, these changes may help the heart keep up with its workload. But eventually, the thickened heart walls become stiff, and the ventricles cannot fill with blood normally. Or the stretched-out chambers, like stretched-out rubber bands, become less able to contract and pump blood. Most people tend to have problems with both filling and pumping to some degree.

Blood clots may form in the heart's stretched-out chambers. Clots are more likely to form when heart failure is advanced or when a person also has another heart disorder, such as an abnormal heart rhythm (arrhythmia) called atrial fibrillation[1] or a heart valve disorder.[2] Part of a clot may break loose, travel through the bloodstream (becoming an embolus), and block an artery elsewhere in the body. If a clot blocks an artery to the brain, a stroke may result.

Causes

Aging alone does not cause heart failure. But changes due to aging, such as slight thickening and stiffening of the heart's walls, make older people more susceptible to heart failure.

In older people, the most common causes of heart failure are high blood pressure and heart attacks (due to coronary artery disease). Other heart disorders, such as heart valve disorders, abnormal heart rhythms, a problem with the heart muscle itself (cardiomyopathy), inflammation of the sac around the heart (pericarditis), and heart infections, can also result in heart failure. A sudden illness, such as pneumonia, can strain the heart, contributing to the development of heart failure.

Drinking large amounts of alcohol and taking certain drugs (such as doxorubicin, a chemotherapy drug) can damage the heart. Then, the heart may be unable to pump forcefully enough,

1. see page 706
2. see page 715

HEART FAILURE:
FILLING AND PUMPING PROBLEMS

Normally, the heart stretches as it fills with blood, then contracts to pump out the blood. Heart failure may develop when the heart does not fill with blood as it normally does or when the heart cannot pump forcefully enough. Problems with filling are called diastolic dysfunction. Problems with pumping are called systolic dysfunction.

The most common reason the heart does not fill normally is that the walls of the heart's lower chambers (ventricles) have stiffened and thickened. Consequently, blood backs up in the upper left chamber (left atrium) and in blood vessels to the lungs. The heart may be able to pump out a normal percentage of the blood it receives, but the amount of blood is still reduced.

Pumping problems usually occur when the heart has become damaged and cannot pump normally. Pressure inside the heart increases because less blood is pumped out. As a result, the ventricles enlarge. Eventually, the ventricles, stretched out like old rubber bands, become even less able to pump, and less blood is pumped to the body.

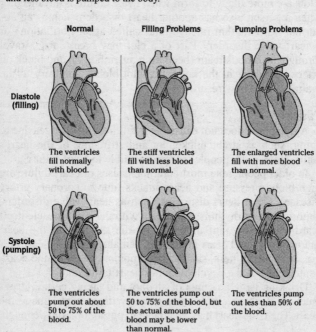

	Normal	**Filling Problems**	**Pumping Problems**
Diastole (filling)	The ventricles fill normally with blood.	The stiff ventricles fill with less blood than normal.	The enlarged ventricles fill with more blood than normal.
Systole (pumping)	The ventricles pump out about 50 to 75% of the blood.	The ventricles pump out 50 to 75% of the blood, but the actual amount of blood may be lower than normal.	The ventricles pump out less than 50% of the blood.

WHAT IS CARDIOMYOPATHY?

Cardiomyopathy means that there is a problem with the heart muscle itself. As a result, the heart does not function normally. The problem may be thickening (hypertrophy) or stiffening of the heart's walls. Or the problem may be stretching (dilation) of the heart's chambers, causing the heart to enlarge.

Cardiomyopathy does not always produce heart failure because the heart may still be able to pump enough blood to meet the body's needs. Whether cardiomyopathy leads to heart failure depends partly on the cause. If an infection is the cause and it can be treated effectively and early, cardiomyopathy may resolve. Drinking too much alcohol can also cause cardiomyopathy in susceptible people. If such people stop drinking alcohol, cardiomyopathy may resolve or not progress. However, cardiomyopathy in older people usually leads to heart failure sooner or later, because the causes are usually chronic disorders. Coronary artery disease and high blood pressure are common causes.

Cardiomyopathy can usually be detected by echocardiography (ultrasonography of the heart). Sometimes more invasive procedures, such as cardiac catheterization, are needed to confirm the diagnosis.

resulting in heart failure. Sometimes the cause of heart failure is unknown.

ADDITIONAL DETAIL

Disorders can cause heart failure in two ways. They can cause problems with the heart's ability to fill with blood or to pump blood out. Among older people, filling problems (called diastolic dysfunction) and pumping problems (called systolic dysfunction) are equally common.

Filling problems usually occur because the walls of the ventricles have become stiff. As a result, the ventricles cannot fill with blood normally, and too little blood is pumped out. As people age, heart muscle tends to become stiffer, making heart failure due to filling problems more likely. High blood pressure or a type of cardiomyopathy called hypertrophic cardiomyopathy can cause filling problems because either disorder can make the heart muscle thicker and stiffer.

Filling problems are not always caused by a stiff heart. They may result from thickening of the sac around the heart (constrictive pericarditis) or fluid accumulation within the sac (pericardial effusion). Either disorder can prevent the heart from expanding and filling normally. In atrial fibrillation (an abnormal heart rhythm), the atria beat rapidly and irregularly. As a result, the atria do not move enough blood into the ventricles. If atrial fibrillation occurs suddenly in older people, heart failure may result.

Pumping problems usually occur when the heart muscle has been damaged. A damaged heart pumps less blood out, causing pressure inside the heart to increase and the heart's chambers to enlarge. The most common cause of heart damage is a heart attack (due to a blockage in an artery that supplies the heart with blood). Other disorders that can damage the heart and cause pumping problems include heart valve disorders, high blood pressure, and certain infections (usually caused by viruses) and inflammatory disorders (such as lupus).

In aortic stenosis (a heart valve disorder), the opening between the left ventricle and the aorta (aortic valve) narrows. As a result, pumping blood out of the heart is harder. Aortic stenosis is a common cause of heart failure in older people.

Kidney and lung disorders can result in heart failure. If the kidneys are not functioning normally (because of a disorder or changes due to aging), they are less able to remove excess fluid and salt from the body. If extra fluid and salt accumulate in the body, the heart may have to work harder. Sometimes heart failure results. If a lung disorder such as emphysema or scarring (pulmonary fibrosis) develops, blood pressure in the lungs increases. As a result, pumping blood to the lungs is harder for the right ventricle.

Symptoms

Symptoms of heart failure may develop slowly, over weeks, months, or years. Or they may occur suddenly, especially if heart failure is due to a heart attack.

The main symptoms are shortness of breath (especially when exercising or lying in bed), fatigue, and swelling in the feet or ankles. A little swelling is not worrisome, but too much swelling in the legs and feet can make the skin fragile (resulting in sores) and make walking difficult. The legs, liver, and abdomen may also swell because of fluid accumulation.

Usually, heart failure does not cause pain. However, it may cause a sensation of fullness or tightness in the chest.

At first, people may feel short of breath only during exercise and other physical activities. Symptoms occur during physical activity because active muscles need more blood and the malfunctioning heart cannot pump enough. Inactive people may have vague symptoms, such as sleepiness, irritability, or confusion.

Symptoms may be triggered by eating salty foods or drinking an excessive amount of fluid in a day, especially if the kidneys are not functioning normally. Salt causes the body to retain fluid, so more fluid accumulates.

As heart failure progresses, shortness of breath occurs with less and less strenuous activity. It may occur when people lie down and be relieved when they sit up. This condition is called orthopnea. Some people wake up suddenly because they have trouble breathing when they lie down. Some people have a chronic cough that becomes worse when they lie down. Lying down causes problems because when a person lies down, fluid tends to accumulate in the lungs.

If heart failure becomes severe, any physical activity, such as going up steps or even walking short distances, may become difficult. Breathing becomes more and more difficult. To sleep, some people with severe heart failure need to sit up or use several pillows.

People may gasp for breath or make gurgling sounds when they breathe. They may feel restless, anxious, and as if they are suffocating. These symptoms occur when a large amount of fluid accumulates in the lungs (a condition called pulmonary edema). The skin may turn pale or bluish (cyanotic), and people may break out in a cold sweat. Blood pressure may become very high or very low. If the brain does not receive enough blood, people may become confused, lose consciousness, or faint.

When heart failure is very severe, people may go into shock. Shock occurs when blood pressure is too low to keep blood flowing to the body's organs. Unless treated quickly, people in shock due to heart failure usually die within a few hours or days.

Diagnosis

Doctors can sometimes diagnose heart failure on the basis of symptoms alone. Older people should tell their doctor if they feel short of breath or unusually tired or if they are no longer able to do their normal activities. Older people may think that these symptoms are unimportant or result from aging. But the symptoms may indicate heart failure.

When doctors suspect heart failure, they perform a physical examination. Using a stethoscope, they listen for abnormal heart and breathing sounds. Listening to the heart may provide clues about the cause of heart failure. Abnormal breathing sounds may mean that fluid has accumulated in the lungs. Doctors check for other signs of fluid accumulation: swollen neck veins, an enlarged liver, and swelling in the abdomen or legs.

Other tests are usually needed to confirm the diagnosis. The chest is x-rayed to see whether the heart is enlarged and whether fluid has accumulated in the lungs. Echocardiography (ultrasonography of the heart) is done to see how well the heart is filling and pumping. Echocardiography also helps doctors determine the cause of heart failure. It can show how well the heart is beating and whether heart valves are functioning normally.

With echocardiography, doctors can measure the ejection fraction and thus evaluate the heart's pumping ability. The ejection fraction is the percentage of blood that the left ventricle pumps out with each heartbeat (some blood remains in the left ventricle). Normally, the ejection fraction is between 50% and 75%.

Other tests that may be done include cardiac catheterization[1] and nuclear scanning.[2] A blood test may be done to measure the level of a protein (called B-type natriuretic peptide) that is released by the heart into the blood when pressure inside the heart increases.

Prevention and Treatment

Prevention and treatment of disorders that can cause heart failure (such as high blood pressure and coronary artery disease) can help prevent heart failure, regardless of a person's

1. see page 132
2. see page 128

age. Being treated promptly and appropriately during a heart attack is particularly important.

Although heart failure is a chronic disorder for most people, much can be done to make physical activity more comfortable, improve the quality of life, and prolong life.

Sometimes treating the disorder causing heart failure can prevent heart failure from worsening and relieve symptoms. For example, high blood pressure may be controlled with antihypertensive drugs. After a heart attack, treatment may consist of drugs, angioplasty, or coronary artery bypass graft surgery. A damaged heart valve can be repaired or replaced. An abnormal heart rhythm can be corrected with drugs, surgery, or use of an artificial pacemaker. Excess fluid in the sac around the heart can be drained.

General measures: Some lifestyle changes can help prevent heart failure from worsening and relieve symptoms. Trying to stay physically fit, even for people who cannot exercise vigorously, is important. People with heart failure should follow an exercise program as prescribed by a doctor.[1] A cardiac rehabilitation program may also be helpful.[2]

Losing excess weight and stopping smoking can help prevent heart failure from worsening. Alcohol consumption should be limited to one or two drinks a day. In people with heart failure, larger amounts of alcohol can cause the heart to function less well and beat abnormally. People with heart failure due to drinking large amounts of alcohol should not drink any alcohol.

Almost everyone with heart failure should avoid using table salt and eating salty foods (such as chips, pretzels, canned soups, and canned vegetables). The salt (sodium) content of packaged foods is listed on the label. The use of salt in cooking should also be limited. Health care practitioners usually give people with severe heart failure specific guidelines for salt consumption, such as no more than 2 grams of sodium a day. Usually, people who limit their salt consumption do not need to limit the amount of fluid they drink. But most people with heart failure should not drink more than six to eight glasses of fluid a day.

Limiting salt consumption may help prevent swelling but

1. see page 911
2. see page 179

does not relieve it. Elevating the legs when sitting can reduce swelling. Some people also need to wear full-length support stockings. When lying down, using several pillows or elevating the head of the bed can help make breathing easier.

Recording body weight every day can help people determine whether they are retaining fluid. Usually, the best time to weigh is in the morning after urinating but before eating breakfast. If weight increases by more than 2 pounds (about 1 kilogram) a day or 5 pounds (about $2\frac{1}{4}$ kilograms) a week, fluid is probably being retained. A decrease of more than 2 pounds a day or 5 pounds a week may mean that too much fluid is being lost. People should report such changes to their doctor, because they may need a change in the dose of a drug.

A yearly influenza (often called flu) vaccination is particularly important for people with heart failure. Influenza can stress the heart and cause heart failure to worsen suddenly. A vaccination to help prevent pneumonia is also important.

People with heart failure should ask their doctor or another health care practitioner to review the drugs they are taking. Some drugs, such as all nonsteroidal anti-inflammatory drugs (NSAIDs) except aspirin, should be used only if recommended by a doctor. NSAIDs tend to make fluid retention worse.

Drugs: The choice of drugs depends on other disorders a person has and on the severity of heart failure.

Angiotensin-converting enzyme (ACE) inhibitors help prevent heart failure from worsening, relieve symptoms for most people, and prolong life. These drugs cause blood vessels to expand (dilate). Then, the heart can pump blood more easily. Angiotensin II receptor blockers have effects similar to those of ACE inhibitors, and they may have fewer side effects. Angiotensin II receptor blockers are often used instead of or in addition to an ACE inhibitor. Other drugs that dilate blood vessels (vasodilators) may be used when people cannot take ACE inhibitors or angiotensin II receptor blockers.

Beta-blockers are often given with ACE inhibitors. Beta-blockers help the heart function better and prolong life. They are especially helpful for people who have had a heart attack. Doctors adjust the dose carefully and monitor the person's response to the drug because these drugs may temporarily worsen symptoms.

Diuretics are used to remove extra fluid from the body and to help prevent fluid from accumulating. If heart failure is very mild, a diuretic may be taken only on days when fluid accumulation is noticeable. If heart failure is more severe, a diuretic is usually taken every day. Bumetanide, furosemide, and torsemide are most commonly used. People with severe heart failure may be given metolazone or a stronger diuretic. Most diuretics cause the body to lose potassium in the urine. For this reason, doctors may recommend increasing the amount of potassium in the diet. Good sources of potassium are bananas, oranges, and other fruits. Alternatively, doctors may recommend a potassium supplement. People who take a diuretic may need to urinate more often and more urgently. If they have urinary incontinence, taking a diuretic may cause problems. However, people can usually time when they take a diuretic so that a bathroom is available when they are likely to need to urinate.

Aldosterone antagonists, such as spironolactone and eplerenone, prevent potassium loss. These drugs are weak diuretics. Spironolactone prolongs life and reduces the need for hospitalization in people with severe heart failure. Eplerenone may prolong life in people with heart failure, particularly if it is due to moderate or severe heart damage after a heart attack.

Sometimes the dose of a diuretic needs to be adjusted. For example, the dose may need to be decreased in hot weather because people sweat more. Or the dose may need to be increased if the body is retaining fluid. Weighing every day helps people notice these changes. The dose of a diuretic must be adjusted by a doctor. However, with experience, many people can learn to adjust the dose of the diuretic with their doctor's supervision.

Digoxin, one of the oldest treatments for heart failure, slightly increases the force of each heartbeat and slows a heart rate that is too rapid. Digoxin helps relieve symptoms, especially if atrial fibrillation is present.

For people who have severe symptoms and have not responded well to the usual treatments, other drugs that help the heart pump more efficiently may be used. These drugs include dopamine, dobutamine, and milrinone. Nesiritide, which causes blood vessels to dilate, may also be given. These drugs are given intravenously and are used for a short time.

Anticoagulants (sometimes called blood thinners), such as warfarin, make blood less likely to clot. They can help prevent clots from forming in the heart's chambers. People who take warfarin must have blood tests periodically to check the blood's ability to clot. If blood is taking too long to clot, bleeding can occur. People who have coronary artery disease or diabetes are often given aspirin, which makes blood clots less likely to form. People who have an abnormal heart rhythm may be given antiarrhythmic drugs.[1]

Oxygen therapy: Some people with severe heart failure need oxygen therapy. It helps relieve shortness of breath. Several devices can be used at home.[2]

Surgery: If heart failure is severe, a pacemaker that stimulates the two ventricles to pump at the same time (biventricular pacemaker) may be implanted. It may help relieve symptoms and enable people to be more physically active. An implanted cardioverter-defibrillator (ICD) may be used to treat people who are likely to have a severe abnormal heart rhythm (such as ventricular tachycardia or ventricular fibrillation).

Emergency treatment: Severe symptoms of heart failure may occur suddenly and require prompt emergency treatment in a hospital. Such treatment can be life saving. The accumulation of fluid in the lungs (pulmonary edema) is often the most serious problem, so oxygen is usually given through a face mask or through short tubes inserted in each nostril (nasal prongs). A diuretic is given intravenously. Nitroglycerin (which dilates blood vessels) may be given intravenously or applied to the skin. Sometimes morphine is given to dilate blood vessels and relieve anxiety. These drugs can produce rapid, dramatic improvement. If needed, a breathing tube may be inserted into the person's airway for a short time. The tube is connected to a mechanical ventilator, which assists breathing.

Outlook

Heart failure usually worsens over time. Although many people with heart failure live for several years, more than three fourths of people die within 10 years. How fast heart failure worsens varies greatly from person to person. People with heart failure may die suddenly and unexpectedly, without symptoms becoming worse. Sudden death is usually caused by a severe abnormal heart rhythm (such as ventricular fibrillation). A per-

1. see table on page 699
2. see page 819

℞ SOME DRUGS USED FOR HEART FAILURE

Type	Drug	Comments
Angiotensin-converting enzyme (ACE) inhibitors	Benazepril Captopril Enalapril Fosinopril Lisinopril Moexipril Perindopril Quinapril Ramipril Trandolapril	ACE inhibitors cause blood vessels to expand (dilate). Thus, they decrease the workload of the heart. They may also have direct beneficial effects on the heart. These drugs are the main-stay of treatment. They prevent heart failure from worsening, relieve symptoms, and prolong life. People who take them are less likely to be hospitalized. Taking these drugs also enables people to function better. ACE inhibitors can cause cough, which some people cannot tolerate
Angiotensin II receptor blockers	Candesartan Eprosartan Irbesartan Losartan Telmisartan Valsartan	Angiotensin II receptor blockers have effects similar to those of ACE inhibitors and may have fewer side effects. However, their effects are still being evaluated in people with heart failure. They may be used with an ACE inhibitor or used alone in people who cannot take an ACE inhibitor because it causes a troublesome cough
Beta-blockers	Acebutolol Atenolol Betaxolol Bisoprolol Carteolol Carvedilol Metoprolol Nadolol Penbutolol Pindolol Propranolol Timolol	Beta-blockers slow the heart rate and reduce the workload of the heart. They are appropriate for most people with heart failure. These drugs are usually used with ACE inhibitors and provide an added benefit. They may temporarily worsen symptoms, but they help the heart function better and prolong life. They also make dying suddenly less likely
Other vasodilators	Hydralazine Isosorbide dinitrate	Vasodilators cause blood vessels to dilate. These vasodilators are usually given if an ACE inhibitor

Table continues on the following page.

Type	Drug	Comments
	Nitroglycerin	or angiotensin II receptor blocker cannot be used or does not relieve symptoms. Nitroglycerin is useful in people who have heart failure and chest pain (angina)
Cardiac glycosides	Digoxin	Cardiac glycosides increase the force of each heartbeat and slow a heart rate that is too fast. They are given to people with moderate to severe heart failure and people with certain abnormal heart rhythms (such as atrial fibrillation). These drugs relieve symptoms. People who take them are less likely to be hospitalized
Loop diuretics	Bumetanide Ethacrynic acid Furosemide Torsemide	These diuretics help the kidneys excrete more fluid and salt in the urine. Taken by mouth, these diuretics are used to treat moderate to severe heart failure. They may be given intravenously as emergency treatment
Thiazide and thiazide-like diuretics	Chlorthalidone Hydrochloro- thiazide Indapamide Metolazone	The effects of these diuretics are similar to but milder than those of loop diuretics. The two types of diuretics are particularly effective when used together. Taken by mouth, these diuretics are sometimes used to treat mild heart failure. Metolazone is also used to treat severe heart failure, especially in people who have a kidney disorder
Aldosterone antagonists	Eplerenone Spironolactone	Aldosterone antagonists help prevent potassium loss. They are weak diuretics. Spironolactone prolongs life in people with severe heart failure and makes them less likely to be hospitalized. Eplerenone may prolong life in people with heart failure, particularly if it is due to moderate

Type	Drug	Comments
		or severe heart damage after a heart attack.
Anticoagulants	Heparin Warfarin	Anticoagulants may be given to prevent clots from forming in the heart chambers.
Opioids	Morphine	Morphine is given to relieve pain. It also helps relieve the shortness of breath and anxiety that often accompanies pulmonary edema.
Positive inotropic drugs (drugs that make the heart contract more forcefully)	Dobutamine Dopamine Milrinone	For people who have severe symptoms, these drugs may be given intravenously to stimulate the heart to contract and help keep blood circulating.
Vasodilators given intravenously	Nesiritide Nitroglycerin Nitroprusside	These vasodilators may be given intravenously to reduce the heart's workload in people who have severe symptoms.

son's outlook depends on the person's age, the cause of heart failure, and other disorders the person has. For example, the outlook is worse for people who have diabetes or a kidney disorder.

Eventually, severe heart failure may make doing daily activities difficult. If the usual treatments have not worked, health care practitioners should be asked to realistically describe what can be expected. Then together, the person with severe heart failure, family members, and practitioners can make decisions about care.

As heart failure progresses, care may focus more on treatments that relieve symptoms (palliative care) and less on treatments that may prolong life, although both types of treatment may be appropriate. Often, treatments to prolong life in people with severe heart failure are uncomfortable and expensive. They often do not improve quality of life. At some point, a decision to stop these treatments and to rely on palliative care may be appropriate.[1]

1. see page 211

Palliative care may involve using opioids (such as morphine) to relieve shortness of breath and tightness or fullness felt in the chest. Antianxiety drugs, such as clonazepam or lorazepam, can be used to relieve anxiety caused by feeling short of breath. Diuretics may be given in high doses to help the body get rid of excess fluid. Palliative care helps reduce suffering, enables a person to have a better quality of life, and helps the person prepare for death. Palliative care can also help family members cope with their grief.

Because people with heart failure often have little or no warning that death is near, they should prepare advance directives.[1] For example, they should decide whether or under what circumstances they want cardiopulmonary resuscitation (CPR) if the heart suddenly stops beating. People should periodically review their advance directives because their wishes may change as heart failure worsens. Making or updating a will is also important.

47

Abnormal Heart Rhythms

An abnormal heart rhythm may be too rapid, too slow, or irregular. The heart may beat abnormally in response to an emotion or event. The heart may seem to skip a beat when a person is excited. It may race when a person is nervous or afraid. These sensations are called palpitations. In such cases, palpitations are usually of no consequence. However, they can be symptoms of a disorder involving abnormal heart rhythm called an arrhythmia.

Normally in older people who are resting, the heart rate (heartbeats per minute) is 60 to 80. It may be slower if the heart is well conditioned by regular physical activity. The heart rate may be faster in people who are physically inactive. The heart beats in a regular rhythm, changing its rate in response to different activities. That is, the heart speeds up or slows down to adjust the amount of blood it pumps in response to the body's needs.

Heartbeats are controlled by the heart's electrical system. Electrical currents are produced and coordinated by the heart's natural pacemaker (sinus or sinoatrial node), located in the upper right heart chamber (right atrium). The electrical currents flow through the heart along specific pathways in the heart and at a controlled speed. They stimulate the heart to contract, producing each heartbeat. Certain hormones and nerve impulses from other parts of the body signal the heart when a change in heart rate is needed.

Arrhythmias are more likely to develop as people age, particularly in those who have other heart disorders. In a few people, an arrhythmia occurs only once. In many other people, arrhythmias occur from time to time (intermittently). Some arrhythmias gradually occur more and more often and may become constant.

For most people, arrhythmias are harmless, although they can cause considerable anxiety if people become aware of them. However, some arrhythmias have serious consequences, such as falls, motor vehicle accidents, heart failure and, occasionally, death without any warning (sudden death). Most arrhythmias can be treated effectively.

Types

Arrhythmias are categorized partly by their speed. Slow arrhythmias are called bradycardias. Fast arrhythmias are called tachycardias. Arrhythmias are also categorized by what type of problem started the arrhythmia. A problem may involve the upper chambers (atria), the lower chambers (ventricles), or the initiation or conduction of electrical currents in the heart. Arrhythmias that result from problems in the atria include premature atrial beats, supraventricular tachycardia, atrial flutter, and atrial fibrillation. Arrhythmias that result from problems in the ventricles include premature ventricular beats, ventricular tachycardia, and ventricular fibrillation. Arrhythmias that result from problems initiating and conducting electrical currents include malfunction of the heart's pacemaker (some cases of sinus bradycardia and sick sinus syndrome) and heart block.

Causes

Arrhythmias are most commonly caused by other heart disorders, particularly coronary artery disease, heart valve disorders, and heart failure.

Many drugs, prescription and nonprescription, can cause or worsen arrhythmias. For example, taking certain drugs used to treat heart disorders (such as beta-blockers, calcium channel blockers, and digoxin) can cause slow arrhythmias. Taking theophylline (used to treat chronic obstructive pulmonary disease, or COPD) and decongestants (such as phenylephrine, pseudoephedrine, and oxymetazoline) can cause fast arrhythmias.

An overactive thyroid gland (hyperthyroidism) may cause fast arrhythmias. An underactive thyroid gland (hypothyroidism) may cause slow arrhythmias. Sometimes no cause for an arrhythmia can be identified.

Certain circumstances may trigger arrhythmias. Fast arrhythmias may be triggered by exercise, emotional stress, excessive alcohol consumption, or smoking. Slow arrhythmias may be triggered by pain, straining to urinate or to have a bowel movement, vomiting, or even swallowing. These circumstances can trigger slow arrhythmias because they may overstimulate the nerve that slows the heart rate (vagus nerve). Most arrhythmias triggered by these circumstances are not serious and resolve on their own.

Symptoms

Often, arrhythmias do not cause any symptoms. Sometimes an arrhythmia causes palpitations. That is, a person may sense that the heart is beating too rapidly, too forcefully, or irregularly.

Arrhythmias may make people feel weak and unable to do their normal activities. They may feel dizzy or faint and lose consciousness because the heart is not pumping enough blood to the brain. If these symptoms occur, people should see a doctor promptly. Arrhythmias that cause such symptoms may have serious consequences. Occasionally, in some people (usually those who have a heart disorder), certain arrhythmias cause death without any warning.

Some arrhythmias, particularly atrial fibrillation, can cause a stroke or sudden pain in an arm or a leg. These problems occur when part of a blood clot in the heart breaks off, travels through the bloodstream, and blocks an artery that carries blood to the brain or to an arm or a leg. A clot that travels through the bloodstream is called an embolus.

Arrhythmias may worsen symptoms of coronary artery disease, heart valve disorders, or heart failure (such as chest pain and shortness of breath).

Diagnosis

Doctors may suspect an arrhythmia on the basis of symptoms. So doctors may ask the following questions:

- Are the palpitations fast or slow?
- Are they regular or irregular?
- Are they brief or prolonged?
- Do they occur at rest or only during strenuous or unusual activity?
- Do they start and stop suddenly or gradually?
- Does the arrhythmia causes any other symptoms?

Doctors also check the person's pulse and blood pressure. All of this information helps doctors determine whether an arrhythmia is present and, if so, what type and how severe it is. However, additional tests are usually needed to be certain.

Electrocardiography (ECG)[1] can often confirm the diagnosis. Usually, ECG is done in the doctor's office, and heart rhythm is recorded for less than a minute. Thus, an intermittent arrhythmia is often missed. So doctors sometimes ask a person to wear a portable ECG (Holter) monitor so that the heart rhythm can be recorded continuously, usually for 24 hours. A person can wear a Holter monitor for days if necessary. Another monitor, called an event recorder, can be worn for a longer period of time. It is similar to a Holter monitor, but it records heart rhythm only when the user or someone with the user activates it by pushing a button. The user is instructed to activate the monitor when

1. see page 661

HOLTER MONITOR: CONTINUOUS ECG READINGS

The small monitor is attached to a strap worn over one shoulder. Through electrodes attached to the chest, the monitor continuously records the electrical activity of the heart.

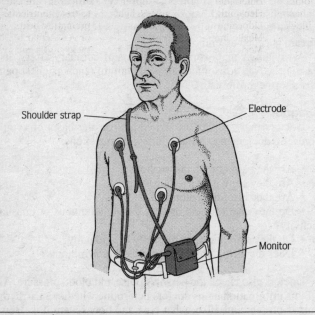

symptoms occur. When wearing either type of monitor, a person may be asked to keep a diary of symptoms and activities. This information helps doctors determine whether the symptoms are caused by an arrhythmia and whether an arrhythmia is more likely to occur during certain circumstances.

If exercise is thought to trigger an arrhythmia, doctors may ask a person to walk on a treadmill while heart rhythm is recorded by ECG (a procedure called exercise stress testing).

If doctors think an arrhythmia could be life threatening, hospitalization is usually necessary. In the hospital, heart rhythm can be continuously recorded and displayed on a television-type monitor by the bedside or nursing station. Thus, any problems can be identified and managed promptly.

℞ SOME DRUGS USED FOR ARRHYTHMIAS

Type	Examples	Possible Side Effects	Comments
Sodium channel blockers	Dofetilide Flecainide Lidocaine Mexiletine Moricizine Phenytoin Procainamide Propafenone Quinidine Tocainide	Digestive upset, dizziness, light-headedness, tremor, retention of urine, increased pressure within the eye in people who have glaucoma, dry mouth, and other arrhythmias (which can be fatal, particularly in people who have another heart disorder)	These drugs are used to treat ventricular premature beats or ventricular tachycardia and to restore atrial fibrillation to a normal rhythm
Beta-blockers	Acebutolol Atenolol Betaxolol Bisoprolol Carteolol Carvedilol Metoprolol Nadolol Penbutolol Propranolol Timolol	An abnormally slow heart rate (bradycardia), heart failure, spasm of the airways (broncho-spasm), changes in blood sugar levels, poor circulation, insomnia, shortness of breath, depression, Raynaud's phenomenon, hallucinations, erectile dysfunction, and fatigue With some	These drugs are used to treat ventricular premature beats, ventricular tachycardia, paroxysmal supraventricular tachycardia, atrial flutter, and atrial fibrillation. People who have asthma should not take these drugs

Table continues on the following page.

Type	Examples	Possible Side Effects	Comments
		beta-blockers, an increase in the triglyceride level	
Potassium channel blockers	Amiodarone Bretylium Ibutilide Sotalol	Scarring in the lungs (pulmonary fibrosis), an underactive thyroid gland (hypothyroidism), low blood pressure, and other arrhythmias For sotalol, which is also a beta-blocker, see previously under beta-blockers	These drugs are used to treat ventricular tachycardia, ventricular fibrillation, atrial fibrillation, and atrial flutter Because amiodarone can be toxic, it is used for long-term treatment only in some people who have serious arrhythmias Bretylium is used only for short-term treatment of life-threatening ventricular tachycardias
Calcium channel blockers	Diltiazem Verapamil	Constipation, low blood pressure, and swollen feet	Only certain calcium channel blockers (such as diltiazem and verapamil) are used to treat atrial flutter, atrial fibrillation, and paroxysmal supraventricular tachycardia
Digoxin		Abnormally slow heart rate, nausea, vomiting, and serious arrhythmias; if the dose is too high, xanthopsia	Digoxin is used to treat atrial flutter, atrial fibrillation, and paroxysmal supraventricular tachycardia

Type	Examples	Possible Side Effects	Comments
		(a condition in which objects appear greenish yellow)	
Adenosine		Spasm of the airways (broncho-spasm) and temporary flushing	Adenosine is used to end episodes of paroxysmal supraventricular tachycardia. People who have asthma should not take this drug

Occasionally, when a serious arrhythmia is suspected, electrophysiologic testing is done to confirm its presence and, if it is present, to determine its characteristics. For this test, a person is given a sedative but is conscious. Then a flexible tube (catheter) is inserted through a vein and threaded into the heart. The catheter contains many small wires with tiny electrodes at their tips. The electrodes stimulate the heart to determine whether a serious arrhythmia can be triggered. Doctors can stimulate specific parts of the heart and thus determine which part is causing the arrhythmia. This test can also help doctors determine the most effective treatment for the arrhythmia.

Treatment

Many arrhythmias do not require specific treatment. Sometimes arrhythmias occur less often or even stop when doctors change a person's drugs or adjust the doses. Limiting or eliminating alcohol and beverages that contain caffeine and stopping smoking may also help. If arrhythmias occur during exercise, a person can talk to a doctor about possible precautions to take during exercise.

Drugs: If an arrhythmia is thought to be serious or causes significant symptoms, antiarrhythmic drugs may be used. These drugs can prevent or control most intermittent arrhythmias. Often, antiarrhythmic drugs must be taken indefinitely. If the cause of the arrhythmia can be eliminated, the drugs may be discontinued. The type of antiarrhythmic drug used depends on which arrhythmia is present.

In older people, the dose of many antiarrhythmic drugs must be reduced, because as people age the body does not eliminate these drugs as quickly. One antiarrhythmic drug, disopyramide, is not usually given to older people. It can cause blurred vision, constipation, or retention of urine. It also tends to make the heart contract more weakly.

Surgery: Two types of electronic devices that are implanted surgically are used to treat serious arrhythmias: artificial pacemakers and implanted cardioverter-defibrillators (ICDs). Sometimes one device that combines the two functions is used. The type of device a person needs depends on the arrhythmia. These devices are permanently implanted under the skin, usually below the left or right collarbone. They are connected to the heart by wires running inside a vein.

Artificial pacemakers are most commonly used to treat slow arrhythmias. When the heart beats too slowly, a pacemaker stimulates the heart to make it beat more rapidly. Occasionally, pacemakers are used to treat fast arrhythmias. Implantable artificial pacemakers act in place of the heart's own pacemaker.

An implanted cardioverter-defibrillator is about the size of a deck of cards. It automatically senses life-threatening fast arrhythmias (ventricular tachycardia or ventricular fibrillation) and delivers an electrical shock to the heart. The shock almost always restores the normal heart rhythm. Most often, this device is used to treat people who might otherwise lose consciousness or die of the arrhythmia.

Sometimes destroying or removing an abnormal area in the heart's electrical system can control or eliminate an arrhythmia. Usually, a catheter with electrodes at its tip is inserted into the heart. Heat from the electrodes destroys the abnormal area. This procedure, called catheter ablation, is successful in most people. Less commonly, the area is destroyed or removed during open-heart surgery.[1]

Occasionally, angioplasty or coronary artery bypass surgery may be done to control arrhythmias due to coronary artery disease.[2]

1. see box on page 721
2. see page 656

KEEPING THE BEAT: ARTIFICIAL PACEMAKERS

Artificial pacemakers are electronic devices that act in place of the heart's natural pacemaker (the sinus or sinoatrial node). They produce electrical impulses that initiate each heartbeat. Pacemakers consist of an impulse generator, a battery, and wires that connect the pacemaker to the heart.

An artificial pacemaker is implanted surgically. A local anesthetic (used to block sensation in a very limited area) is injected to numb the insertion site. Then wires that connect to the pacemaker are usually inserted into a vein near the collarbone (subclavian vein) and threaded into the heart. Through a small incision, the impulse generator (which is about the size of a silver dollar) is inserted just under the skin near the collarbone and connected to the wires. Usually, the procedure takes about 30 to 60 minutes. People may be able to go home shortly afterward or may stay in the hospital for a few days. Pacemakers can be checked in the doctor's office or by telephone. They can be adjusted from outside the body, without surgery. The battery for a pacemaker usually lasts 10 to 15 years. Nevertheless, the battery should be checked regularly. The battery is replaced through a small incision made after a local anesthetic is injected. Replacement takes only a few minutes, and the whole process takes only a few hours, with no overnight stay at the hospital.

Some pacemakers control the heart rate all the time. Others, called demand pacemakers, allow the heart to beat naturally unless it skips a beat or begins to beat at an abnormal rate. Still others, called programmable pacemakers, can do either. Some pacemakers can adjust their rate depending on the wearer's activity. They increase the heart rate during exercise and decrease it during rest.

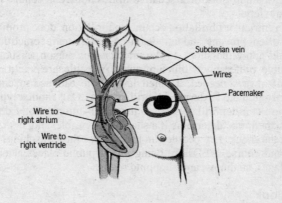

Subclavian vein

Wires

Pacemaker

Wire to
right atrium

Wire to
right ventricle

Emergency treatment: If an arrhythmia develops rapidly and causes severe chest pain, heart failure, or loss of consciousness, emergency treatment is needed.

If the heart is beating too slowly, atropine or other drugs may be given intravenously to stimulate the heart to beat faster. A temporary external pacemaker may be needed. It is connected to the heart by wires inserted into a large vein in the neck or near the collarbone.

If the heart is beating too rapidly but the problem is not life threatening, doctors may ask a person to bear down as if having a bowel movement. Or, doctors may massage the carotid arteries in the neck. These maneuvers sometimes slow the heart rate or return the heart rhythm to normal.

If the heart is beating too rapidly, antiarrhythmic drugs given intravenously can usually restore the normal heart rhythm. However, if drugs do not work, an electrical shock may be applied to the person's chest. One of two procedures is used. Defibrillation is used to restore an irregular fast heart rhythm to normal. Cardioversion is used to restore a regular fast heart rhythm to normal. Devices that can do either, called cardioverter-defibrillators, are often used. For these procedures, a health care practitioner applies two small paddles to the chest. These procedures are safe but cause pain. If conscious, the person is given a small dose of a sedative intravenously to relieve pain and anxiety.

If ventricular fibrillation occurs, defibrillation, done promptly, can often prevent sudden death. A health care practitioner should apply the shock to the unconscious person as soon as possible, preferably within 5 minutes. A health care practitioner is not always needed. Trained lay people can use machines called automated external defibrillators (AEDs), another type of cardioverter-defibrillator. These machines automatically detect the arrhythmia, determine if a shock is advisable, and, if so, deliver the shock. Lay people can learn to use these machines at a first-aid course. AEDs are being put in public places, such as airplanes, stadiums, and shopping malls.

Outlook

In many people, arrhythmias do not have serious consequences and do not require treatment. Whether an arrhythmia has serious consequences depends on how fast the heart beats, which parts of the heart are affected, and how long the arrhythmia lasts. Generally, arrhythmias started by a problem in the ventricles are the most serious. Sometimes an arrhythmia started by a problem in the atria, such as atrial fibrillation, also has serious consequences. The seriousness of an arrhythmia also depends partly on the cause. The outlook tends to be the worst with arrhythmias due to severe, long-standing (chronic) heart disorders. In contrast, in people who do not have a heart disorder, arrhythmias are often harmless.

Symptoms do not reliably indicate how serious an arrhythmia is. Some potentially life-threatening arrhythmias may cause no symptoms, and some otherwise inconsequential arrhythmias cause significant symptoms.

PREMATURE BEATS

Premature beats are extra heartbeats of the atria (atrial beats) or ventricles (ventricular beats).

Premature beats themselves are usually not serious. However, in people whose heart is abnormal in structure or function, premature beats may mean that serious problems are more likely.

Premature beats are more common among older people, including healthy older people. But they are particularly common among people who have coronary artery disease. Premature beats may be triggered or worsened by consuming alcohol or caffeinated beverages (such as coffee or tea) or by using some cold, hay fever, or asthma remedies. Physical or emotional stress may also trigger them.

Premature beats usually cause no symptoms. People may feel them, usually as occasional skipped heartbeats. Some people have bothersome palpitations. In people with a heart disorder (particularly coronary artery disease), premature ventricular beats may lead to ventricular tachycardia or ventricular fibrillation, both of which are life threatening.

Diagnosis and Treatment

Premature beats may be detected during a physical examination and are confirmed by electrocardiography (ECG). Sometimes a portable ECG (Holter) monitor is used. Usually, no treatment is needed. If premature beats occur frequently or cause intolerable palpitations, an antiarrhythmic drug (such as a beta-blocker) may be given.

ATRIAL FLUTTER AND ATRIAL FIBRILLATION

Atrial flutter and atrial fibrillation are very similar. In both arrhythmias, the atria beat much faster than normal. The main difference is that the atria beat regularly in atrial flutter and irregularly in atrial fibrillation.

Normally, the atria contract while the ventricles are resting. This contraction pumps blood into the ventricles. In atrial flutter and atrial fibrillation, the atria do not have time to fill with blood completely, and they do not pump blood into the ventricles in a coordinated way. Thus, the ventricles of the heart cannot fill with blood and pump it out efficiently.

Atrial flutter is usually temporary. Typically, it either goes away (with or without treatment) or changes into another arrhythmia, usually atrial fibrillation. Sometimes atrial fibrillation is intermittent. But it can become constant, with no periods of normal heart rhythm. Both atrial flutter and atrial fibrillation may lead to serious problems, such as blood clots and heart failure.

Atrial flutter and atrial fibrillation are more common among older people. Other than premature beats, atrial fibrillation is the most common abnormal heart rhythm among older people. About 1 out of 10 people over 80 have chronic atrial fibrillation.

In older people, the most common causes of atrial flutter are coronary artery disease and chronic obstructive pulmonary disease (COPD). The most common causes of atrial fibrillation are high blood pressure, coronary artery disease, mitral valve disorders, and heart failure.

In atrial flutter or atrial fibrillation, the ventricles often beat faster than normal. The faster the ventricles beat, the less well they fill with and pump blood. Generally, the faster they beat, the more serious the consequences. Consequences may include chest pain, a heart attack, or heart failure.

Also during these arrhythmias, the left atrium does not empty completely. Clots tend to form in the blood that remains in the atrium. The clots can break off, leave the heart, travel through arteries, and eventually block small arteries elsewhere in the body. As a result, the area that the blocked artery normally supplies with blood does not get enough blood. Atrial fibrillation is more likely to cause clots than atrial flutter. The risk of blood clots is high for older people with atrial fibrillation.

Symptoms

Symptoms of atrial flutter or atrial fibrillation depend largely on how fast the heart rate is. With a heart rate up to about 120 beats per minute, some older people have no symptoms, but a few develop heart failure. With a faster rate, many people have unpleasant palpitations or chest discomfort. People with atrial flutter tend to have a fast but regular pulse. Those with atrial fibrillation tend to have a fast, irregular pulse. If the conduction of electrical currents in the heart is also abnormal, the pulse may remain normal or may even be slower than normal, despite flutter or fibrillation.

People who have atrial flutter or atrial fibrillation may feel weak, faint, and short of breath. They may develop chest pain or heart failure. Sudden pain or cramping in a leg or an arm may develop if atrial fibrillation causes blood clots to form in the atrium and part of one breaks off and blocks an artery in the leg or arm. A stroke may occur if a blood clot blocks an artery to the brain.

Diagnosis and Treatment

Doctors may suspect atrial flutter or atrial fibrillation on the basis of symptoms. Sometimes one of the arrhythmias is detected during a routine examination in a person who has no symptoms. Electrocardiography (ECG) can confirm the diagnosis. If the arrhythmia is intermittent, a portable ECG (Holter) monitor or event recorder may be needed. Sometimes transesophageal echocardiography (ultrasonography of the heart) is done to determine whether clots have formed in the heart. For this test, an imaging device is passed down the person's throat into the esophagus. This test is safe but can cause gagging and anxiety. Therefore, doctors usually give the person a sedative beforehand.

In an emergency—when atrial flutter or atrial fibrillation results in chest pain or shock—doctors usually use a cardioverter-defibrillator to try to restore a normal rhythm quickly. For this procedure, an electrical shock is applied to the chest with two small paddles.

In nonemergencies, when blood pressure is adequate and no chest pain is felt, an antiarrhythmic drug is given intravenously to slow the fast heart rate so that the heart pumps blood more efficiently. For people who also have heart failure, digoxin is often used first. For other people, a drug such as diltiazem, verapamil, or propanolol may be used. Sometimes one of these drugs is given with digoxin. Although these drugs slow the rapid heart rate, they do not usually restore heart rhythm to normal. Other drugs, such as procainamide, ibutilide, or dofetilide may be given intravenously to restore heart rhythm back to normal very quickly. If the heart rhythm returns to normal and if atrial flutter or atrial fibrillation is unlikely to recur, the drugs may be discontinued. People are then monitored periodically by their doctor to check for recurrences of the arrhythmia.

If atrial fibrillation persists, antiarrhythmic drugs (such as amiodarone, propafenone, sotalol, or quinidine) may be given by mouth to restore the heart rhythm to normal. Some people may be given drugs such as diltiazem, verapamil, or propranolol (with or without digoxin) to control the heart rate, rather than trying to restore heart rhythm to normal. In either case, warfarin (an anticoagulant) may also be given to help prevent blood clots from forming. However, taking warfarin increases the risk of bleeding, especially for older people. For example, minor bumps may cause bleeding under the skin (bruises), cuts may bleed longer, and bleeding after surgery may be excessive. To keep this risk as low as possible, doctors periodically do blood tests to measure how long blood takes to clot and adjust the dose of warfarin accordingly. Warfarin is not given to people who have bleeding disorders and may not be given to people who are at high risk of falling.

In some people who have taken antiarrhythmic drugs for a few weeks, the heart rhythm returns to normal. If it does not, an electrical shock is often applied to the chest to restore a normal heart rhythm. This procedure may cause a clot to be dislodged from the heart and thus increases the risk of a stroke. Taking warfarin for 3 weeks before the procedure helps reduce the risk of blood clots. Warfarin is continued for several weeks after the electrical shock is applied and may be continued indefinitely in people at high risk for recurrence of atrial fibrillation.

In some people, an electrical shock does not restore a normal heart rhythm. In other people, an electrical shock returns heart rhythm to normal for several weeks or months, then atrial flutter or atrial fibrillation recurs. Some people do not wish to have an electrical shock applied to the chest. In all of these situations, most people must take antiarrhythmic drugs and warfarin for the rest of their life. If palpitations are uncomfortable despite the continued use of drugs or if heart failure develops, a procedure called catheter ablation may be recommended. In this procedure, part or all of the electrical connection between the atria and ventricles is destroyed. If all of the connection is destroyed, a permanent artificial pacemaker must be implanted.

VENTRICULAR TACHYCARDIA

In ventricular tachycardia, the heart beats regularly but too rapidly. Sometimes the heart beats too rapidly for a few seconds, then returns to a normal rate. If the heart beats too rapidly for more than 30 seconds, the disorder is called sustained ventricular tachycardia.

Sustained ventricular tachycardia is more common among older people. Most commonly, it is caused by coronary artery disease (often by a heart attack), heart failure, or use of digoxin or certain other antiarrhythmic drugs in doses that are too high (causing toxicity). If sustained ventricular tachycardia is triggered by such an event and does not recur within the next few days, it is unlikely to recur.

In sustained ventricular tachycardia, the ventricles cannot fill adequately or pump blood normally. Thus, ventricular tachycardia often leads to dizziness, loss of consciousness, or heart failure. It sometimes leads to ventricular fibrillation, which causes death unless promptly corrected.

Most people with ventricular tachycardia notice palpitations. People may feel dizzy or faint because blood pressure tends to fall. Occasionally, ventricular tachycardia causes few symptoms, even at rates of up to 200 beats per minute, but it is still extremely dangerous.

Diagnosis and Treatment

Electrocardiography (ECG) is used to diagnose ventricular tachycardia and to help determine whether treatment is needed. A portable ECG (Holter) monitor may be used to record heart rhythm over a 24-hour period.

If ventricular tachycardia causes low blood pressure or fainting or is sustained (even without causing symptoms), treatment is needed immediately. Antiarrhythmic drugs (such as lidocaine, procainamide, amiodarone, or bretylium) may be given intravenously. If these drugs do not promptly restore a normal heart rhythm, cardioversion (an electrical shock applied to the chest) is used. After cardioversion, an antiarrhythmic drug (such as amiodarone or sotalol), given by mouth, is often prescribed to prevent recurrences. Such a drug may not be prescribed if sustained ventricular tachycardia was triggered by an event such as a heart attack and is unlikely to recur.

If ventricular tachycardia recurs despite treatment with antiarrhythmic drugs, electrophysiologic testing or exercise stress testing may be done while the person is given different antiarrhythmic drugs. These tests are likely to trigger the arrhythmia. Then doctors can determine which drug is most effective in preventing and treating the arrhythmia.

Alternatively, an implantable cardioverter-defibrillator (ICD)[1] may be used. It detects ventricular tachycardia and delivers an electrical shock to correct it. Less commonly, catheter ablation or open-heart surgery is done. These procedures are used to destroy the small abnormal area in the ventricles that is usually responsible for sustained ventricular tachycardia.

VENTRICULAR FIBRILLATION

In ventricular fibrillation, the left ventricle contracts so irregularly, rapidly, and weakly that it quivers.

Different parts of the ventricle contract at different times. As a result, little if any blood is pumped from the heart. Thus, ventricular fibrillation is a form of cardiac arrest (when the heart suddenly stops pumping). Unless treated within 4 to 6 minutes,

1. see page 702

ventricular fibrillation usually results in permanent brain damage or death within several minutes after it begins.

The most common cause of ventricular fibrillation is coronary artery disease, particularly a heart attack. Other causes include severe heart failure, electrical shock, a dangerously low body temperature (hypothermia), near drowning, and very low levels of potassium in the blood (hypokalemia). Certain antiarrhythmic drugs used to treat other arrhythmias can, on occasion, cause ventricular fibrillation.

Ventricular fibrillation causes loss of consciousness within seconds. A person suddenly collapses, turns deadly white, has very dilated pupils, and has no detectable pulse, heartbeat, or blood pressure. Vital organs (such as the heart, brain, and kidneys) do not receive enough blood. Without treatment, the person dies within minutes.

Diagnosis and Treatment

Ventricular fibrillation is suspected when a person suddenly collapses and does not have a pulse or blood pressure. The diagnosis is confirmed by electrocardiography (ECG).

Ventricular fibrillation must be treated as an extreme emergency. Cardiopulmonary resuscitation (CPR) must be started within a few minutes. It must be followed by defibrillation (an electrical shock delivered to the chest) as soon as the equipment is available. Antiarrhythmic drugs may then be given to help maintain the normal heart rhythm.

When ventricular fibrillation is treated within a few minutes (before lack of oxygen damages the brain or other vital organs), some people recover completely. However, people who are successfully resuscitated from ventricular fibrillation due to coronary artery disease are at high risk of another episode. They should usually be evaluated with cardiac catheterization (coronary angiography) or electrophysiologic testing.

If possible, the disorder causing ventricular fibrillation is treated. Otherwise, a defibrillator is surgically implanted. Alternatively, antiarrhythmic drugs are given to prevent recurrences. People who have severe coronary artery disease and poor heart pumping function are less likely to survive, even when defibrillation is promptly done.

SINUS BRADYCARDIA AND SICK SINUS SYNDROME

In sinus bradycardia, the heart beats regularly but more slowly than usual (less than 60 beats per minute). Sick sinus syndrome is malfunction of the heart's natural pacemaker (sinus or sinoatrial node) that causes heart rhythm to vary randomly. Heart rhythm may be too slow or too fast.

A slow heart rate may be a sign of good physical condition. But it may also result when the heart's natural pacemaker (sinus node) malfunctions. If the heart's pacemaker malfunctions, other areas of the heart can produce electrical currents so that the heart continues to beat but more slowly than normal.

The heart's pacemaker is more likely to malfunction in older people. Usually, no serious problems result. However, sometimes the slow heart rate causes blood pressure to become so low that the brain does not get enough blood. Then, a person may feel dizzy or even faint.

Sinus bradycardia may be caused by a heart attack, a dangerously low body temperature (hypothermia), an underactive thyroid gland (hypothyroidism), or increased pressure within the skull (which can result from a hemorrhagic stroke). Conditions that briefly but strongly stimulate the vagus nerve (which controls heart rate) can temporarily slow the heart rate. Examples are vomiting or straining during a bowel movement or urination. Drugs given to slow the heart rate, such as beta-blockers and the calcium channel blockers verapamil and diltiazem, frequently cause sinus bradycardia.

The bradycardia-tachycardia syndrome is a type of sick sinus syndrome. In this disorder, slow heartbeats (bradycardia) alternate with fast heartbeats (tachycardia), such as atrial fibrillation and atrial flutter. Whether sick sinus syndrome causes any serious problems depends on the disorder causing it and the severity of the bradycardia or tachycardia.

The most common causes of sick sinus syndrome are coronary artery disease and scarring of the heart's electrical system.

Symptoms

Sinus bradycardia usually causes no symptoms. If the heart rate is less than 40 beats per minute, a person may feel weak and tired. If the rate is lower, the person may faint, because the brain does not get enough blood.

People with bradycardia-tachycardia syndrome may feel palpitations when the heart beats rapidly. When the heart beats slowly, they may feel dizzy. When the heart switches from beating rapidly to beating slowly, they may faint.

Diagnosis and Treatment

Doctors can often diagnose severe sinus bradycardia or sick sinus syndrome on the basis of symptoms and the results of electrocardiography (ECG). They may ask the person to wear a portable ECG (Holter) monitor to record the heart rhythm for 24 hours.

Many people with sinus bradycardia do not need treatment. If symptoms occur when straining during a bowel movement or urination, avoiding straining may prevent recurrences. If a beta-blocker or calcium channel blocker is the cause of a slow heart rate, discontinuing the drug or reducing the dose may relieve symptoms. If bradycardia causes symptoms and the cause cannot be corrected, a permanent artificial pacemaker is often implanted to speed up the heart rate. People with bradycardia-tachycardia syndrome may also need drugs to slow the rapid heart rate. After a pacemaker is implanted, a beta-blocker or a calcium channel blocker is often used to slow the heart rate and prevent tachycardia.

HEART BLOCK

In heart block, the electrical currents that pass through the tissues between the atria and ventricles are delayed or blocked.

Depending on its severity, heart block may cause no problems or serious problems, such as loss of consciousness or fainting. Heart block is classified as first, second, or third degree based on its severity. Heart block is more common among older people. Electrocardiography (ECG) is needed to make the diagnosis.

In **first-degree heart block,** the electrical currents flowing between the atria and ventricles are slightly delayed. First-degree heart block may occur in healthy people. But it may be caused by rheumatic fever, disorders that damage the heart's electrical system, and other heart disorders. It may also be caused by drugs, particularly those that slow the heart rate (such as beta-blockers, diltiazem, verapamil, and amiodarone). This disorder produces no symptoms. No treatment is needed.

In **second-degree heart block,** the electrical currents are sometimes (intermittently) blocked. The heart may beat slowly, irregularly, or both. Common causes include heart attack, scarring of the heart's electrical system, heart infections (myocarditis), and use of digoxin or other drugs that slow the heart rate in doses that are too high. Second-degree heart block may cause dizziness and fainting. Sometimes second-degree heart block progresses to third-degree heart block. If second-degree heart block causes symptoms and its cause cannot be eliminated, an artificial pacemaker is usually implanted.

In **third-degree (complete) heart block,** the electrical currents flowing between the atria and ventricles are completely blocked. Another part of the heart then acts as a pacemaker. This substitute pacemaker is slower than the heart's normal pacemaker and is often irregular and unreliable. Common causes include heart attack, scarring of the heart's electrical system, and toxicity due to digoxin or other drugs that slow the heart rate. Third-degree heart block commonly causes fatigue, dizziness, and fainting. It is a serious disorder that can affect the heart's ability to pump. Heart failure can result. Third-degree heart block can cause death if the substitute pacemaker is too slow or if the heart stops beating.

In an emergency, third-degree heart block may be treated with a temporary external pacemaker until a permanent one can be implanted. A temporary pacemaker may also be used when doctors think that heart rhythm is likely to return to normal after the cause of the heart block resolves—for example, after a person recovers from a heart attack or after digoxin is discontinued. For nearly all other people with third-degree heart block, a permanent artificial pacemaker is needed.

48

Heart Valve Disorders

Heart valves control blood flow through the four chambers of the heart. A heart valve consists of an opening guarded by flaps (cusps or leaflets). The leaflets of each valve open and close like one-way swinging doors to make sure that blood flows in only one direction. A heart valve disorder may involve narrowing (stenosis) of a valve's opening, interfering with blood flow through the valve. Or a heart valve disorder may involve backward leakage (regurgitation) of blood through a valve. Stenosis and regurgitation may affect the same valve.

The more severe the narrowing or leakage becomes, the harder the heart has to work and the more likely symptoms are to occur. If heart valve disorders are not diagnosed and treated, blood pressure may increase. Or blood may begin to back up in the heart, and the heart may become unable to pump enough blood to the body. Serious disorders such as heart failure, stroke, abnormal heart rhythms (arrhythmias), and infection of the heart valves (endocarditis) can result.

A heart valve disorder can develop in any of the four heart valves (mitral, aortic, tricuspid, or pulmonary valves).[1] The mitral valve controls blood flow from the left upper chamber of the heart (atrium) to the left lower chamber (ventricle). The aortic valve controls blood flow from the left ventricle into the aorta, the artery that carries oxygen-rich blood to the body. The tricuspid valve controls blood flow from the right atrium into the right ventricle. The pulmonary (pulmonic) valve controls blood flow from the right ventricle into the arteries that carry blood to the lungs (pulmonary arteries). Among older people, disorders of the aortic valve and the mitral valve are the most common.

1. see art on page 658

UNDERSTANDING STENOSIS AND REGURGITATION

A heart valve can malfunction in two ways. Its opening can narrow, causing stenosis. Or a heart valve can leak, causing regurgitation. Stenosis and regurgitation can affect any heart valve. Below, they are shown at the mitral valve.

Normal Valve Mechanisms

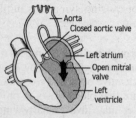

Aorta
Closed aortic valve
Left atrium
Open mitral valve
Left ventricle

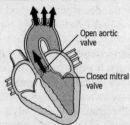

Open aortic valve
Closed mitral valve

Normally, when the left ventricle relaxes (after it contracts), the aortic valve closes, the mitral valve opens, and blood flows from the left atrium into the left ventricle. Then the left atrium contracts, pumping more blood into the left ventricle.

As the left ventricle contracts, the mitral valve closes, the aortic valve opens, and blood is pumped into the aorta.

Mitral Stenosis

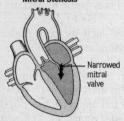

Narrowed mitral valve

Mitral Regurgitation

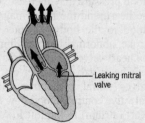

Leaking mitral valve

In mitral stenosis, the opening of the mitral valve is narrowed. As a result, blood flows from the left atrium into the left ventricle with more difficulty. Pressure in the left atrium increases.

In mitral regurgitation, the mitral valve leaks when the left ventricle contracts. As a result, some blood flows backward into the left atrium.

Causes

Among older people, several disorders can cause heart valves to malfunction. Calcium may accumulate in a valve (a disorder called degenerative calcification). This disorder affects about one third of people over 70. Certain hereditary disorders can cause the valves to deteriorate over time. The most common one, myxomatous degeneration, can cause the valves to become floppy and thus leak. A valve may be defective at birth. Such a valve may deteriorate, sometimes not causing symptoms until late in life. A heart attack or an infection of the heart valve may damage the structures that support the valve. Leakage may result. Less commonly, a heart valve disorder may be caused by rheumatic fever (a now rare childhood illness that can develop after strep throat if it is not treated).

Symptoms

Symptoms vary depending on which valve is malfunctioning, how quickly the disorder develops, and whether the valve is narrowed or leaking. Some heart valve disorders cause few or no symptoms. Some cause severe symptoms that occur suddenly.

The most common symptom is shortness of breath during physical activity. Shortness of breath usually occurs because the heart has to work harder to pump the same amount of blood. And during physical activity, the heart is already working harder because the heart needs more oxygen. Chest pain may occur if the heart does not get enough oxygen. Lack of oxygen may damage the heart. The damage may prevent the heart from pumping enough blood for the body's needs.

Some people with a heart valve disorder feel their heart beating rapidly and irregularly (a feeling called palpitations). They may feel weak or faint. These symptoms may be due to an abnormal heart rhythm called atrial fibrillation. Atrial fibrillation may develop when blood backs up in and stretches the left atrium, causing the heart to enlarge.

If a heart valve disorder worsens, people may also feel short of breath during rest. This symptom indicates that heart failure is developing. Heart failure develops as the heart works harder and harder to pump blood to the rest of the body. At first, as the heart tries to pump harder, its walls thicken and its chambers enlarge. But eventually, the heart cannot keep up with the extra work. Then blood backs up in the veins that carry blood to the left atrium from the lungs. Pressure in the blood vessels of the lungs increases. Fluid may leak out of blood vessels and accumulate in the lungs, interfering with breathing.

Blood clots tend to form when blood backs up in the atrium. Clots do not cause symptoms unless part of the clot breaks off, travels through the bloodstream, and blocks an artery elsewhere in the body. If an artery that carries blood to the brain is blocked, a stroke may result.

Diagnosis

Heart valve disorders are often first suspected during a routine physical examination. Doctors may detect abnormal heart sounds (murmurs) when they use a stethoscope to listen to the heart. Heart murmurs occur because blood does not flow through the valve normally. The pulse may be fast and irregular. A chest x-ray may show an enlarged heart.

Echocardiography (ultrasonography of the heart) is an accurate way to detect a heart valve disorder. This test helps doctors confirm the diagnosis and determine which heart valve disorder is present and how severe it is. Echocardiography can also detect evidence of heart damage, such as weak pumping of the heart. For the procedure, a hand-held device that emits and records ultrasound waves is placed on the chest. This procedure is safe and painless. If a closer look at the heart is needed, an ultrasound device is passed down the throat into the esophagus. This method (called transesophageal echocardiography) is safe but sometimes causes gagging and anxiety. So before the procedure, doctors usually give people a drug to calm them.

Treatment

For many older people with a heart valve disorder, drugs are effective. The drugs used depend on the type of disorder.

Antihypertensive drugs may be used. These drugs are typically used to lower blood pressure. However, they are also used to treat some heart valve disorders because these drugs reduce the amount of work the heart has to do. Two types of antihypertensive drugs—calcium channel blockers and angiotensin-converting enzyme (ACE) inhibitors—reduce the heart's workload by causing arteries to widen (dilate).

Beta-blockers (another type of antihypertensive drug) are used to treat some heart valve disorders. Beta-blockers slow the

REPLACING A HEART VALVE

A damaged heart valve may be replaced with a mechanical valve made of metal or with a valve made of tissue, usually from pigs or cows, placed in a synthetic ring. With a mechanical valve, the risk of blood clots is higher. But tissue valves do not last as long. Which type is used depends on individual circumstances and preferences. Older people who need a heart valve replaced should discuss with their doctor which type is best for them. A St. Jude valve is an example of a mechanical valve.

For heart valve replacement, a general anesthetic is given. Usually, open-heart surgery using a heart-lung machine is done. The damaged valve is removed, and the replacement valve is sewn in place. The operation takes 2 to 5 hours.

After surgery, the person is monitored in an intensive care unit for a day or two, before being moved to a regular unit. The length of the hospital stay varies from person to person. Full recovery takes 6 to 8 weeks.

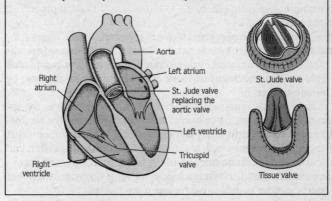

Aorta
Left atrium
Right atrium
St. Jude valve replacing the aortic valve
Left ventricle
Tricuspid valve
Right ventricle

St. Jude valve

Tissue valve

heart rate so that the blood has more time to flow through the narrowed valve opening. These drugs lessen palpitations and other symptoms.

People who also have atrial fibrillation may be given digoxin (commonly used to treat heart failure). This drug slows the heart rate when it is too rapid.

If the left atrium is stretched and enlarged, warfarin (an anticoagulant) is used to prevent clots from forming. However, warfarin increases the risk of bleeding, especially for older people. For example, minor bumps may cause bleeding under the skin (bruises), cuts may bleed longer, and bleeding after surgery or an injury may be excessive. To keep this risk as low as possible, doctors instruct a person to periodically have blood tests that measure how long blood takes to clot. The dose of warfarin can be adjusted based on the test results. Warfarin is not given to people who have bleeding disorders. It may not be given to people who are at high risk of falling.

If symptoms of heart failure develop, diuretics are sometimes used. They increase the amount of fluid and salt excreted by the kidneys. However, doctors carefully adjust the dose and monitor the use of these drugs because symptoms may worsen if the kidneys excrete too much fluid.

If symptoms develop or if tests detect permanent heart damage, repair or replacement of the valve may be recommended. Age does not affect the decision to perform such a procedure. However, the presence of other disorders and the person's overall condition (for example, being very frail) may make a procedure inadvisable.

If possible, the abnormal valve is repaired. In one type of repair, excess valve tissue is removed, and a supporting ring is implanted. If an abnormal valve cannot be repaired, it is replaced with a metal (mechanical) valve or a valve made of pig, cow, or human tissue.

Heart valve repair or replacement is very effective. Symptoms may resolve, often completely, and life can often be prolonged. Valve repair or replacement usually requires open-heart surgery. Sometimes new techniques using a small incision can be used. These techniques result in fewer problems, and recovery may be faster. Having a kidney or lung disorder or another heart disorder makes valve replacement riskier.

Risks of valve repair or replacement include breathing problems, abnormal heart rhythms, bleeding, stroke, and death. The risks are higher for older people but are usually less than the risks of not having the valve repaired or replaced.

People who have a heart valve disorder or who have had a heart valve replaced must take antibiotics before certain surgical, dental, or medical procedures. This precaution helps prevent endocarditis. Such people should talk with their doctor about what their risk of developing endocarditis is, what to do to prevent it, and what its early symptoms are.

Outlook

Sometimes heart valve disorders are mild, require no treatment, and do not shorten life. In other cases, drugs or surgery can effectively control symptoms or even cure the disorder. But having another chronic disorder may make the outlook worse or may even make treatment of a heart valve disorder inadvisable. Then, life may be shortened, and the focus shifts to improving quality of life and relieving symptoms.

For people with a heart valve disorder, death is often due to heart failure[1] or an abnormal heart rhythm.[2] In either case,

---

OPERATING ON THE HEART: OPEN-HEART SURGERY

Many older people worry that they are too frail to go through open-heart surgery. Such surgery seems drastic. An incision is made in the chest, and the breastbone is cut and separated. The heart is exposed, and its beating is usually stopped. However, this surgery can mean a difference between life and death. In general, open-heart surgery is recommended if it has less serious risks than the disorder without the surgery. Most often, open-heart surgery is done to replace a malfunctioning heart valve or to bypass blocked coronary arteries.

When the heart's beating is stopped, a heart-lung (cardiopulmonary bypass) machine does the work of the lungs and heart. It puts oxygen into the blood and pumps blood to the body. A tube connects the atria to the machine. (The atria are the heart chambers that receive blood from the body.) This tube carries blood from the heart into the machine. Another tube connects the machine to the aorta, which carries blood to the body. Thus, the heart is clear of blood and is still, making the work of the surgeon easier. After the work on the heart is completed, the surgeon restarts the heart. Occasionally, open-heart surgery leads to problems, such as a stroke, a heart attack, confusion, or blood clots, or even death.

After surgery, people recover in a special coronary or intensive care unit. There, they are hooked up to many tubes, which are used to give drugs, monitor the heart, help with breathing, and drain fluids. A temporary external pacemaker may be connected to the heart with wires inserted into veins. These tubes and wires are removed as people recover. The incision is painful, and the nose and throat are sore from insertion of tubes. However, the pain can usually be relieved. People usually stay in the hospital for 5 to 7 days. Recovery and rehabilitation take about 6 to 8 weeks. Rehabilitation programs begun in the hospital help speed recovery.

---

1. see page 680
2. see page 694

death may occur without warning. Consequently, preparing advance directives is important.[1]

AORTIC STENOSIS

In aortic stenosis, the opening of the aortic valve narrows.

Aortic stenosis is the most common heart valve disorder among older people. In this disorder, the heart—specifically, the left ventricle—has to work harder to pump blood through the valve into the aorta and to pump enough blood to the brain and other vital organs. Pressure increases in the left ventricle. Conditions that lower blood pressure, such as dehydration,[2] can make pumping enough blood even harder. Aortic stenosis develops gradually. It can lead to serious heart problems and, if untreated, to death.

Causes

In older people, the most common cause of aortic stenosis is the accumulation of calcium (calcification) on a normal valve or on a valve that was mildly defective at birth. For example, an aortic valve may have two leaflets (called bicuspid) rather than the usual three. Calcium makes the valve stiff and narrows the opening.

Sometimes calcium accumulates on the aortic valve but does not interfere with blood flow. This disorder is called aortic sclerosis.

Symptoms and Diagnosis

Many people with aortic stenosis do not have symptoms. When symptoms develop, they may be mild at first and may be mistakenly attributed to getting older.

Usually, symptoms first occur during physical activity, when the demands on the heart are greater. People may become short of breath, feel faint, or actually faint. They may also have a feeling of tightness, heaviness, or pain in the chest (angina). Severe aortic stenosis can lead to heart failure and sometimes death without warning.

1. see page 953
2. see page 249

Doctors usually base the diagnosis on abnormal heart sounds, abnormalities in the pulse, and the results of echocardiography. Echocardiography can help doctors determine how narrow the valve's opening is.

Treatment and Outlook

Usually, if aortic stenosis does not cause any symptoms, people do not need treatment. However, they should see their doctor regularly and avoid overly stressful physical activity. They should also avoid becoming dehydrated. The doctor uses echocardiography to monitor the progression of the disorder.

If the valve's opening has become greatly narrowed or if symptoms develop, doctors almost always recommend surgery to replace the aortic valve. In these cases, the risk of surgery is almost always less than the risk of not having surgery. Before surgery in older people, cardiac catheterization is usually done to determine whether coronary artery disease is also present. If it is, coronary artery bypass graft (CABG) surgery is done at the same time.

If surgery is done, symptoms are greatly relieved or even eliminated. People can function much better and can usually avoid further hospitalization.

WHAT IS AORTIC SCLEROSIS?

Sometimes calcium accumulates on the aortic valve, and the valve thickens. But the thickening does not interfere with blood flow through the valve. This disorder is called aortic sclerosis. About 1 out of 4 people over 65 have this disorder.

Aortic sclerosis does not cause symptoms. It may cause a soft heart murmur, heard by a doctor through a stethoscope. Aortic sclerosis may not make a person feel any different, but it increases the risk of a heart attack and death. Consequently, identifying and eliminating or controlling risk factors for coronary artery disease are important for people with aortic sclerosis. These risk factors include smoking, high blood pressure, abnormal cholesterol and triglyceride levels, and diabetes.

AORTIC REGURGITATION

In aortic regurgitation, some blood that has already been pumped out of the heart and into the aorta leaks backward into the heart.

A leak may develop gradually (over months or years) or quickly (over hours or days).

Causes

In people with aortic stenosis or aortic sclerosis, valves may not close completely, resulting in aortic regurgitation.

Aortic regurgitation may result when the aorta enlarges, often because of high blood pressure. When the aorta is enlarged, the valve may not close completely. As a result, blood leaks backward through the valve into the heart.

Aortic regurgitation may occur quickly if a tear in the lining of the aorta (aortic dissection) or a bulge that forms in a weakened area of the aorta (aortic aneurysm) affects the aortic valve. Infection of the heart valves (endocarditis) may also cause aortic regurgitation to occur quickly.

Symptoms and Diagnosis

If regurgitation develops gradually, it may cause no symptoms, or symptoms may develop slowly. Usually, symptoms do not appear until years after the regurgitation started. At first, people may tire more easily or feel short of breath during physical activity. If regurgitation worsens, people also feel short of breath during rest. This worsening means that heart failure is developing.

If regurgitation occurs quickly, symptoms may develop quickly and become severe. People may feel short of breath and as if their heart is racing. Severe heart failure may develop quickly. Death may occur without warning.

Doctors usually suspect the diagnosis on the basis of abnormal heart sounds, abnormalities in the pulse, and the results of a chest x-ray. However, echocardiography is much more accurate. Echocardiography can usually detect aortic regurgitation and the heart damage that may result from regurgitation. Usually, no other tests are needed.

Treatment and Outlook

If regurgitation develops gradually, most people do not need treatment at first. But when regurgitation becomes moderate to severe, even if it does not cause symptoms, most people are given a drug to reduce the amount of work the heart has to do. The drug may be an angiotensin-converting enzyme (ACE) inhibitor or a calcium channel blocker. These drugs may postpone the development of symptoms and thus the need for valve replacement. However, if symptoms develop or if echocardiography detects substantial heart damage (even if no symptoms are present), the aortic valve is replaced.

If regurgitation occurs quickly, the aortic valve is usually replaced as soon as possible. If the cause is endocarditis or aortic dissection, the valve may be repaired instead.

Without treatment, aortic regurgitation tends to worsen over time. The outlook is worse for older people, partly because many of them also have coronary artery disease. If heart failure develops, the outlook is also worse. After heart valve replacement, people over 75 tend to continue to have heart problems (including heart failure) and are more likely to die.

MITRAL STENOSIS

In mitral stenosis, the opening of the mitral valve becomes narrow.

When mitral stenosis develops, blood flow from the left atrium into the left ventricle is impaired. Pressure in the left atrium increases, stretching and enlarging it. These changes commonly result in an irregular, fast heart rhythm called atrial fibrillation.[1] Also, blood clots may form in the atrium. Part of a clot may break off and block an artery elsewhere in the body. Occasionally, a stroke results.

Severe mitral stenosis tends to be diagnosed and treated in younger people. Thus, mitral stenosis in older people is uncommon and tends to be milder.

1. see page 706

Causes

Mitral stenosis almost always results from rheumatic fever, a childhood illness. Rheumatic fever is now rare in regions where antibiotics are widely used to treat strep throat and thus prevent rheumatic fever. Less commonly, mitral stenosis develops in older people when calcium accumulates on the valve.

Symptoms and Diagnosis

Mild mitral stenosis causes few or no symptoms. If the disorder is moderate or severe, people may notice an irregular, fast heartbeat (indicating atrial fibrillation). At first, they may feel short of breath only during physical activity. But if the disorder worsens, they may feel short of breath during rest (indicating that heart failure is developing). Some people can breathe comfortably only when propped up with pillows or sitting upright. Some people cough up blood.

Mitral stenosis is more likely to cause atrial fibrillation and blockages due to blood clots in older people than in younger people.

Doctors usually suspect the diagnosis based on symptoms, abnormal heart sounds, and the results of echocardiography. Occasionally, mitral stenosis is first diagnosed in people who have had a stroke due to a blood clot.

Treatment and Outlook

Most people with mild to moderate mitral stenosis can be treated with drugs, such as beta-blockers, and thus avoid surgery. Heart failure and atrial fibrillation, if present, are treated. Warfarin (an anticoagulant) is usually given to prevent clots from forming.

If mitral stenosis causes symptoms and is worsening, the mitral valve may be repaired or replaced. The outlook for people with mitral stenosis depends on the severity of the disorder. If heart failure develops, the outlook is worse. When the valve is repaired or replaced, symptoms are generally relieved, and people can function much better.

MITRAL REGURGITATION

In mitral regurgitation, blood leaks backward through the mitral valve each time the left ventricle contracts to pump blood into the aorta.

In older people, mitral regurgitation usually develops gradually (over months or years). But it may develop quickly (over hours or days). Most older people have mild mitral regurgitation, which does not require treatment.

Causes

In older people, mild mitral regurgitation slowly develops when calcium accumulates at the base of the mitral valve. Severe mitral regurgitation may be caused by heart attacks, degeneration of the valve (myxomatous valve disease), or infection of the heart valves (endocarditis). Regurgitation can develop quickly if the structures that support the valve tear because a heart attack occurs or because the structures have weakened over time.

Symptoms and Diagnosis

Mild mitral regurgitation may cause few or no symptoms. People may tire easily and feel short of breath only during physical activity. If the disorder worsens, people may notice an irregular, fast heartbeat (indicating atrial fibrillation). Heart failure may develop.

If regurgitation develops quickly, symptoms may develop and become severe quickly. Breathing becomes very difficult, and people feel as if their heart is racing. Severe heart failure may develop.

Doctors usually suspect the diagnosis on the basis of abnormal heart sounds, abnormalities in the pulse, and the results of echocardiography. Transesophageal echocardiography [1] is needed only when regurgitation is severe and valve repair or replacement may be needed.

Treatment

Most people with mitral regurgitation are given warfarin (an anticoagulant) to prevent clots from forming. Other disorders (such as heart failure or atrial fibrillation) that are causing mitral regurgitation are treated. If regurgitation is mild, such treatment may make surgery unnecessary.

If symptoms are severe or if echocardiography detects substantial heart damage (even if no symptoms are present), the

1. see page 718

mitral valve may be repaired or replaced. Repair or replacement is usually recommended if heart failure has developed. The valve is repaired if possible. Repair of the mitral valve is safer than replacement of the valve, and people are likely to live longer and have fewer symptoms.

Many people with mild mitral regurgitation have a good outlook. However, mitral regurgitation may worsen, causing symptoms and eventually heart failure. Getting regular checkups, which may include echocardiography, is important.

49

Blood Disorders

Blood consists of a liquid (plasma) that contains red blood cells, white blood cells, platelets, and other components. A blood disorder can develop when there are too many or too few of these components or when they are abnormal.

Each component of the blood has an important function. Red blood cells (erythrocytes) carry oxygen to the body's tissues and carry carbon dioxide (a waste product) from the tissues. If there is a problem with red blood cells, the body's tissues do not get enough oxygen, and tissues and organs may malfunction. People with too few red blood cells (anemia) often feel tired. White blood cells (leukocytes) help fight infection and cancer. If there is a problem with white blood cells, infections and cancer are more likely to develop. Platelets (thrombocytes) and clotting factors help blood clot. If there is a problem with platelets or clotting factors, excessive bleeding or excessive clotting may occur. The inner part of bone (bone marrow) contains immature, unspecialized cells, called stem cells, that develop into white blood cells, red blood cells, or platelets. If there is a problem with bone marrow, too many or too few of these components may be produced.

Some blood disorders are more common among older people. However, sometimes blood disorders are not detected promptly because the symptoms, such as weakness, fatigue, and shortness of breath, are mistakenly attributed to aging itself. Certain cancers that affect the blood's components, such as multiple myeloma and leukemia, are relatively common among older people.[1]

ANEMIA

In anemia, the number of red blood cells (red blood cell count) is low. In some types of anemia, red blood cells are also abnormal in size or shape.

Anemia, although common among older people, is never normal. Anemia can have serious causes and consequences and should always be evaluated by a doctor.

Red blood cells contain a protein called hemoglobin, which contains a tiny amount of iron. Hemoglobin enables red blood cells to carry oxygen from the lungs and deliver it to the body's tissues. Every cell in the body needs oxygen to produce energy for the cell's activities. When energy is produced, carbon dioxide is given off as a waste product. Red blood cells carry carbon dioxide away from the tissues and back to the lungs to be breathed out. In anemia, there is not enough hemoglobin because there are not enough red blood cells or because less hemoglobin is produced. In some anemias, hemoglobin is also abnormal. Thus, in anemia, blood cannot carry enough oxygen to the body's tissues or remove enough carbon dioxide.

A hormone called erythropoietin helps the body maintain a normal number of red blood cells. When tissues are not getting enough oxygen, the kidneys produce erythropoietin. Erythropoietin stimulates the inner part of bones (bone marrow) to produce more red blood cells.

To produce red blood cells, the body needs many nutrients. The most critical ones are iron, vitamin B_{12}, and folic acid. When the body does not get enough of these nutrients, the bone marrow does not produce enough red blood cells, and the ones produced may be abnormal. If iron is lacking, red blood cells

1. see page 765

may be abnormally small. If vitamin B_{12} or folic acid is lacking, red blood cells may be abnormally large.

Causes

Anemia may be caused by abnormal bleeding. Anemia develops when the bone marrow cannot produce enough red blood cells to replace those lost through bleeding. Bleeding is not always obvious. Sometimes it is gradual and slow and goes unnoticed. For example, a stomach ulcer, a polyp in the large intestine, or cancer of the kidneys, bladder, or digestive tract can cause bleeding that may not be noticed. Iron—a critical nutrient for red blood cell production and a component of hemoglobin—is also lost when bleeding occurs. Iron deficiency anemia, usually due to abnormal bleeding, is the most common anemia among older people.

Another cause of anemia is reduced production of red blood cells. To produce red blood cells, the body needs enough vitamin B_{12}, folic acid, and iron. Consuming too little of one of these nutrients or being unable to absorb one of them can result in anemia. For example, in pernicious anemia, the body is not able to absorb vitamin B_{12}. Consuming too little iron can result in iron deficiency anemia. However, in the United States, anemia rarely results from consuming too little iron because supplemental iron is added to many foods.

Certain chronic disorders—such as infections, inflammation (as occurs in rheumatoid arthritis), cancer, and kidney disorders—can reduce red blood cell production. The type of anemia that results is called anemia of chronic disease. In some disorders, abnormal cells invade and replace much of the bone marrow, where red blood cells are produced. These disorders include cancer that has spread to bone (metastatic cancer), leukemia, multiple myeloma, and lymphoma. Other problems in the bone marrow, including aplastic anemia and myelodysplastic syndrome, may result in anemia. In some kidney and other chronic disorders, the kidneys do not produce enough erythropoietin, which stimulates red blood cell production.

Less commonly, the cause of anemia is destruction of more red blood cells than can be produced. This type of anemia is called hemolytic anemia. In older people, the cause of hemolytic anemia is often unknown. However, hemolytic anemia may result from many disorders and from use of certain drugs.

Sometimes hemolytic anemia results from an autoimmune reaction: The immune system mistakes red blood cells for foreign invaders and produces antibodies to destroy them. Why this reaction occurs is unknown.

PROBLEMS IN THE BONE MARROW

Stem cells are immature or unspecialized cells that can develop into different types of cells. They remain unspecialized until signaled by the body to change. They replace cells that are worn out, damaged, or diseased. Some disorders, such as aplastic anemia, myelodysplastic syndrome, and myeloproliferative disorders, affect stem cells in the bone marrow and thus interfere with the production of red blood cells, white blood cells, and platelets.

In aplastic anemia, the bone marrow does not have enough stem cells and thus cannot produce enough red and white blood cells and platelets. Aplastic anemia is relatively rare but is more common among older people. Aplastic anemia is commonly caused by malfunction of the body's immune system, causing the body to attack its own tissues (autoimmune disorder). Other causes include exposure to radiation and use of certain chemotherapy drugs, the antibiotic chloramphenicol, and drugs used to treat seizures (anticonvulsants). Sometimes the cause is unknown. People with aplastic anemia must be treated immediately, or they will die. Transfusions are given and may have to be continued indefinitely. Stem cell or bone marrow transplantation can cure aplastic anemia, but older people can rarely withstand this taxing treatment. Drugs that may help include corticosteroids, such as prednisone, and drugs that suppress the immune system (immunosuppressants), such as antithymocyte globulin and cyclosporine. Drugs that stimulate production of the blood's components may be used: a synthetic version of erythropoietin or darbepoietin for red blood cells, colony-stimulating factors for white blood cells, and thrombopoietin for platelets.

In myelodysplastic syndrome, the bone marrow has enough stem cells, but they do not mature normally into red blood cells, white blood cells, and platelets. Myelodysplastic syndrome affects mostly older people. Usually, its cause is unknown, but it can be caused by use of certain drugs or alcohol or by toxic substances in the environment, such as lead. Erythropoietin, given by injection, is sometimes useful. It increases the blood cell count.

In myeloproliferative disorders, the immature cells (called stem cells) that develop into blood cells or platelets increase too much, or the fibrous tissue that supports the cells increases too much. Primary thrombocythemia, polycythemia vera, and myelofibrosis are myeloproliferative disorders. In a few people, a myeloproliferative disorder progresses or transforms into a cancer such as leukemia.

Anemia may result from hereditary disorders, which are usually detected early in life. Examples are sickle cell anemia and thalassemias.

Symptoms

Typically, anemia causes fatigue and weakness. It also makes people look pale. Older people are less likely to look pale, although the gums and other tissues in the mouth may be paler. Older people with anemia, even when mild (when the red blood cell count decreases only slightly), are more likely to become confused, depressed, agitated, or listless than younger people. They may also become unsteady and have difficulty walking. However, some older people with mild anemia have no symptoms at all, particularly when anemia develops gradually, as it often does in older people. Other people experience symptoms only when the body's tissues require more oxygen quickly, for example, during physical activity.

As the red blood cell count decreases further, anemia may cause light-headedness, sweating, a rapid pulse, and rapid breathing. These symptoms may occur even during rest. When tissues do not get enough oxygen, anemia may cause painful lower leg cramps during exercise, shortness of breath, and chest pain (angina), especially in people who have peripheral arterial disease or certain types of lung or heart disorders. Symptoms tend to be more severe when anemia develops rapidly.

If anemia is due to vitamin B_{12} deficiency, symptoms may develop because the nerves malfunction. People may feel tingling in the feet and hands and lose sensation in the legs, feet, and hands. The feet and legs are affected earlier and more often than the hands and arms. People may lose the ability to sense vibration and to know where their arms and legs are (position sense). Weakness in muscles may be slight or moderate, and reflexes may be lost. Walking becomes difficult. Some people become irritable and depressed. Mental function may be impaired in a way that resembles dementia. Some of these symptoms may occur before the anemia develops. They may be permanent, even if the deficiency is treated and the anemia resolves.

If anemia is due to slow bleeding in the urinary tract, blood may appear in the urine. If bleeding occurs in the digestive tract, blood may appear in the stool.

If anemia is due to sudden, excessive bleeding, two problems

TAKING A SAMPLE OF BONE MARROW

For a bone marrow biopsy, the skin and tissue over the bone are numbed with a local anesthetic. Then, the sharp needle of a syringe is inserted into the bone, usually the hip bone. The doctor pulls back on the plunger of the syringe and draws out a small amount of the soft bone marrow. The marrow can be spread on a slide and examined under a microscope.

Usually, a person feels a slight jolt of pain, followed by minimal discomfort. The procedure takes only a few minutes.

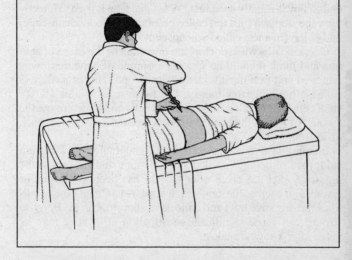

can result: Blood pressure falls because the amount of fluid left in the blood vessels is insufficient, and the body's oxygen supply is drastically reduced because the number of oxygen-carrying red blood cells has decreased so quickly. Either problem may lead to a heart attack, a stroke, kidney failure, or death.

Diagnosis

Sometimes anemia is detected before a person notices symptoms, when routine blood tests are done. If the amount of hemoglobin and the percentage of red blood cells in the blood (hematocrit) is low, anemia is diagnosed. Also, blood tests can usually help doctors determine the type and cause of the anemia. Doctors look at the size and appearance of red blood cells. They measure the levels of newly formed red blood cells, iron, ferritin (the protein that carries iron when it is outside of red blood cells), vitamin B_{12}, folic acid, and substances produced when red blood cells are destroyed. Other tests to determine the cause are also done.

Even if abnormal bleeding is not obvious, it is usually assumed to be the cause of iron deficiency anemia. In either case, the stool and urine are tested for blood to try to identify the source of the bleeding. If the digestive tract is the likely source, endoscopy is usually done first.[1] A flexible tube is used to directly view the stomach (in a test called esophagogastroduodenoscopy) and colon (in a test called colonoscopy).

Occasionally, when doctors are uncertain of the cause of anemia and think it could be serious, a sample of bone marrow is removed and examined under a microscope. This procedure is called a bone marrow biopsy. The purpose is to evaluate the stem cells that develop into red blood cells and to determine the amount of iron in the bone marrow, where the body stores much of its iron.

Imaging tests (such as computed tomography[2] or a barium study) are sometimes needed. For a barium study, x-rays of the digestive tract are taken after barium has been swallowed or given as an enema. Barium, which appears white on x-rays, outlines the digestive tract and collects in abnormal areas. Because barium can cause significant constipation, a laxative may be given after x-rays are taken.

Treatment

Treatment depends on the severity and cause of the anemia. If the anemia is mild, no treatment may be necessary. If the anemia is severe, red blood cells must be replaced by giving blood transfusions. Otherwise, treatment focuses on the cause of the anemia.

If the cause is abnormal bleeding, treatment involves locating the source of the bleeding and correcting the problem. Typically, iron supplements, usually tablets, are taken for several months to replace iron that is lost when blood is lost.

Anemia due to a deficiency of iron, vitamin B_{12}, or folic acid is treated by taking supplements of the deficient nutrient. Iron

1. see art on page 117
2. see page 124

supplements are usually taken by mouth for about 6 months. Sometimes iron supplements are given by injection. Vitamin B_{12} supplements are often given by injection. Injections are given daily or weekly for several weeks, then once a month. Vitamin B_{12} supplements can also be taken as tablets. Almost everyone who has anemia due to vitamin B_{12} deficiency must take these supplements for life. Folic acid supplements are usually taken as one tablet daily.

If anemia is caused by a chronic disorder, treatment involves treating the disorder. Taking iron or vitamin supplements does not help. Drugs that may be causing or contributing to the anemia are discontinued if possible. Sometimes injections of erythropoietin (a synthetic version of the hormone produced by the body) or darbepoietin help, particularly if the disorder cannot be cured. These drugs stimulate the production of red blood cells.

Sometimes blood transfusions are given for a short time. For example, they are given when blood loss is rapid or massive or when other treatments cannot quickly and effectively relieve serious symptoms, such as very low blood pressure or angina. Transfusions may be given when the red blood cell count is so low that a heart attack, a stroke, or kidney failure is likely to occur. Blood transfusions may be needed indefinitely when anemia persists and no other treatment is effective.

People who have anemia due to kidney failure or some other chronic disorder may benefit from injections of erythropoietin.

LOW PLATELET COUNT

A low platelet count (called thrombocytopenia) refers to an abnormally low number of platelets, the particles in blood that help with clotting. As a result, blood does not clot normally.

Usually, the platelet count is about 150,000 to 350,000 platelets in a microliter of blood. In people with a low platelet count, bleeding is more likely to occur, even after a slight injury. When the platelet count is very low (below 20,000), massive bleeding may occur even when there is no injury. Bleeding may be life threatening.

Causes

The platelet count may decrease if the bone marrow does not produce enough platelets. Leukemia, lymphomas, infection with human immunodeficiency virus (HIV, which causes AIDS), and a variety of other bone marrow disorders[1] can have this effect. Or the platelet count may decrease if the spleen enlarges and traps platelets. Thus, fewer platelets are in the bloodstream. Myelofibrosis and some forms of cirrhosis can have this effect.

The body may use or destroy too many platelets. HIV infection, lupus (systemic lupus erythematosus), idiopathic thrombocytopenic purpura, thrombotic thrombocytopenic purpura, and hemolytic-uremic syndrome can have this effect. Some drugs, such as heparin and certain antibiotics, also have this effect.

In idiopathic thrombocytopenic purpura, the immune system produces abnormal antibodies that destroy the body's platelets. Why the antibodies develop is unknown. The bone marrow produces more platelets to compensate but cannot keep up with the demand.

Taking heparin may cause a low platelet count. Heparin is a drug that makes blood less likely to clot (anticoagulant). But paradoxically, it sometimes stimulates clot formation. Then the platelet count decreases because so many platelets are used up.

Drinking alcohol may result in a low platelet count by damaging the bone marrow. Aspirin, nonsteroidal anti-inflammatory drugs (NSAIDs), and antihistamines may interfere with how platelets function, although the platelet count remains normal.

Symptoms

Bleeding in the skin may be the first sign that the platelet count is low. Often, many tiny red dots appear in the skin on the lower legs. People may bruise easily. Slight injuries sometimes cause small scattered bruises. The gums may bleed, and blood may appear in the stool or urine. Bleeding due to injuries may be hard to stop.

Bleeding worsens as the platelet count decreases. When the count is below 20,000, bleeding in the digestive tract or brain

1. see box on page 731

may occur even when there is no injury. This bleeding may be life threatening.

Diagnosis

Doctors suspect a low platelet count when people bruise easily and bleed excessively. Blood tests are done to determine the platelet count and thus confirm the diagnosis. Using an electronic counter to count platelets helps determine how low the platelet count is. The time blood takes to clot (bleeding time) may also be measured. Sometimes a low platelet count is detected when blood tests are done for other reasons. People who have a disorder that can reduce the platelet count should periodically have blood tests.

Doctors try to identify the cause, so that appropriate treatments can be used. Symptoms may suggest a cause. A fever suggests an infection. An enlarged spleen, felt during a physical examination, suggests a disorder that causes the spleen to enlarge.

A sample of bone marrow may be removed and examined under a microscope. This procedure, called a bone marrow biopsy, may be done to determine whether the bone marrow is producing enough platelets.

Treatment

If the platelet count is below 20,000, people are usually treated in a hospital or advised to stay in bed to avoid injury. They are usually given a transfusion of platelets. If the platelet count is 20,000 to 30,000 and excessive bleeding occurs, platelets are usually transfused.

Treating a disorder that has reduced the platelet count often restores the count to normal. If taking heparin is the cause, it is usually discontinued.

For some disorders such as idiopathic thrombocytopenic purpura, a corticosteroid such as prednisone may be used to temporarily prevent antibodies from destroying platelets. Then the platelet count increases. After the corticosteroid is discontinued, the count may decrease again. In such cases, people may need to continue a corticosteroid for the rest of their life, or one of several other treatments may be tried.

If the spleen is trapping too many platelets, the spleen may be surgically removed. This procedure (splenectomy) increases the platelet count.

CLOTTING DISORDERS

In clotting disorders, blood becomes more likely to clot when clotting is not needed.

A blood clot (thrombus) may form in a blood vessel (vein or artery) and block it. Or a clot may form in an artery or in the heart, travel through the bloodstream, and block an artery elsewhere (embolus). In most clotting disorders, veins are blocked more often than arteries. Veins in the legs are most commonly affected. If a critical blood vessel is blocked, the consequences may be serious. Examples are deep vein thrombosis, pulmonary embolism, strokes, heart attacks, and gangrene.

As people age, particularly after age 55 for men and age 60 for women, blockages in arteries and veins become more common. The reason for the increase is unclear. Atherosclerosis, which becomes more common as people age, may partly explain the increase of blockages in arteries, but not that in veins.

Normally, blood clots in response to injury. Clots form to plug breaks in blood vessels and prevent blood from leaking out of the blood vessels. Platelets are crucial to clotting. When a blood vessel breaks, platelets are activated. They become sticky and change from rounded to spiny. These changes enable platelets to stick to the broken blood vessel wall and to each other, helping form a plug at the break. At the same time, platelets release proteins and other substances that promote further clotting. These substances activate proteins called clotting factors, such as fibrinogen. Until activated, clotting factors are dissolved in the blood. When fibrinogen is activated, it is converted to fibrin, which consists of long strands. The strands are interwoven in the platelet plug and radiate from it. They form a net that entraps more platelets and red blood cells and thus help strengthen the clot. Platelets also release substances that cause the blood vessel to contract (constrict). This effect also helps reduce the bleeding.

After an injured blood vessel heals, other reactions help stop the clotting process and dissolve clots. These reactions also involve proteins dissolved in the blood. Without this control system, minor blood vessel injuries could trigger widespread clotting throughout the body, which occurs in some disorders.

Causes

Not moving around sufficiently can slow blood flow and cause blood to pool in the veins of the legs.[1] Then, blood clots are more likely to form, particularly in the deep veins of the legs. Clots may form when people are paralyzed or have to stay in bed for a long time—for example, after surgery or a heart attack. Even sitting for a long time, especially in confined spaces as in a car or an airplane, can make clots more likely.

Certain disorders cause blood to clot more readily because the clotting factors become overactive. These disorders include disseminated intravascular coagulation and the antiphospholipid syndrome.

• **Disseminated intravascular coagulation** is usually triggered by surgery, severe injuries, or a substance that enters the bloodstream. For example, some types of bacteria release harmful substances (toxins) into the bloodstream, and many kinds of cancer cells release substances that stimulate clotting. Disseminated intravascular coagulation can cause both excessive clotting and excessive bleeding. The disorder usually begins with small blood clots developing throughout the bloodstream. A clot may block a vein deep in the leg, causing deep vein thrombosis.[2] As more and more clots form, clotting factors, which help control bleeding, are used up. Then bleeding occurs.

• In **antiphospholipid syndrome,** abnormal proteins appear in the blood. The most common are anticardiolipin antibodies and lupus anticoagulant. Despite the name, lupus anticoagulant is really the opposite of an anticoagulant. Rather than make blood less likely to clot, lupus anticoagulant makes blood clot more readily, especially in arteries.

In some hereditary disorders, blood tends to clot more readily. Many people with such a disorder do not have symptoms until they are in their 60s. In some hereditary disorders, the body does not produce enough of a protein that helps control

1. see page 649
2. see page 649

clotting, or one of these proteins is ineffective. These proteins include protein C, protein S, and antithrombin III. In all of these disorders, the production of fibrin, which helps clots form, increases. In activated protein C resistance (factor V Leiden mutation), one clotting factor does not respond when protein C signals to stop clotting. About 3% of people have this disorder. In another hereditary disorder (prothrombin G20210A polymorphism), production of prothrombin, another clotting factor, is increased, leading to increased clotting.

A high level of homocysteine in the blood (hyperhomocysteinemia) makes the blood in veins and especially arteries more likely to clot. A high level may result from a hereditary disorder or a deficiency of vitamin B_6, vitamin B_{12}, or folic acid. Chronic kidney failure and the use of certain drugs can also result in a high homocysteine level. These drugs include methotrexate (used to treat cancer), the anticonvulsants phenytoin and carbamazepine, some cholesterol-lowering drugs such as fibric acid derivatives and niacin, and the antibiotic isoniazid.

Sometimes the bone marrow produces too many platelets, making blood more likely to clot. This disorder is called thrombocythemia.[1]

Atherosclerosis, polyarteritis nodosa, and giant cell arteritis make blood more likely to clot in arteries. These disorders cause inflammation of or injury to arteries, stimulating clot formation.

Heart failure increases the risk of clots. Because the heart cannot pump blood adequately, blood backs up in the heart and blood vessels. Clots are more likely to form when blood is not moving (stagnates) or is moving too slowly. Atrial fibrillation also increases the risk of clots. The reason is similar to that for heart failure. In atrial fibrillation, one of the heart's chambers (left atrium) does not empty completely because the heart beats irregularly and too fast. So clots tend to form in the blood that remains in the atrium.

Obesity increases the risk of clots because it puts pressure on veins, slowing the flow of blood.

The use of tamoxifen (used to treat breast cancer) or estrogen can make blood clot more readily. Also, people with cancer are more likely to develop blood clots.

1. see page 744

Symptoms

Symptoms depend on which blood vessels are blocked by the clots. For example, an arm or a leg may swell or become painful and red. If a leg remains severely swollen, the skin on the lower leg may become itchy and turn a reddish brown. This skin is easily injured, often resulting in an ulcer. These symptoms may result when clots permanently damage the deep veins in a leg (a disorder called chronic venous insufficiency). [1] Less commonly, the abdomen or face swells.

People with disseminated intravascular coagulation can have symptoms related to both clotting and bleeding. Shortness of breath may develop as small blood vessels of the lungs leak or clots form in them. The skin, lining of the mouth, and whites of the eyes (sclera) may become yellowish (jaundice) if clotting and bleeding occur in the liver. Often, many tiny red dots appear in the skin on the lower legs. People may bruise easily. The gums may bleed, and blood may appear in the stool or urine. Small blackened areas may develop in the fingers and toes if fibrin, a component of clots, is deposited in the blood vessels there. Gangrene can result.

When disseminated intravascular coagulation appears suddenly (as it may after surgery), it can cause uncontrollable, life-threatening bleeding. If it develops more slowly (as it may in people with cancer), clots in veins are more common than bleeding. This form is milder and tends to be chronic.

Diagnosis and Treatment

A blood clot may be detected when it causes symptoms or when a routine examination is done. An imaging test is usually needed to confirm the presence of clots. If clotting in veins is suspected, ultrasonography is useful for confirming clotting and for locating the clots. Magnetic resonance imaging (MRI) may be done if ultrasonography results are unclear. If results are still unclear, venography may be needed. For this test, special x-rays are taken after contrast dye is injected into a vein. When clotting in arteries is suspected, clotting may be confirmed using blood tests or arteriography. For arteriography, special x-rays are taken after contrast dye is injected into arteries.

1. see page 649

WHEN A CLOT BLOCKS A BLOOD VESSEL

Location of Blockage	Symptoms
Veins near the surface of legs or arms	Pain and inflammation (redness, swelling, and warmth) in legs or arms (due to superficial thrombophlebitis)
Veins deep in a leg	Swelling and aching of a leg (due to deep vein thrombosis)
Vein to the liver	Sudden, intense pain in the abdomen or coughing up or vomiting of blood (due to portal vein thrombosis)
Major arteries to the lungs	Shortness of breath, chest pain, or loss of consciousness (due to pulmonary embolism)
Arteries to the brain	A transient ischemic attack or stroke
Arteries to the heart	Chest pain (angina) or a heart attack
Arteries in an arm or a leg	A pale, cool arm or leg and if the clot persists, gangrene

The cause must be identified. Blood tests can help. The amount and activity of different proteins that control clotting are measured. The platelet count and the time blood takes to clot may be determined. These tests are usually done after a blood clot has been treated.[1]

If the cause is another disorder or a drug, the clotting problems may subside when the disorder is treated or the drug is discontinued.

If a hereditary disorder is the cause, people who have had one or more clots are often advised to take the anticoagulant warfarin for the rest of their life. Sometimes people who have had only one clot are advised to take warfarin or another anticoagulant, heparin, only when the risk of clots is high. For example,

USING DRUGS TO CONTROL CLOTTING

Sometimes drugs are needed to keep blood from clotting too readily. If blood clots too readily, life-threatening clots may form in arteries of the heart, brain, or lungs. As a result, the risk of a heart attack, a stroke, or pulmonary embolism is increased. Several different types of drugs can help control clotting.

Antiplatelet drugs make platelets less sticky and thus less likely to clump together and block a blood vessel. The most commonly used antiplatelet drug is aspirin. Other antiplatelet drugs include clopidogrel, dipyridamole, abciximab, and tirofiban.

Anticoagulants make blood less likely to clot. Although sometimes called "blood thinners," anticoagulants do not really thin the blood. Instead, they inhibit the activity of proteins in the blood that help blood clot (clotting factors). Commonly used anticoagulants are heparin and warfarin. Heparin is injected under the skin or given intravenously for a short time, usually in a hospital. Warfarin is given by mouth, usually for a longer time after discharge from the hospital.

The effects of these drugs must be closely monitored. If the dose is too high, excessive bleeding can occur. If the dose is too low, it may not prevent clots. So people who take them must have blood tests periodically. These tests measure how long blood takes to clot. The dose of the drug is adjusted on the basis of test results. A new type of anticoagulant, low-molecular-weight heparin, does not have to be monitored as much. It is injected under the skin. Lepirudin and argatroban are a new type of anticoagulant that specifically inhibits the activity of one activated clotting factor called thrombin. Thrombin helps in the formation of fibrin, an integral part of a clot. These drugs are used instead of heparin if heparin causes the platelet count to become low.

Thrombolytic (fibrinolytic) drugs can help dissolve a blood clot. Thrombolytic drugs, such as streptokinase and tissue plasminogen activator, are sometimes used when blood clots cause a heart attack or stroke. These drugs may save lives, but they also increase the risk of severe bleeding.

they should take an anticoagulant when they need bed rest for a long time. Because taking anticoagulants increases the risk of excessive bleeding, people who take them must have blood tests periodically to check whether blood is taking too long to clot. Doctors then adjust the dose of the anticoagulant if needed.

People with a high homocysteine level may be advised to take vitamin supplements with folic acid, vitamin B_6, and vitamin B_{12}, which may lower the homocysteine level.

Clotting in arteries may be treated with a drug that makes platelets less likely to clump and thus makes blood clots less likely to form. These drugs, called antiplatelet drugs, include aspirin, clopidogrel, and dipyridamole. If a clot is still present or if a person has atrial fibrillation, heparin or warfarin is used.

If a clot causes blood pressure to fall dangerously low or blocks blood flow to the brain or other vital organs, emergency treatment is needed. Treatment may involve giving drugs to dissolve clots (thrombolytic drugs) or, rarely, performing surgery to remove a clot from a blood vessel. However, these treatments can have dangerous, even life-threatening side effects, especially in older people.

If disseminated intravascular coagulation develops suddenly, it requires emergency treatment for clotting and bleeding. If bleeding is severe, transfusions of red blood cells, platelets, and clotting factors are given to replace those that are used up and to stop the bleeding. If clotting is more of a problem than bleeding, heparin may be given.

THROMBOCYTHEMIA

In thrombocythemia, too many platelets are produced. Excessive clotting or bleeding may result.

Thrombocythemia usually develops between the ages of 50 and 70. This rare disorder is more common among women.

In the bone marrow, the cells that become platelets increase in number (proliferate). Why the cells proliferate is unknown. But the result is too many platelets. If there are too many platelets, blood clots can form spontaneously. Clots may block blood vessels, especially small ones. Sometimes in thrombocythemia, platelets do not function normally. Then, excessive bleeding may occur.

Causes

Usually, no cause can be identified. This form is called primary (essential) thrombocythemia. Sometimes thrombocythemia is a reaction to another disorder or condition. This form is called secondary thrombocythemia. For example, too many platelets may be produced during an infection, after surgery or chemotherapy, or in response to excessive bleeding or tissue damage, which can occur during a heart attack. Other disorders that can cause thrombocythemia include iron deficiency anemia, cancer that has spread (metastasized), leukemia, lymphoma, polycythemia vera, and rheumatoid arthritis.

Symptoms

Most people do not have symptoms. About one third of people have symptoms due to blockages in small blood vessels. The hands and feet may tingle or feel as if they are burning. The fingertips may feel cold. Sometimes the legs become painful and red because clots block veins near the surface of the legs (a disorder called superficial thrombophlebitis).[1] Vision may be distorted. Other symptoms include headaches, weakness, and dizziness.

Less commonly, symptoms result from blockages in larger blood vessels, including crucial blood vessels. People who also have another disorder such as atherosclerosis are more likely to have a blockage in a crucial blood vessel.

Occasionally, the abdomen swells if too many platelets accumulate in the spleen, causing it to enlarge, or if blood clots cause the liver to enlarge.

If bleeding occurs, it is usually mild. Some people have nosebleeds, or the gums bleed slightly. Some people bruise easily. In a few people, usually those who are taking aspirin or another nonsteroidal anti-inflammatory drug (NSAID), bleeding occurs in the digestive tract.

Diagnosis

Thrombocythemia is usually diagnosed when a routine blood test detects too many platelets. In essential thrombocythemia, the platelet count is usually 2 to 4 times higher than normal.

Doctors must determine whether thrombocythemia is caused by another disorder. Blood tests can help. Sometimes a bone marrow biopsy is necessary. A sample of bone marrow is removed and examined under a microscope for characteristic changes caused by disorders that can increase the platelet count.

1. see page 648

Treatment and Outlook

Aspirin and similar drugs such as clopidogrel or dipyridamole are sometimes recommended, because they help control
symptoms such as headache and burning or tingling in the
hands and feet. These drugs make platelets less likely to stick
together and blood clots less likely to form. However, they increase the risk of bleeding.

A drug that suppresses platelet production is occasionally
used. These drugs include the chemotherapy drug hydroxyurea,
anagrelide (a drug that specifically suppresses platelet production), and interferon-alpha (a drug that affects the immune system). Treatment is typically started when the platelet count
becomes very high or when bleeding or clotting problems
occur. The dose is adjusted so that the platelet count decreases
to a number that is unlikely to increase the risk of clotting. The
dose is decreased if the platelet count decreases too much or if
the red and white blood cell count decreases. These drugs also
suppress production of other blood cells. Because hydroxyurea
may increase the risk of leukemia, anagrelide and interferon-
alpha may be preferred. These drugs may have side effects, but
most older people tolerate the drugs fairly well.

If a drug does not slow platelet production quickly enough,
plateletpheresis may be done. In this procedure, blood is withdrawn from one arm into a tube attached to a blood cell separa-
tor machine. The machine removes the platelets, then returns
the blood minus the platelets through a tube attached to the
other arm.

If thrombocythemia is due to another disorder, that disorder
is treated. If treatment is effective, the platelet count usually returns to normal.

Thrombocythemia is usually not life threatening. However,
older people are more likely to have a blockage in a crucial
blood vessel. Occasionally, primary thrombocythemia changes
into a more serious disorder, such as polycythemia vera or certain types of leukemia.

POLYCYTHEMIA VERA

**In polycythemia, too many red blood cells are produced.
Polycythemia vera is polycythemia with no identifiable**

cause. The blood becomes thicker, blood flows less easily through small blood vessels, and blood clots are more likely to form.

Polycythemia vera is relatively uncommon. The average age at which the disorder is diagnosed is 60. Polycythemia vera is more common among men.

In many people with polycythemia vera, too many platelets and too many white blood cells are also produced. Sometimes excess blood cells are produced by the spleen and liver as well as by the bone marrow. As a result, these organs enlarge. Polycythemia vera makes the spleen enlarge in another way. Normally, the spleen removes abnormal, old, or damaged red blood cells. In polycythemia vera, the spleen has to remove more and more red blood cells from the bloodstream.

Polycythemia vera progresses slowly. After many years, it may progress to myelofibrosis. Rarely, it progresses to leukemia. If not treated, polycythemia vera can become life threatening.

The cause of polycythemia vera is, by definition, unknown. If the cause of polycythemia can be identified, it is called secondary polycythemia.

Symptoms

Many people do not have any symptoms for many years. Usually, the first symptoms are weakness, fatigue, headache, light-headedness, shortness of breath, and night sweats. Vision may be affected. People may have blind spots or see flashes of light. The gums may bleed, and small cuts may bleed more than expected. The skin, especially the face, often looks red. People may itch all over, particularly after bathing or showering. The hands and feet may tingle or feel as if they are burning. Rarely, pain is felt in the bones.

The abdomen may feel uncomfortably full because the liver and spleen enlarge. Abdominal pain may result if thickened blood or blood clots interfere with blood flow to the lining of the stomach and causes it to erode. This erosion may lead to ulcers.

Other symptoms can result if a clot blocks a large or crucial blood vessel.

POLYCYTHEMIA WITH AN IDENTIFIABLE CAUSE

Sometimes the body produces too many red blood cells, and no cause can be identified. This disorder is called polycythemia vera. When a cause can be identified, the disorder is called secondary polycythemia.

Secondary polycythemia can result from the following:

• **Conditions that prevent the body's tissues from getting enough oxygen.** Examples are smoking, spending time at a high altitude, and having a severe lung disorder or heart failure.

• **Conditions that reduce the amount of fluid (plasma) in the blood.** In such cases, the percentage of red blood cells in the blood (hematocrit) increases even though the number is normal. These conditions include burns, vomiting, diarrhea, and use of drugs that increase the amount of salt and water excreted by the kidneys (diuretics). Not drinking enough fluids can also reduce the amount of plasma in the blood.

• **Cysts in the kidneys or tumors in the kidneys, liver, or brain that produce erythropoietin.** Erythropoietin is a hormone that stimulates the bone marrow to produce red blood cells. These cysts and tumors are rare.

Symptoms of secondary polycythemia are similar to those of polycythemia vera but are usually much milder.

If possible, the condition causing polycythemia is corrected or treated. Depending on the cause, oxygen given by nasal prongs, phlebotomy, or fluids given by mouth or intravenously may be appropriate. Smokers are advised to stop smoking and are offered specific treatment to help them. People who live at high altitudes may be advised to move to lower altitudes if possible.

Generally, the outlook for people with secondary polycythemia is much better than for those with polycythemia vera. Secondary polycythemia, unlike polycythemia vera, does not progress to leukemia.

Diagnosis

Polycythemia may be diagnosed during routine blood tests, even before a person has any symptoms. The percentage of red blood cells in the blood (hematocrit) and the amount of hemoglobin, which is the protein that carries oxygen in red blood cells, are abnormally high. The platelet and white blood cell count may also be high.

A high hematocrit usually indicates polycythemia. However, another test to confirm the diagnosis is occasionally needed. In this test, red blood cells are withdrawn, labeled with a very small amount of a radioactive substance, and injected back into the body. The total number of red blood cells in the body (red blood cell mass) can be calculated by checking for radioactive cells in a sample of blood withdrawn after a certain time.

Once polycythemia is diagnosed, doctors determine whether the disorder is polycythemia vera or secondary polycythemia. The person's medical history may help, but sometimes additional tests are needed. For example, blood tests to measure the level of erythropoietin may be done. The level is very low in polycythemia vera but is normal or high in secondary polycythemia. A bone marrow biopsy may also be done.

Treatment and Outlook

Polycythemia vera cannot be cured. But treatment can control it and reduce the risk of problems, such as the formation of blood clots.

Treatment focuses on reducing the number of red blood cells. The usual way is to remove blood from the body in a procedure called phlebotomy. The procedure is similar to donating blood. A pint of blood is removed every other day until the hematocrit reaches a normal level. The level is kept normal by removing blood every few months, as needed.

Phlebotomy may increase the platelet count, which is often already high because of the polycythemia, and does not reduce the size of an enlarged liver or spleen. So people who undergo phlebotomy may also need drugs to suppress production of platelets. The chemotherapy drug hydroxyurea, given by mouth, is often used. It lowers the platelet count and thus reduces the risk of clots. If hydroxyurea has bothersome side effects or reduces the white blood cell count too much, anagrelide may be used instead. It also lowers the platelet count and reduces the risk of clots.

If phlebotomy is ineffective, interferon-alpha (a drug that affects the immune system) may be given as injections.

Other drugs can help control some of the symptoms. For example, antihistamines can help relieve itching. Aspirin can relieve burning sensations in the hands and feet as well as bone pain. Bathing in water that is warm rather than hot and patting rather than rubbing dry may help.

Without treatment, most people who have polycythemia vera live less than 2 years. Death usually results from blockage of a crucial blood vessel. When treated, most people live at least 10 to 15 years.

MYELOFIBROSIS

In myelofibrosis, fibrous tissue in the bone marrow grows too much and crowds out the immature cells (called stem cells) that develop into blood cells.

Myelofibrosis is rare. It usually affects people between the ages of 50 and 70.

Anemia develops and worsens progressively. Many of the red blood cells in the blood are immature or misshapen. White blood cells and platelets may also be immature. As myelofibrosis progresses, the white blood cell count may increase or decrease, and the platelet count typically decreases. The liver and spleen often enlarge as they make more blood cells. Thus, they try to compensate for the inadequate production of blood cells in the bone marrow.

This disorder often results in death in 3 to 5 years. However, for some people, stem cell transplantation cures the disorder.

Causes

The cause of myelofibrosis may be unknown. In such cases, it is called idiopathic. Myelofibrosis may accompany other blood disorders, such as chronic myelocytic leukemia, polycythemia vera, thrombocythemia, multiple myeloma, and lymphoma. It may also accompany tuberculosis or bone infections. Exposure to certain toxic substances, such as benzene and radiation, increases the risk of developing myelofibrosis.

Symptoms and Diagnosis

Many people have no symptoms for years. As the anemia becomes more severe, people feel weak, tired, and generally unwell. They may lose weight and have a low-grade fever and night sweats. They are more likely to get infections because the white blood cell count is low. They are more likely to bleed because the platelet count is low.

The abdomen may feel uncomfortably full or pain may occur because the liver and spleen enlarge. Blood pressure in veins of the liver may become abnormally high (a disorder called portal hypertension). Varicose veins in the esophagus may bleed (a disorder called esophageal varices).

Myelofibrosis is suspected when a person has anemia and when the red blood cells, viewed under a microscope, are misshapen and immature. However, a bone marrow biopsy is needed to confirm the diagnosis.

Treatment and Outlook

Stem cell transplantation is the only treatment available that may cure myelofibrosis. But because this treatment is so taxing, it is rarely recommended for people over 75. People who are younger than 75 and who are in otherwise good health can undergo this treatment if an appropriate donor is available. Usually, stem cells are removed from bone marrow in the donor's hip bone with a syringe after the donor is given a general anesthetic. Sometimes stem cells can be obtained from blood. Five years after treatment, about half of people who receive a transplant are alive, and about one fourth have no sign of the disorder. However, transplantation has significant risks, such as graft-versus-host disease, serious infections, and death.

Other treatments may be able to delay or relieve symptoms. The combination of male sex hormones (androgens) and the corticosteroid prednisone lessens the severity of the anemia in about one third of people with myelofibrosis, but the effect lasts for only 6 to 18 months. However, men who have prostate cancer cannot take male sex hormones. In women, these hormones may have masculinizing side effects, such as a lower voice and increased body hair.

Alternatively, blood transfusions are used to treat the anemia. Erythropoietin (a synthetic version of the hormone produced by the body) or darbepoietin are effective in a few people. These drugs stimulate the bone marrow to produce red blood cells. Infections are treated with antibiotics.

The chemotherapy drug hydroxyurea or interferon-alpha (a drug that affects the immune system) may reduce the size of the liver or spleen. However, either drug may worsen the anemia, because they suppress production of blood cells. Rarely, when the spleen becomes extremely large and painful, it is removed or treated with radiation therapy.

On average, people with myelofibrosis live 3 to 5 years after the disorder is diagnosed. Some people live only a year or two. People who are older than 70, have severe anemia, have an enlarged liver, or lose weight do less well. Having a very high or very low white blood cell count or a very low platelet count is also likely to shorten life. Because myelofibrosis is progressive, people who have it should decide on and write down advance directives.[1]

50

Finding and Living With Cancer

Cancer is one of the most feared diseases. Some types of cancer can be treated successfully in older people; a true cure—or at least a very prolonged remission—can sometimes be achieved. Thus, a diagnosis of cancer is not necessarily an imminent death sentence. Even when cancer is advanced, most symptoms usually can be effectively managed, although it remains true that most older people with advanced cancer will die from their cancer.

A cancer is a group of cells (usually coming from a single cell) that has uncontrolled growth. Healthy cells are transformed into cancerous cells in a complex way. The first step is called initiation, in which a change in the cell's genetic material sets the stage for the cell to become cancerous. Initiation may be caused by any number of cancer-causing agents (carcinogens), such as tobacco, radiation, or chemicals. The second step, called promotion, allows a cell that has been initiated to become cancerous. Promotion may be caused by substances in the environment.

Cancer can begin anywhere in the body, but certain cancers are more common than others. Cancer can also develop at any age but is much more common in older people. Over half of all

---

1. see page 953

TALKING ABOUT CANCER

Term	Meaning
Aggressiveness	The degree to which (or speed at which) a tumor grows and spreads
Anaplasia	A lack of differentiation. Thus, an anaplastic cancer is highly undifferentiated and usually very aggressive
Benign	A description of an abnormal growth of cells (tumor) that is not cancerous
Carcinoma-in-situ	Cancerous cells that are still contained within the tissue where they have started to grow and that have not yet become invasive or spread to other parts of the body
Cure	Complete elimination of the cancer with the result that the specific cancer will not grow back
Differentiation	The extent to which the cancerous cells resemble normal cells—less resemblance means the cancer is less differentiated and usually more aggressive
Invasion	The process that occurs when a cancer infiltrates and destroys surrounding tissue
Malignant	A description of a tumor that is cancerous
Metastasis	Spread of cancerous cells to a completely new location
Neoplasm	General term for a tumor, whether cancerous or noncancerous
Recurrence (relapse)	Cancerous cells return after treatment, either in the

Table continues on the following page.

Term	Meaning
	primary location or as metastases (spread)
Remission	Absence of all evidence of a cancer after treatment
Survival rate	The percentage of people who survive for a given time period after treatment (for example, the 5-year survival rate is the percentage of people who survive 5 years)
Tumor	Abnormal growth or mass

cancer diagnoses and half of cancer deaths occur in people over age 65. Lung, breast, prostate, and colon cancer are especially common in older people.

Cancer is more common in older people for a number of reasons. The longer people are alive, the longer they are exposed to cancer-causing agents. The cells of the immune system, which help protect against cancer, become less active with increasing age. Also, the body's ability to repair damage to genetic material inside the cell declines with aging, allowing for more opportunities for cancer cell initiation. Yet, there is evidence that certain types of cancer are less aggressive in older people.

Cancers harm people in a number of ways. As cancers grow, they may invade and damage nearby parts of the body. Cancers may also interfere with the function of organs and tissues simply by pressing up against them. They can spread to distant tissues, producing collections of cells (called metastases) that may invade and damage tissues and blood vessels in these new areas. Cancers can also produce hormones or similar chemical substances, which can travel through the bloodstream to cause unwanted effects throughout the body.

SCREENING

Doctors are best able to treat cancer when it is found early. However, in early stages, cancer rarely causes symptoms, making it difficult to find cancer early. Early diagnosis of cancer is helped by regular screening. Screening in older people is often different in terms of benefits and risks. Little may be gained from detecting a slow-growing cancer that would never cause harm within the person's predicted life expectancy. Moreover, the screening procedures and any additional tests and treatments may carry risks without benefits.

Types of screening tests vary, depending on the cancer. Some simple self-screening measures can be carried out, with the assistance of a family member or friend if necessary. For instance, to check for colon cancer, a person can collect small samples of stool on special cards, which are then sent to a health care practitioner and analyzed for the presence of blood. A woman may be able to detect breast cancer at an early stage by examining her breasts monthly (although regular breast examination by a doctor and mammography are also needed). Regularly examining the skin can help detect skin cancer. However, because most people cannot see all of their skin, help from a family member or friend should also be sought from time to time, and a doctor should perform an annual total body examination. This way, areas that are difficult to see, such as the back, can be checked.

In general, doctors recommend that older people be screened for several types of cancer. For some cancers, such as those of the breast and colon, screening has been proven to reduce the risk of dying from that cancer. However, screening is not as effective for all cancers, and experts disagree about which people benefit most from some screening tests. For example, many experts agree that older men should have regular rectal examinations to test for prostate cancer and rectal cancer. By contrast, the prostate-specific antigen (PSA) test is controversial. Sometimes the PSA level in the blood is elevated in men with prostate cancer, but the PSA level can also increase in men with a noncancerous condition called benign prostatic hyperplasia, and it may be normal in men with prostate cancer. Moreover, screening may not reduce the risk of older men dying from prostate cancer. Thus, PSA screening is commonly omitted in men whose life expectancy is less than 10 years (due to their age and the diseases they have).

RECOGNIZING THE WARNING SIGNS

Warning signs of cancer are often vague or very general, particularly in the early stages. Many symptoms of cancer can also be caused by other conditions. Nonetheless, even vague symptoms may provide an early warning—and an early warning means a better chance of a cure. Some of these vague symptoms include fatigue, night sweats, and new or persistent pain. A person who experiences such symptoms should be examined by a doctor. Certain symptoms are common in many cancers. These include pain, bleeding, enlarged lymph nodes, unexplained weight loss, and nausea. However, each type of cancer has its own warning signs, such as breast lumps in breast cancer, difficulty swallowing in esophageal cancer, and yellowish skin (jaundice) in pancreatic cancer.

Pain: As a cancer grows, it eventually presses on or invades surrounding tissues, often causing pain. However, many other conditions also cause pain. All cancers are initially painless and some may remain so, even after growing quite large. One should not have faith in the misconception that "all cancers produce pain" and ignore other symptoms that may occur in the absence of pain.

Bleeding: Cancer cells are not bound strongly to each other, and cancers therefore tend to be fragile and bleed easily. Cancers can also cause bleeding by growing into blood vessels, causing them to bleed. The location of bleeding depends on where the cancer is. Colon cancer usually causes blood to be detectable in the stool, and cancer of the kidney usually causes blood to be detectable in the urine. However, bleeding can have many causes other than cancer. Often bleeding is not evident, particularly if bleeding is internal. Unusual fatigue that is not improved by rest may indicate internal bleeding. Bleeding and easy bruising are typical of leukemia, but leukemia causes bleeding by a different means. The platelets in the bloodstream become fewer in number as the bone marrow (where platelets are made) produces cancer cells instead. People with low platelet levels tend to bleed easily.

Enlarged lymph nodes: Certain cancers spread initially to nearby lymph nodes. Affected lymph nodes become large and feel hard and may be difficult or impossible to move about. They are usually painless, unlike enlarged nodes from infections.

Weight loss: Some weight loss is usual in early stages of cancer; severe weight loss (cachexia) often occurs as the cancer advances. In response to the cancer, the body may release chemicals called cytokines (two such cytokines are tumor necrosis factor and interleukin 6). The release of cytokines can cause weight loss. Weight loss may also result from side effects of cancer treatment, such as nausea or vomiting. A person may be unable to eat or to digest food because of abnormalities resulting from the cancer, such as blockage of the throat, esophagus, or intestine. Weight loss may also occur because the person is depressed or just too tired to eat.

Nausea: Nausea may result from changes in the levels of substances in the blood (such as increased levels of calcium, decreased levels of sodium, or high levels of urea in the blood). The spread of cancer (metastasis) to the liver or brain can also cause nausea. Many people who take chemotherapy drugs or powerful pain relievers, such as the opioids used to treat cancer pain, experience nausea as a side effect.

Other symptoms: Cancers may be found because of symptoms created by the original (primary) tumor. They may also be found because they have spread to another part of the body and caused symptoms there. For example, bone pain may result from a cancer that has spread to bone. However some bone pain, such as pain in joints, is common in old age and usually does not signify cancer. Weakness or altered sensation in one part of the body can result from cancer that has spread to the brain. But identical symptoms can be caused by a stroke.

A cancer may release substances that act as hormones. For example, some cancers release a substance that mimics the effects of parathyroid hormone. This substance causes the level of calcium in the blood to increase and thereby leads to such symptoms as abdominal pain, muscle weakness, diarrhea, and even mental confusion. Another substance released by a cancer can cause effects similar to those of cortisol, producing a very full, chubby facial appearance and stretch marks in the skin.

CONFIRMING THE DIAGNOSIS AND STAGING

A screening test is performed before a doctor has any real suspicion that a person has cancer. A diagnostic test is performed when a doctor suspects cancer. Some tests help ensure that the diagnosis is correct. Then, other tests determine whether the cancer has spread and to which areas, a procedure called staging. The tests ordered vary with the type of cancer but generally include blood tests, imaging studies (such as x-rays, computed tomography [CT], or magnetic resonance imaging [MRI]), and a biopsy. With a biopsy, a small piece of tissue is removed from a suspicious area for examination under a microscope. Sometimes an excisional biopsy is carried out, in which all of the suspicious tissue is removed and examined. Biopsy of nearby lymph nodes is often done to see if the cancer has spread.

GUIDELINES FOR TREATMENT

In many cases, doctors hope to completely eliminate the cancer from the body, thus curing it. Other times, cure is not possible, yet treatment still aims to slow the growth of the cancer so that a person might live longer. Sometimes, treatment is likely to cause more harm than good, and treatment aims only to reduce symptoms that would otherwise cause pain and suffering (palliative treatment).

The earlier a cancer is found, the more likely cure is possible. Advanced cancers and those that recur after initial treatment indicate that the cancer has spread. Cure is then unlikely.

The main types of treatment for cancer are surgery, radiation therapy, and drugs. Surgery is used when possible to completely remove the cancer or partially remove ("de-bulk") it, so that other therapies have a better chance of success. Surgery can also be used to stop bleeding or relieve pressure on a particular structure or organ.

Radiation therapy is directed at a tumor to destroy it or at least to reduce its size. Not all cancers respond to radiation therapy.

QUESTIONS TO ASK WHEN DIAGNOSED WITH CANCER

- What type do I have?
- At what stage is it?
- What is the outlook for people with this type of cancer at this particular stage?
- What are the treatment options, and how might they affect my outlook?
- Am I eligible to participate in a clinical trial?
- What are the options for palliative care and end-of-life care if my doctors determine that the type and stage of my cancer means that treatment is unlikely to alter the outlook?

Several types of drugs are used to treat cancer. Chemotherapy involves drugs that kill cancer cells. Chemotherapy drugs work by many mechanisms, always targeting something that is unusual about the cancer cells. However, chemotherapy drugs always kill some normal cells as well, and the drugs often cause side effects that can make people feel very ill. Other drugs suppress certain hormones that stimulate cancers to grow and thereby suppress cancer growth. Some newer drugs attack cancerous cells in novel ways, resulting in their death. An example is imatinib for chronic myelocytic leukemia. This drug attaches to and prevents leukemia cells from functioning, thereby resulting in their death.

Immunotherapy stimulates the immune system to attack a cancer or uses antibodies that attach themselves to cancer cells. Such antibodies can be combined with chemotherapy drugs or radioactive agents, so that the drugs go (target) exactly where they are needed, to the cancer cells.

Having other diseases and conditions can complicate cancer treatment. For example, heart failure or impaired kidney function may limit the choices and dosages of chemotherapy drugs usually used to treat certain types of cancer. Chronic liver disease can make the use of chemotherapy drugs more challenging by increasing toxic side effects of several of the drugs. Chronic obstructive pulmonary disease (COPD) can limit the use of radiation that might otherwise be used to treat lung cancers, due to the potentially harmful effects of the radiation to lung tissue already damaged by COPD. However, treatment of a cancer is usually possible in spite of other diseases and conditions.

Some cancers caught early enough can be removed surgically. However, cancers are sometimes located in places that surgery cannot reach, such as deep in the brain. Some cancers have already spread, so that removing the original tumor does not offer cure. Therefore, doctors may give additional therapy, such as radiation therapy to eliminate cancer cells in nearby lymph nodes or chemotherapy or hormone therapy to eliminate cancer cells throughout the body. This therapy, termed "adjuvant therapy," is commonly used in breast, colon, and head and neck cancers.

If a cancer is known to have spread, surgery is much less likely to improve survival. Instead, the cancer may be treated by radiation therapy and by chemotherapy. Such treatment is less likely to achieve a cure, but it may lengthen survival or at least effectively treat many symptoms.

Often, people with cancer are treated at regional centers that specialize in cancer. Such centers are staffed with doctors and other health care practitioners with expertise in treating cancer. The centers often offer drugs and treatment programs at the forefront of research on possible new treatment approaches.

Some people may participate in a clinical trial, a research study that tests how well new medical treatments work. Although these treatments may still be experimental, they are carefully monitored by review boards of the universities and hospitals involved. Such safety oversight means that people must usually receive care at a hospital or medical center in order to participate in a clinical research trial.

Sometimes, people with cancer decide to seek alternative medicine or a combination of alternative and conventional medicine. Although some alternative therapies may be helpful, people should not rely on them to the exclusion of established effective therapies. People who seek alternative therapies should be sure to discuss them with their doctor.

Some older people with cancer decide not to undergo any treatment other than relief of pain and other suffering. Such a decision is often appropriate when the cancer cannot be cured and the treatment is likely to cause side effects. A person may choose to travel or otherwise get involved in enjoyable activities while feeling well, rather than feeling ill due to treatments. Such decisions must be made with full information about the risks and benefits of treatment and require careful consultation and discussion with a knowledgeable doctor.

LIVING WITH CANCER

With treatment, people with cancer may live for many years after diagnosis. However, the treatment of cancer can also have side effects, such as nausea and fatigue. Cancer symptoms, and those symptoms that occur as side effects of cancer treatment, can often be relieved, at least for a time (such as by drugs to prevent nausea). Controlling such symptoms can greatly improve quality of life. Many people find that they can carry out most of their usual activities while they are being treated for cancer.

Pain: Many people with cancer are concerned that they will have a lot of pain. However, cancer pain can often be controlled very well. A variety of pain relievers can be used, depending on the severity of the pain. For mild pain, nonsteroidal anti-inflammatory drugs (NSAIDs), such as ibuprofen, may be sufficient. For severe pain, opioids, such as morphine and hydromorphone, may be necessary. Some opioids can provide relief for several hours or even days. Some can be applied as patches. In addition, antidepressants, anticonvulsants, and local anesthetics can be given along with pain relievers to offer more relief.[1]

Many people fear that they will become dependent on strong pain relievers. However, such concerns are not valid. There is no reason why a person should have to live with pain. In addition, failure to use pain relievers with sufficient regularity and at sufficient doses can allow pain to reappear; such pain then requires higher doses of pain relievers than would otherwise be required.

However, some side effects occur routinely with opioid use. Almost every older person will develop constipation. Constipation from opioids must be treated with a stimulant laxative.[2] Many older people who take opioids will have difficulty emptying their bladder. All opioids make people tired, especially when they are just starting to take an opioid. Sometimes doses can be adjusted or different opioids can be tried to help reduce these side effects.

Nausea: Nausea, often accompanied by vomiting, can be a symptom of cancer and a side effect of treatment. Several new drugs are available to lessen nausea and vomiting.

Weight loss: The use of anti-nausea drugs has made weight loss associated with use of chemotherapy drugs less common. Food supplements can help prevent and treat weight loss. Drugs to increase muscle mass may also be given, such as dronabinol (which also can be used to reduce nausea) or megestrol. Many people with advanced cancer lose weight, in part due to loss of appetite. When cancer is advanced, weight loss is often seen as acceptable, especially when compared with the alternative of

1. see also page 339
2. see page 338

potential side effects and discomfort that may develop when drugs or feeding tubes are used to treat weight loss.

Hair loss: Some chemotherapy drugs can cause hair loss. Some people find this side effect distressing. Many people purchase wigs before beginning cancer treatment so that the wig can be made to look similar to their own hair. Other people choose to wear hats and scarves or even to leave their heads uncovered. The most important consideration is that the person be comfortable with the choice.

Fatigue: Fatigue may be related to the cancer itself or to the effects of treatment. For example, radiation therapy can cause fatigue. Many chemotherapy drugs affect the rapidly dividing cells of the bone marrow, leading to a low level of red blood cells, which results in anemia and fatigue. In some people, a drug that increases the body's production of red blood cells can reduce fatigue. People experiencing fatigue may need to adjust their activities. Some experts recommend a daily schedule that includes frequent rest periods. Activities that require a lot of energy can be planned for parts of the day when energy level is highest.

Depression: People may feel hopeless or overwhelmed by the diagnosis of cancer or by the stress of navigating the health care system. Also, the metabolic and hormonal effects of the cancer itself can contribute to depression. A cancer diagnosis is frightening, and depression can be compounded by agitation due to the fear or an attempt to hide the fear and depression. Opioids can cause or worsen depression. Regardless of the cause, antidepressant drugs can be very helpful.

Evidence has shown that a positive attitude and resilient hope are important parts of therapy. Sometimes, people benefit from sharing their concerns with others in similar situations. Support groups can provide members with advice and encouragement. Other people with depression may benefit from counseling with a psychiatrist or psychologist.

Potential challenges while living with cancer: Cancer treatment may go on for several months. Social service agencies can help coordinate the many health care services needed. They can assist with transportation to and from treatments and in arranging home health services. They can also direct people to additional sources of help. Organizations devoted to helping people with cancer, such as the American Cancer Society, can provide additional information.

People may need assistance with insurance forms, and they may also want financial and legal advice. It is important that older people with cancer update a will and prepare an advance medical directive.[1] They may want to discuss their concerns about care with their doctors and family members. Knowing when a person with cancer is moving from living with the disease to dying from the disease is often very difficult. However, exploring options for palliative care and end-of-life care[2] is well worth considering when the outlook for the cancer is unlikely to be altered by treatment.

1. see page 953
2. see page 211

Canoeing rivers in Alaska didn't start for me until my mid-40s. Our son started a business selling kayaks and accessories. As the business grew, I became more and more involved. We went from a small-scale retail shop to a full summer season of instruction and guided trips.

I became the CEO. I did all the reservations, planned and prepared meals for the trips, packed and unpacked gear for the classes and trips, instructed on water from my canoe, guided clients in camping skills. My favorite group of clients was from the Elderhostel program. Once a year 16 clients from all over the United States came to float the Chena River for a week. I was the lead guide and had others who came along to assist.

It was hard for some of our men clients to understand how a woman, indeed one with gray hair, could be so in love with this outdoor, rugged activity. I feel a thrill when maneuvering a canoe through a boulder garden. I love the surrounding beauty of the land and a feeling of solitude when traveling a remote river. The community feeling around the campfire and the simplicity of camp life give me pleasure.

The commitment required for a full-time summer schedule caused us to sell the business to be more spontaneous with our time. It was hard for me to hang up my hat to full-time canoe instruction and guided trips. We continue to do extensive canoe trips with friends. I miss being in charge. The friends we travel with have their independence and don't look to me for guidance. I can still carry gear and canoes over the portage; I can paddle the river for 6 to 8 hours a day. I can still accomplish the physical labor of camp set up and take down. My good health allows me to continue paddling my canoe at the age of 70. My 30 years of experience leading others to skillfully maneuver the swift, cold waters of Alaskan rivers gives me the confidence to continue doing what I love.

Mary Lou Davis

51

Cancers

A cancer (malignancy) is a cell or a group of cells that become abnormal and grow without any of the body's usual controls. Cancers move into normal tissues and can spread to adjacent tissues (invade locally) or spread through blood vessels or lymph vessels (part of the body's immune system) to more distant tissues (metastasize). Cancers can develop from any tissue within any organ.

Leukemias and lymphomas are cancers of blood and blood-forming tissues. With leukemias, most of the cancerous cells are in the bone marrow and blood. With lymphomas, the cancerous cells are in lymph nodes, the bone marrow, the spleen, and the liver. Lymphoma cells usually form clumps as they grow, resulting in a solid mass. A collection of cancerous cells is called a tumor.

Carcinomas and sarcomas are types of cancers that always form solid masses. Carcinomas are cancers of epithelial cells, cells that cover the surface of the body, produce hormones, or make up glands. Cancers of the skin, lung, colon, stomach, breast, prostate, and thyroid gland are carcinomas. Carcinomas occur more often in older than in younger people. Sarcomas are cancers of mesodermal cells, which are cells that form muscles and connective tissue. Examples of sarcomas are leiomyosarcoma (cancer of smooth muscle that is found in the walls of digestive organs) and osteosarcoma (bone cancer). Sarcomas occur more often in younger than in older people.

Some of the most common cancers in older people are breast cancer, chronic lymphocytic leukemia, colorectal cancers (cancers of the colon and the rectum), lung cancer, mouth, head, and neck cancers, multiple myeloma, prostate cancer, skin cancer, and vulvar cancer.

BREAST CANCER

Breast cancer is the second most common cancer among women after skin cancer. Most breast cancers occur in women over 60. Although rare, men can develop breast cancer, and their risk also increases with age.

Women who have had breast cancer are at high risk of developing cancer in the other breast. Having a close relative with breast cancer increases a woman's risk by two to three times. Women who had their first menstrual period at a young age, those in whom menopause occurred at a later age, and those who have never had children or who had their first child after 40 have an increased risk of developing breast cancer. Taking estrogen after menopause slightly increases the risk of breast cancer. The risk of breast cancer is also somewhat higher in women who are obese or who drink more than moderate amounts of alcohol.

Symptoms

The earliest symptom of breast cancer is often a lump or thickening in the breast or under the arm. In the early stages, the lump may move freely beneath the skin when it is pushed with the fingers. In more advanced stages, the lump may adhere to the chest wall or to the skin over it and cannot be moved. A change in the size, shape, or contour of the breast or in the appearance of the skin of the breast or nipple can be a symptom of breast cancer. Sometimes the skin may appear puckered or dimpled. The lump may be painful, but pain is an uncommon and unreliable sign. A discharge from the nipple may occur. Sometimes the breast becomes red and swollen.

Sometimes the breast feels normal, but the lymph nodes in the underarm feel like hard small lumps and may be slightly tender.

Screening

Because breast cancer has few symptoms in its early stages and because breast cancer is more easily cured if it is detected early, experts recommend that all older women be screened regularly for breast cancer. Women are encouraged to examine their breasts each month. They should examine their breasts on the same day each month, picking a date that is easy to remember.

A breast examination is a routine part of a physical examination. Experts recommend that women over 40 have an annual breast examination. A health care practitioner observes each breast for irregularities in the contour and the skin of the breast or nipple, feels (palpates) each breast to check for lumps or thickening of breast tissue, and checks the underarms for enlarged lymph nodes.

A mammogram is an x-ray of the breast. It detects many cancers that are too small to feel. However, because mammography is designed to be sensitive enough to detect the possibility of breast cancer at an early stage, it may identify a "suspected" cancer when none is present (a false-positive result). If the mammogram is not completely normal, magnetic resonance imaging (MRI) may be done. MRI is sometimes more sensitive for identifying small cancers. However, MRI is even more likely to produce false-positive results.

Having a mammogram can reduce the rate of death due to breast cancer in women over 50. Most experts agree that women aged 50 or older should have a mammogram every year or every other year. There is no upper age limit after which women can safely stop having mammograms. Women who are expected to live for at least 3 to 5 more years should continue to receive annual mammograms.

Diagnosis

When a lump or some other suggestive change is noted during breast self-examination or an examination by a health care practitioner, additional tests are needed to diagnose breast cancer.

Mammography is done to pinpoint the location of a lump found during an examination and to determine if there are other abnormalities in the same breast or the other breast. Ultrasonography may be used to determine if the lump is fluid-filled (cyst) or solid. Cysts are usually not cancerous. If the lump is solid, a biopsy is performed. In aspiration biopsy, a needle is used to remove some cells from the lump. A piece of tissue from the lump (incisional biopsy) or the entire lump (excisional biopsy) can be examined instead.

The tissue sample is examined under a microscope to determine whether cancer is present. Because a needle biopsy can miss some tumors, a negative result requires further testing. If cancer is detected, the sample is analyzed to determine the characteristics of the cancer cells and whether the cancer has spread. Understanding the characteristics allows the doctor to develop a profile of the cancer that guides the selection of treatment approaches.

Types and Staging

Breast cancer is described as in situ (not invasive), locally invasive, regionally invasive, or metastatic (distant). Cancers may also be described as glandular or ductal. A glandular cancer begins in the tissue that produces milk. A ductal cancer begins in the milk ducts, the tiny tube-like structures that channel milk to the nipple. Paget's disease of the breast is a type of ductal cancer. It often appears first as a crusty or scaly nipple sore or a discharge from the nipple. Another type is inflammatory breast cancer. Cancer cells in the skin block the lymphatic vessels in the breast, causing the breast to appear red, warm, and swollen. Inflammatory breast cancer often grows rapidly and has a poor outcome.

The stage of breast cancer is determined according to how much it has spread and is designated by a number (0 through 4) or described with a specific term. For example, carcinoma in situ is the earliest stage of breast cancer. In this stage, the cancer has not spread at all. Locally invasive cancer has spread into adjacent breast tissue. It may or may not extend into nearby lymph nodes or the chest wall. Metastatic cancer is cancer that has spread from the breast to other parts of the body. Breast cancer can spread to any area of the body, but it most often spreads to bones, liver, or the lungs, and sometimes even to the brain.

Breast cancer cells may or may not have receptors for the hormone estrogen, which stimulates the cancer to grow. Cancers that have receptors are called estrogen receptor–positive cancers. Estrogen receptor–positive breast cancers are most common among postmenopausal women, and outlook for cancer control is usually good. Similarly, some breast cancer cells have receptors for progesterone. The outlook is even better for breast cancers that are both estrogen receptor– and progesterone receptor–positive.

Another characteristic of breast cancer is the status of HER-2/

neu receptors, which are found on all breast cancer cells. In about one third of breast cancers, the number of HER-2/*neu* receptors is increased (amplified or over-expressed). These cancers are faster growing and therefore more malignant than those with a normal level of HER-2/*neu* receptors. When doctors determine the profile of a breast cancer, they also include the cancer's proliferative index, which helps determine how rapidly the cancer cells are growing. A measure of the p53 gene or its product helps doctors determine how poorly the growth of the cancer is regulated. New tests for interpreting altered genes are improving the ability to determine who is at higher risk of recurrence and the likelihood of responding to treatments.

Treatment

A woman's preferences play an important role in determining treatment options. However, treatment options also depend on the type and stage of breast cancer and the woman's overall health.

Treatment almost always involves surgery. Depending on the size of the tumor and how many lymph nodes contain cancer cells, radiation therapy, chemotherapy, or both may be used after surgery. Sometimes, if a tumor is large, chemotherapy is given before surgery to reduce the size of the tumor. Treatment may include the use of hormone-blocking drugs or biologic preparations, such as antibodies, which help the body fight cancer. Often, a combination of therapies is used.

Surgery: There are two approaches used for surgery: breast-conserving surgery and mastectomy. In breast-conserving surgery, the surgeon removes the cancerous tumor and some surrounding tissue but leaves as much of the breast intact as possible. Surrounding tissue is removed to help improve the likelihood that the cancer will be cured. However, removing less tissue preserves more of the breast, allowing the woman to heal faster and keep more of the natural appearance of her breasts.

There are three types of breast-conserving surgery. A lumpectomy removes the least amount of surrounding tissue. A partial mastectomy (also called wide excision surgery) and a quadrantectomy remove the tumor and some additional surrounding tissue. Lymph nodes may be removed as well. Breast-conserving surgery is usually followed by radiation therapy to reduce the likelihood of recurrence in the remaining breast tis-

SURGERY FOR BREAST CANCER

What type of breast cancer surgery is done depends on how large the tumor is and how far cancer cells have spread. For breast-conserving surgery, only the tumor and an area of normal tissue surrounding it is removed. There are three types of breast-conserving surgery. Lumpectomy consists of removing only a small amount of surrounding normal tissue. Wide excision (partial mastectomy) consists of removing a somewhat larger amount. Quadrantectomy consists of removing one fourth of the breast.

For mastectomy, all breast tissue is removed. There are different types of mastectomies. They vary in whether other tissues, such as the lymph nodes and the muscle under the breast, are also removed.

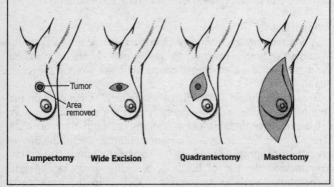

Tumor
Area removed

Lumpectomy **Wide Excision** **Quadrantectomy** **Mastectomy**

sue. In early-stage breast cancer, results of breast-conserving surgery plus radiation therapy are equivalent to the results of mastectomy. However, mastectomy is usually done when the cancer is so widespread that all of the cancer cannot be removed unless the whole breast is removed.

A simple mastectomy involves removing the breast. In a modified radical mastectomy, the surgeon also removes the lymph nodes in the underarm area. In a radical mastectomy, the surgeon removes not only the lymph nodes in the underarm area but also the muscle under the breast.

Surgery to reconstruct the breast can be done at the time of the initial surgery or several months later. The decision depends on the nature and site of the cancer. Decisions regarding reconstructive surgery are very personal, and a woman should discuss the possibilities with her doctor. Because immediate reconstruction prolongs the length of the initial operation, an important factor in the decision is the woman's general health.

To determine whether the cancer has spread, doctors examine lymph nodes under the arm (sentinal lymph nodes). Contrast dye or a radioactive marker is injected into the breast at or near the cancer. The doctor identifies the lymph node (or nodes) where the dye or marker accumulates, so that they can be examined for evidence of cancer. This procedure has reduced the need for extensive surgery of the underarm area and the subsequent risk of long-term arm swelling (lymphedema). Knowing whether the cancer has spread is critical in determining what additional therapy is needed.

When a woman with breast cancer has one or more other life-threatening diseases that shorten her life expectancy, doctors may not recommend treatment to cure the cancer. However, they usually recommend a lumpectomy to prevent the cancer from causing sores or ulcers in the remaining breast tissue, which would be painful and reduce the woman's quality of life.

Radiation therapy: Radiation therapy is usually used after a woman undergoes surgery to remove the cancer. The goal is to kill cancer cells remaining at the site from which the tumor was removed and from surrounding areas. Radiation therapy is usually given over a period of several weeks. Swelling in the breast, reddening and blistering of the skin, and fatigue are common after radiation therapy, but these effects usually disappear after several months. The rate of breast cancer recurrence in the area where surgery was performed seems to decrease with age, so some experts do not recommend radiation therapy in all older women.

Chemotherapy: Chemotherapy is used to kill cancer cells that were not removed during surgery or killed by radiation therapy. Chemotherapy is generally recommended when staging tests suggest that the cancer has spread beyond the area of the breast.

The choice of chemotherapy drugs depends on several factors, including the type and stage of cancer. Chemotherapy drugs are usually given intravenously, but some can be taken by mouth. Commonly used drugs include cyclophosphamide, doxorubicin, epirubicin, fluorouracil, methotrexate, docetaxel, paclitaxel, and vinorelbine. Most women experience side effects, such as nausea and vomiting, fatigue, and hair loss, re-

HOW LYMPH NODE STATUS INFLUENCES SURVIVAL

Lymph Node Status	Chances of Surviving 5 Years	Chances of Surviving 10 Years	Chances of Surviving 10 Years Without Recurrence*
No cancer in any node	Better than 90%	Better than 80%	Better than 70%
Cancer in one to three nodes	About 60 to 70%	About 40 to 50%	About 25 to 40%
Cancer in four or more nodes	About 40 to 50%	About 25 to 40%	About 15 to 35%

*More intensive therapy is gradually helping to reduce the recurrence rates.

gardless of the drugs used, but the severity of the side effects depends on which drugs are used.

Trastuzumab, which is an antibody, is used primarily for treatment of more advanced breast cancers. However, increasingly, it is being used earlier in the treatment of cancers with increased HER-2/*neu* receptors.

Drugs that block the actions of estrogen and progesterone may be used when cancer cells have receptors for these hormones. Hormone-blocking drugs work better to control cancers that are positive for both estrogen and progesterone receptors than they do for breast cancers that are positive for only one or the other. Tamoxifen is the most commonly used estrogen-blocking drug. This drug increases the likelihood of survival in women whose cancers are estrogen receptor–positive. There are other newer drugs that block the effects of hormones. These so-called aromatase inhibitors have proven effectiveness and are now frequently being used before tamoxifen. Anastrozole, one such aromatase inhibitor, may improve survival and result in fewer side effects than tamoxifen does.

Outlook

Doctors regularly monitor women who have been treated for breast cancer to ensure that the cancer has not returned. Breast cancer that has spread beyond the lymph nodes is rarely cured. However, treatment may relieve symptoms, improve survival, and afford a good quality of life.

CHRONIC LYMPHOCYTIC LEUKEMIA

Chronic lymphocytic leukemia (CLL) is a slowly progressing disease in which mature lymphocytes (a type of white blood cell) become cancerous and gradually replace normal cells in lymph nodes.

CLL is one of the four main types of leukemia and is the most common type in older people. The other three are acute lymphocytic leukemia, acute myelocytic leukemia, and chronic myelocytic leukemia. Most people who develop CLL are older than 60. CLL affects men two to three times more often than women.

Almost always, the cause of CLL is unknown. CLL begins with cancerous mature lymphocytes in the bone marrow, blood, and lymph nodes. The cancerous cells in the bone marrow crowd out normal cells, resulting in a decreased number of red blood cells, normal white blood cells (which help fight infection), and platelets (which are needed for blood clotting). Cancerous lymphocytes spread to the liver and spleen, both of which begin to enlarge. The levels of antibodies, proteins that help fight infections, also decrease. The immune system, which ordinarily defends the body against foreign organisms and substances, sometimes becomes impaired, reacting to and destroying normal body tissues, including red blood cells and platelets.

Treatment of CLL can relieve most symptoms for a very long time. However, for some people, complications develop that cause quality of life to deteriorate, and the potential benefit for further treatment becomes extremely limited.

Symptoms and Diagnosis

In early stages of CLL, most people have no symptoms. Gradually, people may see or feel bumps under the skin where lymph nodes have enlarged. Other later symptoms may include fatigue, loss of appetite, weight loss, shortness of breath when exercising, and a sense of abdominal fullness resulting from an enlarged spleen. As CLL progresses, people may appear pale and bruise easily. Symptoms that may indicate infection, such as fever, tend to occur late in the course of the disease as the body's susceptibility to invading bacteria, viruses, and fungi increases.

Sometimes CLL is discovered accidentally when white blood

cell counts done for some other reason show an increased number of lymphocytes. Specialized tests, performed on the cells in the blood to characterize the lymphocytes, usually confirm the diagnosis of CLL. Blood tests also may show that the person has a decreased number of red blood cells, platelets, and antibodies. A biopsy of the bone marrow is occasionally needed if the diagnosis remains uncertain.

Treatment

Because CLL progresses slowly, some people never require treatment. For many others, treatment may not be needed for years—when the number of lymphocytes begins to steadily increase, the lymph nodes begin to enlarge, or the number of red blood cells or platelets decreases.

Drugs used to treat the leukemia help relieve symptoms and reduce the size of the enlarged lymph nodes and spleen, but these drugs do not cure the disease. Initial treatment for many people with CLL includes chemotherapy drugs such as chlorambucil or fludarabine. Either drug can control CLL for months to many years. Eventually CLL becomes resistant to either or both of these drugs, and other drugs or antibodies (such as alemtuzumab) may be used to control symptoms.

Anemia due to a decreased number of red blood cells is treated with blood transfusions and occasionally with injections of erythropoietin or darbepoietin (drugs that stimulate the formation of red blood cells). Low platelet counts are treated with platelet transfusions. Infections are treated with antibiotics, antiviral drugs, or antifungal drugs, depending on the type of microorganism. Radiation therapy is sometimes used to shrink enlarged lymph nodes or an enlarged liver or spleen if the enlargement is causing discomfort and chemotherapy is ineffective.

Finally, for some people, bone marrow (stem cell) transplantation may produce long-term disease control (and possibly a cure). Transplantation involves collecting stem cells from the person's blood before high doses of chemotherapy drugs are administered. Stem cells are unspecialized cells that transform into immature blood cells, which eventually mature to become red blood cells, white blood cells, and platelets. The collected stem cells are then returned (transplanted) to the person after the high-dose treatment. Generally, stem cell transplantation is so taxing that it is usually reserved for people who are younger than 75.

Outlook

CLL usually progress slowly. At the time CLL is diagnosed, the doctor determines how far the disease has progressed (staging) to predict how long the person is likely to survive. Staging is based on such information as number of lymphocytes in the blood and bone marrow, size of the spleen and liver, presence or absence of anemia, and platelet count.

Many people with CLL survive 10 to 20 years or longer after the diagnosis is made and usually do not need treatment in the early stages. Some may die of other causes and never need treatment for their CLL. However, among people who are anemic or who have a low number of platelets at the time CLL is diagnosed, more immediate treatment is needed, and the outlook even with treatment is less favorable. Some people with CLL develop other cancers, such as skin or lung cancers. CLL can also transform into a more aggressive type of lymphoma. Eventually, in some people with CLL, death occurs when the bone marrow can no longer produce a sufficient number of normal cells to carry oxygen, fight infections, and prevent bleeding.

COLORECTAL CANCER

Colon cancer begins in the colon; rectal cancer begins in the rectum. "Colorectal cancer" is a more general term that encompasses cancers that begin in either the colon or the rectum. Although colon and rectal cancers are similar, there are some differences in how they develop and are treated. Each year about 130,000 people are diagnosed with colorectal cancer. Most of the people who develop colorectal cancer are over 50. Women are more likely to develop cancer of the colon, and men are more likely to develop cancer of the rectum.

In addition to age, the following are risk factors for colorectal cancer: a history of polyps (growths that protrude into the colon or rectum), a family history of colorectal cancer, a history of ulcerative colitis or Crohn's disease, and a diet high in fat and low in fiber. To help prevent colorectal cancer, people should eat a diet low in fat and high in fiber, avoid drinking excessive amounts of alcohol, maintain a healthy weight through diet and exercise, and take an aspirin daily. Many colon cancers start in polyps, so doctors help prevent colorectal cancer by removing polyps when they find them.

Symptoms

In early colorectal cancer, a person may be free of any symptoms or have slight bleeding in the stool. Other symptoms include:

- A change in bowel habits, such as prolonged constipation or diarrhea or bowel (fecal) incontinence (the unintentional release of stool)
- Blood in the stool
- Unusual stomach or gas pains
- Unexplained weight loss
- Fatigue
- Vomiting

Having these symptoms does not necessarily mean that a person has colorectal cancer. However, because colorectal cancer that is detected early can be cured, a doctor should be consulted if any of these symptoms occur.

Screening and Diagnosis

Many experts recommend regular screening for colorectal cancer beginning at age 50. Several screening methods are available. One approach is to undergo a digital rectal examination (in which a doctor inserts a gloved finger into the rectum and feels for any abnormalities) and a test to detect hidden blood in the stool (fecal occult blood testing) every year. Some experts also suggest that the colon and rectum be examined with sigmoidoscopy, or preferably with colonoscopy, at age 50. Sigmoidoscopy allows the doctor to examine the lower portion of the colon; colonoscopy allows examination of the entire colon. Any polyps found are removed, and the examination is repeated in a year. If no polyps are found, testing can be repeated in 5 to 10 years.

"Virtual colonoscopy" is a term being used to describe screening that uses computed tomography (CT) scanning without actual

STAGING COLON CANCER

Stage 0: Cancer is limited to the inner layer (lining) of the colon over the polyp. More than 95% of people with cancer at this stage survive at least 5 years.

Stage 1: Cancer spreads to the space between the inner layer and muscle layer of the colon. (This space contains blood vessels, nerves, and lymphatic vessels.) More than 90% of people with cancer at this stage survive at least 5 years.

Stage 2: Cancer invades the muscle layer and outer layer of the colon. About 55 to 85% of people with cancer at this stage survive at least 5 years.

Stage 3: Cancer extends through the outer layer of the colon into nearby lymph nodes. About 20 to 55% of people with cancer at this stage survive at least 5 years.

Stage 4 (not shown): Cancer spreads to other organs, such as the liver, lungs, or ovaries, or to the membrane (called the peritoneum) lining the abdominal cavity, the space that holds the digestive organs. Fewer than 1% of people with cancer at this stage survive at least 5 years.

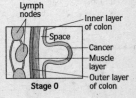

Stage 0

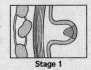

Stage 1

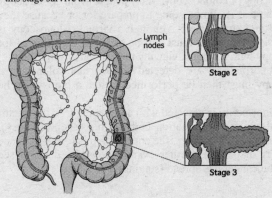

Stage 2

Stage 3

UNDERSTANDING COLOSTOMY

A colostomy is done to provide a new exit for stool from the colon to the outside. A new exit may be needed temporarily to give a damaged part of the colon time to heal. Or a new exit may be needed permanently because the rectum and anus have been removed, usually because of cancer.

For a colostomy, the colon is cut. The part that remains connected to the small intestine and stomach is brought through an opening that has been formed in the tissues of the abdomen to the surface of the skin. This part of the colon is then stitched to the skin. Stool passes through the opening and into a disposable bag.

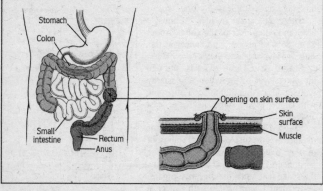

sigmoidoscopy or colonoscopy. Many people avoid colonoscopy because the test is cumbersome to prepare for or because they fear the examination itself. Although a virtual colonoscopy is less intrusive, the colon must still be cleansed the same as for colonoscopy with a flexible viewing tube called a colonoscope.[1] And if abnormalities are detected with virtual colonoscopy, colonoscopy must then be performed so that a biopsy can be done.

If an abnormality is detected with a screening test, the doctor removes tissue for examination under a microscope (biopsy). If the abnormality is a polyp, the entire polyp is removed. Once a cancer is diagnosed, further examinations are done to see whether the cancer has spread (staging).

1. see page 134

Treatment

Treatment depends on how far the cancer has spread. Usually, the first step is surgery to remove the cancer and the area around it.

The type of surgery depends on the area where the cancer is and how far it has spread. Partial colectomy involves removing the part of the colon where cancer is located and then attaching the ends of the remaining colon to each other. Usually, bowel habits return to normal or almost normal after this type of surgery.

If the cancer is more extensive, larger parts of the colon and rectum may need to be removed. Doctors have to create an opening in the skin of the abdomen so that stool can be eliminated from the body. This opening is called a stoma or an ostomy. Because the colon is involved, the opening is called a colostomy. A colostomy may be temporary (until the surgical site has healed) or permanent.

If the cancer has spread outside the colon or rectum, chemotherapy, radiation therapy, or both may be used to ensure that cancer cells are killed. Chemotherapy with fluorouracil may prolong survival if colon cancer has spread to nearby lymph nodes. If colon cancer has spread more widely, to organs such as the liver, chemotherapy with fluorouracil or irinotecan does not improve survival but it may help improve symptoms. However, chemotherapy can cause many side effects. Radiation therapy may help reduce pain in some people with colon cancer that has spread widely. Chemotherapy and radiation therapy may help prolong survival in some people with rectal cancer that has spread beyond the rectum, but both may cause many side effects.

Outlook

The outlook after surgery for colorectal cancer very much depends on the stage of the cancer at diagnosis.[1] However, it also depends on how well the person responds to treatment and the person's general health. More than 90% of people with colorectal cancer that is limited to the inner lining of the colon or rectum or that has grown no further than the layer of tissue just under the inner lining will live at least 5 years after treatment.

1. see art on page 777

However, if the cancer extends into nearby lymph nodes or has spread to other organs, the likelihood of living at least 5 years after treatment is greatly decreased.

Even after successful treatment, colorectal cancer recurs in about one third of people within 3 to 5 years. Chemotherapy and radiation therapy after surgery have reduced the likelihood of recurrence for many people, but both can cause many side effects. Regular examinations by a doctor are important. Doctors recommend that most people undergo blood tests to look for carcinoembryonic antigen (CEA), an indicator of some kinds of cancer cells, every 2 to 3 months for 2 to 5 years after treatment.

Colonoscopy should be performed every 2 to 3 years to look for evidence that the cancer has recurred and for new tumors or polyps.

LUNG CANCER

Lung cancer is one of the most common types of cancer, and it causes the most deaths from cancer in both men and women. The chance of developing lung cancer increases with age. Lung cancer is more common in men than in women, but the frequency is increasing in women because more women are smoking.

Lung cancer that begins in the lungs is called primary lung cancer; cancer that begins elsewhere in the body and spreads to the lungs is called metastatic lung cancer. Metastatic cancers spread to the lungs most commonly from breast, colon, and prostate cancers.

Most primary lung cancers develop in the larger airways (bronchi). A few develop in the air sacs (alveoli). The two main types of primary lung cancers are small cell cancers and non-small cell cancers. Other types of lung cancers include bronchial carcinoids and sarcomas. Cancer of the lymphatic system (lymphoma) may also start in the lungs.

Causes

Cigarette smoking causes most lung cancers. Cigar and pipe smoking can also cause lung cancer. The more a person has smoked and the longer a person has smoked, the greater is the risk of developing lung cancer. About 10% of smokers eventually develop lung cancer.

Much less often, lung cancer is caused by substances such as asbestos and arsenic. The risk of developing lung cancer is especially high in people who have been exposed to these substances and who also smoke. Air pollution and exposure to radon gas in homes may cause a small number of lung cancers. Occasionally, lung cancers develop in people whose lungs have been scarred by other diseases, such as tuberculosis.

Symptoms

The symptoms of lung cancer depend on its type and location and the way it spreads. A very common symptom, and often the first to develop, is a persistent cough. People who have chronic bronchitis or another lung disease that produces coughing often notice their coughing becoming worse if lung cancer develops. Sputum may be streaked with blood. If lung cancer grows into a blood vessel, it may cause severe bleeding.

Lung cancer may cause wheezing, either by growing inside an airway or by growing very near an airway and compressing it. The airway may become partially or completely blocked. Blockage of an airway can lead to collapse of part of the lung, a condition called atelectasis. A blocked airway may also cause shortness of breath and pneumonia, with coughing, fever, and chest pain.

Symptoms of lung cancer that usually develop later include fatigue, weakness, loss of appetite, and weight loss. Severe shortness of breath may develop if cancer spreads widely within the lungs. Fluid may accumulate around the lung (pleural effusion) if the cancer spreads into the space between the lungs and the chest wall (pleural space). Pleural effusions can produce shortness of breath.

Persistent chest pain may develop if lung cancer grows into the tissues of the chest wall. Lung cancer may also grow into certain nerves in the neck, causing a condition called Horner's syndrome. Symptoms of Horner's syndrome include a droopy eyelid, a pupil that cannot dilate (stays small) in the dark, a sunken appearance of the eye, and decreased sweating on one side of the face. Cancers at the top of the lung (the portion closest to the collar bone) may grow into the nerves that supply the arm, making the arm painful, numb, and weak—this combination of symptoms is called Pancoast syndrome. The voice can become hoarse if cancer compresses and damages the nerves of the voice box.

Difficulty swallowing may develop if lung cancer grows into or very near the esophagus. Occasionally, lung cancer causes an abnormal channel (fistula) to develop between the esophagus and an airway. Such a fistula can cause severe coughing during swallowing, because food and fluid enter the lungs.

Lung cancer may grow into the heart, causing abnormal heart rhythms, blocking blood flow through the heart, or causing fluid to build up in the sac that surrounds the heart (pericardium). The cancer may grow into or compress the superior vena cava, the large vein in the chest that carries blood back to the heart. Blockage of this vein causes blood to back up in other veins of the upper body; this condition is called superior vena cava syndrome. The blood causes the face, neck, and upper chest wall to swell; sometimes shortness of breath, headache, impaired vision, dizziness, and drowsiness occur.

Lung cancer can spread through the bloodstream to the liver, brain, adrenal glands, spinal cord, bones, and other parts of the body. The spread of lung cancer may occur early in the disease, especially with small cell cancer. Symptoms—such as headache, confusion, seizures, and bone pain—may develop even before lung problems become noticeable.

Screening and Diagnosis

There is no good way to screen for lung cancer. People with a very high risk of developing it may undergo periodic tests, but most lung cancers are missed anyway.

A doctor suspects lung cancer when a person, especially a smoker, has a persistent or worsening cough, shortness of breath, or coughed-up sputum tinged with blood. Sometimes a shadow on a chest x-ray taken to evaluate cough or some other symptom provides the first clue, although such a shadow is not proof of cancer.

Computed tomography (CT) may show small nodules that are not apparent on chest x-rays. Positron emission tomography (PET)[1] and a certain type of CT called spiral CT may improve the ability to detect small cancers. CT can also reveal whether the lymph nodes are enlarged; a biopsy of enlarged lymph

1. see page 126

nodes is often needed to determine if cancer is the cause of the enlargement.

Doctors usually need to examine sputum or a sample of lung tissue to confirm the diagnosis. A flexible viewing tube called a bronchoscope can be used to look inside airways and obtain tissue for examination under a microscope. If the cancer is too deep in the lung to be reached with a bronchoscope, a doctor can usually obtain a sample of tissue by inserting a needle through the skin while using CT to guide movements of the needle. This procedure is called a needle biopsy. Sometimes, a specimen can be obtained only through an opening in the chest wall, in a procedure called a thoracotomy.

A CT scan of the abdomen or head may be done to determine if lung cancer has spread, especially to the liver, adrenal glands, or brain. A bone scan may show that it has spread to the bones. In people with small cell cancer, a bone marrow biopsy is sometimes done, because this type of cancer tends to spread to the bone marrow.

Cancers are categorized based on how large the tumor is, whether it has spread to nearby lymph nodes, and whether it has spread to distant organs. The different categories are called stages. The stage of a cancer suggests the most appropriate treatment and enables a doctor to estimate the person's outlook.

Prevention and Treatment

Prevention of lung cancer includes quitting smoking and avoiding exposure to potentially cancer-causing substances in the environment.

Surgery is the best treatment for nonsmall cell lung cancers that have not spread beyond the lungs. However, surgery is unlikely to be helpful if the cancer has spread beyond the lungs, if the cancer is too close to very large airways (the trachea or its two main branches), or if the person has another potentially life-threatening disorder (such as severe coronary artery disease or chronic obstructive pulmonary disease).

Before surgery, a doctor estimates how much lung tissue needs to be removed and how much lung tissue will be left. Depending on how far the cancer has spread, the amount varies from a small part of a lung to an entire lung. Tests are then done to determine if the amount of lung tissue estimated to be left after surgery will be enough to ensure adequate lung function. If these tests indicate that removing the cancerous part of the lung will result in inadequate lung function, surgery is not possible.

Removal of the cancer does not always result in a cure. The extent of cancer in the lung and identification of all areas where a cancer has spread cannot always be determined. Therefore, many people who undergo surgery eventually die from their cancer, either in the lung or at another site. Survivors must have regular checkups, including periodic chest x-rays and CT scans.

For nonsmall cell lung cancers, results of surgery may be improved by chemotherapy and radiation therapy given before and after surgery.

Radiation therapy may also be given to people who choose not to have surgery, who cannot undergo surgery because they have another serious condition, or whose cancer has spread. Although radiation therapy usually only partially shrinks the cancer or slows its growth, it may halt growth for a prolonged period in 10 to 15% of them. Combining chemotherapy with radiation therapy may provide further benefit. Radiation therapy is also useful for controlling symptoms that develop from complications of lung cancer, such as coughing up blood, bone pain, superior vena cava syndrome, and pressure on nerves.

The effectiveness of chemotherapy alone for nonsmall cell lung cancer is not very good. If nonsmall cell lung cancer has spread, some people live several more months when given chemotherapy.

Chemotherapy, sometimes coupled with radiation therapy, is the treatment of choice for small cell cancer because the cancer has almost always spread to other parts of the body by the time it is diagnosed. In about 25% of people, chemotherapy substantially prolongs survival and may occasionally cure these people. Without chemotherapy, only half of the people with small cell cancer survive 4 months. However, chemotherapy often causes many side effects that can make people feel very ill. People with small cell cancer who have been responding well to chemotherapy may benefit from radiation therapy to the head to treat cancer that may have spread to the brain. Sometimes lung cancer spreads to the brain early enough that no symptoms are apparent and nothing abnormal can be seen on a CT or MRI scans of the head.

Other treatments are often needed to relieve symptoms. Because many people with lung cancer have a decrease in lung function, oxygen therapy and bronchodilators (drugs that widen the airways) may help breathing. Advanced lung cancer may cause such intense pain and difficulty in breathing that many people require large doses of opioids in the weeks or months before their death. Fortunately, opioids can control pain if adequate doses are used.

Outlook

Lung cancer has a poor outlook. On average, people with untreated lung cancer survive little more than 6 months. Overall, even with therapy, fewer than 15% of people survive for 5 or more years. Because small cell cancer has almost always spread beyond the lung at the time of diagnosis, its outlook is worse than for other types of lung cancer.

MOUTH, HEAD, AND NECK CANCERS

Cancer of the mouth (oral cancer) and cancers of the head and neck area are common, and they are among the most deadly cancers known. The great majority of oral, head, and neck cancers occur in people over the age of 50. Unfortunately, these cancers tend to spread early, so many people are diagnosed at late stages when the outlook for responding to treatment is poor.

Causes

Oral, head, and neck cancers have three major risk factors: older age, tobacco use, and alcohol consumption. Tobacco is responsible for the large majority of these cancers. Several other factors may play a role, including heredity, exposure to certain chemicals that can cause cancer, and viruses. Sun exposure can cause lip cancer. A diet low in fruits and vegetables increases a person's risk of developing oral cancer.

Symptoms and Diagnosis

Early cancers frequently produce no symptoms. Cancers in the larynx and throat may cause hoarseness and a feeling of fullness, as if something is stuck in the throat.

Many early oral cancers appear as white, red, or a mixture of red and white sores or ulcers. Sores or ulcers that do not disappear after 3 to 4 weeks should be examined by a dentist or doctor. Cancers can occur as lumps in the mouth, on the tongue, in the back of the throat, and in the neck. Pain does not occur until cancers become larger, and the neck may not swell until oral cancers have spread to lymph nodes in the neck.

Diagnosis is made by tissue biopsy. CT or MRI scanning is then done to determine the exact location of the cancer and to determine if the cancer has spread.

Treatment

Doctors treat small oral, head, and neck cancers with surgery. If the entire cancer is removed and there is no evidence of spread, no further treatment may be needed other than careful follow-up by a doctor for many years. Because recurrence is much more likely with continued tobacco use and alcohol consumption, these should be discontinued.

With large oral, head, and neck cancers, surgery is required to remove the tumor as well as nearby lymph nodes. Because these lymph nodes are located in the neck, surgery involves removing extensive portions of one or both sides of the neck. About 4 weeks after surgery, the person then undergoes radiation therapy. Radiation therapy is usually given five times per week for 5 to 7 weeks. Doctors direct the radiation to the areas from which cancerous tissue was removed, as well as to other areas in the head and neck that are at risk for cancer spread. Radiation therapy is commonly combined with chemotherapy. Chemotherapy may help improve survival, but only if the cancer has not spread (metastasized) to other parts of the body. Chemotherapy may help if the cancer has already metastasized. In such instances, the chemotherapy is used without radiation therapy, to help slow the cancer's growth while preserving the function of structures such as the vocal cords, which can be damaged by radiation therapy.

Outlook

The outcomes for oral, head, and neck cancer depend on the severity of the disease and the type of treatment. In general, more than 80% of people with small cancers and no lymph node involvement live 5 years or longer. But fewer than 20% of people with large cancers that have spread to nearby lymph nodes live more than 5 years.

Surgery for oral, head, and neck cancer can cause significant problems. People may experience numbness; pain; and difficulty eating, chewing, speaking, swallowing, and tasting, depending on which parts of the mouth, head, and neck were removed in the surgery. If surgery involves the face or neck, disfigurement can be expected.

Radiation therapy can cause oral sores and ulcers (mucositis) to develop during and immediately after therapy. Permanent mouth dryness also develops because the radiation frequently destroys salivary glands. Problems associated with a dry mouth[1] develop, putting people at high risk for dental cavities and oral infections (particularly fungal infections). Radiation to the face and neck can lead to difficulty opening the jaw, moving the neck, and swallowing.

Before and after treatment for oral, head, or neck cancer, the person should be examined by a dentist. Any problems such as tooth decay or periodontal disease should be treated, and a program of careful oral hygiene should be begun under the dentist's direction.

MULTIPLE MYELOMA

Multiple myeloma is a cancer of plasma cells. Plasma cells develop from a type of white blood cell called B lymphocytes. Normal plasma cells produce antibodies that help the body to fight infections. Multiple myeloma cells grow uncontrollably in the bone marrow and occasionally in other parts of the body.

Multiple myeloma most often occurs in people 60 or older. Although its cause is not certain, the increased occurrence among close relatives indicates that heredity plays a role. Exposure to radiation is a possible cause, as is exposure to benzene and other chemicals. Infection with a type of herpes virus may play a role.

In multiple myeloma, the overabundance of cancerous cells in the bone marrow suppresses development of normal white blood cells, red blood cells, and platelets. In addition, the cancerous cells almost always produce a large amount of a single type of antibody accompanied by a markedly reduced amount of all other types of normal antibodies.

1. see page 566

Often, collections of cancerous plasma cells develop into tumors that destroy bone tissue, most commonly in the pelvic bones, spine, ribs, and skull. Infrequently, these tumors develop in areas other than bone, such as the lungs, liver, and kidneys.

Symptoms

Because plasma cell tumors often invade bone, pain may occur, often in the back, ribs, and hips. Plasma cell tumors cause loss of bone density (osteoporosis), which weakens bones, making fractures more likely. Calcium is released from the bones, which may result in abnormally high levels of calcium in the blood. High calcium levels can affect the heart, kidneys, and brain, possibly causing constipation, increased frequency of urination, weakness, and confusion.

The reduced production of red blood cells often leads to anemia, which causes fatigue and weakness and may lead to heart problems. The reduced production of white blood cells leads to repeated infections, which may cause fever and chills. The reduced production of platelets impairs the blood's ability to clot and results in easy bruising or bleeding.

Pieces of monoclonal antibodies, known as light chains, frequently end up in the kidneys, sometimes permanently damaging them and causing kidney failure. These antibody pieces are called Bence Jones proteins. The increased number of cancerous cells can lead the body to produce too much uric acid. Excess uric acid is excreted in the urine, which can lead to kidney stones. Deposits of antibody pieces in the kidneys or other organs can lead to amyloidosis.[1]

In rare instances, multiple myeloma interferes with blood flow to the skin, fingers, toes, nose, kidneys, and brain because the blood thickens (hyperviscosity syndrome).

Diagnosis

Multiple myeloma may be discovered even before a person has symptoms, when an x-ray performed for another reason shows a loss of bone density. Bone loss may be widespread or limited to scattered punched-out areas of a few bones.

Multiple myeloma is sometimes suspected because of symptoms, such as back pain or bone pain of other sites, fatigue,

1. see box on page 399

fevers, and bruising. Blood tests performed to investigate such symptoms may reveal that a person has anemia, a decreased white blood cell count, a decreased platelet count, or kidney failure.

The two most useful blood tests are serum protein electrophoresis and immunoelectrophoresis. They detect and identify an overabundance of a single type of antibody found in most people who have multiple myeloma. Doctors also measure the different types of antibodies, especially IgG, IgA, and IgM.

A bone marrow biopsy is almost always performed to confirm the diagnosis. Other blood tests are useful in determining the overall outlook for the person. Higher levels of certain proteins in the person's blood when the disease is diagnosed usually indicate a poorer outlook and are likely to affect treatment decisions.

Treatment and Outlook

Multiple myeloma remains incurable despite recent advances in therapy. Treatment is aimed at preventing or relieving symptoms and complications, destroying abnormal plasma cells, and slowing progression of the disease.

The most consistently helpful drugs for multiple myeloma are corticosteroids, such as prednisone or dexamethasone. In addition, chemotherapy slows the progression of multiple myeloma by killing the abnormal plasma cells. Because chemotherapy kills normal cells as well as abnormal ones, the blood cells are monitored and the drug doses are adjusted if the number of normal white blood cells and platelets decreases too much.

Melphalan, and less often cyclophosphamide, are the chemotherapy drugs most often given with corticosteroids. Vincristine and doxorubicin are also effective and may have less severe side effects, particularly on the bone marrow, than melphalan and cyclophosphamide. For people who have a good response to chemotherapy, the drug interferon-alpha may prolong the response somewhat but has little impact on survival.

Thalidomide and new drugs called proteosome inhibitors are being used as alternatives to the chemotherapy drugs that are usually given. Because these treatments are also toxic to normal blood cells made in the bone marrow, stem cells are collected from the person's blood before the high-dose chemotherapy is administered. Stem cells are unspecialized cells that transform into immature blood cells, which eventually mature to become red blood cells, white blood cells, and platelets. The collected stem cells are then returned (transplanted) to the person after the high-dose treatment. Generally, this procedure is so taxing that it is usually reserved for people who are younger than 75.

Strong analgesics and radiation therapy directed at the affected bones can help relieve bone pain. Radiation therapy may also prevent the development of fractures. Monthly intravenous administration of pamidronate or the more potent zoledronic acid (both are bisphosphonates, drugs that decrease the rate of bone loss) can reduce the likelihood of fractures. Most people with multiple myeloma receive pamidronate or zoledronic acid as part of their treatment forever. Staying active is also important; prolonged bed rest tends to accelerate bone loss and makes the bones more vulnerable to fractures. Most people can enjoy a normal lifestyle that includes most activities. Drinking plenty of fluids dilutes the urine and helps prevent dehydration, which can make kidney failure more likely.

People who have symptoms of infection—fever, chills, cough that produces sputum, or reddened areas of the skin— should seek attention from a doctor promptly because they may need antibiotics. Erythropoietin or darbepoietin, drugs that stimulate red blood cell formation, may adequately treat anemia. Those who have severe anemia may need transfusions of red blood cells. High levels of calcium in the blood can be treated with intravenous fluids and often require intravenous bisphosphonates. People who have high levels of uric acid in the blood may benefit from allopurinol, a drug that blocks the body's production of uric acid.

Treatment slows disease progression in more than 60% of people. The average survival is more than 3 years after the disease is diagnosed, but survival time varies widely depending on the symptoms and complications at the time of diagnosis and the response to treatment. Importantly, advances in treatment and better pain relievers have greatly improved quality of life. Occasionally, people who survive for many years after successful treatment of multiple myeloma develop leukemia or irreversible loss of bone marrow function. These late complications may result from chemotherapy and often lead to severe anemia and an increased susceptibility to infections and bleeding.

Because multiple myeloma is ultimately fatal, people with multiple myeloma are likely to benefit from discussions of end-of-life care.[1] They may also want to have an advance directive in place.[2]

PROSTATE CANCER

In the United States, prostate cancer is one of the most common cancers in men and the second most common cause of cancer death (exceeded only by lung cancer). The chance of developing prostate cancer increases with aging. More than three fourths of men with prostate cancer are 65 or older when cancer is diagnosed. The risk is highest among African Americans and Hispanics and among men whose close relatives had prostate cancer.

The cause of prostate cancer is not known. Prostate cancer commonly begins as a small lump in the prostate gland. Male hormones, especially testosterone, stimulate the growth of prostate cancer. The cancer usually grows very slowly and may take decades to produce symptoms. In many men, prostate cancer never produces symptoms. Many men die from some other cause without ever knowing that they had prostate cancer. But in some men, the cancer is more aggressive so that it grows rapidly and spreads outside the prostate.

Prostate cancer can spread directly to nearby structures, such as the urethra or bladder. When the cancer spreads beyond the region of the prostate, it most commonly spreads to bones, especially vertebrae and ribs; it may spread to the brain.

Symptoms

Prostate cancer usually causes no symptoms until it reaches a late stage. Sometimes, symptoms similar to those of benign prostatic hyperplasia (BPH) develop,[3] including difficulty starting or continuing urination and a need to urinate frequently or urgently. However, these symptoms do not develop until the

1. see page 211
2. see page 953
3. see page 886

cancer is large enough to compress the urethra and partially block the flow of urine or irritate the bladder muscle. Some men have bloody urine.

Sometimes, symptoms develop after the cancer spreads. Pain develops when prostate cancer spreads to bone. Bones may weaken enough to easily fracture. Cancer that spreads to vertebrae can compress the spinal cord, resulting in pain, numbness, leg weakness, or incontinence. Cancer that spreads to the skull can compress brain tissue, resulting in seizures, confusion, headaches, and weakness, among other symptoms. When cancer spreads to bone marrow, production of red blood cells decreases, resulting in anemia, with symptoms such as fatigue and weakness.

Screening

Because prostate cancer is common, many doctors check for it in men with no symptoms (screening). However, experts disagree about the role of screening. Screening seems to offer the advantage of finding more prostate cancers early—when they are most likely to be curable. However, because prostate cancer may grow very slowly in many men, screening may find many cancers that might never cause symptoms or death. Treating a slow-growing cancer might be more damaging than leaving the cancer untreated. Newer tests are being developed to help doctors identify cancers that are more likely to grow quickly.

Screening tests are not foolproof. They may suggest the possibility of prostate cancer in men who do not actually have prostate cancer. In other words, they may give false-positive results. Tests, such as biopsies, are then done to try to find the cancer. These tests can be stressful and carry some risk.

To screen for prostate cancer, a doctor performs a digital rectal examination. A gloved finger is inserted into the man's rectum to feel the surface of the prostate gland. If the man has prostate cancer, a doctor sometimes feels a hard bump in the prostate. Another screening test involves measuring the level of prostate-specific antigen (PSA) in a sample of blood. PSA is a substance that is usually higher in men with prostate cancer. PSA levels tend to increase with aging, but cancer increases the PSA levels even more. Also, PSA levels are higher than normal in men with BPH or inflammation and infection of the prostate (prostatitis). Unfortunately, because some prostate cancers do not produce PSA, screening with only a PSA test is unreliable.

Diagnosis

If the results of a digital rectal examination or PSA test suggest prostate cancer, a biopsy is done. In a biopsy, tissue samples from the prostate are taken and examined under a microscope.[1] Usually, a doctor first obtains images of the prostate by inserting an ultrasound transducer, or probe, into the rectum (transrectal ultrasound). Then tissue samples are taken from the prostate using a needle inserted through the probe. This procedure takes only a few minutes. A local anesthetic helps control pain.

Two features help a doctor determine the likely course and the best treatment of the cancer: how distorted (malignant) the cells look under a microscope (grading) and how far the cancer has spread (staging).

Grading usually involves microscopic examination and biochemical tests of the tissue samples. Doctors look to see how distorted the overall gland is and how abnormal the cancer cells appear and determine the Gleason score. The score helps rate the aggressiveness of prostate cancer. Those cancers that are most distorted tend to grow and spread quickly and have a higher Gleason score (8 or higher). Those that are less likely to grow quickly and spread have a lower Gleason score (5 or lower). This is true regardless of the man's age.

Staging involves tests to assess how far the cancer has spread. Doctors perform an examination to determine whether the cancer has spread within the prostate, to lymph nodes in areas near the prostate, or to organs far from the prostate. Testing may not be necessary when the likelihood of spread beyond the prostate is extremely low. Results of the digital rectal examination, ultrasound scan, and biopsy reveal how far the cancer has spread within the prostate. Computed tomography (CT) or radiolabeled antibody nuclear scans of the pelvis help detect spread to the lymph nodes. A bone scan reveals spread to bone. If doctors suspect that cancer has spread to certain sites, CT or MRI may be done.

1. see page 140

Treatment

Choosing among treatment options can be complicated and often depends on the man's lifestyle preferences and life expectancy. Current treatments are not without side effects, which may affect quality of life. For example, surgery to remove the prostate, radiation therapy, and hormone therapy can result in involuntary loss of urine (urinary incontinence) and erectile dysfunction (impotence). When choosing among treatment options, men need to weigh the advantages and disadvantages.

Treatment strategies: Treatment for prostate cancer usually involves one of three strategies: watchful waiting, curative treatment, or palliative therapy.

• **Watchful waiting** foregoes treatment until symptoms develop, if they develop at all. This strategy is best for men whose cancers are unlikely to spread, cause symptoms, or affect life expectancy. For example, most low grade cancers confined to a small area within the prostate grow very slowly. These cancers usually do not spread for many years. Men over 80 years of age are most likely to choose watchful waiting, particularly if they have other medical problems, because older men are far more likely to die of other diseases before such cancers cause symptoms. During watchful waiting, symptoms can be treated if necessary. Periodic testing may be done to see if the cancer is growing rapidly or spreading. The man may later decide to pursue curative treatment if testing shows growth or spread.

• **Curative treatment** is a common strategy for men with cancers confined to the prostate that are likely to cause troublesome symptoms or death. Curative treatment approaches are surgery or radiation. High grade or rapidly growing cancers are more commonly treated. Curative treatment may also help men with small, slowly growing cancers (even though symptoms from such cancers may not develop until a decade later) if the man expects to otherwise live many years. Curative treatment for cancers that have spread outside the prostate is difficult unless the extent of the spread can be clearly identified. For example, cancers confined or adjacent to the prostate are more likely to be successfully treated. Side effects of curative treatment, which may include urinary incontinence and erectile dysfunction, can affect quality of life. Incontinence and erectile dysfunction are sometimes permanent.

• **Palliative therapy** aims at treating the symptoms rather than the cancer itself. This strategy is best suited to men with widespread prostate cancer that is not curable. The growth or spread of such cancers can usually be slowed or even temporarily reversed, relieving symptoms. Because these treatments cannot cure the cancer, symptoms eventually worsen. Death from the disease eventually follows.

Four forms of treatment are used in curative or palliative strategies for prostate cancer: surgery, radiation therapy, hormone-blocking therapy, and chemotherapy. Combinations and sequential use of these treatments are common.

Surgery: Surgical removal of the prostate (prostatectomy) is useful for cancer confined to the prostate. Surgery is less effective in curing fast-growing cancers, because they are more likely to have already spread by the time the cancer is diagnosed. Prostatectomy requires general anesthesia, a hospital stay, and a surgical incision, but only one procedure is needed.

There are two types of surgery to remove the prostate: radical prostatectomy and nerve-sparing prostatectomy. In radical prostatectomy, the entire prostate, the seminal vesicles, and part of the vas deferens are removed. Radical prostatectomy causes erectile dysfunction in many men, and urinary incontinence in some, yet it is more likely to cure prostate cancer. Men over 65 are less likely to have radical prostatectomy because they have a greater likelihood of having chronic diseases that shorten their life expectancy.

In nerve-sparing prostatectomy, some of the nerves needed to achieve erection are preserved, reducing the risks of erectile dysfunction (and incontinence). This procedure can be used if the surgeon sees that the cancer has not invaded the nerves and blood vessels. Nerve-sparing radical prostatectomy can be done using a type of endoscope (a flexible viewing tube) called a laparoscope. Alternatively, the surgery can be performed with computer-controlled robotic arms. Laparoscopic and robot-assisted techniques require a smaller incision and produce less postoperative pain, but they are offered only at major referral centers.

Radiation therapy: Radiation therapy can cure cancers that are confined to the prostate, as well as some cancers that have invaded nearby tissues. Radiation therapy cannot cure cancer that has spread to distant organs, including bone. However, radiation therapy can relieve pain that results from the spread of prostate cancer to bone.

Whereas surgery is accomplished in one procedure, radiation therapy usually requires many separate treatment sessions over the course of several weeks. During traditional radiation therapy (external beam radiation), a machine sends beams of radiation to the prostate and surrounding tissues. Treatments are usually given 5 days per week for 5 to 7 weeks.

Although erectile dysfunction can develop after radiation therapy, it is slightly less likely than after surgery. Urinary incontinence occasionally results. Urethral strictures—scars that narrow the urethra and interfere with the flow of urine—can develop. Other troublesome but usually temporary side effects of traditional radiation therapy include burning during urination, having to urinate frequently, blood in the urine, irritation and inflammation of the rectum and diarrhea (radiation proctitis), and sudden urges to defecate.

With recent technical advances, doctors can more precisely focus the radiation beam on the cancer (a procedure called three-dimensional conformal radiotherapy). Conformal radiotherapy causes fewer temporary side effects, particularly radiation proctitis.

Radiation can also be delivered by inserting radioactive implants into the prostate (brachytherapy). Implants are placed using images obtained from ultrasound or CT scans. Brachytherapy offers some advantages: it can deliver high doses of radiation to the prostate while sparing healthy surrounding tissues and producing fewer side effects. Brachytherapy can be performed in a few hours, does not require repeated treatment sessions, and uses only spinal anesthesia. Brachytherapy is not appropriate for all men. Combined treatment with brachytherapy and traditional radiation therapy is sometimes recommended.

Hormone-blocking therapy: Because prostate tissue tends to grow more quickly in the presence of testosterone, reducing testosterone levels tends to slow cancer growth. Hormone-blocking therapy can be effective in men in whom surgery and radiation therapy have failed. Hormone-blocking therapy is also effective when used before radiation therapy, and it is now routinely used this way. It is not effective when used before surgery. Hormone-blocking therapy is not curative, and cancer recurs in all men in whom other therapies have failed.

Hormone-blocking drugs used to treat prostate cancer in the United States include leuprolide and goserelin, which prevent the pituitary from stimulating the testes to make testosterone. A doctor injects these drugs periodically, usually for the rest of the man's life. Other drugs that block testosterone's effects (such as flutamide, bicalutamide, and nilutamide) may also be used. These drugs are taken daily by mouth.

Testosterone levels can also be reduced by surgically removing the testes. This treatment is very effective, but many men do not want to undergo such a body-altering treatment.

Low testosterone levels that result from hormone-blocking drugs can produce hot flashes, thinning and weakening of bones, loss of energy, reduced muscle mass, fluid retention, reduced libido, reduced body hair, erectile dysfunction, and breast enlargement (gynecomastia). In an effort to reduce these symptoms, hormone-blocking therapy is sometimes given intermittently instead of continuously.

Chemotherapy: Chemotherapy may be used for cancers that have spread beyond the prostate. Treatment that combines chemotherapy with other approaches improves survival in men with aggressive, later-stage cancers.

The introduction of bisphosphonate therapy (zoledronic acid) has greatly improved care for men in whom prostate cancer has spread to bones. Bisphosphonates interfere with cells (osteoclasts) in bones that are activated by cancer cells, thereby reducing bone destruction and the likelihood of fractures.

SKIN CANCER

Skin cancer is the most common type of cancer, affecting hundreds of thousands of people each year. Skin cancer occurs in the outer layers of the skin. People who have light-colored skin and those who have spent a lot of time in the sun are most at risk. Because sun exposure is a risk factor for skin cancer, skin cancer is most likely to occur on the face (including the lips and ears), the neck, and the arms.

Skin cancer is classified by the type of skin cells in which it develops: basal cells or squamous cells. A third type, melanoma, develops in the pigment-containing cells deep in the skin. Melanoma is far less common but far more serious than basal or squamous cell cancers. Although the diagnosis and treatment of basal and squamous cell cancers are similar, the approach to melanoma is more complex.

Symptoms and Diagnosis

The earliest sign of skin cancer is a change in the skin. A person may notice a new mole or a change in an existing mole. A smooth, shiny, or waxy looking lump or an area of skin that is red or reddish brown or rough or scaly looking may be a sign of skin cancer. A sore or rash that will not heal is another sign.

Because skin cancer that is found early is usually curable, a person who notices a change in the appearance of his skin should be checked by a doctor. The doctor examines the skin and performs a biopsy.[1] Usually, the biopsy can be done in the doctor's office.

Prevention and Treatment

Skin cancer most often results from many years of exposure to the sun, but it is never too late to protect the skin. People should use sunscreens with a high skin protection factor (SPF) on all exposed areas of the skin when they are outside. Wearing long-sleeved shirts, long pants, and wide-brimmed hats is also helpful.

People should examine their skin about every 3 to 4 months, and they should be examined by a doctor if they notice changes. Because it is difficult to see all areas of the skin, especially if movement is hampered by some other condition (such as arthritis), a family member should be asked to examine hard-to-see areas. Older people should have all areas of their skin examined every year by a doctor.

Sometimes a doctor detects a patch of skin that is likely to become cancerous. The patch is called actinic keratosis. Doctors usually recommend removing actinic keratosis when it is found rather than waiting for cancer to develop. To remove actinic keratosis, a doctor may apply liquid nitrogen or a chemical.

Treatment of skin cancer depends on the type, location, and extent of the cancer, as well as the person's general health. Most often, a skin cancer is removed with surgery, along with some

1. see page 141

of the skin around it. For melanomas, a wider area of tissue must be removed, and nearby lymph nodes must also be examined for evidence of spread.

The person may have a scar after the cancer is removed. In some areas, such as the face, the surgery is done using a microscope (Mohs' surgery) to minimize the amount of tissue removed. If a large area of tissue is removed, a skin graft may be used to help the site heal. In a skin graft, healthy tissue from another area of the body is used to cover the site from which the cancer was removed. Sometimes additional surgery can be performed after the area has healed to improve the appearance of the scar.

Skin cancer in some sites may be treated with radiation therapy.

Outlook

Most basal cell and squamous cell skin cancers can be cured but, if left until late, can cause significant disfigurement. Melanomas are curable if treated early but are often fatal if not. People treated for skin cancer should be re-examined by a doctor regularly so that cancer can be detected early if it returns.

VULVAR CANCER

Cancer of the vulva (the area of the external female genitals) most often occurs after menopause. The average age at which vulvar cancer is diagnosed is 70 years.

The risk of developing vulvar cancer is higher in women who have persistent itching of the vulva, have or had genital warts due to human papillomavirus (HPV), or had cancer of the vagina or cervix.

The large majority of vulvar cancers are skin cancers that develop near or at the opening of the vagina. Squamous cell carcinomas are the most common. Melanomas and basal cell carcinomas are much less common. Rare types include Paget's disease and cancer of Bartholin's glands (the small glands adjacent to the opening of the vagina that secrete fluid for lubrication during intercourse).

Vulvar cancer begins on the surface of the vulva. Most of these cancers grow slowly, remaining on the surface for years. However, some grow quickly. Untreated, vulvar cancer can eventually extend more deeply, sometimes invading the vagina, urethra, or anus. Vulvar cancer may also spread to nearby lymph nodes.

Symptoms and Diagnosis

Patches of vulvar skin may turn white, brown, or red before cancer develops. Such patches may indicate that cancer is likely to develop. Once a cancer is present, the involved skin may have sores that never seem to heal. In other instances, the cancer can be felt as a lumpy area. Sometimes the involved skin is scaly or discolored. The surrounding skin may seem to tighten and pucker. Itching is common. Eventually, the area may bleed or produce a watery discharge.

A sample of the abnormal skin must be removed to determine if cancer is present, and if so, to identify the type of cancer. Sometimes doctors apply stains to the abnormal skin to help locate the best place to obtain a sample of tissue. Doctors may also use an instrument with magnifying lenses (a colposcope) to examine the abnormal skin and to pinpoint the best place to obtain a sample.

Treatment and Outlook

The woman's preferences play an important role in determining treatment options. However, treatment options also depend on the type and stage of cancer and the woman's overall health. Because some vulvar cancers spread quickly, especially squamous cell carcinomas and melanomas, surgery is almost always needed to remove the cancer. For very small cancers that do not extend deeply, surgery may involve removal of only the skin. Alternatively, in a limited number of women with small cancers, treatment may consist of using a beam of light to remove the abnormal tissue (laser surgery), application of an ointment containing a chemotherapy drug, such as fluorouracil, or radiation therapy.

Larger cancers and any that have invaded deeper tissues require more extensive surgery that involves removing all or at least part of the vulva. Radiation therapy, chemotherapy, or both may be used to shrink large cancers before surgery. Sometimes the clitoris must be removed. Nearby lymph nodes may also be removed. Sexual intercourse is usually possible after removal of all or part of the vulva.

Because basal cell carcinomas rarely spread (metastasize) to distant sites, surgery usually involves removing only the cancer. The whole vulva is removed only if the cancer is extensive.

If vulvar cancer is detected early, most women remain free of any sign of cancer for at least 5 years after treatment (although cancer may recur in a small number even after 5 years). If the cancer has invaded nearby lymph nodes, less than one third of women survive for 5 years.

> *"Yesterday is History. Tomorrow is a Mystery.*
> *Today is a Gift."*

This phrase from Dr. Robert Schuller of the Crystal Cathedral has made an impact on my perspective on aging.

As a child we had our heroes and heroines—a person we wanted to be like, a movie star, a sports figure, a role model—the magical era of make believe. But then, in our young adult years, we were very busy raising a family, experiencing World War II, and not focusing on the childhood dream of wishing to be someone else. We all had challenges and survived them. That is History.

Today is a Gift. I am very fortunate in my profession as a weekly TV hostess to confront many aging issues, bring to light the many contributions seniors are making, i.e., volunteering, mentoring the young, and taking on health issues with a positive and informative outlook.

Personally, I had cataract surgery on television to encourage viewers. Also, when I learned of seniors having a fear of a colonoscopy, I had mine done on my TV show—long before Katie Couric. The feedback from the medical community has been very rewarding. Many viewers have responded by requesting these procedures as some of their concerns have been alleviated. Presently, I am fighting breast cancer while sharing the whole procedure with my viewers to demonstrate strength, determination, and courage. The doctors told me they will do 70 percent, but I have to do 30 percent.

So being a "role model" to the viewers has been a gratifying experience. You don't have to have a TV show to be a role model to others. One of the blessings is the love, understanding, and awareness the younger generation has come to recognize in the aging population.

Keep a good sense of humor. Have faith in God. Live every day to its fullest. Don't worry about tomorrow. Tomorrow is a Mystery.

Eileen Jensen-Kercheval

52

Pneumonia and Influenza

Pneumonia and influenza, long considered scourges of old age, are among the most common health problems that confront people in their later years. Pneumonia and influenza are infections that are often far more serious in older people. Frail older people are at greatest risk. Pneumonia, for example, used to be called "the old man's friend," a quick way to death for an older person whose health was failing. Today, doctors try to prevent pneumonia and influenza and generally treat them aggressively—and successfully—in all but the most ill people.

PNEUMONIA

Pneumonia is infection of the small air sacs of the lungs (alveoli) and surrounding tissues.

The infection causes inflammation and deterioration of lung function. The lungs become unable to easily transfer oxygen to the blood, increasing the work of breathing.

Pneumonia occurs in people of all ages. However, it occurs far more commonly in older people, in whom it tends to be far more serious. Younger people with pneumonia can often be treated at home, whereas most older people with pneumonia must be hospitalized because the infection tends to worsen quickly.

Pneumonia often affects only a portion of a single lung but can affect an entire lung or even both lungs. In many older people, the lung infection spreads beyond the lungs. The infection can enter the blood (sepsis).

When pneumonia occurs among people living in houses or apartments within a community, it is called community-acquired pneumonia. However, pneumonia is even more likely among older people who are hospitalized (hospital-acquired pneumonia) or living in institutional settings, such as nursing homes (nursing home–acquired pneumonia). Older people in hospitals or institutions often have weakened defenses against infection. Further, infections spread more efficiently in a closed environment.

Causes

Bacteria are the most common microorganisms that cause pneumonia. However, viruses and fungi cause pneumonia as well. These microorganisms are everywhere and are inhaled into the lungs all the time. Yet pneumonia does not occur every time these microorganisms are inhaled. Pneumonia develops only when these microorganisms gain a foothold in the tiny air sacs of the lungs.

Normally, several defense mechanisms help prevent microorganisms from reaching the air sacs. Specialized cells lining the airways have microscopic hairlike projections that constantly sweep anything that does not belong in the lungs up and out. Coughing is another way the lungs rid themselves of microorganisms. If microorganisms do reach the air sacs, the immune system, which normally helps defend the body against infection, is usually able to destroy the microorganisms before pneumonia develops.

Certain characteristics and conditions make older people more likely to develop pneumonia. First, the system of cleansing the airways is not as effective as in younger people. Weakness may make coughing less vigorous. And, with aging, the immune system is weakened.

Among all older people, those at greater risk of developing pneumonia include the following:

• Those whose lungs have been damaged by smoking or chronic obstructive pulmonary disease (smoking irritates the lining of the lungs and paralyzes the cells that normally sweep and cleanse the airways)

• Those whose lungs have recently been irritated by a mild infection, such as a cold or, especially, influenza

• Those who have poor cough reflex or who are too weak (or

who are in pain from recent surgery or an accident) to cough vigorously

• Those who are less able to fight off infections, such as those who are undernourished

• Those who are taking certain drugs, such as corticosteroids

• Those who have certain diseases, such as heart failure or diabetes

• Those who have cancer in or near the airways of the lungs (the cancer may block the airways and trap any microorganisms that have reached the air sacs)

• Those who are paralyzed (for example, by a spinal injury or stroke)

• Those who are unconscious (in part because they are unable to cough)

Microorganisms that produce pneumonia can end up in air sacs in several ways. In some cases, people inhale microorganisms (which are present in tiny droplets) when they are near someone already infected. Spread in hospitals and nursing homes often occurs this way. More common among older people, however, is the presence of bacteria in their throat (colonization). These bacteria may remain there harmlessly or suddenly cause pneumonia if mucus or food is inhaled into the airway (aspiration) instead of passed into the esophagus. When aspiration occurs, the food or mucus can make its way into the lungs, carrying the bacteria from the throat along for the ride. Rarely, microorganisms from elsewhere in the body reach the lungs by traveling through the bloodstream.

Streptococcus pneumoniae (pneumococcus) is the most common bacterial cause of community-acquired pneumonia. Other common bacterial causes include anaerobic bacteria (which grow in the absence of oxygen), *Haemophilus influenzae,* and *Legionella pneumophila* (which causes a type of infection called Legionnaires' disease). Influenza virus and respiratory syncytial virus can also cause community-acquired pneumonia in older people, as can *Mycobacterium tuberculosis,* the microorganism causing tuberculosis. Although fungi can cause community-acquired pneumonia, they more commonly cause pneumonia in hospitalized patients who may be sick or debilitated (for example, cancer patients receiving chemotherapy).

Staphylococcus aureus, Klebsiella, Proteus, Escherichia

coli, and *Pseudomonas aeruginosa* are bacteria that often cause pneumonia that develops in hospitalized or institutionalized people, such as those in nursing homes. Outbreaks of influenza and respiratory syncytial virus infection are also common in nursing homes. Tuberculosis occurs in this setting as well.

Symptoms and Diagnosis

The most common symptom is a cough that produces mucus (sputum). Many minor viral infections cause cough; the difference is that pneumonia causes thick sputum that is usually yellow or green. It may be tinged with blood or have a rusty color.

Fever is common, and chills, chest pain, and shortness of breath may develop. Symptoms vary depending on how extensive the pneumonia is and on which microorganism is causing the infection.

A doctor checks for pneumonia by listening to the person's chest with a stethoscope. Pneumonia usually produces distinctively abnormal sounds in the lungs. These sounds are caused by narrowing of the airways or filling of the air sacs of the lung with inflammatory cells and fluid.

In most cases, the diagnosis is confirmed with a chest x-ray. Doctors usually obtain a sample of blood. They may try to obtain a sample of mucus that has been coughed up. The laboratory tries to make a preliminary identification of the microorganism (smear or stain) and to grow (culture) the microorganisms present in the samples. Knowing the exact type of microorganism usually helps doctors choose better treatment options. However, despite these tests, the precise microorganism cannot be identified in up to half of the people who have pneumonia. When the person is severely ill and is not helped by initial therapy, doctors can try to obtain better samples, often by inserting a long flexible tube (bronchoscope) into the airways.

Prevention

Pneumonia caused by the pneumococcus bacterium or by the influenza virus can often be prevented with a vaccine. The pneumococcal vaccine is given once to people 65 or older. Even if the vaccine does not prevent pneumococcal pneumonia, it usually lessens the infection's severity. People at high risk of becoming infected with this type of bacteria (for example, patients with chronic obstructive pulmonary disease or heart failure) may need the pneumococcus vaccine every 6 years.

Older people who are at risk of pneumonia from aspiration due to difficulty chewing and swallowing because of conditions such as a stroke need to take special precautions. They may be given food that is finely chopped or in the form of soft solids or thickened liquids. They should be as upright or erect as possible while eating and should remain upright for at least an hour after eating.

For those who cannot cough vigorously, exercises that encourage breathing deeply and therapy to clear mucus may help. These exercises often use a small inspirometer that requires deep breathing to raise a ball in a tube. These exercises are particularly important for those who have had chest or abdominal surgery or who smoke.

Quitting smoking is an essential part of prevention in smokers.

Treatment

The vast majority of older people with pneumonia are hospitalized, where they can be treated with intravenous antibiotics. Older people can get very sick very fast from pneumonia and tend to respond less well to oral antibiotics.

Treatment of pneumonia depends first on whether the cause is a bacteria, a virus, or a fungus. The mainstay of treating bacterial pneumonia is antibiotics. Most viral pneumonia gets better without specific treatment. Pneumonia caused by unusual microorganisms, such as tuberculosis, also requires drugs that kill the organisms.

Doctors usually give antibiotics immediately whenever they suspect bacterial pneumonia, even before the bacteria are identified. Prompt treatment with antibiotics helps reduce the severity of pneumonia and the chance of developing complications, some of which are fatal.

When choosing an antibiotic, doctors try to predict which type of bacteria is likely to be the cause. The doctor often changes the antibiotic later if the type of bacteria is identified and its susceptibility to various antibiotics becomes known.

People who are short of breath or whose blood is low in oxygen are given supplemental oxygen. Although rest is an important part of treatment, moving often and getting out of bed and into a chair are encouraged.

INFLUENZA

Influenza (often called flu) is infection with one of the influenza viruses. Influenza infection affects the entire body but is most evident in what it does to the airways and lungs.

Influenza virus is categorized as type A or type B. Within each type are many different subtypes (strains). Although some people blame influenza for every cold they develop, real influenza is caused by a very different virus than the common cold and produces much more severe symptoms.

Every year outbreaks of influenza occur during late autumn or winter, although the exact timing of these outbreaks varies throughout the world. Influenza occurs primarily in epidemics, in which many people get sick all at once. In each epidemic, usually only one strain of influenza virus is responsible.

Influenza affects people of all ages. In older people, influenza is particularly serious. Indeed, in a typical year it leads to more than 20,000 deaths in the United States, with older people accounting for more than 80% of those deaths.

If influenza were merely an infection in the throat, it might be regarded as little more than an annoyance. However, influenza may lead to other problems, particularly in older people, especially those with chronic obstructive pulmonary disease, heart failure, diabetes, or other chronic diseases. Influenza frequently irritates the trachea and bronchi, leading to tracheitis and bronchitis. In some older people, influenza leads to pneumonia, either by the virus itself or, more commonly, from a bacterial infection. Pneumonia is the main cause of most deaths resulting from influenza infection.

Rarely, inflammation of muscles (myositis) or of the sac surrounding the heart (pericarditis) complicates influenza. Inflammation of the brain (encephalitis), the spinal cord (transverse myelitis), or nerves that branch off from the spinal cord (Guillain-Barré syndrome) may also develop. These complications may be the result of the body's immune system being overstimulated from fighting the influenza virus.

Causes

The influenza virus enters the airways and reaches the lungs when the person inhales tiny droplets containing the virus that have been coughed or sneezed out by an infected person. A person can also develop influenza by touching a surface or object that has been touched, coughed on, or sneezed on by an infected person and then touching his nose or mouth.

Symptoms

The illnesses produced by the two different types and multiple strains of influenza virus are similar in most ways. However, type A influenza tends to produce more severe symptoms than those of type B influenza.

Symptoms usually start within a day or two after the person becomes infected. Symptoms can begin very suddenly. At first the symptoms mimic a cold but quickly become much more severe. Chills are often the first indication of influenza. The person may begin to feel very tired and weak and lose his appetite. Fever is common during the first few days, with body temperature sometimes reaching 102° to 103° F. Muscle aches and pains throughout the body are common, but they tend to be most noticeable in the back and legs. Headaches occur frequently, with aching around and behind the eyes.

The throat very often becomes scratchy and sore. A runny nose, a burning sensation in the chest, and a dry cough may develop. Later, the cough can become severe, and the person may bring up mucus (sputum). The skin may be warm, and the person may appear flushed, especially on the face. The throat may redden, the eyes may water, and the whites of the eyes may become reddened and irritated.

Most symptoms begin to decrease after 2 or 3 days if the person does not develop complications. However, fever sometimes lasts for several more days, and cough may persist even longer, sometimes for a few weeks. Tiredness and weakness may also persist, occasionally for several weeks.

A person with influenza may seem to be getting better but then develop shortness of breath and a worsened cough that may produce bloody mucus if bronchitis or pneumonia develops. Rarely, muscle pain occurs if inflammation of the muscles develops, or chest pain develops with inflammation of the sac surrounding the heart. Confusion and headaches may indicate inflammation of the brain. Loss of sensation and weakness or even paralysis develops if inflammation occurs in the spinal cord or in the nerves that branch off from the spinal cord.

Diagnosis

A doctor usually diagnoses influenza on the basis of the symptoms and on the physical examination findings in the setting of a known influenza outbreak. These findings may include enlarged, tender lymph nodes on one or both sides of the neck and intense redness on the nose and on the back of the throat. The severity of the illness and the presence of a high fever and body aches help distinguish influenza from a cold.

If other cases of influenza have recently been diagnosed in the area, the doctor's diagnosis is reinforced, because influenza occurs mainly in epidemics. However, if there are no other cases of influenza and there is lingering doubt about the diagnosis, the doctor can order tests on samples of blood or mucus from the lungs that can identify the influenza virus.

Prevention

Vaccination is the best way to avoid contracting influenza. The vaccine prevents influenza in most people, although it may be less effective in very old people. Vaccination also significantly decreases the risk of pneumonia, hospitalization, and death. A new vaccine is produced and given each year, because the strain of the influenza virus causing outbreaks continually undergoes changes. Changes in the virus strain render the influenza vaccine used in a previous year ineffective against the newest strain.

The traditional injectable form of influenza vaccine is very safe. Some people receiving the vaccine experience soreness at the injection site. Rarely, the vaccine produces a slight fever for a day or less. People who are allergic to chickens' eggs are usually not vaccinated, because the vaccine contains very tiny amounts of egg protein.

In the United States, the vaccine is usually available in late September or early October. Most assisted living facilities and nursing homes urge every resident to be vaccinated because of the high risk of outbreaks for people living in close quarters. Vaccination in the fall is best, so that people are protected during the winter months, when epidemics of influenza are most likely to peak. However, people can still benefit from receiving the vaccine during the winter months. For most people, about 2 weeks is needed for the vaccination to provide protection against influenza.

A new nasally administered influenza vaccine is now available, but it is not recommended for people 50 or older.

Several antiviral drugs can also be used to prevent infection with influenza virus. Doctors may prescribe these drugs when they know a person has recently been exposed to someone with influenza. In addition, these drugs may be used during an outbreak in a nursing home to protect unvaccinated people who are at high risk of developing influenza, even if they have not yet been exposed to anyone with influenza. Amantadine and rimantadine are older antiviral drugs that offer protection against influenza type A but not influenza type B. These drugs can cause stomach upset, nervousness, sleeplessness, and other side effects, especially in older people. Rimantadine tends to cause fewer side effects than amantadine. Two new drugs, oseltamivir and zanamivir, can prevent infection with both types of influenza virus. These drugs produce minimal side effects.

Treatment and Outlook

The main treatment for influenza is to rest, drink plenty of fluids, and avoid exertion. Fever and aches are sometimes treated with acetaminophen or nonsteroidal anti-inflammatory drugs (NSAIDs, such as aspirin or ibuprofen). Other measures that are used to treat the common cold, such as decongestants and steam inhalation, may help relieve some symptoms.

Amantadine, rimantadine, oseltamivir, and zanamivir are antiviral drugs helpful in treating influenza. However, these drugs work only if they are taken in the first day or two after the person becomes ill. They help to shorten the duration of symptoms for many people. Most doctors now recommend zanamivir and oseltamivir, which work against both influenza type A and type B. If doctors suspect a complication such as bronchitis or bacterial pneumonia, they prescribe antibiotics.

Most people with uncomplicated influenza recover fully and can remain at home. Some people with influenza begin to resume normal activities a day or two after body temperature returns to normal and muscle aches diminish. However, influenza can be very debilitating in other people, making it difficult to care for themselves. Recovery may take several days or even a few weeks in such people. They may neglect eating properly, which compounds the seriousness of the illness. Older people with influenza who live alone should consider staying with family or friends.

Influenza with a complication such as pneumonia is a more serious illness and is fatal for many older people. Even so, most people with complicated influenza do recover fully with time and treatment. However, treatment requires careful attention and usually hospitalization. Any older person with influenza who is having trouble breathing, has high fevers, or becomes confused should seek emergency medical treatment.

53

Chronic Obstructive Pulmonary Disease

Chronic obstructive pulmonary disease (COPD) is the collective name for two diseases—emphysema and chronic bronchitis. Both diseases decrease air movement in the lungs because of blockage in the airways. Unlike asthma, in which the blockage comes and goes, in COPD, the blockage persists.

Emphysema is the form of COPD in which abnormal air-filled spaces form among the millions of tiny air sacs (alveoli) in the lungs. These air-filled spaces develop when the thin walls that make up and separate clusters of alveoli and that hold the airways open are destroyed. Destruction of these walls leads to partial or complete obstruction of the small airways. The obstruction makes it difficult for air to move out of the lungs when a person exhales. Some air is trapped so that more air remains in the lungs after exhaling than would in a person with healthy lungs.

The number of tiny blood vessels (capillaries) in the walls of the alveoli decreases. Having fewer blood vessels and obstructed airways means that movement of oxygen and carbon dioxide between the alveoli and the blood is impaired. As a result, the level of oxygen in the blood may decrease while the level of carbon dioxide may increase. A lower oxygen level in the blood, if severe enough, causes shortness of breath, high blood pressure in the lungs, and strain on the right side of the heart. The strain can eventually lead to heart failure. A low oxygen level in the blood may also stimulate the body to produce more red blood cells, a condition called secondary polycythemia.

Chronic bronchitis is the form of COPD that affects the airways rather than the alveoli. Chronic bronchitis is characterized by a persistent cough that produces sputum. Chronic bronchitis differs from acute bronchitis, which usually begins with an infection and typically lasts no more than a few weeks; chronic bronchitis lasts 3 months or more during 2 successive years. Obstruction in chronic bronchitis is caused by swelling of the walls of the airways, spasm of muscle tissue in the walls of the airways, and formation of excess mucus, which is coughed up as sputum.

In the United States, about 16 million people have COPD. COPD is especially common among people over age 55. It is a very common cause of death and is becoming increasingly so. Fortunately, treatment can help control symptoms and improve the quality of life of most people with this disease.

Causes

Cigarette smoking is the most common cause of COPD. Almost all people with COPD are or have been smokers. Pipe and cigar smokers are at lower risk than cigarette smokers but are still at greater risk of COPD than are people who do not smoke tobacco in any form.

People exposed to smoke from nearby cigarette smokers (secondhand, or passive, smoke exposure) and people who have worked or lived in an environment polluted by chemical fumes or dust are also at a slightly increased risk of developing mild COPD. Thus, some nonsmokers develop mild COPD.

HOW AIRWAYS BECOME OBSTRUCTED

The airways of the lungs may become obstructed because of a muscle spasm, swelling in the wall of the airways, accumulation of mucus, or a combination of these. Spasm causes the same sort of narrowing that swelling causes and so looks very much the same. The differences between spasm and swelling occur at a level that can be seen only with a microscope.

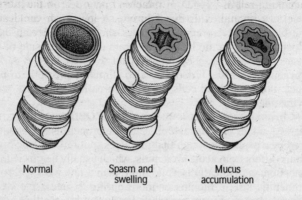

Normal | Spasm and swelling | Mucus accumulation

Symptoms

A mild cough that produces clear sputum is frequently an early symptom of COPD. The person usually has this cough when first getting out of bed in the morning. Gradually, shortness of breath develops as the obstruction slows airflow and increases the effort of breathing. At first, the shortness of breath may be noted only with physical exertion. Or, the shortness of breath may be noted only with a chest cold (acute bronchitis).

As the disease progresses, shortness of breath with exertion becomes more troublesome. The person may hear himself wheeze. Severe shortness of breath may even occur at rest. Shortness of breath while performing everyday activities, such as going to the bathroom, washing, and dressing, may persist after recovery from even a minor cold. More serious infections, such as pneumonia, become more common and cause symptoms more severe than in people with healthy lungs.

When COPD becomes more severe, some people lose weight because, among other reasons, shortness of breath makes eating difficult, and the overworked breathing muscles consume more energy. Commonly, the legs swell, which may be due to heart failure. People with more severe COPD may intermittently cough up blood even when they have mild lung infections. Coughing up blood also raises concern about the possibility of lung cancer, which occurs more frequently among people with smoking-related COPD. Headaches may occur in the morning because breathing worsens during sleep, which can lead to higher levels of carbon dioxide in the blood and decreased delivery of oxygen to the brain.

As COPD progresses, some people, especially those who have emphysema, develop altered breathing patterns. Some breathe out through pursed lips. Others are more comfortable standing over a table with their arms outstretched and their weight on their palms, a position that helps them breathe more easily. Some people gradually develop a barrel-shaped chest as their lungs expand because of trapped air. The skin, fingernails, or lips may turn bluish (cyanosis) if the level of oxygen in the blood is very low.

Occasionally, sudden pain develops on one side of the chest and shortness of breath worsens if an overexpanded area of the lung tears the lung's surface. The tear allows air to leak from the lung into the space between the lung and the rib cage (pleural space). This condition is called a pneumothorax. A pneumothorax can make breathing very difficult and usually requires emergency care.

Many people experience flare-ups, with a noticeable worsening of their cough, an increase in the amount of sputum, and increased shortness of breath. These flare-ups may be due to a viral infection, a bacterial infection, or exposure to inhaled substances that irritate the airways. During a flare-up, sputum color tends to change from white to yellow or green, and fever and body aches may occur. Shortness of breath may worsen, becoming a problem even when the person is at rest.

Diagnosis

Emphysema is diagnosed on the basis of the medical history and physical examination as well as on tests that measure lung function during inhalation and exhalation (pulmonary function tests). The doctor tries to determine, by measuring lung function, the severity of airflow obstruction and whether airflow improves in response to drugs. Chronic bronchitis is diagnosed solely on the basis of a history of a persistent cough that produces sputum.

When COPD is in an early stage, the doctor may find nothing during a physical examination. As the disease progresses, the doctor may hear wheezing through a stethoscope and may notice that exhalation takes longer than expected. The doctor may also notice that as the person breathes, the chest moves less and the muscles in the neck and shoulders contract. With severe disease, it may be difficult for the doctor to hear breath sounds at all with the stethoscope because less air is moving in and out of the air spaces and there is less lung tissue to transmit breath sounds to the chest wall.

In early COPD, results of a chest x-ray are usually normal. As COPD worsens, the chest x-ray shows over-expansion of the lungs.

Oxygen in the blood can be measured by taking a sample of blood from an artery or by using a clip attached briefly to an ear or a finger (pulse oximetry). Oxygen is often at low levels at rest or with exercise. Occasionally, a blood test shows an abnormally high number of red blood cells (polycythemia). Increasing the production of red blood cells is one way the body tries to overcome a decreased level of oxygen in the blood. When COPD is severe, high levels of carbon dioxide can be detected in blood samples taken from arteries.

Treatment

The most important treatment for COPD is to stop all forms of smoking, including cigarettes, cigars, and pipes. Ex-smokers should avoid inhaling secondary smoke, which may mean avoiding bars and restaurants that allow smoking or asking a family member who smokes to do so only outside the house. Stopping smoking when obstruction of airflow is minimal or even moderate often lessens cough, reduces the amount of sputum produced, and slows the progression of shortness of breath. Stopping smoking at any point can be beneficial. Reducing exposure to other irritants in the air, including secondhand smoke and air pollution, is also recommended. Many people with COPD benefit from staying in air-conditioned spaces.

If the person develops the flu (influenza) or pneumonia, the shortness of breath that accompanies COPD usually worsens suddenly. Therefore, people with COPD are advised to receive the influenza vaccine every year and the pneumococcal vaccine at the time of diagnosis. Revaccination with the pneumococcal vaccine is often recommended every 6 years.[1] At the first sign of a cold, a person with COPD should consult a doctor. Often, the doctor provides a plan for such occasions so that the patient can begin treatment on his own.

Treatment of symptoms: Treatment aims to relieve symptoms of wheezing and shortness of breath by reducing airflow obstruction. Obstruction due to emphysema is irreversible, so treatment is not very helpful for the emphysema component of COPD. But other changes in the airways of people with COPD are to some degree potentially reversible, including muscle spasm and increased mucus and swelling of the walls of the airways. Therefore, treatment that targets these components can be helpful in reducing airflow obstruction.

Many drugs used to treat COPD are taken through an inhaler, which is a device that allows the user to spray very tiny droplets of a drug into the lungs via the mouth and throat. These droplets can then be inhaled deeply into the lungs. An inhaler that provides a specific and consistent dose is called a metered-dose inhaler. Ipratropium, which helps open (dilate) obstructed airways by reducing muscle spasm, can be taken up to four times daily. A short-acting beta-adrenergic agonist drug, such as albuterol, relieves shortness of breath more rapidly. A combination of ipratropium and albuterol, taken through an inhaler, is also available.

Salmeterol, a long-acting beta-adrenergic agonist drug, is taken every 12 hours with a small disc-shaped device that contains the drug in powder form. After pulling a small lever on the device, the person places his mouth around a small opening and inhales the salmeterol in a single breath. Salmeterol provides prolonged relief of symptoms for some people, especially at night, but does not begin working for at least 15 minutes after use.

For people who have difficulty using metered-dose inhalers or who do not get enough relief from them, other options are available. A delivery device called a spacer can be used with a metered-dose inhaler. Ipratropium and albuterol may also be

HOW TO USE A METERED-DOSE INHALER

- Shake the inhaler after removing the cap.
- Breathe out for 1 or 2 seconds.
- Put the inhaler in the mouth and start to breathe in slowly, as if sipping hot soup.
- Press the top of the inhaler as soon as a breath is started.
- Breathe in slowly until the lungs are full. (Breathing in should take about 5 or 6 seconds.)
- Hold the breath for 4 to 6 seconds.
- Breathe out and repeat the procedure.

If pressing the inhaler's top and breathing in at the same time is difficult, a spacer can be used. Attach the spacer to the inhaler and press the inhaler's top. Put the mouthpiece in the mouth and breathe in as with the inhaler. A spacer holds the dose of drug sprayed by the inhaler. The dose can then be breathed in from the spacer in two or three slow, deep breaths after pressing the inhaler's top only once. The spacer helps get more of the dose into the lungs instead of losing some in the air or mouth. Repeat the procedure.

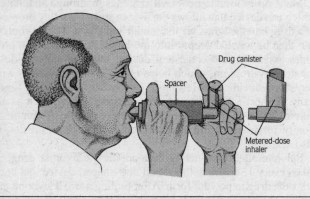

Drug canister

Spacer

Metered-dose inhaler

taken with the aid of a nebulizer. A nebulizer is a portable machine that creates a mist of drug, and its use does not have to be coordinated with breathing. It requires a power source, such as household current, a battery, or a car's cigarette lighter. Therapy with a nebulizer is reserved for people who have severe disease.

Theophylline is often taken by people who respond minimally or not at all to other drugs. This drug is taken in pill form. The dose is adjusted by the doctor based on levels of theophylline in the blood, which are measured periodically. The short-acting form is usually taken four times a day, but long-acting forms of theophylline can be taken once or twice daily.

Corticosteroids may be helpful for people whose symptoms cannot be controlled by the other drugs. Corticosteroids lessen symptoms and help reduce the frequency of flare-ups. Corticosteroids are available in inhalers or as pills. Recently, a combination of salmeterol and a corticosteroid in powder form has been developed. This combination of drugs is taken with a disc-shaped device. After pulling the small lever on the device, the person places his mouth around a small opening and inhales both drugs in a single breath.

Because inhaled corticosteroids go directly into the lungs, they produce fewer side effects than corticosteroids taken as pills. However, high doses of inhaled corticosteroids taken for several years may also have side effects, such as osteoporosis. Corticosteroids taken as pills are largely restricted to people with COPD flare-ups or those who have severe symptoms from airflow obstruction despite undergoing other therapy.

No reliable therapy is available to thin the mucus so that it can be coughed up more easily. However, drinking enough to avoid dehydration may prevent thick mucus accumulation. When COPD is severe and mucus is excessive, respiratory therapy may help loosen mucus in the chest.

Treatment of flare-ups: A doctor treats flare-ups as soon as possible. About half of flare-ups are due to viruses and half to bacterial infections.

If a viral cause is suspected, the doctor usually recommends rest, plenty of fluids, and, occasionally, corticosteroids for several days. If treatment fails, hospitalization may be needed.

If a bacterial infection is suspected, the doctor usually prescribes an antibiotic. Many doctors give people who have moderate or severe COPD a supply of an antibiotic and advise them to start taking the drug early in a flare-up. There are many options for antibiotics that can be taken by mouth. Antibiotics do not prevent flare-ups. Sometimes corticosteroids are taken by mouth for about 10 to 14 days to help reduce the severity and length of flare-ups due to bacterial infections.

Oxygen therapy: Oxygen therapy prolongs life and improves quality of life for people with severe COPD and severely reduced oxygen levels in their blood. Although round-the-clock therapy is best, using oxygen at least 12 hours a day also has some benefits. This therapy often improves mental functioning and helps relieve shortness of breath, high blood pressure in the lungs, and heart failure caused by COPD.

Different devices are available for providing oxygen therapy. People who are homebound can use electrically powered oxygen concentrators. The use of compressed oxygen in small tanks permits trips outside the home. Liquid oxygen systems are more expensive but are preferable for active people, because liquid oxygen permits longer trips away from home. A special valve called a demand valve can be attached to the portable oxygen delivery device to increase the length of time that the unit can be used before a refill is needed. Oxygen therapy cannot be used near open flames or while smoking.

Surgery: Lung volume reduction surgery, which involves removing areas where air is persistently trapped, may help relieve severe symptoms.

Pulmonary rehabilitation: Pulmonary rehabilitation can help most people feel better. Programs include education about the disease, exercise, nutrition, and counseling. These programs can improve the person's independence and quality of life, decrease the frequency and length of hospital stays, and improve the ability to exercise. Exercise programs can be carried out in the clinic and at home.[1] Stationary bicycling, stair climbing, and walking are used to exercise the legs. Weight lifting is used for the arms. Often, oxygen is used during exercise. However, gains are quickly lost if the person stops exercising. Special techniques are taught for decreasing shortness of breath during such strenuous activities as exercise and sexual activity. For example, the person can be taught to keep his lips partly closed, as if whistling, during exhalation (pursed-lip breathing). Pulmonary rehabilitation, however, does not improve lung function or prolong survival.

Outlook

As airway obstruction worsens, the outlook becomes progressively worse, with an increased risk of death. Death may result from respiratory failure, pneumonia, pneumothorax, heart rhythm abnormalities (arrhythmias), or blockage of the arteries that lead to the lungs (pulmonary embolism). Cigarette smokers

1. see also page 911

lose lung function more rapidly than nonsmokers do. If a person stops smoking, lung function improves minimally. Continued smoking, however, virtually ensures that symptoms will worsen. People with COPD have a risk of lung cancer beyond that due to their use of cigarettes.

People in late stages of COPD are likely to need considerable help adhering to their recommended medical care and with performing everyday activities. Some older people find that staying at home becomes too difficult because of fatigue, shortness of breath, the need for oxygen, and the complexities of taking prescribed drugs. Such people may move to a nursing home to obtain the care they need.

People with end-stage disease who develop flare-ups or pneumonia may need to have a tube put down their throat and be temporarily supported with mechanical ventilation in an intensive care unit. The period of mechanical ventilation may be short or long, and some people remain dependent on the ventilator until death. People on a ventilator cannot eat or talk, thus quality of life is greatly diminished. It is important for people to consider and discuss with their doctors and loved ones whether they wish to have this kind of therapy. Some people choose another alternative—hospice care. The best way of ensuring that one's wishes are carried out is to discuss them with loved ones and to have completed an advance directive, such as a living will or a durable power of attorney for health care.[1]

1. see page 953

54

Swallowing and Reflux Disorders

When eating, people hope to enjoy a good taste in their mouth, followed by a comfortable feeling of fullness in their stomach. But for many older people, food does not always move from the mouth, down the throat (pharynx), to the stomach, and onward as expected. Problems in the mouth, throat, or esophagus (which connects the throat and the stomach) may interfere. Furthermore, after food reaches the stomach and mixes with digestive acid, it sometimes flows backward (refluxes) into the esophagus—a disorder called gastroesophageal reflux disease (GERD).

Difficulty moving food down the throat may seem like a minor problem. Taking smaller bites, chewing more thoroughly, or eating more slowly may solve the problem. But sometimes these simple fixes do not work. Difficulty moving food from the mouth to the stomach may be the sign of a problem that can have serious consequences. Consequences include undernutrition, weight loss, dehydration, aspiration pneumonia, and even death.

Normally, wavelike contractions of the esophagus (called peristalsis) move food from the throat down the esophagus to the stomach. At the upper and lower ends of the esophagus are ring-shaped muscles called sphincters. During swallowing, the sphincters relax and open up so that food can pass through. When the esophagus is not in use, the sphincters contract, preventing food and stomach acid from flowing backward from the stomach to the mouth.

As people age, several changes may affect the ability to swallow. Slightly less saliva is produced.[1] As a result, food is soft-

MOVING FOOD TO THE STOMACH AND ONWARD

The process of moving food from the mouth to the stomach and keeping it moving in the right direction is complex, and many things can go wrong.

The process begins with chewing. The tongue moves food around, breaking it into smaller pieces and mixing it with saliva. Then, food can be swallowed more easily. The tongue pushes the food to the back of the mouth, triggering the swallowing reflex. Swallowing moves food to the throat. When food enters the throat, the voice box (larynx) moves up and a flap of tissue (epiglottis) covers its opening tightly so that food does not enter the airway and lungs. At the same time, the food triggers a ring-shaped muscle at the upper end of the esophagus (upper esophageal sphincter) to relax and allow food to pass through. After food passes through the sphincter, it contracts again to prevent food from moving backward. This sphincter remains contracted, until food triggers it to relax.

The esophagus contracts rhythmically to move food along. At the lower end of the esophagus, food triggers another ring-shaped muscle (lower esophageal sphincter) to relax and allow food to pass into the stomach. The sphincter then contracts again, preventing food from moving backward.

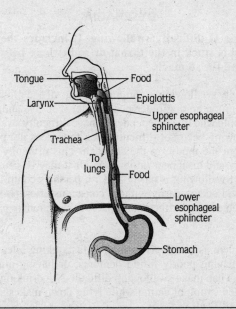

ened (macerated) less well and is drier before it is swallowed. The muscles in the jaws and throat may weaken slightly, making chewing and swallowing less efficient. Also, older people are more likely to have conditions that make chewing and swallowing difficult. For example, they are more likely to have loose teeth or to wear dentures.

As people age, the contractions that move food through the esophagus become weaker. This change is very slight and usually has little effect on moving food to the stomach. But if older people try to eat while lying down or lie down just after eating, food may not easily move to the stomach. If reflux develops, the aging esophagus may be slower to move refluxed stomach acid back into the stomach. Some older people have a hiatal hernia. A hiatal hernia occurs when part of the stomach bulges upward through the opening for the esophagus in the diaphragm.[1] A hiatal hernia may contribute to reflux.

DYSPHAGIA

Dysphagia is difficulty swallowing. It includes the feeling that food is stuck in the throat or somewhere between the throat and the stomach.

Difficulty swallowing is common among all age groups but is more common among older people. Between 5% and 10% of older people who live independently have difficulty swallowing.

Swallowing becomes difficult when food does not pass normally from the mouth to the stomach. This difficulty may be temporary and disappear on its own. Or it may be caused by a disorder. Swallowing is partly under a person's control (is voluntary) and occurs partly without conscious effort (is involuntary). Problems can affect either part of the action.

Causes

A problem as simple as eating too fast, taking bites that are too big, having poorly fitting dentures, or having missing or loose teeth can make swallowing difficult. Not drinking enough water when eating or eating while lying down makes swallowing more difficult.

1. see box on page 830

People with dementia may not chew food adequately or may forget to swallow it.

Disorders that damage any part of the body that is involved in swallowing—muscles, nerves, or brain—may cause difficulty swallowing. A stroke is the most common example among older people. Almost 30% of people who have had a stroke have difficulty swallowing. Parkinson's disease, myasthenia gravis, pseudobulbar palsy, systemic sclerosis, and amyotrophic lateral sclerosis (Lou Gehrig's disease) can also cause difficulty swallowing. Some drugs, especially phenothiazines (a type of antipsychotic drug), can cause difficulty swallowing because they affect the throat muscles.

Some disorders interfere with normal contractions of the esophagus. Then food cannot move through the esophagus into the stomach as it normally does. The esophagus contracts, but the contractions do not move food. This abnormal contraction can cause esophageal spasm. In about one third of people with spasms, the lower esophageal sphincter does not open normally and does not contract in coordination with the rest of the esophagus. As a result, the movement of foods and fluids into the stomach may be delayed, causing a feeling that food is stuck.

Uncommonly, the nerves that control the lower esophageal sphincter and the esophagus are abnormal, resulting in achalasia. In achalasia, the esophagus does not contract, and the lower esophageal sphincter does not relax normally to allow food to pass into the stomach. The cause of achalasia is unknown. It usually begins, almost unnoticed, between the ages of 20 and 60, then progresses gradually over many months or years. At first, people have difficulty swallowing solid foods, but eventually they also have difficulty swallowing liquids.

Swallowing may become difficult because the esophagus is narrowed or completely blocked. Progressive damage to the esophagus can cause scar tissue to form. This inflexible scar tissue (called a stricture) narrows the esophagus and restricts the movement of food through it.

The esophagus is not easily damaged. However, it can be damaged gradually by the repeated backward flow of acid from the stomach (gastroesophageal reflux) over months to years. Taking certain drugs can damage the lining of the esophagus (causing erosion) or cause deeper sores (ulcers). These drugs include bisphosphonates (used to treat osteoporosis), aspirin, other nonsteroidal anti-inflammatory drugs (NSAIDs), some antibiotics (such as doxycycline, tetracycline, and clindamycin), and potassium or iron supplements. Damage by drugs is more common among older people. Part of the reason may be that the esophagus does not contract normally or that older people do not drink enough water when they take the drug.

An abnormal ring of tissue may narrow the esophagus. The most common type is Schatzki's ring, which is located near the stomach. What causes these rings to form is unclear, but they may result from damage due to reflux, abnormal contractions of the esophagus, or the use of certain drugs. These rings intermittently cause difficulty swallowing. Usually, difficulty occurs when solid foods are eaten rapidly. The solid food most commonly caught in a ring is poorly chewed meat. The result is severe pain. Because this problem often occurs when dining out, it is sometimes called steakhouse syndrome.

Thin sheets of tissue (webs) may form across the interior of the esophagus, partially blocking it. Rarely, webs may result from severe iron deficiency that is not treated. Esophageal webs are more common among older people. A few people are born with esophageal rings or webs, which do not cause symptoms until later in life. Webs, like rings, cause difficulty swallowing solid foods, not liquids.

A pouch (diverticulum) that develops just above the upper esophageal sphincter or in the wall of the esophagus may make swallowing difficult. Food is caught in the pouch, causing discomfort. If the pouch is filled, it can block the passage of food. Sometimes pouches form in response to injury or irritation. They may form if the contractions of the throat and upper sphincter are not coordinated. Sometimes the cause is unknown. The most common type is Zenker's diverticulum, which forms just above the upper esophageal sphincter. Zenker's diverticulum usually develops after age 50.

Food and foreign bodies may block the esophagus. The esophagus can be partially or completely blocked by a noncancerous (benign) or cancerous (malignant) tumor in the esophagus. Esophageal cancer rarely causes difficulty swallowing, but many people still fear that possibility.

Several disorders can block the esophagus by putting pressure on it from outside. For example, a heart disorder may cause part of the aorta or heart to enlarge and press on the esophagus. Cancer (most commonly, lung cancer), an aortic aneurysm, enlargement of the thyroid gland, or excessive growth of bones in the spine (vertebrae) can also put pressure on the esophagus.

Symptoms

Most people who have difficulty swallowing have difficulty swallowing solids, particularly breads and meats. After eating, people may feel as if they have a lump in their throat or tightness in their chest. They may have to swallow several times before the food feels as if it has gone down. Much later, swallowing liquids may become difficult. Some people have difficulty swallowing solids and liquids from the beginning.

People with difficulty swallowing may regurgitate food through the mouth or nose. When they lie down at night, they may cough or spit up food swallowed many hours before. They may inhale (aspirate) food into the windpipe (trachea), then cough. Aspirating food can lead to lung disorders, including airway infections and a form of pneumonia called aspiration pneumonia.

Depending on the cause of dysphagia, people may have chest pain when they eat. Chest pain may be caused by spasms of the esophagus. This pain is often described as a squeezing pain under the breastbone (sternum). The pain resembles chest pain due to coronary artery disease (angina), so the two are sometimes confused. Some people feel pain in the throat when they swallow. This pain may be caused by an infection or, rarely, cancer.

People with Zenker's diverticulum may have bad breath because food collects in the pouch. The pouch can also interfere with taking pills. Pills can become stuck in the pouch and thus are not absorbed into the bloodstream. Occasionally, the pouch causes pressure or swelling in the neck.

If people continue to have difficulty swallowing, they may lose weight and become undernourished and dehydrated.

Diagnosis

If difficulty swallowing lasts more than a few days, the person should see a doctor promptly. The doctor tries to identify the cause. Symptoms provide some clues to the cause. So the doctor usually asks whether the person has difficulty swallowing both solids and liquids, whether pain is felt, and, if so, where and when. Whether the person has vomited blood or seen blood in stool is also a concern. The throat is examined, and the person is asked to swallow to see if the throat is working normally.

Usually, tests are needed to identify the cause. Most often, the esophagus is examined with a flexible viewing tube (endoscope) that is passed down the throat.[1] To rule out cancer, doctors may take a sample of tissue with instruments threaded through the tube. Some disorders, such as esophageal rings or webs, can be treated at the same time.

A barium study may be done before endoscopy. Or it may be done afterward if endoscopy does not provide enough information. A barium study involves swallowing a barium solution or food coated with barium. Barium can be seen on x-rays. X-rays are taken continuously as the barium passes down the throat and esophagus to the stomach (in a procedure called fluoroscopy). This study is painless, and the barium passes through the digestive system and out of the body, causing no harm. A barium study can detect esophageal webs and rings, other blockages, and pouches. It can also detect tumors, ulcers, and evidence of spasm. This study helps doctors assess the function of the nerves and muscles involved in swallowing. Thus, doctors can determine whether a disorder that affects these muscles or nerves, such as a stroke, could be the cause.

Additional tests may be done, depending on the suspected cause. If the cause could be abnormal contractions of the esophagus (such as esophageal spasm), pressures in the esophagus may be measured with a tube placed in the esophagus. This test is called manometry. During the test, a person is asked to swallow water or a semisolid material or is given an injection of edrophonium, a drug that may trigger a spasm. This test helps doctors determine whether the pain is caused by spasms.

Treatment

Treatment focuses on helping the person swallow safely (including how to avoid aspiration) and on treating the disorder causing the problem if possible. Effective treatment enables a

1. see art on page 117

person to eat enough types of foods to get a well-balanced, adequate diet. Sometimes simple measures are the only treatment needed. For example, chewing food thoroughly and then sipping water can help prevent symptoms. Sitting upright while eating can help. Foods with certain textures, such as thick creamed soups or pureed fruits, may be easier to swallow. The best consistency is often found by trial and error. Using appropriate eating utensils may help. For example, using a small straw or small spoon can limit the amount of food put in the mouth. A smaller amount is easier to swallow.

If the cause is a disorder that impairs the muscles or nerves involved in swallowing, speech therapists may suggest exercises to strengthen the muscles or improve coordination and techniques to use when eating.[1] If the cause is esophageal spasms or achalasia, drugs that relax the muscles of the esophagus may help relieve symptoms. Examples are nitroglycerin, long-acting nitrates, and calcium channel blockers (such as nifedipine). Some of these drugs—those with anticholinergic effects (such as dicyclomine)—are rarely used for older people because of side effects.[2]

Usually, achalasia requires additional treatment. Doctors may inject botulinum toxin into the lower esophageal sphincter. Botulinum toxin paralyzes the sphincter, enabling it to relax and allow food to pass through. This treatment may provide more sustained symptom relief for older people than for younger people. The effects usually last 6 to 24 months, so injections need to be repeated. After two to three injections, they usually become ineffective. So injections cannot be used indefinitely. Alternatively, doctors may widen the passageway with a balloon dilator (called a bougie). This dilator is a tube with a deflated balloon attached to one end. It is passed down the throat to the lower esophageal sphincter, then inflated and deflated once. This procedure may provide long-lasting relief, sometimes permanently. If symptoms recur, the procedure can be repeated.

When these treatments are ineffective or symptoms are substantial, surgery may be done to correct achalasia. For this procedure (called myotomy), the muscular fibers in the lower esophageal sphincter are cut. As a result, the abnormal tightness

1. see page 179
2. see box on page 58

POUCHES AND BULGES IN THE DIGESTIVE TRACT

Abnormal pouches or bulges in the digestive tract can interfere with the movement of food from the mouth to the stomach and onward. A pouch called Zenker's diverticulum may form just above a ring-shaped muscle at the upper end of the esophagus (upper esophageal sphincter). Zenker's diverticulum may make swallowing uncomfortable or difficult.

Part of the stomach may bulge upward through the opening (hiatus) in the diaphragm, the muscle that separates the chest from the abdomen. This abnormal bulge, called a hiatal hernia, may cause the sphincter at the lower end of the esophagus to malfunction. Then acid and enzymes produced by the stomach may flow backward (reflux) into the esophagus. Reflux can cause indigestion and may damage the esophagus. In the most common type (sliding hiatal hernia), the top part of the stomach sometimes slides up through the hiatus.

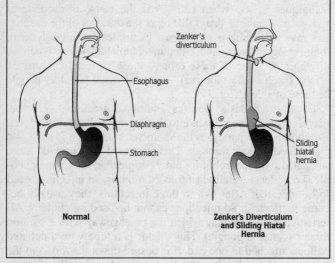

Normal

Zenker's Diverticulum and Sliding Hiatal Hernia

of the sphincter is relieved. Myotomy can often be done with instruments threaded through a viewing tube called a laparoscope. The laparoscope is inserted through a small incision in the abdomen. This procedure is successful in most people. If needed, surgery to prevent reflux is usually done at the same time. Before surgery is done, a specialist is usually consulted.

If an esophageal web is due to iron deficiency, treating the deficiency usually results in disappearance of the web. For other esophageal webs and esophageal rings, an endoscope or dilators are used to clear or widen the esophagus.

If Zenker's diverticulum is large and causes symptoms, surgery to eliminate the pouch is usually recommended. Surgery may be done through an incision in the neck (open surgery) or through an endoscope inserted through the mouth. Using an endoscope may be preferred because it is faster, relieves symptoms equally well, and may not require an overnight stay in the hospital.

GASTROESOPHAGEAL REFLUX

In gastroesophageal reflux (gastroesophageal reflux disease, or GERD), acid and enzymes produced by the stomach flow backward into the esophagus.

Reflux causes indigestion and heartburn. Occasional reflux, often the result of a dietary indiscretion, is usually bothersome but not serious. However, repeated reflux can result in inflammation of the esophagus (esophagitis), open sores (ulcers) in the lining of the esophagus, formation of scar tissue, and narrowing of the esophagus (strictures). After years, reflux can lead to esophageal cancer. Most of the time, reflux can be treated effectively with changes in lifestyle and with drugs.

About 1 out of 10 people has reflux every day, and about half of people have it at least once a month. Reflux affects old and young alike. It is more common among men.

The acid and enzymes produced by the stomach are designed to break down or digest food, but they can also break down some of the body's tissues. The stomach has a lining that protects it, but the esophagus does not. Thus, if stomach acid and enzymes flow backward into the esophagus, it can be damaged.

Normally, the ring-shaped muscle at the lower end of the esophagus (lower esophageal sphincter) remains contracted to prevent the contents of the stomach from flowing backward. The sphincter is triggered to relax when there is food in the esophagus, so that food can pass through to the stomach. After food passes into the stomach, the sphincter contracts again, closing off the esophagus.

A thin muscle called the diaphragm separates the chest from

the abdomen. To get to the stomach, the esophagus passes through a small opening in the diaphragm called the hiatus. Like the lower esophageal sphincter, this opening also contracts and relaxes in response to food and may help prevent reflux.

Causes

Reflux occurs when the lower esophageal sphincter malfunctions. The sphincter may relax at the wrong time (when the stomach is full). Or the sphincter may be weak and unable to contract tightly enough. In either case, the stomach's contents can flow backward into the esophagus and can even reach the mouth.

Lying down soon after eating contributes to reflux. Thus, older people who go to sleep or take a nap very soon after eating often have reflux symptoms.

A hiatal hernia may contribute to reflux. In the most common type of hiatal hernia, the top part of the stomach sometimes slides up and bulges through the opening in the diaphragm (hiatus). This type is called a sliding hiatal hernia. A hiatal hernia may cause the lower esophageal sphincter to malfunction or refluxed material to remain in the esophagus longer (making damage more likely).

Reflux may be triggered or worsened by diet or lifestyle choices. Drinking alcohol or caffeinated beverages such as coffee stimulates acid production, making the symptoms of reflux worse. Being obese may make reflux worse because of what or how much is eaten. Also, the extra weight puts pressure on the stomach. Smoking and eating certain foods (such as chocolate and peppermint) tend to weaken the sphincter muscle. For some people, eating fatty foods and foods with a high acid content (such as citrus fruits) makes reflux symptoms worse.

Certain drugs (such as drugs with anticholinergic effects, some antidepressants, calcium channel blockers, and nitrates) tend to weaken the sphincter muscle. Some disorders, such as diabetes, and some drugs, such as opioids, delay the emptying of the stomach. Then, the stomach's contents increase, and more material is available for reflux.

Symptoms

The most obvious symptom of reflux is burning pain behind the breastbone (heartburn). Sometimes the pain extends to the neck, throat, and face. People with reflux may have a bitter, sour, or salty taste in the mouth, caused by regurgitated material from the stomach. The regurgitated material may stimulate saliva production. Often, symptoms occur after people eat or when they lie down.

Reflux does not always cause regurgitation or heartburn. In some people, reflux may cause squeezing chest pain similar to chest pain due to coronary artery disease (angina). Squeezing pain due to reflux, like heartburn, is usually felt behind the breastbone or just below it.

If reflux continues, swallowing solid foods may become more and more difficult. After eating, people may feel as if they have a lump in the throat. Swallowing becomes difficult when repeated irritation from the reflux causes scar tissue to form in the esophagus. The inflexible, tight scar tissue narrows the esophagus.

People who have difficulty swallowing may inhale (aspirate) food into the windpipe (trachea). Aspiration can result in lung disorders, including bronchitis and a form of pneumonia called aspiration pneumonia.

Sometimes blood is vomited up or appears in the stool. Blood in the stool usually appears dark and tarry. The blood appears because the inflamed esophagus may bleed. Bleeding is usually slight but can be massive.

Reflux may cause sore or bleeding gums, hoarseness, sore throat, inflamed sinuses (sinusitis), and earaches. These symptoms develop if continued reflux irritates the tissues of the mouth, throat, and nose.

When reflux repeatedly irritates the lower part of the esophagus for a long time, the cells lining the esophagus may change. This disorder is called Barrett's esophagus. This disorder may cause no other symptoms. However, the abnormal cells are precancerous (that is, they may develop into cancer). Having Barrett's esophagus greatly increases the risk of developing cancer called adenocarcinoma of the esophagus.

Diagnosis

People should see their doctor if reflux symptoms last longer than 2 weeks. In most people, reflux can be diagnosed based on symptoms, and treatment can be started without diagnostic tests. Tests are usually necessary only when the diagnosis is unclear or symptoms persist despite treatment.

When a test is needed, a doctor usually examines the esophagus with a flexible viewing tube (endoscope).[1] This procedure, called endoscopy, is used to check for inflammation, Barrett's esophagus, and esophageal cancer. Occasionally, barium studies are done. X-rays are taken after a person consumes a barium solution or food coated with barium and lies down with the head lower than the feet. X-rays can show the reflux of barium from the stomach into the esophagus. A doctor may press on the person's abdomen to increase the likelihood of reflux. This test can also detect ulcers and narrowed areas in the esophagus.

Doctors may measure the strength of the lower esophageal sphincter. This test, called manometry, helps determine whether a sphincter is functioning normally and whether surgery is appropriate.

The pH (acidity) of the esophagus may be measured continuously, usually for 24 hours. In this test, a thin, flexible tube with a sensor probe on the tip is inserted through the nose and into the esophagus (near the lower esophageal sphincter). The other end of the tube is attached to a monitor on the person's belt. The monitor records the acid levels in the esophagus. Alternatively, a small probe is placed in the esophagus using a tube inserted through the mouth or nose. The probe is attached to the esophagus, and the tube is removed. The probe sends information about pH data to a small receiver worn by the person. The probe remains in place for almost 48 hours, then detaches and passes through the digestive tract and out of the body. A pH test can determine how much reflux is occurring. It also helps doctors pinpoint when symptoms occur in relation to reflux. The esophageal pH test is done whenever surgery for reflux is being considered.

Treatment

For many people with gastroesophageal reflux, lifestyle changes may be the only treatment needed. Raising the head of the bed about 6 inches can prevent acid from flowing into the esophagus when a person is lying down. Using blocks under the head of the bed is more effective than extra pillows. Waiting for

1. see art on page 117

several hours after eating before lying down and eating smaller meals may lessen symptoms. Losing weight, if needed, can help. Foods (including fatty foods) and beverages (such as caffeinated beverages and alcohol) that make reflux worse should be eaten in limited amounts or eliminated. Smoking, which tends to weaken the sphincter muscle, should be stopped. Not wearing clothes that are tight around the middle of the body and avoiding unnecessary bending may help. If drugs are contributing to reflux, doctors may be able to substitute another drug or reduce the dose.

If symptoms persist, certain drugs are effective.

Doctors often recommend taking antacids at bedtime to relieve symptoms, such as heartburn and the pain due to ulcers in the esophagus. Antacids are most likely to be helpful when symptoms occur only occasionally. Antacids that are available without a prescription are often recommended. Antacids make stomach acid less acidic (that is, they neutralize the acid). These drugs do not cure reflux or help ulcers heal.

Histamine-2 (H_2) blockers and proton pump inhibitors reduce acid production. H_2 blockers include cimetidine, famotidine, nizatidine, and ranitidine. Some H_2 blockers are available without a prescription. Proton pump inhibitors are usually the most effective treatment for gastroesophageal reflux, because they reduce acid production the most. Proton pump inhibitors are especially helpful when symptoms occur very frequently. Examples are esomeprazole, lansoprazole, omeprazole, pantoprazole, and rabeprazole. Omeprazole is available without a prescription. H_2 blockers and proton pump inhibitors may quickly relieve most symptoms of reflux, but they must be given for 4 to 12 weeks for ulcers to heal completely. If symptoms recur, these drugs are started again. Some people have to take these drugs continuously.

Drugs with cholinergic effects (such as bethanechol or metoclopramide) can stimulate muscles in internal organs to contract. They may help the lower esophageal sphincter close more tightly and help the stomach empty its contents into the small intestine more quickly. However, these drugs have side effects that greatly limit their use.

If other treatments do not relieve symptoms or if inflammation persists, surgery may be done. Surgery may be preferable for people who do not want to take drugs for many years. Surgery may be done using a laparoscope in a minimally invasive procedure. This procedure is usually safe for older people. However, it causes problems in some people. The most common problems are difficulty swallowing, a sensation of bloating or abdominal discomfort after eating, and loss of the ability to belch or vomit.

Dogs have always played an important part in my life—but even more now that I am in the twilight years.

For one thing, I have never been a "morning" person and didn't particularly enjoy talking to anyone, family or friends, until mid-morning. Now that I have retired I have two dogs and so feel obliged to get up early to walk them; otherwise half the day can fly by while you are lingering over breakfast! I have had both knees replaced with titanium joints so I am inclined to be stiff when I get up; however, after walking the dogs my joints feel as though they have been oiled, and I really enjoy the fresh air and exercise in all weathers.

I live in a rural area, and I appreciate the seasons so much more than when I was working. I never identified the songs of birds in my younger days. One is never lonely when one has a dog—they seem to understand one's feelings so much more than many people. There is also a feeling of security, and I am not afraid to walk down a country lane with two protective and alert dogs. All dogs are not the same, of course, but the Tibetan breeds are particularly aware of anyone near, either in front of or behind you, and that is reassuring.

I meet many people on my walks—people of all ages and nationalities. Some people stop for a brief chat, and it is refreshing to hear different viewpoints on world news and also about different lifestyles. I meet foreigners who are visiting the area. I may never see them again, but it is surprising what pearls of wisdom I pick up. I am absolutely certain that if I didn't have a dog, I would be sitting in a chair most of the day—watching the world go by and feeling stiff and useless. It's early evening and we are all going out to take a walk and to watch the sun setting.

Eleanor MacDougall

55

Bowel Movement Disorders

Bowel function varies tremendously, not only from one person to another but also for any one person at different times. The large intestine (which comprises the colon and the rectum) is taken for granted when things are running smoothly. But when things go awry—for example, when stool passes too slowly or too quickly—the large intestine becomes the focus of attention.

CONSTIPATION

Constipation is a condition of infrequent or uncomfortable bowel movements.

People often disagree over what is meant by "infrequent." Many people believe they are constipated if they do not have several bowel movements every day. However, even daily bowel movements are not normal for everyone. Having less frequent bowel movements does not necessarily indicate a problem unless the frequency has decreased noticeably. For many older people, constipation means straining with bowel movements; passage of small, hard stools; or a sense that they have not emptied their rectum completely.

Constipation sometimes develops suddenly and lasts briefly. Among older people, however, constipation more often begins gradually and persists for months or years. Fortunately, constipation usually responds well to treatment.

Causes

Constipation most commonly occurs when the waste (stool) that forms after food is digested moves too slowly (slow transit) as it passes through the digestive tract. Dehydration, changes in diet and activity, and certain drugs are frequently to blame for slow transit of stool. When stool moves slowly, too much water is absorbed from the stool, and it becomes hard and dry. Gradual enlargement of the rectum and impaired coordination of the pelvic and anal muscles sometimes contribute to or cause constipation. Sometimes a combination of these processes occurs. A fourth cause, bowel obstruction, is serious but very uncommon.

Slow transit of stool: When transit of stool slows, more water is pulled from the stool, resulting in hard and dry stools that are difficult to pass.

Dehydration slows transit, because the body's response to dehydration is to remove additional water from stool in an effort to conserve its supply of water. Similarly, changes in diet, particularly eating foods low in fiber, can slow transit, because fiber helps hold water in the stool and increases its bulk. Stool that contains less water moves more slowly through the digestive tract.

The decline in physical activity that often accompanies aging may slow transit, because physical activity stimulates the intestines to move stool along.

Many drugs slow transit of stool through the large intestine. These include iron; opioids; certain drugs taken for high blood pressure or coronary artery disease, such as calcium channel blockers; drugs with anticholinergic effects (for example, certain antihistamines, sedatives, and antidepressants); antacids that contain calcium or aluminum hydroxide; and some drugs used to relieve nausea (serotonin antagonists).

Certain disorders can slow intestinal transit, including an underactive thyroid gland (hypothyroidism), high blood calcium levels (hypercalcemia), and Parkinson's disease. Diabetes can damage nerves that normally help control intestinal transit. Nerve or spinal cord injury may also slow transit. Abdominal surgery may slow transit as well, because bands of fibrous tissues (adhesions) that can gradually form after surgery can slow or even block (obstruct) movement of stool through the digestive tract. Noncancerous (benign) and cancerous (malignant) tumors can obstruct the digestive tract. Chronic pain and certain mental health disorders, especially depression, can also slow transit by interfering with the digestive tract's ability to move stool.

Rectal enlargement: In some older people, the rectum enlarges for no obvious reason. As the rectum enlarges, it becomes less able to sense accumulating stool, and its contractions weaken. As rectal contractions weaken, stool is not expelled as effectively. Constipation results as more and more stool accumulates. This accumulating stool may be putty-like or may harden. Impaction results when the rectum can no longer empty the stool that accumulates. Once enlargement and weakened contractions have begun, added fiber (the indigestible part of food) in the diet or fiber taken in a laxative preparation can worsen constipation and promote impaction. Delaying bowel movements habitually can also contribute to enlargement of the rectum and impairment of rectal contractions.

Impaired coordination of pelvic and anal muscles: A normal bowel movement involves relaxation of the pelvic support muscles (the muscles that support the bladder, uterus, and rectum) and of the circular band of muscle that keeps the anus closed (anal sphincter). Contraction and relaxation of pelvic support muscles and anal muscles are coordinated by the brain, the spinal cord, and certain nerves. If coordination of the pelvic and anal muscles is impaired, the person may sense the need to have a bowel movement, but the pelvic support muscles and the anal sphincter do not relax. This faulty coordination leads to constipation.

Symptoms

In addition to infrequent bowel movements, a person with constipation may describe having to strain to have a bowel movement. Hemorrhoids can develop from increased pressure created by straining. Some people report passing stools that are hard or small and feeling as if the rectum has not been completely emptied after a bowel movement. Constipation involving impaction of stool in the rectum may be accompanied by loss of control of bowel movements or by leakage and soiling (fecal incontinence).

When constipation is caused by worsening obstruction, the person may first have a decreased appetite, followed by nausea and vomiting.

Diagnosis

A doctor usually relies on the person's account of constipation when making a diagnosis. But the doctor also examines the rectum with a gloved finger and, if stool is present, determines the amount and consistency. The person's symptoms and an examination are often all that are needed to confirm a diagnosis of constipation and to determine the likely cause.

When the cause remains unclear, blood tests may be done. The doctor may also recommend an examination with a flexible viewing tube, either of just the lower part (rectum and sigmoid colon) of the large intestine (sigmoidoscopy) or of the entire large intestine (colonoscopy). This examination is important if the constipation developed suddenly or if it is worsening noticeably.

Occasionally, other tests are needed to determine the cause. A plain x-ray may show evidence of bowel obstruction or suggest another cause. Another test involves swallowing several capsules containing tiny rings that can be seen on x-rays. An x-ray is taken several days later. If more than 20% of the rings remain in the digestive tract 5 days after they have been swallowed, transit time through the intestine is slow. Another type of test involves use of x-rays after a dye (barium) has been instilled into the rectum. X-rays are taken while the person tries to move his bowels and pass the barium.

Treatment

Constipation with impaction: When stool is impacted, tap water enemas are commonly used. Although people receiving an enema can be placed in a variety of positions, usually they are positioned so that they are lying on their left side, with knees flexed and drawn up toward the chest. About 5 to 10 ounces of water at body temperature are gently instilled into the rectum and sigmoid colon. The water is instilled through a tube with a bulb that is squeezed to draw the water up and then squeezed again to push the water out. When the water is expelled from the rectum, the impacted stool is expelled with it. Nonprescription prepackaged enemas containing sodium biphosphate can be used in place of tap water but offer no advantages.

If enemas fail to work, a health care practitioner may need to remove the stool manually using a gloved finger. The person is then sometimes asked to drink a solution containing dissolved salts (electrolytes) and polyethylene glycol, which cleanses the digestive tract.

After the impaction has been removed, the person may be told to add fiber to the diet or to use laxatives to prevent constipation. Small amounts of polyethylene glycol–containing solution may be given daily as well. Laxatives may be used every 2 to 3 days to stimulate bowel contractions if a bowel movement does not occur spontaneously.

Constipation without impaction: If the stool is not impacted, several options are available for treating constipation.

Diet and physical activity are often the most important treatment considerations. Increasing the intake of fluids and fiber is often the first step. Vegetables, fruits (especially prunes), whole-grain breads, and high-fiber cereals are excellent sources of fiber. Bran is an alternative source. Some people find it helpful to sprinkle 2 or 3 teaspoons of unrefined miller's bran on high-fiber cereal or fruit 2 or 3 times a day. Miller's bran also mixes well with applesauce, which also contains fiber. To work well, fiber must be consumed with plenty of fluids. Increased physical activity is also helpful because it stimulates contractions in the intestine, which helps move stool along.

Treatment of an underlying disease that is causing constipation may relieve the problem. Likewise, when a drug contributes to or causes constipation, a doctor may lower the dose or substitute another drug.

Laxatives and stool softeners are sometimes needed if changes in diet, physical activity, and drugs are insufficient. Most laxatives are safe for long-term use, whereas others should be used only occasionally. Some are better for preventing constipation, whereas others can be used for treating it. All laxatives must be used with caution, however, because overzealous use can lead to diarrhea, dehydration, or abdominal cramps.

Bulking agents, such as psyllium and methylcellulose, are laxatives that help hold water in the stool and add bulk to it. The increased bulk stimulates the natural contractions of the large intestine. Bulkier stools are softer and easier to pass. Bulking agents act slowly and gently. These agents generally are taken in small amounts at first. The dose is increased gradually until regularity is achieved. People who use bulking agents should always drink plenty of fluids.

℞ DRUGS AND AGENTS USED TO PREVENT OR TREAT CONSTIPATION

Drug/ Type	Agent	Selected Side Effects	Comments
Bulking agents	Calcium polycarbophil Methylcellulose Psyllium	Flatulence (gas), bloating	Bulking agents generally are used to prevent or control chronic constipation
Osmotic agents	Lactulose Magnesium salts (magnesium hydroxide, magnesium citrate) Polyethylene glycol Sorbitol	Cramps, flatulence (lactulose, sorbitol)	Osmotic agents are better for treating constipation than for preventing it
Stimulant agents	Bisacodyl Cascara Castor oil Senna	Abdominal pain (cramps)	Stimulant agents are not used if there is a possibility of an intestinal obstruction. They are particularly helpful for treating constipation caused by drugs, such as opioids.
Stool softeners	Docusate	Nausea (especially with syrup or liquid formulation)	Used alone, stool softeners are unlikely to be helpful for treating constipation.

Osmotic agents are laxatives that pull large amounts of water into the large intestine, making the stool soft and loose. The excess fluid also stimulates contractions. These laxatives consist of salts or sugars that are poorly absorbed. They may cause fluid retention in people with kidney disease or heart failure, especially if used frequently or in larger-than-recommended doses.

Some contain magnesium and phosphate, which can be partially absorbed into the bloodstream, resulting in harm to people with kidney failure.

Stimulant laxatives contain substances that directly stimulate the walls of the large intestine (such as senna, cascara, and bisacodyl), causing them to contract. Taken by mouth, stimulant laxatives generally cause a semisolid bowel movement in 6 to 8 hours. However, stimulant laxatives may cause cramping. Some are available as suppositories. When taken as suppositories, these laxatives often work in 15 to 60 minutes. The body can become dependent on stimulant laxatives if they are not used correctly. For these reasons, stimulant laxatives are best used only for brief periods. If longer use is needed, they should be used no more often than every third day and under a doctor's supervision. They can help prevent constipation in people who are taking drugs that almost always cause constipation, such as opioids.

Stool softeners, such as docusate, help water to penetrate the stool more easily and soften the stool. Some people find the softened nature of the stool unpleasant. Used alone, stool softeners are unlikely to be helpful. Softeners are most helpful when taken together with laxatives for people who must avoid straining because they have hemorrhoids or have recently undergone surgery.

Prevention

A combination of an adequate intake of fluids, adequate exercise, and a high-fiber diet best prevents constipation. Laxatives are sometimes a helpful addition to these measures. For

THE LAXATIVE HABIT

Laxatives have a place in the treatment of constipation but are only one among many options. Not surprisingly, many people who get relief from constipation after taking a laxative turn to them the next time constipation becomes a concern. Many laxatives are easy to take, and the taste of some may even be appealing.

The temptation is strong for some people to set a goal of moving their bowels at least once every day and to think that laxatives are the best way to achieve that goal. But daily bowel movements are not necessary for good health. The laxative habit is one that is more easily prevented than broken.

example, when a person needs to take a potentially constipating drug, a stimulant laxative along with increased intake of dietary fiber and fluids helps prevent constipation.

DIARRHEA

Diarrhea is the passage of loose or watery bowel movements.

Bowel movements usually occur more frequently, but an increase in the frequency of stool without a change in the consistency is not diarrhea. People who eat large amounts of vegetable fiber, for example, may move their bowels three to five times a day, but the stool in such cases is usually firm and well formed.

Diarrhea is a common problem among older people. Most often, diarrhea begins suddenly. Although diarrhea is always likely to be annoying, fortunately it typically lasts for a brief period and resolves on its own. However, persistent diarrhea can cause dehydration and requires treatment.

Causes

Diarrhea is the result of the stool containing too much liquid. The excess liquid is primarily water. The amount of water remaining in the stool can become excessive if too little is absorbed from material moving through the digestive tract or if the body adds more water to the material.

Sometimes the excess liquid consists of more than just water. Among people who cannot absorb fats or carbohydrates adequately, excess fats or carbohydrates remain in the stool in addition to excess water, resulting in diarrhea. Among people whose large intestine becomes inflamed or infected, diarrhea can involve a combination of excess water and blood, mucus, and tissue from the lining of the large intestine.

Diarrhea that develops suddenly and lasts briefly is most often caused by an infection resulting from a virus, bacteria, or parasites. Sometimes bacteria produce diarrhea by releasing a toxin. The toxin can end up in the digestive tract even in people who do not have an infection, for example, when food contaminated with the substance is eaten. Other times bacteria that have already infected the intestine release the toxin from within the digestive tract. When diarrhea is caused by microorganisms or ingestion of chemical toxins, it is sometimes referred to as gastroenteritis. Outbreaks of gastroenteritis can occur in sites where people live close together and have frequent contact, such as nursing homes. Alternatively, when diarrhea is caused by food contaminated with microorganisms or toxins, it may be referred to as food poisoning. In some cases, the cause of sudden, brief diarrhea is a new drug, an increase in the dose of a drug, or a change in diet (such as drinking more juice or eating more fruit or dairy products). Rarely, the cause is ischemia of the colon, if the colon's blood supply is suddenly decreased due to a blockage in an artery.

Diarrhea that persists can have a variety of causes. Infection can cause persistent diarrhea. Overgrowth of bacteria normally present in the small intestine is another cause. *Clostridium difficile* is a type of bacteria that commonly causes such an overgrowth. Overgrowth with *C. difficile* or with other types of bacteria may occur after treatment with antibiotics.

Eating foods that contain hexitol, sorbitol, and mannitol can also cause persistent diarrhea. Inability to absorb certain nutrients, such as lactose (milk sugar) and fructose, can result in diarrhea. People who have difficulty digesting fatty foods may develop diarrhea. Certain drugs can cause diarrhea, including antacids that contain magnesium. People who have had a portion of their intestines removed may develop persistent diarrhea. Rarely, abnormal growths in the digestive tract, such as polyps and tumors, cause persistent diarrhea.

Symptoms

In diarrhea, the consistency of stool can be anything from soft and pasty to completely watery. The color can range from brown to clear. Black stools may indicate bleeding in the digestive tract, although some drugs used to treat diarrhea (those containing bismuth subsalicylate) turn the stools black. When a black color is caused by blood (melena), the stools usually appear tarry and are foul smelling. Rarely, stools are loose and red from blood (for example, if hemorrhoids are present or if ischemia of the colon develops).

Crampy pain and excessive flatulence (gas) may occur. People with diarrhea often feel an urgency to move their bowels. Some people experience nausea, with or without vomiting, especially if the diarrhea is caused by an infection. Fever may develop if the diarrhea is caused by an infection.

Light-headedness and weakness may occur if diarrhea leads to dehydration, which in turn can cause blood pressure to drop. Blood pressure can drop enough to cause fainting (syncope) or heart rhythm abnormalities (arrhythmias). Rapid breathing or shortness of breath, loss of appetite, nausea, and fatigue may occur, causing blood and other body fluids to be too acidic (a condition called metabolic acidosis).

Diagnosis

Diarrhea should be evaluated by a doctor if it is accompanied by light-headedness or blood in the stool or in any case in which it lasts for more than 3 days. A doctor first tries to determine whether the diarrhea began suddenly and has been present for a short time or whether it has been persistent (lasting more than 3 weeks).

When diarrhea is not severe and has lasted less than 1 week, the symptoms and physical examination alone are often enough to determine the cause and necessary treatment. The doctor tries to determine whether changes in drugs or diet may be the cause; whether the person has other symptoms, such as a fever or pain; and whether the person has been exposed to people with an infection.

When diarrhea persists longer than 3 weeks, stool samples may be examined. Examination of stool samples reveals if the stool is formed or watery and if it contains fat, blood, or other substances. The volume of stool over 24 hours may also be determined. Samples can be tested for infectious organisms, including certain bacteria and parasites. The doctor may examine the lining of the anus and rectum using sigmoidoscopy. Sometimes a biopsy (removal and microscopic examination of tissue) of the rectal lining is performed.

Treatment

Treatment of diarrhea depends on its cause. Most people with diarrhea only have to remove the cause and suppress the diarrhea until the body heals itself. For example, diarrhea is sometimes cured when a person eliminates foods that have recently been added to the diet. If diarrhea develops while taking a certain drug, the diarrhea may be cured if the drug can be discontinued or replaced with another drug. If diarrhea is caused by a viral infection, it generally resolves by itself in 24 to 48 hours. Diarrhea caused by a bacterial infection may resolve by itself, but sometimes it requires treatment with an antibiotic. Diarrhea caused by a parasitic infection is treated with antiparasitic drugs.

Many prescription and nonprescription drugs are available for the treatment of diarrhea. Nonprescription drugs include adsorbents (for example, kaolin-pectin), which adhere to chemicals, toxins, and some infectious organisms. Some adsorbents can also help firm up the stool. Bismuth helps many people with diarrhea. One side effect of bismuth is that it turns the stool black. Another nonprescription drug used is loperamide.

Prescription drugs used to treat diarrhea include opioids, codeine, and diphenoxylate. Bulking agents used for chronic constipation, such as psyllium and methylcellulose, can sometimes help relieve chronic diarrhea as well.

Diarrhea tends to cause dehydration if it lasts more than a day or two. As long as the person is not vomiting and does not feel nauseated, drinking fluids containing a balance of water, sugars, and salts can be very effective. One example of such a fluid is 8 ounces of fruit juice mixed with a teaspoon of corn syrup or honey and a pinch of salt, followed by 8 ounces of water mixed with a half-teaspoon of baking soda (sodium bicarbonate).

If, however, the person is vomiting or is unable to drink enough fluids to remain hydrated, hospitalization and treatment with water and salts given intravenously may be necessary.

FECAL INCONTINENCE

Fecal incontinence is the uncontrolled passage of bowel movements.

Losing control over bowel movements and becoming incontinent is humiliating for most people. Older people who become incontinent of stool (feces) often fear that others will view them as helpless and dependent. Fortunately, fecal incontinence can often be cured or controlled with treatment.

Causes

Fecal incontinence has a variety of causes. Some causes, such as sudden diarrhea from an infection, stroke, and injuries to the anus or spinal cord, can suddenly turn a continent person into an incontinent person. Other causes, such as constipation with impaction, rectal prolapse (protrusion of the inside lining of the rectum through the anus), dementia, and damage to nerves from diabetes, gradually interfere with control of bowel movements until incontinence develops. Once incontinence develops, it may resolve and not return. Alternatively, incontinence may persist but occur sporadically or persist and occur frequently.

Symptoms and Diagnosis

Fecal incontinence can range from a small amount of staining on underclothing to loss of a large amount of stool. When stool is lost, it may be entirely liquid, entirely solid, or a mixture of both.

A doctor examines the anus and rectum, checking the extent of sensation of the skin around the anus and how tightly the anus closes. The doctor usually examines the inside of the anus and rectum using either a very short rigid viewing tube (anoscopy) or a longer flexible viewing tube (sigmoidoscopy). If the cause remains unclear, more specialized tests may be needed. These tests include x-rays to determine how the rectum functions after a barium dye is instilled into it or measurements of nerve and muscle function of the anus and rectum (manometry).

Treatment

If fecal incontinence is caused by impacted stool in the rectum, the impaction must be removed. Options for removal include the use of enemas or manual removal of the impacted stool with a gloved finger. Once the impaction is removed, the large intestine is emptied with laxatives or by drinking a polyethylene glycol–containing solution.

Treatment of fecal incontinence involves establishing a regular pattern of bowel movements that results in well-formed stools. Dietary changes often help. In people without impaction, adding foods with a high fiber content to the diet increases the bulk of stools and the regularity of bowel movements. If fecal incontinence is due to persistent diarrhea, the cause of the diarrhea is addressed. A drug that slows bowel movements, such as loperamide, may be beneficial.

Exercising the circular muscle that keeps the anus closed (anal sphincter) by squeezing and releasing it increases its tone and strength and helps prevent fecal incontinence from recurring. Biofeedback can help a person learn to control this muscle when a bowel movement is imminent. Biofeedback involves electrical monitoring and display of muscle contractions so that the person can directly observe muscle activity. Biofeedback can also improve the person's response to the presence of stool in the rectum. About 70% of motivated people benefit from biofeedback.

Surgery may benefit a small number of people—for instance, when the cause is an injury to the anal sphincter. As a last resort, a colostomy (the surgical creation of an opening between the large intestine and the abdominal wall) may be performed. The anus is sewn shut, and bowel movements are diverted into a removable plastic bag attached to an opening in the abdominal wall. A colostomy does not always have to be permanent.

I was raised in a rural fishing community on Prince Edward Island. I attended a one-room school. At 16, I started my career as a fisherman. There were no hydraulics or electronics; we manually lifted and pulled. For 46 years, you'd find me on the water fishing.

At age 50, I was approached to become a member of the New London Fire Department. After some thought, I decided to become a volunteer firefighter. Over the years, I was instructed in first aid and CPR, trained to go through a burning building looking for survivors or pets, bringing a person out an upstairs window and down a ladder, and all other necessary training.

Even when I retired, I continued with the fire department. My role changed from active duty to ground duty. This includes unrolling and rolling up hoses, directing traffic, cleaning the trucks and the fire hall, or whatever ground work has to be done. Fire fighting has gotten into my blood and I can't get clear of it. I've continued with the fire department even though I no longer respond to the emergency location. Instead, when a call comes over the pager, I rush to the fire hall, a distance of 3 miles, and man the phone and radios. When the pager goes, be it day or night, I always try to get to the fire hall. Good people are depending on me.

Keeping active keeps me in good health. I suggest that everyone who is able to get out and move around should keep going. Take up some hobby and keep active. Most days, you can find me in my workshop, building and repairing projects. Some of my upholstery items can be found in homes throughout the community. I visit the wharf regularly to meet and talk with old friends and to keep up with community happenings.

Arnold Meek

56

Urinary Tract Infections

The urinary tract is normally free of infectious microscopic organisms (microorganisms). But microorganisms sometimes manage to get into the urinary tract and cause infections. An infection anywhere along the urinary tract is called a urinary tract infection (UTI).

Urine is produced by the two kidneys. Each kidney has a collection area for urine, called the renal pelvis. Each renal pelvis drains into a ureter, which channels the urine to the bladder. The bladder empties into a single tube called the urethra. The urethra channels urine outside of the body. In a man, the opening of the urethra is at the tip of the penis. In a woman, the opening is in the vulva.

UTIs are usually confined to the bladder (cystitis). Much less often, microorganisms move up one of the ureters from the bladder, resulting in an infection of the kidney (pyelonephritis).

UTIs are very common in older people. Women are affected more often than men, although this difference narrows with aging. Most UTIs, at their worst, are annoying and distressing. However, pyelonephritis may be more serious. Occasionally UTIs spread into the bloodstream (sepsis), causing serious problems and even death. Fortunately, most UTIs respond very well to treatment.

Causes

Microorganisms that cause UTIs almost always come from the skin at or near the opening of the urethra. Microorganisms that enter the urinary tract through the opening of the urethra are usually washed back out by the flushing action of urine. However, some manage to spread upward, where they can cause a UTI.

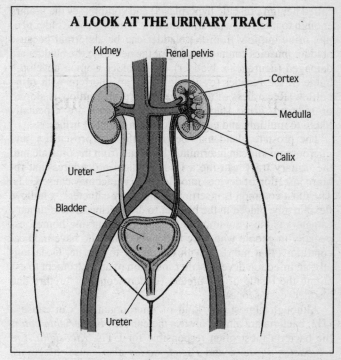

A LOOK AT THE URINARY TRACT

Kidney

Renal pelvis

Cortex

Medulla

Calix

Ureter

Bladder

Ureter

Very rarely, microorganisms from an infection elsewhere in the body pass from the blood into the kidneys, causing a kidney infection. Also very rarely, a process such as cancer in the colon or rectum can cause a passageway to form between the intestine and the bladder (vesicoenteric fistula), through which bacteria can travel to cause infection. Microorganisms are then able to move into the urinary tract, resulting in a UTI. In women, an infection in the vagina can cause a passageway to form between the vagina and the bladder (vesicovaginal fistula).

Older women are especially prone to UTIs. Women have a shorter urethra than men, thus microorganisms have a shorter distance to travel to reach the bladder. Also, the drop in estrogen level with menopause leads to thinning and inflammation of the urethra's lining, weakening its defense against infection.

In older men, the prostate gland grows larger (a condition

called benign prostatic hyperplasia) and compresses the urethra enough to interfere with urine outflow.[1] Among some older people, urine outflow from the bladder can be abnormal because bladder muscles contract weakly or the nerves to the bladder are damaged (neurogenic bladder). Some older women develop a bulge in the bladder (cystocele) that can interfere with urine outflow. Regardless of the cause, when urine outflow is slowed or reduced, urine stagnates. Microorganisms are especially likely to multiply and cause infection in stagnant urine.

The prostate gland may become infected (prostatitis), and microorganisms can intermittently spread from the prostate into the urinary tract, causing a UTI. Medical procedures that require insertion of devices into the urinary tract may cause UTIs. The most common is insertion of a urinary catheter—a hollow, flexible tube placed in the bladder to drain urine. Use of urinary catheters is most common in hospitals and nursing homes, especially in people who have had surgery or who have medical conditions that interfere with the ability to urinate. Occasionally, an infection develops after insertion of an instrument to examine the inside of the ureters (ureteroscope) or urethra and bladder (cystoscope).

Although almost any kind of microorganism can cause a UTI, bacteria are almost always the culprits. *Escherichia coli* is the bacteria most often responsible for UTIs. *Klebsiella, Enterobacter, Proteus,* and *Pseudomonas* also cause infections. Less often, other bacteria, such as *Enterococcus* and *Staphylococcus,* cause UTIs. Fungi (such as *Candida*) and viruses rarely infect the urinary tract.

Symptoms

Cystitis, an infection in the bladder, often results in a painful burning sensation (dysuria) and in a need to urinate frequently, often at night (nocturia) and urgently. The urgent need to urinate may cause an uncontrollable loss of urine (incontinence).[2]

Fever is uncommon unless the infection has spread to become an upper UTI or spread to the blood (sepsis). Flank pain may result from an infected kidney (pyelonephritis). Confusion can develop, especially if the UTI involves a high fever.

1. see page 886
2. see page 859

The urine may smell especially foul or appear cloudy or bloody. In the very rare instance of a vesicoenteric and vesico-vaginal fistula, air may pass through the urethra with urine (pneumaturia), producing bubbles.

Sometimes bacteria get into the bladder and remain there for varying amounts of time without causing any symptoms (sometimes called asymptomatic bacteriuria). This process is most likely to occur in a person whose bladder is not emptying adequately because of nerve damage and virtually always occurs after several weeks in a person who has a permanently placed catheter.

Diagnosis

A doctor suspects cystitis on the basis of the symptoms alone. Tests on a urine sample confirm the diagnosis.

A urine sample is obtained by first cleansing the skin surrounding the urethra with an antiseptic wipe, then urinating into a sterile container. If the person is unable to manage because of limited dexterity or an inability to understand instructions, a health care practitioner may need to assist. Occasionally, the urine in the container contains microorganisms that were not cleansed from the skin by wiping before urination. In these instances, a urine sample can be obtained by inserting a catheter into the bladder.

The urine is examined under a microscope to check for the presence of white blood cells and microorganisms. The urine may also be sent to the laboratory to grow and identify the microorganism (urine culture).

The urine is sometimes tested with strips (dip sticks) to check for the presence of nitrites (substances released by bacteria) and leukocyte esterase (a protein found in white blood cells) whose function is to fight infection. These substances indicate that an infection may be present in the urinary tract.

A complete blood count test is often done to check for a high white blood cell count, a possible sign of infection. Blood can also be tested to grow and identify any microorganisms that may have spread from the urinary tract into the bloodstream.

Additional tests are rarely needed but may be done in people who have frequent UTIs. One such test is a measurement of the amount of urine remaining in the bladder after urination is complete (residual urine). Frequent UTIs may also be evaluated by examining the anatomy of the urinary tract with imaging tests, such as an ultrasound, CT scan, cystoscopy, or ureteroscopy.

Prevention

Improvement of personal hygiene may help prevent UTIs. Antibiotics are sometimes used to prevent infections.

In people who have had a urinary catheter inserted, the catheter is removed as soon as possible to prevent infection.

Treatment

UTIs that produce symptoms are treated with antibiotics. If fungi are causing the infection, antifungal drugs are used. If a person has a UTI but does not have any symptoms, treatment is not necessary. Drug therapy for a person who does not have symptoms is costly and can cause unwanted side effects. In addition, such therapy can be harmful, because it may allow the microorganism causing the infection to become resistant to the drug that is being given.

Antibiotics are usually taken by mouth. Common choices include trimethoprim-sulfamethoxazole, amoxicillin, ampicillin, cephalexin, ciprofloxacin, levofloxacin, and nitrofurantoin. Other antibiotics are also effective. For the treatment of pyelonephritis, antibiotics are sometimes given through a tube inserted into a vein (intravenously) until symptoms subside. Antibiotics are often taken for 3 days in women and 7 days in men for the treatment of cystitis; pyelonephritis is treated for 7 to 14 days. People with diabetes, a weakened immune system, or an abnormality blocking the flow of urine may need prolonged antibiotic treatment to eradicate the infection.

In conjunction with antibiotics, other drugs are occasionally taken to speed relief of symptoms. Dicyclomine provides temporary relief from the bladder spasms that cause the sensation of urgent urination. Phenazopyridine reduces the burning pain on urination.

Surgery or other procedures (such as insertion of a cystoscope or ureteroscope that includes special instruments) may be necessary to relieve physical blockages to the flow of urine or to correct structural abnormalities in the urinary tract. Draining urine from a blocked area can help control the infection and prevent kidney damage.

Outlook

UTIs usually respond well to drug therapy. However, a subsequent UTI may develop if the microorganism was not eliminated from the urinary tract during treatment. A second infection caused by the same microorganism is called a relapse infection. Alternatively, infection by one type of microorganism may be followed quickly by an infection caused by a different microorganism. One possible cause of a relapse or recurrent infection is failure to take antibiotics long enough or in a large enough dosage to eliminate the microorganism from the urinary tract. Recurrent infections can occur when abnormalities persist in the urinary tract.

I began making meals at an early age. Before I was asked to cook, I made mud pies for my country-made dolls, but a wish came true. My early years on the farm cooking were the highlight of farm work for me. We ate mostly vegetables that we grew. We took whatever was ripe from the fields and put it in a pot. I call it dump cooking. I made herb medicines—syrups, teas, and greasy rubs—from the yard bushes, field herbs, and trees. There was always a tea or tonic brewing on the stove. I still feel that I need some herb tonic with my prescribed medicine.

I never in one of my timeless dreams believed I would have my own restaurant. A miracle it is. Folks come from all over. My recipes remind them of the fresh foods they ate when they were growing up. I like to cook and grow vegetables and flowers. I am happy working at 74 years.

Being one of the aging, whom I call the experienced citizens, I have a lot to offer after helping to build America with bare hands and with grass roots experience, like most of the aging who worked domestic farm and other jobs when the pay was low. I serve on the local board on aging. It is necessary to care for the health and well-being of the older population. It is sometimes hard for us to understand technology and confusing paperwork, especially when all the children have left home and the years keep rolling. Working to me is being active doing what I love doing. But for some, depression and loneliness take a toll, causing fear in the lives of us elderly. Seeing to their needs is important to me. One day I will retire. I have cooked for all but 11 years of my life.

Mildred Council

57

Urinary Incontinence

Urinary incontinence is the uncontrollable loss of urine.

Urinary incontinence is common, affecting about 1 out of 3 older people. The condition is more common among women than among men until after the age of 85, when it tends to affect both sexes equally. Some people are incontinent every time they urinate, whereas many others are incontinent intermittently. Many people live with incontinence without seeking medical help because they fear that it indicates a more serious illness or they are embarrassed by it. Others mistakenly believe incontinence to be a normal part of aging and assume that nothing can be done for it. On the contrary, urinary incontinence is never normal and, when it does occur, is often treatable and curable.

Urinary incontinence is not only a problem in itself but also can lead to many other problems and complications, particularly among older people. For example, incontinence can cause a person to avoid activities and interactions with others, which can lead to isolation and depression. In addition, incontinence can increase the risk of skin rashes and pressure sores (from urine irritating the skin) as well as falls (from attempts to reach the toilet quickly).

Control of Urination

The kidneys produce urine continuously. Urine is carried from each of the two kidneys through tubes (the ureters) to the bladder, which stores the urine. The lowest portion of the bladder connects with a channel (the urethra) that carries urine out of the body. In women, the urethra is short and exits the body through the area where the external genitals are located (vulva). In men, the urethra is much longer and exits the body through the penis. In both men and women, a muscle (the urinary sphincter) encircles the connection between the lowest part of the bladder and the urethra. The urinary sphincter remains closed (contracted) most of the time to prevent urine from leaving the bladder.

When the bladder is full, nerves in the bladder wall send messages to the spinal cord; the messages are then relayed to the brain, and the person becomes aware of the urge to urinate. A person who has control over urination can then decide whether to urinate or to wait. When the decision is made to urinate, the urinary sphincter relaxes, allowing urine to flow out through the urethra. At the same time, the muscle in the bladder wall (detrusor muscle) contracts to push urine out. Muscles in the abdominal wall and in the pelvis may contract as well to increase the pressure on the bladder, helping it to empty.

Causes and Symptoms

Aging itself does not cause urinary incontinence, but changes that occur with aging can increase the risk of developing urinary incontinence by interfering with a person's ability to control urination.[1] For example, the maximum amount of urine that the bladder can hold (bladder capacity) decreases. The ability to postpone urination decreases. More urine remains in the bladder after urination (residual urine), partly due to less effective squeezing of the bladder muscle. In postmenopausal women, the urinary sphincter does not hold back urine in the bladder as effectively, because the decrease in estrogen levels after menopause leads to shortening of the urethra and thinning and fragility (atrophy) of its lining. Also, urine flow through the urethra slows. In men, urine flow through the urethra may be impeded by an enlarged prostate gland, eventually leading to bladder enlargement.

Urinary incontinence has many possible causes. Some causes, such as a bladder infection, a broken hip, or delirium, can bring on incontinence suddenly and abruptly. Other causes, such as an enlarged prostate in men or dementia, gradually interfere with control of urination until incontinence results. Incontinence may resolve and never recur. Alternatively, it may persist, recurring sporadically or, in some cases, frequently.

1. see also page 19

Many experts try to categorize incontinence according to the basic cause of the problem. The categories or types that most experts agree on are urge incontinence, stress incontinence, overflow incontinence, functional incontinence, and mixed incontinence.

Urge incontinence: Urge incontinence is an abrupt and intense urge to urinate that cannot be suppressed, followed by an uncontrollable loss of urine. The amount of urine lost may be small or large. People with urge incontinence usually have very little time to get to the bathroom before they have an "accident." The sense of needing to rush to get to the bathroom is especially disturbing and potentially dangerous for people who have a disorder that limits their mobility or stability, such as arthritis or Parkinson's disease. Most people with urge incontinence urinate more frequently, not only during the day but also at night (nocturia). The combination of urgency, increased frequency of urination, and increased urination during the night is often referred to as an overactive bladder, whether or not the combination leads to incontinence.

Some people with urge incontinence also have poor squeezing ability of the bladder muscle. In such people, even though the bladder is overactive, the contractions are less effective at emptying the bladder.

Urge incontinence is the most common type of persistent incontinence in older people. The cause of bladder overactivity and urge incontinence is usually unknown. Stroke, dementia, or other disorders that affect the ability of the brain or spinal cord (for example, lumbar spinal stenosis) to inhibit bladder contractions when there is no opportunity to urinate contribute to urge incontinence. Conditions that irritate the bladder, such as atrophic vaginitis in women, prostate enlargement in men, or severe constipation, can also contribute to urge incontinence.

Stress incontinence: Stress incontinence is the uncontrollable loss of small amounts of urine when coughing, straining, sneezing, or lifting heavy objects or during any activity that suddenly increases pressure within the abdomen. This increased pressure overcomes the resistance of the closed urinary sphincter. Urine then flows into and through the urethra. Stress incontinence is common in women but uncommon in men.

Any condition or event that weakens and reduces resistance

DRUGS THAT MAY CAUSE OR WORSEN URINARY INCONTINENCE

Type of Drug	Examples	Effects
Alcohol	Beer, wine, liquor	Increases urination by increasing urine production
Alpha agonists	Nasal decongestants containing pseudoephedrine	Tighten the urinary sphincter; can cause urine to be retained in the bladder and uncontrollable leakage of small amounts of urine (overflow incontinence)
Alpha blockers	Doxazosin, prazosin, tamsulosin, terazosin	Relax the urinary sphincter and urethra; can cause incontinence when coughing, straining, sneezing, lifting heavy objects, or putting any other pressure on the abdomen (stress incontinence)
Angiotensin-converting enzyme (ACE) inhibitors	Benazepril, captopril	Can cause cough and worsen stress incontinence
Antidepressants	Amitriptyline, desipramine, nortriptyline	Interfere with bladder contraction and worsen constipation; can cause urine to be retained in the bladder and overflow incontinence
Antihistamines	Chlorpheniramine, diphenhydramine	Interfere with bladder contraction and worsen constipation; can cause urine to be retained in the bladder and overflow incontinence
Antipsychotics	Haloperidol, risperidone thioridazine, thiothixene	Can slow mobility and cause abrupt urge to urinate followed by uncontrollable loss of

Type of Drug	Examples	Effects
		urine (urge incontinence)
Caffeine	Coffee, cola, tea, some nonprescription headache remedies	Increases urination by increasing urine production
Calcium channel blockers	Diltiazem, verapamil	Interfere with bladder contraction and worsen constipation; can cause urine to be retained in the bladder and overflow incontinence
Diuretics	Furosemide, thiazides	Increase urination by increasing urine production
Opioids	Morphine	Interfere with bladder contraction and worsen constipation; can cause urine to be retained in the bladder and overflow incontinence
Sedatives	Diazepam, flurazepam, lorazepam	Can slow mobility and worsen urge incontinence

of the urinary sphincter or urethra can cause stress incontinence. Childbirth, for example, can weaken the urinary sphincter, as can surgery involving organs or structures in the pelvis, such as the uterus (for example, hysterectomy). If a portion of the bladder loses its support of fibrous connective tissue and bulges into the wall of the vagina (a condition called cystocele), the lowest part of the bladder changes shape. If the shape of the bladder changes, the position of the urethra can change where it connects with the bladder, which then interferes with and weakens the urinary sphincter. In postmenopausal women, a lack of estrogen weakens the urinary sphincter's ability to hold back urine flow by allowing the lining of the urethra to become thinner and more fragile, a condition called atrophic urethritis. In men, stress incontinence may follow prostate surgery if the urinary sphincter is injured. In both men and women, obesity can cause or worsen stress incontinence because extra weight adds additional pressure on the bladder.

Some older people with severe stress incontinence have nearly constant urine loss (sometimes referred to as total incontinence). This condition usually occurs because the urinary sphincter does not close adequately.

Overflow incontinence: Overflow incontinence is the uncontrollable leakage of small amounts of urine, usually caused by some type of blockage or by weak contractions of the bladder muscle. When urine flow is blocked or the bladder muscle can no longer contract, urine is retained in the bladder (urinary retention), and the bladder enlarges. Pressure in the bladder continues to increase until small amounts of urine dribble out. The increased pressure in the bladder can also damage the kidneys.

In older men, an enlarged prostate can block the urethra. Less commonly, scar tissue narrows or sometimes even blocks the lowest part of the bladder, where it connects to the urethra, or blocks the urethra itself (urethral stricture). Such narrowing or blockage may occur after prostate surgery. In men and women, severe constipation or stool impaction can cause overflow incontinence if stool fills the rectum to the point of putting pressure on the lower portion of the bladder, the urinary sphincter, or the urethra. Nerve damage that paralyzes the bladder (a condition commonly called neurogenic bladder) can also cause overflow incontinence. Stroke and diabetes mellitus can paralyze the bladder, leading to overflow incontinence.

Functional incontinence: Functional incontinence refers to urine loss resulting from the inability (or sometimes unwillingness) to get to a toilet. The most common causes are conditions that lead to immobility, such as stroke or severe arthritis, and conditions that interfere with mental function, such as dementia due to Alzheimer's disease. In rare cases, people become so depressed that they do not go to the toilet (psychogenic incontinence).

Mixed incontinence: Mixed incontinence involves more than one type of incontinence. The most common type of mixed incontinence occurs in older women, who often have a mixture of urge and stress incontinence. Urge incontinence and functional incontinence occur together in people with severe dementia, Parkinson's disease, stroke, and other disabling neurologic disorders.

Diagnosis

The information collected by asking about urination and incontinence can help doctors determine the type, severity, and cause of the problem and develop an appropriate treatment plan. Doctors often ask the following questions:

- How long has incontinence been occurring?
- With episodes of incontinence, are undergarments typically just damp, or are they soaked?
- Before urination or episodes of incontinence, is there an abrupt and intense urge to urinate? How much time typically passes before urination begins after feeling an urge to urinate?
- Do certain events or actions seem to trigger a need to urinate (such as the sound of running water, washing hands, exercise)?
- Do episodes of incontinence occur with laughing, coughing, sneezing, or bending?
- What is the frequency of urination or episodes of incontinence during a typical day? A typical night?
- How difficult is it to start urinating? Once urination begins, is the urine flow interrupted?
- Does there seem to be a relationship between urination and taking drugs or drinking alcohol or caffeinated beverages?
- How has incontinence affected the ability to carry out daily activities?

A person with urinary incontinence may be asked to keep a diary in which urinary habits are recorded for at least 3 days. This diary can help the doctor evaluate how often incontinence occurs and how much urine is being lost during episodes of incontinence. The diary may also help the doctor determine the cause of incontinence.

A physical examination can provide valuable information. A rectal examination can confirm whether the person is severely constipated or if stool is impacted. Nerve damage contributing to or causing incontinence may be detected by an examination of sensation and reflexes in the lower body. In women, a pelvic examination can help identify problems that may contribute to or cause incontinence, such as atrophy of the lining of the urethra and dropping down of the bladder into the vagina. Stress incontinence is sometimes diagnosed simply by observing the loss of urine while the person is coughing or straining. The amount of urine left in the bladder after urination (residual urine) can be measured with ultrasound. Alternatively, the amount of residual urine can be measured with a small tube (catheter) that is placed into the bladder (urinary catheterization). A large amount of residual urine may indicate overflow incontinence, the result of urine flow being blocked or the bladder not contracting adequately. Examination of the urine with a microscope (a urinalysis) can help determine whether an infection is present.

Special tests performed during urination (urodynamic evaluation) are helpful in some cases. These tests measure the pressure in the bladder at rest and when filling. A catheter is inserted through the urethra into the bladder, and water is passed through the catheter while the pressure within the bladder is recorded. Normally, the pressure increases slowly and steadily. In some people, pressure increases in spurts or rises too sharply before the bladder is completely filled. The pattern of pressure change helps the doctor determine the type of incontinence and the best treatment. The rate of urine flow can also be measured; this measurement can help determine whether urine flow is obstructed and whether the bladder muscle can contract strongly enough to expel the urine. In some cases, a doctor may look into the bladder with a flexible viewing tube called a cystoscope.

Treatment

Treatment varies according to the type and cause of incontinence. In most cases, incontinence can be cured or reduced considerably.

Sometimes treatment involves only education and some simple behavioral changes. The person learns about bladder functioning and the effects of drugs and fluid intake. The person also learns how to establish bladder and bowel habits that promote control over urination, such as being patient and not rushing urination and bowel movements. The person is advised to avoid fluids that may irritate the bladder, such as caffeinated beverages, or to reduce intake. Drinking six to eight 8-ounce glasses of noncaffeinated fluids a day is recommended to prevent the urine from becoming too concentrated—which can irritate the bladder as well.

If specific disorders or drugs are causing or contributing to incontinence, treatment involves an effort to eliminate or minimize these factors. Drugs that reduce squeezing of the bladder muscle often can be discontinued. For people taking diuretics, the timing of the dose can be adjusted so that the person can be close to a bathroom when the drug takes effect.

Urge incontinence: People with urge incontinence are encouraged to urinate at regular intervals—typically about every 2 to 3 hours—before the urge occurs. They are often encouraged to urinate when it is convenient, such as before leaving home to go shopping. If a diary of urinary habits was kept to help the doctor evaluate the incontinence, the diary may be helpful for establishing the time interval for urination. This type of training, sometimes called habit or bladder training, keeps the bladder relatively empty, thus reducing the likelihood of incontinence. Another approach involves learning to resist urination for gradually longer periods once an urge to urinate is felt. The goal is urination every 3 to 4 hours without incontinence.

Performing pelvic muscle exercises (Kegel exercises) can be very helpful. These exercises involve repeatedly contracting the pelvic muscles many times a day to build up strength. The person learns to use these muscles properly in situations that cause incontinence, such as listening to running water, coughing, and standing with a full bladder.

Drugs that relax the bladder by reducing muscle contractions may help. The two most commonly used drugs are oxybutynin and tolterodine. The long-acting forms of these drugs can be taken once a day. Although these drugs can help by reducing the strong urge to urinate, they have potential side effects, such as dryness of the mouth and constipation. Some drugs that relax the bladder increase the amount of urine remaining in the bladder after urination, so frequency and amount of urination must be monitored for any noticeable decrease when these drugs are first taken or when the dose is increased. People who take diuretics may need to time their dose to be close to a bathroom when the drug takes effect. Recently, the use of a pacemaker whose wires are implanted into the spinal cord has proved useful in some people who have multiple episodes of urge incontinence (more than 50 per day).

KEGEL EXERCISES: SQUEEZE AND RELAX

Kegel exercises help strengthen the pelvic muscles, primarily those around the vagina, urethra, and rectum. Women who perform these exercises regularly can help improve sexual function and prevent or reduce the involuntary loss of urine (urinary incontinence) or stool (fecal incontinence).

To perform these exercises, a woman squeezes the muscles used to stop the flow of urine for about 10 seconds, and then relaxes them for about 10 seconds. The exercise is repeated 10 to 20 times in a row at least three times a day. Muscle tone usually improves in 2 to 3 months. Kegel exercises can be performed anywhere, whether a woman is sitting, standing, or lying down.

Finding the right muscles to squeeze can be difficult. The muscles can be identified by inserting a finger into the vagina and squeezing or by trying to stop the flow of urine. If pressure is felt around the finger or urine flow stops, the right muscles are being squeezed.

The exercises should not be performed while urinating. If improvement is not noticed within 3 to 4 months, referral to a physical therapist who uses biofeedback training may help. Electrodes temporarily attached to the skin near the anus and the vagina transmit signals that create displays of muscle activity. Thus, by allowing the woman to visualize the effects of her efforts at contracting certain muscles, she is better able to identify and contract the appropriate muscles.

Stress incontinence: People with stress incontinence, like those with urge incontinence, are encouraged to urinate about every 2 to 3 hours to avoid a full bladder. Pelvic muscle exercises (Kegel exercises) are usually helpful.

In women whose stress incontinence seems to be due to atrophy of the urethra, applying estrogen cream inside the vagina or to the area immediately surrounding the opening of the urethra may help. Estrogen cream is more likely to help if other drugs that help tighten the urinary sphincter, such as pseudoephedrine, are also taken.

Many people with severe stress incontinence that does not respond to treatment benefit from surgery. Surgery may involve lifting up the bladder and strengthening the part that connects with the urethra. Injections of collagen around the urethra are effective in some cases. In rare cases, surgery may be performed to insert an artificial sphincter in place of a urinary sphincter that does not close adequately.

Overflow incontinence: When the cause is a blockage of urine flow, the incontinence is treated whenever possible by eliminating or reducing the blockage. Drug therapy is sometimes helpful for overflow incontinence in men if the incontinence is due to a partial blockage of urine flow by an enlarged prostate. Drugs that relax the urinary sphincter, such as terazosin and tamsulosin, quickly counteract some of the blockage caused by the enlarged prostate. Finasteride, when taken over a period of months, can reduce the size of the prostate or stop its growth.[1] Saw palmetto, an herbal agent,[2] may also help to control symptoms due to an enlarged prostate gland in some men. Alternatively, men with overflow incontinence caused by an enlarged prostate can undergo surgery to remove all or part of the prostate.[3]

When the cause of overflow incontinence is weakness of bladder muscle contractions, simple approaches may help. Gentle pressure can be applied to the bladder to promote emptying of the bladder. With hands placed over the lowest part of the abdomen or pelvis (the area over the bladder), pressure is applied by squeezing and pressing. In addition, some people benefit from trying to urinate again following a brief pause just after they feel they have emptied their bladder as well as they can (double urination, sometimes referred to as double voiding). Drugs usually are not helpful, though a small number of people benefit from the use of bethanechol.

Regardless of the cause, in some cases of overflow incontinence, a catheter must be inserted into the bladder to drain it and to prevent complications such as recurring infections and kidney damage. Insertion and removal of a catheter several times a day (intermittent catheterization) is recommended rather than a catheter that remains in place indefinitely (permanent indwelling catheterization). Intermittent catheterization is less likely to cause infection. People can insert a catheter themselves (intermittent self-catheterization) but must be capable of remembering to do it and have good hand dexterity.

People who are unable to catheterize themselves may still be able to have intermittent catheterization if another person is able to learn and maintain a schedule.

Functional incontinence: People with functional inconti-

1. see page 890
2. see page 84
3. see page 890

nence often benefit from training that involves reminders to urinate on a regular schedule (prompted urination). People who have difficulty getting to the toilet, undressing and dressing, and getting on or off the toilet are likely to need assistance along with reminders. Railings, grab bars, and elevated toilet seats can be helpful.

People who are incontinent primarily at night may benefit from improvements in lighting so that they are better able to find the toilet. A bedside commode or a hand-held urinal or bedpan may be helpful.

Incontinence of any type: For incontinence of any type, specially designed pads and undergarments can protect the skin and enable people to remain dry, comfortable, and socially active. Many of these items are unobtrusive and readily available. However, a person should not rely solely on these items unless other approaches do not help.

Outlook

Untreated urinary incontinence can greatly detract from a person's quality of life. Caregivers often name incontinence as an important reason for moving a loved one into a long-term care facility, such as a nursing home, because of the substantial burden it places on them.[1] But when people with urinary incontinence let their doctor in on the problem, a satisfactory solution often can be reached.

1. see box on page 192

58

Female Genital and
Sexual Disorders

Women experience many changes as they pass through middle age. These changes, many the result of menopause, help
set the stage for transition into older adulthood. Menopause is
a natural process that typically begins a few years before a
woman's last menstrual period. As women age, the ovaries produce smaller and smaller amounts of estrogen, progesterone,
and testosterone—the sex hormones. Eventually, menstrual periods end and pregnancy is no longer possible. These changes
certainly do not bring an end to sexual activity and pleasure.

Menopause has its price: It puts women at greater risk of developing heart disease, osteoporosis, and genital and sexual
disorders. However, not all genital and sexual disorders experienced by older women are caused exclusively by the changes of
menopause.

Female Reproductive System
The female reproductive system consists of both external and
internal genitals.

The external genitals consist of the labia majora, labia minora, Bartholin's glands, clitoris, and vestibule. The area containing these organs is called the vulva. The external genitals
have three main functions: enabling sperm to enter the body,
protecting the internal genitals from infectious organisms, and
providing sexual pleasure.

The labia majora are folds of tissue that enclose and protect
the other external genitals. The labia majora contain sweat and
sebaceous glands, which produce lubricating secretions. The
labia minora lie just inside the labia majora. During sexual
stimulation, increased blood flow causes the labia minora to

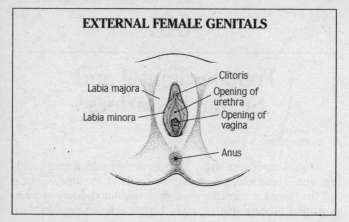

EXTERNAL FEMALE GENITALS

Clitoris

Labia majora

Opening of urethra

Labia minora

Opening of vagina

Anus

swell and become more sensitive to stimulation. The surface of the labia minora is kept moist by fluid secreted by specialized cells.

The two Bartholin's glands, located just inside the vaginal opening, secrete lubricating fluid during sexual intercourse.

The clitoris, located between the labia minora, is a small protrusion that is very sensitive to sexual stimulation. Stimulating the clitoris can result in an orgasm.

The vestibule is the tissue between the labia minora, including the openings to the vagina and the urethra (which carries urine from the bladder to the outside of the body). The vestibule is highly sensitive and is prone to inflammation.

The internal genitals consist of the vagina, uterus, cervix, fallopian tubes, and ovaries.

The vagina connects the external genitals with the uterus. The lower third of the vagina is surrounded by muscles that provide support to the vagina, bladder, and rectum and sometimes contract rhythmically during orgasm.

The lining of the vagina is highly sensitive to estrogen, which allows the vagina to be kept moist by fluids secreted from cells on its surface and by secretions from glands in the cervix (the lower part of the uterus). These fluids may pass to the outside of the body as a vaginal discharge, which is normal.

The uterus is situated behind the bladder and in front of the

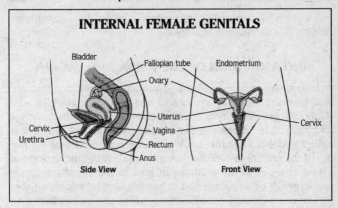

INTERNAL FEMALE GENITALS

Side View / Front View

rectum. The main function of the uterus is to sustain a fetus. The opening to the uterus is called the cervix.

The ovaries produce the female sex hormones (estrogen and progesterone) as well as male sex hormones (testosterone). In women of reproductive age, the ovaries produce and release eggs into the fallopian tubes.

With aging, the ovaries produce smaller and smaller amounts of estrogen, progesterone, and testosterone. The changes in a woman's reproductive organs that occur with aging are due mostly to the effect of lower levels of estrogen and progesterone after menopause. The uterus and the ovaries both become smaller and firmer (atrophy). The labia lose fat, connective tissue, and elasticity. The skin of the labia thins, as do the walls of the vagina. In addition, blood flow to the vagina decreases dramatically, causing the vagina to become shorter, narrower, and drier. All of these changes may make sexual intercourse uncomfortable.

The acidity of the vagina decreases with aging, making the genitals more susceptible to irritation and infection. The muscular support structures in the pelvis weaken, which can lead to collapse of any of the pelvic organs (the bladder, intestines, uterus, and rectum) into the vagina. The level of testosterone becomes proportionately higher because lower levels of female sex hormones are being produced. As a result, women may begin to develop very mild characteristics usually associated with men, such as hair loss and growth of facial hair. Within 5 to 10 years of menopause, testosterone levels drop as well, resulting in a decrease in sex drive.

INFLAMMATION OF THE VULVA AND VAGINA

Inflammation of the vulva and vagina is a condition that can lead to many annoying symptoms and problems. Lack of adequate estrogen is the most common cause in older women; vulvar and vaginal inflammation that results from lack of estrogen is called atrophic vaginitis. Lack of estrogen often causes the lining of the urethra to become thin and fragile (atrophic urethritis). These changes in the urethra can lead to increased frequency and urgency of urination and in many cases an uncontrollable loss of urine (urinary incontinence), which can irritate the vulva and worsen existing inflammation.

Use of perfumes and scented laundry detergents, fabric softeners, and soaps can also cause inflammation. Other causes include allergic reactions (allergic vaginitis); changes in the concentration of normal bacteria (bacterial vaginosis) and yeast (*Candida*) in the vagina; and trichomonal or other infections. Candidal (yeast) infections are especially common in older women with diabetes.

Symptoms and Diagnosis

Inflammation, especially if it results from lack of estrogen, causes vaginal and vulvar dryness, itching, burning, and pain. A watery vaginal discharge is sometimes present. A thicker discharge is much more common when infection is present. All of these changes may lead to discomfort or pain during sexual intercourse.

A doctor performs a physical examination to diagnose inflammation. During the examination, the doctor takes a sample of the vaginal discharge to identify bacteria or other organisms.

Treatment

Treatment depends on the cause. Inflammation due to low estrogen levels is treated with estrogen cream. Estrogen cream can be applied directly to the vulva or inserted into the vagina with a plastic applicator. Alternatively, tablets or plastic rings containing time-released estrogen can be inserted into the vagina. Tablets are inserted 2 to 3 nights per week. Rings need to be replaced only once every 3 months. Low-dose estrogen inserted into the vagina is not significantly absorbed into the bloodstream, so women concerned about the possible adverse effects of estrogen have little to worry about.

Inflammation caused by irritants or allergies subsides with avoidance of perfumes and scented soaps and with the use of loose-fitting cotton underwear and clothes. Bacterial infections are treated with antibiotics, and candidal infection is treated with antifungal cream or pills. Corticosteroid creams may provide temporary relief for some women but may initially worsen the burning sensation.

Many older women benefit from using moisturizers, especially just before sexual intercourse. It is best to avoid any that contain perfumes or other unnecessary chemicals that might cause irritation.

VULVAR PAIN

Some older women develop chronic pain of the vulva without obvious signs of inflammation (vulvodynia). The pain occurs most commonly at the vulvar vestibule (vulvar vestibulitis). The condition is diagnosed when pain is limited to the vulva or vestibule and when usual causes of inflammation are absent on examination and testing.

The cause of vulvar pain is unknown but is thought to be due to irritation of the vulva and vestibule by substances in the urine. Treatment includes avoiding foods that contain oxalates (irritating salts formed from a strong acid called oxalic acid), such as chocolate, nuts, berries, and leafy vegetables like spinach. Calcium citrate tablets may be taken to reduce the excretion of oxalates in the urine. In addition, estrogen cream and anesthetics can be applied to the skin.

SKIN DISORDERS OF THE VULVA

Skin disorders of the vulva may cause significant discomfort and can lead to painful scarring. Although these disorders are easily confused with cancer of the vulva,[1] most are not cancers.

Lichen sclerosus, the most common type of vulvar skin dis-

1. see page 799

order, is characterized by white, shiny patches of parchment-like skin on and around the labia. The patches sometimes extend to the area around the anus. The cause is unknown.

Lichen sclerosus sometimes causes intense itching. However, some women have no symptoms, some have only vague discomfort of the vulva, and still others have discomfort that progressively worsens. The patches of skin affected by lichen sclerosus can bleed easily when scratched or rubbed, making sexual intercourse uncomfortable. Without treatment, the disorder can cause scarring and fusing of the labia, making sexual intercourse impossible. Lichen sclerosus can also cause deep cracks around the anus, resulting in painful bowel movements and bleeding. Skin changes caused by lichen sclerosus may increase the risk of vulvar cancer.

A doctor diagnoses lichen sclerosus by performing a biopsy. Treatment helps prevent disease progression and therefore is recommended regardless of whether the disorder is causing discomfort. A corticosteroid cream applied to the affected areas generally provides relief. Testosterone ointment can also be used. Occasionally, treatment involves retinoid drugs (drugs similar to vitamin A), which help reduce breakdown and damage of connective tissue. Antihistamines may relieve itching but can cause confusion and sedation in older women. Surgery may be necessary if the disorder leads to scarring and fusing of the labia.

Squamous hyperplasia is characterized by discrete, thick, white elevations of skin on the vulva. The cause is unknown. Squamous hyperplasia causes itching limited to the affected skin. A doctor performs a biopsy to make a diagnosis. Treatment involves maintaining good vulvar hygiene and using corticosteroid creams. Squamous hyperplasia does not increase the risk of developing cancer of the vulva.

Other skin disorders affect the vulva but may appear on other areas of the body as well. Lichen planus can cause an itchy rash or scarring ulcers in the mouth, in the vagina, or on the vulva. It is occasionally caused by drugs and is treated with estrogen and corticosteroid creams. Psoriasis and seborrheic dermatitis can affect various parts of the body.

Prevention of skin disorders of the vulva involves good vulvar hygiene, which includes avoiding irritating soaps and perfumes. Periodic self-examination of the vulva is also recommended, as is an annual doctor's examination for detection of skin changes that could signal cancer. Women who are unable to see well enough or who lack the flexibility to examine themselves can ask a spouse, partner, or caregiver to do it for them. Without such help, annual doctor's visits may not catch the progression of skin changes in women with a history of previous abnormalities.

VAGINAL BLEEDING

Many older women experience unexpected vaginal bleeding months or even years after their last regular period. Any vaginal bleeding that occurs after the onset of menopause is considered abnormal, even though it is relatively common. Such bleeding can signify pre-cancer or cancer, including cancer of the uterus or vagina, and so should never be ignored. But bleeding has many other causes. A postmenopausal woman may experience vaginal bleeding because the low estrogen levels after menopause make the vaginal tissue thin and fragile. Thickening of the uterine lining usually is caused by estrogen replacement therapy. Other noncancerous causes of vaginal bleeding include growths protruding from the cervical or uterine lining (cervical or uterine polyps), growths in the uterine wall (fibroids), and infections.

Symptoms

Often, vaginal bleeding occurs without any other symptoms. Symptoms that may accompany vaginal bleeding include abdominal or pelvic cramping or discomfort. Such symptoms cannot generally help distinguish cancer from other causes of vaginal bleeding.

Diagnosis

Vaginal bleeding is usually obvious, but its causes may not be. In making a diagnosis, a doctor first performs a physical examination of the vulva, vagina, uterus, and ovaries (a pelvic examination). A Papanicolaou (Pap) test, in which cells from the surface of the cervix are collected, is then performed to identify vaginal or cervical cancer. A biopsy is performed if an abnormal growth is found during the pelvic examination.

If the physical examination and Pap test do not reveal a cause, a biopsy of the uterine lining (endometrial biopsy) is usually performed to rule out cancer of the uterus. This type of biopsy can be done quickly and safely without anesthesia in a doctor's office. Alternatively, an ultrasound of the uterus can be performed to measure the thickness of the lining. If the lining has thickened, fluid can be infused into the uterus during the ultrasound to identify any polyps or fibroids. If none are identified, a biopsy is then performed.

Another way to identify polyps, fibroids, or cancerous tissue is by hysteroscopy, in which a flexible viewing tube is inserted through the vagina and cervix and into the uterus. Hysteroscopy can be performed in the doctor's office or operating room.

Blood tests to assess the blood count may also be useful if bleeding is heavy or has occurred for a long time.

Treatment

Treatment of vaginal bleeding depends on the cause. Bleeding due to estrogen deficiency is treated with estrogen supplements. If a woman taking estrogen or progesterone develops bleeding, the dosage of either can be altered. For example, estrogen can be given in a lower dose. Occasionally, dilation and curettage (D and C) is necessary if bleeding does not respond to dosage changes. Hysteroscopy can be used to remove abnormal tissues. Alternatively, laser, electricity, or heat can be used through the tip of the hysteroscope to destroy the lining of the uterus. Polyps and fibroids can also be removed surgically. A woman whose fibroids are growing larger may need to have them or the entire uterus surgically removed to ensure against the possibility of cancer. Another possible treatment, once it is determined that cancer or other abnormal growths are not the cause of bleeding, is insertion of a progesterone-containing intrauterine device (IUD). A suspected infection of the uterus can be treated with antibiotics. Endometrial and cervical cancer can be treated with a combination of surgery, radiation, and drugs.[1]

1. see page 758

PELVIC SUPPORT DISORDERS

Pelvic support disorders occur when weakened support allows the bladder, rectum, intestines, or uterus to drop down (prolapse) and, in some cases, protrude into the vaginal wall or even protrude through the opening of the vagina.

Causes

Pelvic support disorders occur because the muscles, connective tissue, and ligaments that keep the organs in place weaken over time. Lack of estrogen, damage to the pelvic muscles and nerves from childbearing and prolonged labor, chronic constipation, heavy lifting, and frequent coughing and sneezing can also cause pelvic support disorders. Obesity may be a factor as well.

Symptoms

Symptoms generally include a sense of pelvic or vaginal heaviness or pressure, a feeling of something bulging or protruding into or through the vagina, and discomfort when walking. Symptoms tend to subside when lying down and worsen when standing.

Other symptoms depend on which tissues are affected and which pelvic organ has lost its support. Weakened support that allows the bladder to drop and protrude into the wall of the vagina (cystocele) may cause pelvic pressure, difficulty starting urination, incomplete bladder emptying, uncontrollable loss of urine (urinary incontinence), and recurring urinary infections. Weakened support that allows the rectum to drop and sometimes protrude into the wall of the vagina (rectocele) may cause constipation and a sense of incomplete emptying during bowel movements. Relaxation of the small intestine that allows the small intestine to drop behind the wall of the vagina (enterocele) causes a feeling of fullness and low back pain. Uterine relaxation that allows the uterus to drop and protrude into the vagina (uterine prolapse) may cause low back pain. In general, multiple symptoms may occur when two or more organs (the bladder, rectum, small intestine, and uterus) drop down at the same time.

The most severe of the pelvic support disorders occurs when the uterus and vagina both drop down and protrude completely

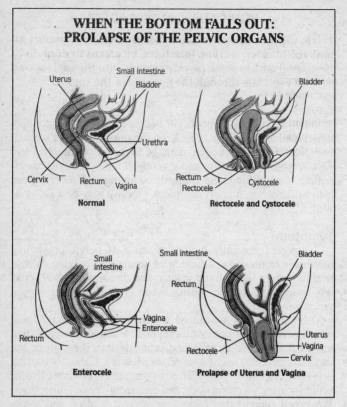

WHEN THE BOTTOM FALLS OUT: PROLAPSE OF THE PELVIC ORGANS

Normal

Uterus — Small intestine — Bladder — Urethra — Cervix — Rectum — Vagina

Rectocele and Cystocele

Bladder — Rectum — Rectocele — Cystocele

Enterocele

Small intestine — Vagina — Enterocele — Rectum

Prolapse of Uterus and Vagina

Small intestine — Rectum — Bladder — Uterus — Vagina — Cervix — Rectocele

through the vaginal opening (procidentia). Symptoms may include a combination of all of the above sensations along with bleeding due to breakdown and development of ulcers in the lining of the exposed vagina and cervix.

Diagnosis and Treatment

Pelvic support disorders are detected during a physical examination, which the doctor may perform with the woman lying or standing. Urine tests, including insertion of a catheter to measure how much urine is left in the bladder, may be useful when a woman has symptoms of bladder relaxation.

Treatment depends on the severity of the disorder. Pelvic relaxation that causes no or only minimal symptoms requires only avoidance of activities that could worsen the disorder—such as heavy lifting and straining during bowel movements—and exercises to strengthen the pelvic muscles (Kegel exercises). [1]

Pelvic relaxation that causes more severe symptoms or that results in prolapse of the uterus and vagina outside the body can be treated in one of two ways: with a pessary or with surgery. A pessary is a latex or silicone support device—often in the shape of a ring, disk, or doughnut—that is inserted into the vagina to support the pelvic structures and relieve symptoms. It is safest when used with estrogen cream to protect the walls of the vagina. Ideally, a woman removes the pessary 1 or 2 nights per week and reinserts it in the morning. For those people who cannot themselves remove or insert the pessary, it should be removed and cleaned after being worn for 4 to 6 weeks. Pessaries are most appropriate when there are reasons to avoid surgery.

Surgery is extremely effective for all pelvic support disorders and in some cases can be performed without general anesthesia. In older women who no longer desire sexual activity, surgery that results in complete closure of the vagina is safe, causes few side effects, and is extremely effective for every form of pelvic support disorder. In sexually active women, reconstructive surgery involves replacement of the pelvic organs into their original positions. The goal of this surgery is to restore normal bladder, bowel, and sexual function. The surgery can be performed either through the vagina or through the abdomen, depending on the type and severity of the problem. Because repositioning the bladder can lead to urinary incontinence, bladder testing may be needed before surgery. This testing, called urodynamics, involves inserting a thin tube (catheter) into the bladder to evaluate the function of the bladder while it is filled and then emptied, during urination, during coughing, and with other maneuvers. In addition, a procedure to prevent incontinence may be needed during surgery.

DECREASED SEXUAL DRIVE

The main sexual disorder affecting older women is a decrease in sexual drive (libido). Decreased libido does not affect

1. see box on page 868

all older women and is not an inevitable result of aging. But it does affect many women. Decreased libido may cause conflict in an important relationship, such as occurs if a woman's desire for sex is much less than her partner's or if it causes a woman to be less sexual than she would like to be.

Causes

Decreased libido has many causes. The low estrogen and testosterone levels that occur with menopause can decrease sexual drive as well as decrease the blood supply to and lubrication of the tissues of the vulva and vagina. This, in turn, can cause pain with intercourse or even with touch and lead the woman to avoid sex. Depression, a condition common among older women, can decrease libido as well. Body changes caused by medical disorders, surgery, or aging itself may decrease libido in many women. Anxiety about body image or performance inhibits some older women, as do beliefs that sexual desire and fantasy are improper or shameful at an older age. In many cases, an older woman has a healthy sexual appetite that may be slowly extinguished if her partner no longer responds to her desire.

The diagnosis of decreased libido is often suspected by the woman herself, but many women do not think to talk to their doctor about the condition and others feel they cannot or should not. Decreased libido can have many treatable causes, however, and generally should be brought to a health care practitioner's attention.

Treatment

Treatment depends on the cause. Communication with a partner about both desire and dissatisfaction is always important. Problems originating in a male partner should be addressed with a doctor trained to treat male sexual problems.

Romantic and sexual experimentation may help the woman overcome boredom. Direct, prolonged stimulation of the clitoris by the woman herself during masturbation or by her partner may help her re-experience desire. Generous use of water-based lubricants may reduce physical discomfort and inhibition.

Hormonal therapy can play an important role. When sexual intercourse is uncomfortable because of atrophic vaginitis, low doses of estrogen can be applied in the vagina. The estrogen can be applied as a cream or tablet or may be contained in a plastic ring that allows it to slowly and steadily leak out into the vagina. Estrogen applied in these ways does not enter the bloodstream in significant amounts, yet the estrogen can maintain tissues of the vagina, keeping them thicker and well lubricated. Testosterone can be supplemented. It is available in pill form, combined with estrogen, and can be obtained in a gel form.

Some drugs used to treat sexual dysfunction in men are currently being studied in women.

I always loved teaching. In high school, I tutored. In college, I joined groups of fellow students who taught each other. I became a teacher of medicine with an emphasis on endocrinology and geriatrics. Finally, as I became geriatric myself, I could teach my contemporaries to maintain health.

Although I was more popular as a lecturer when I spoke with the decisiveness of youth, I think I was better able to teach people as I aged. Why? I think that one's perspective inevitably changes with age and one can take advantage of the change to become more helpful. We learn from experience and thereby become more expert on the subject of life.

Older people, my contemporaries or even older, may have a hard time. Art Linkletter's book on the subject was appropriately titled *Old Age Is Not for Sissies*. As a result of the many assaults of aging, there is a sense of insecurity, of loss of control over what is left of life, and a wealth of questions about how to handle this difficult phase. Yet, there is much to enjoy. When we are old, there is no longer an inhibition against "telling it like it is." We're free to illustrate advice with experiences from our own life. We are not ashamed of being human and subject to the frailties thereof. We no longer compete with contemporaries. Thus, we older people can help each other.

Therein lies the fun side of aging. Having the title "geriatrician" makes it easier, but it is not essential. Any of us can help any other one of us. We can teach from our experiences; we can use the perspective of aging to make aging happier for others; we can share whatever wisdom we've acquired. In this way, we can develop meaningful late-life friendships, companionships, and loves. Transfer of wisdom goes both ways; I learned more from my patients than they learned from me. Now that I am retired, I miss conversations with patients, but I have found that I continue to practice "wisdom-sharing" with family, friends, and neighbors. Aging has its plusses.

David H. Solomon, MD

59

Male Genital and
Sexual Disorders

A man's genitals—the prostate gland, penis, scrotum, and testicles—are responsible for the physical aspect of sexual function. Collectively, these organs are known as the male reproductive system. The prostate gland and the penis have double duty. Because urine passes through them, they are inevitably involved in how the urinary system functions. Thus, problems with the genitals can affect sexual function or, particularly if the prostate gland or penis malfunctions, urination.

Many older men retain the ability to achieve erections, have orgasms, and ejaculate (release semen at orgasm). Nonetheless, aging itself gradually affects sexual function. Erections occur less often, do not last as long, and are less rigid. The penis becomes less sensitive to touch. After orgasm, the penis becomes limp more rapidly, and having another erection takes longer. The volume of fluid ejaculated usually decreases, and ejaculation can occur with little forewarning. Sex drive may decrease, because the level of testosterone (the main male sex hormone) decreases.

Problems with sexual function can result from disorders of the genitals, other disorders, or mental and emotional factors (such as anxiety, fear, or stress). Many sexual problems result from a combination of these factors. Men sometimes feel pressure (from themselves or a partner) to perform well sexually, and they become distressed when they cannot. This feeling is called performance anxiety. Performance anxiety can further reduce a man's ability to enjoy sexual activity.

Benign prostatic hyperplasia, prostatitis, prostate cancer,[1] inguinal hernia, erectile dysfunction (impotence), a decreased sex

1. see page 791

drive, and ejaculation abnormalities become more common with aging. Except for prostate cancer and, very rarely, benign prostatic hyperplasia, these disorders are not life threatening. However, they can cause distress and threaten a man's self-esteem. Men may find talking about these disorders difficult and embarrassing. They may feel that the subject is off-limits for discussion, even with their doctor. But men should not let these feelings prevent them from talking with a doctor, because many of the disorders can be effectively treated.

BENIGN PROSTATIC HYPERPLASIA

Benign prostatic hyperplasia (BPH) is a noncancerous (benign) enlargement of the prostate gland.

The prostate gland is located just under the bladder and surrounds the tube that carries urine from the bladder out of the body (urethra). The prostate gland produces fluid that nourishes sperm. As men age, the prostate gland, which is usually the size of a walnut, enlarges, usually because of BPH. The longer a man lives, the more likely BPH is to develop. The precise cause of BPH is unknown. But changes stimulated by hormones, especially testosterone, are probably involved.

BPH is very unlikely to shorten life. However, as BPH progresses, the urethra can become squeezed (compressed) and partially blocked. The enlarged prostate may prevent the bladder from emptying completely and interfere with the flow of urine. Thus, BPH may cause bothersome symptoms and ultimately damage the bladder and kidneys. Nonetheless, how large the prostate gland is does not always predict how severe the symptoms are. BPH can be effectively treated with drugs and surgery.

Symptoms

When BPH first develops, starting to urinate may be difficult. After urination, the bladder may not empty completely. So shortly thereafter, men may feel the need to urinate again. They may have to urinate more frequently, often at night (a symptom called nocturia). Frequent trips to the bathroom interrupt sleep, sometimes causing irritability and difficulty concentrating during the day. Also, the need to urinate becomes more urgent. The volume and force of the urine flow may decrease noticeably, and urine may dribble after urination is finished.

If the bladder does not empty completely, urine can stagnate there. Then, bladder stones and urinary tract infections are more likely to develop. The urine that remains in the bladder can stretch the bladder too much. Eventually, such stretching leads to uncontrollable leakage of small amounts of urine (overflow incontinence).[1] The bladder can become overactive, leading to an uncontrollable urge to urinate followed by loss of urine (urge incontinence). If urine flow is blocked for a long time, urine backs up in the ureters and the kidneys, which may be damaged.

Symptoms due to BPH can become worse if certain drugs are used. If men with BPH take certain nonprescription drugs, they may be temporarily unable to urinate at all (a condition called urinary retention). These drugs include nonprescription antihistamines (which are in almost all nonprescription sleeping aids, cold remedies, and allergy drugs) and nasal decongestants.

Diagnosis

During a rectal examination, a doctor feels (palpates) the prostate gland to determine whether it is enlarged. The doctor inserts a gloved, lubricated finger into the rectum. The prostate gland can be felt just in front of the rectum. A prostate gland affected by BPH feels enlarged and smooth. But palpation does not cause pain.

For men 50 or over, the doctor may recommend a blood test to measure the level of prostate-specific antigen (PSA). The purpose is to check for prostate cancer.[2] An increase in the PSA level may result from prostate cancer, BPH, or inflammation of the prostate (prostatitis). Nonetheless, PSA measurements may help distinguish between these disorders. The higher the PSA level and the faster it is increasing, the more likely that cancer is the cause. PSA measurements are usually not recommended for men whose life expectancy is less than 10 years because of their age or disorders they have.

If the doctor suspects that the bladder is not emptying completely, a small flexible tube (catheter) may be passed through

1. see page 864
2. see page 791

WHAT HAPPENS WHEN THE PROSTATE GLAND ENLARGES?

In benign prostatic hyperplasia, the prostate gland enlarges. Normally the size of a walnut, the prostate gland may become as large as a tennis ball. The enlarging prostate gland squeezes the urethra, which carries urine out of the body. As a result, urine may flow through more slowly, or less urine may flow through.

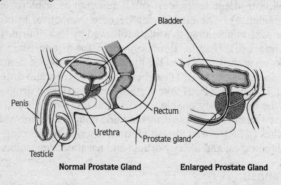

Normal Prostate Gland   **Enlarged Prostate Gland**

the urethra and into the bladder. This procedure (called urinary catheterization) is done after a person urinates as completely as possible. The catheter is used to drain the urine left in the bladder and is then removed. The amount is measured and compared with the range that is considered normal.

A doctor may also take a blood sample, which can be used to assess kidney function. Levels of creatinine and blood urea nitrogen (BUN), both waste products, are measured. Levels are high when the kidneys cannot remove waste products from the blood as they normally do. Thus, high levels indicate kidney damage.

Treatment

For men with BPH, taking extra time to empty the bladder completely when urinating can help prevent infections, bladder stones, and kidney damage. After men urinate once, urinating a second time almost immediately (double voiding) can help empty the bladder. Gently pressing the lower abdomen with the hand may also help. Men who urinate frequently at night should not consume foods or fluids that contain caffeine or excessive amounts of fluids during the hours before sleep.

Treatment is not necessary unless BPH causes bothersome symptoms or blood test results suggest kidney damage.

Alpha-blockers (such as alfuzosin, terazosin, doxazosin, or tamsulosin) relax the urinary sphincter (the band of muscle around the opening between the bladder and the urethra) and the urethra. Thus, urine may flow through more easily. 5-Alpha reductase blockers (such as finasteride and dutasteride) block male hormones from stimulating the prostate gland to grow. The enlarged prostate gland gradually becomes smaller, helping delay the need for surgery or other treatments. However, finasteride or dutasteride may need to be taken for 3 months or more before symptoms are relieved. Saw palmetto, a medicinal herb, appears to relieve symptoms in some men.[1]

If drugs are ineffective, surgery can be performed. Surgery provides the greatest relief of symptoms but can cause problems.

The most common procedure is transurethral resection of the prostate gland (TURP). After an anesthetic is given, a doctor passes a viewing tube (endoscope) through the urethra. Attached to the endoscope is a surgical instrument used to remove part of the prostate gland. TURP can cause infection and bleeding. Some men have urinary incontinence afterward, but it is usually temporary. A few men develop permanent erectile dysfunction (impotence). Occasionally, urine flow becomes blocked again, and TURP must be repeated.

Other surgical procedures provide less symptom relief than TURP, but most are less likely to cause problems. In most of these procedures, an instrument is inserted into the urethra. On the end of the instrument is an attachment used to destroy prostate tissue. Depending on the procedure, the attachment may generate microwave heat, ultrasound waves, electricity, or laser beams. Or the attachment may be a needle.

If a problem such as urinary retention or infection is already present when BPH is diagnosed, the problem may need to be treated before BPH can be treated. Urinary retention can be treated by draining the bladder with a catheter inserted through the urethra.[2] Infections can be treated with antibiotics.

1. see page 84
2. see page 869

PROSTATITIS

Prostatitis is inflammation of the prostate gland. It typically causes pain and swelling.

Prostatitis is common among men of all ages. Usually, prostatitis develops slowly and recurs. This type is called chronic prostatitis. Prostatitis can also develop rapidly. This type is called acute prostatitis. Occasionally, prostatitis causes a collection of pus (abscess) to form in the prostate gland.

Treatment often relieves the symptoms of prostatitis effectively. But prostatitis is sometimes difficult to cure.

Causes

Why chronic prostatitis develops is usually unknown. Sometimes it results from an infection. Acute prostatitis almost always results from an infection. Infections that cause prostatitis are often bacterial. They are rarely fungal, viral, or protozoal.

Symptoms and Diagnosis

Prostatitis causes pain in the area between the scrotum and anus (perineum), in the lower back, and often in the penis and testes. A man may need to urinate frequently and urgently. Urinating may cause pain or burning. Prostatitis may make achieving an erection or ejaculating difficult or even painful. Constipation can develop, making bowel movements painful. Acute bacterial prostatitis commonly causes fever, difficulty urinating, and blood in the urine. These symptoms occasionally occur in other types of prostatitis.

The diagnosis is usually based on the man's symptoms and results of a physical examination. A doctor feels (palpates) the prostate gland by inserting a gloved, lubricated finger into the rectum. The prostate gland may feel swollen and tender when palpated. With the finger still inserted, the doctor may exert gentle pressure (massage) on all parts of the prostate gland. Massaging the prostate gland causes a feeling of pressure but is usually not painful. To confirm the diagnosis, the doctor may ask for a urine sample, which may contain any fluids released when the prostate gland is massaged. The urine sample and fluids are then checked for signs of infection, such as a high white blood cell count or bacteria.

Treatment

Relieving symptoms is an important part of treatment. Frequent ejaculation and sitting in a warm bath can help. Relaxation techniques may relieve pain.

Stool softeners can relieve constipation so that bowel movements are not painful. Pain relievers (analgesics) may be effective. Alpha-blockers, such as doxazosin, terazosin, and tamsulosin, may help relieve symptoms by relaxing the urinary sphincter (the band of muscle around the opening between the bladder and the urethra) and the urethra.

For chronic bacterial prostatitis, antibiotics are the traditional treatment. But their benefit is unclear. An antibiotic that can penetrate prostate tissue, such as ofloxacin, levofloxacin, ciprofloxacin, or trimethoprim-sulfamethoxazole, is taken by mouth for 4 to 6 weeks.

Acute bacterial prostatitis can usually be cured with antibiotics. The same antibiotics used to treat chronic bacterial prostatitis are taken for 2 to 3 weeks.

If an abscess develops in the prostate gland or in the urinary system, it must be drained by making a surgical incision.

INGUINAL HERNIA

An inguinal hernia is the bulging of a loop of intestine through an opening in the wall that surrounds the organs in the abdomen (abdominal wall).

The loop bulges into the inguinal canal. The inguinal canal surrounds the vas deferens, the tube that carries sperm from the testes to the urethra. The loop may bulge into the groin and often extends into the scrotum.

The opening in the abdominal wall may be present from birth. Or it may develop later in life, when the tissues eventually tear after years of being stretched.

If the loop of intestine can be easily pushed back through the opening into the abdomen, the hernia is said to be reducible. A reducible inguinal hernia may slide back and forth as pressure on the abdomen changes. Rarely, the loop of intestine swells and becomes too large to slide back through the opening. Then the loop is trapped outside of the abdomen (incarcerated). If a

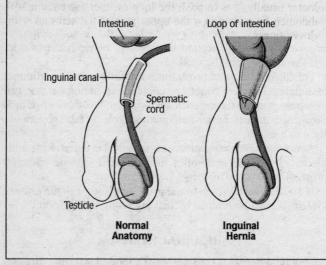

WHAT IS AN INGUINAL HERNIA?

In an inguinal hernia, a loop of intestine bulges through an opening in the abdominal wall into the inguinal canal. The inguinal canal contains the spermatic cord, which consists of the vas deferens, blood vessels, nerves, and other structures.

Intestine

Loop of intestine

Inguinal canal

Spermatic cord

Testicle

Normal Anatomy

Inguinal Hernia

hernia is incarcerated, the loop may be so tightly wedged in the opening that its blood supply is cut off. Such a hernia is said to be strangulated. The affected tissues are deprived of oxygen, which is carried to tissues by blood. Without oxygen, the tissues die within hours, and the intestine is damaged. Gangrene can result. Intestinal gangrene can cause severe infections in the abdomen (peritonitis) and in the blood (sepsis).

Symptoms and Diagnosis

An inguinal hernia usually produces a painless bulge in the groin or scrotum. If the hernia can slide back and forth, the bulge may enlarge when a man stands or strains. The bulge may get smaller or disappear when the man lies down. If the hernia is incarcerated, the bulge does not get smaller or disappear. Strangulated hernias usually become very painful within minutes or hours.

To diagnose an inguinal hernia, a doctor examines the groin and the area around it. For the examination, a man may have to stand and cough or strain. Coughing or straining produces pressure in the abdomen and makes a hernia more obvious. To determine whether the hernia is reducible or incarcerated, the doctor usually tries to push the loop of intestine back into the abdomen by pushing on the upper part of the scrotum with a gloved finger.

Treatment

If the loop of intestine cannot be readily pushed back into the abdomen, the doctor may try another maneuver to temporarily relieve symptoms. The man lies with his head lower than his body. Sometimes an ice pack is placed on the hernia. The doctor then tries to push the loop of intestine back again. The pushing may be continued for what seems to be a long time.

For some hernias, surgery is needed. If a reducible inguinal hernia causes bothersome symptoms, surgery can be done to close the opening in the abdominal wall. Large hernias are often surgically repaired because they are likely to become incarcerated. Incarcerated hernias are almost always repaired because they can become strangulated. For these procedures, men who are in good general health may need only a local anesthetic. They can usually go home the same day.

If a hernia is strangulated, surgery is needed immediately. Damaged parts of the intestine are usually removed. Then the healthy parts are connected.

Outlook

Most inguinal hernias are merely a nuisance, causing an embarrassing bulge in the groin and mild discomfort. However, the bulge and discomfort may gradually worsen. If a hernia becomes strangulated, life-threatening infections can develop within hours.

ERECTILE DYSFUNCTION

Erectile dysfunction (impotence) is difficulty achieving or maintaining an erection.

Occasionally, every man has difficulty achieving an erection. Erectile dysfunction occurs when the problem is frequent or

---

MENTAL AND EMOTIONAL CAUSES OF SEXUAL DYSFUNCTION

- Anger toward a partner
- Anxiety
- Depression
- Discord or boredom with a partner
- Fear of dependence on another person
- Fear of losing control
- Feelings of detachment from sexual activities
- Guilt
- Inhibitions or ignorance about sexual behavior
- Performance anxiety (worrying about performance during intercourse)
- Previous traumatic sexual experiences, such as sexual abuse or previous sexual dysfunction

---

continuous. Erectile dysfunction becomes more common with aging. Although about half of men aged 65 or over and three fourths of men aged 80 or over have erectile dysfunction, it is not a normal part of aging.

For erections to occur during sexual activity, there must first be interest in sexual activity. Such interest requires enough testosterone as well as stimulation by sexual thoughts, sights, smells, or touch. Men also need enough energy to participate. Blood must be able to get to the penis (through arteries). Muscles at the base of the penis must contract, squeezing (compressing) the veins there and thus preventing blood from leaving the penis. Blood then fills the fibrous tissue in the penis (corpora cavernosa), causing the penis to become larger (called engorgement). As a result, the penis becomes rigid. Involuntary (autonomic) nerves control the process. Aging itself does not prevent the process from working.

Causes

Erectile dysfunction may be caused by mental or emotional factors or by physical disorders. It can also result from taking certain prescription or nonprescription drugs or drinking too much alcohol.

ADDITIONAL DETAIL

Anything that decreases a man's energy level (such as illness, fatigue, or stress) can make erections difficult. Mental and emotional factors that can interfere with erections include depression, worrying about performance during intercourse (performance anxiety), guilt, stressful relationships, a change of sex partner, and fear of intimacy.

Disorders that damage any of the body parts involved in producing erections can cause erectile dysfunction. These disorders are much more common among older men.

- **Arteries:** Atherosclerosis and diabetes can damage arteries, causing them to become gradually blocked. Then arteries may not be able to carry enough blood to the penis, and the penis cannot become rigid.
- **Veins:** Some conditions make the veins of the penis drain blood back to the body too rapidly during erections. Then an erection cannot be maintained. These conditions include Peyronie's disease, injuries (including those that may occur during surgery), and scarring in the penis. As men age, scarring becomes more likely. But aging alone does not cause scarring.
- **Nerves:** If the nerves of the penis are damaged, control of blood flow in and out of the penis may be disrupted. Such damage may be due to a stroke, a spinal disorder, peripheral neuropathy, diabetes, or multiple sclerosis. The nerves can be damaged by some surgical procedures, particularly those used to treat prostate gland disorders. Examples are transurethral resection of the prostate gland (TURP) and removal of the prostate (prostatectomy, usually used to treat prostate cancer).
- **Hormones:** Infrequently, a low level of testosterone causes erectile dysfunction.

Drugs can interfere with erections. Examples are antihypertensive drugs, antidepressants, antipsychotics, certain sleep aids, cimetidine, digoxin, and lithium. Drinking too much alcohol can cause temporary erectile dysfunction. Shakespeare commented on this effect of alcohol: "It provokes the desire, but it takes away the performance."

Symptoms and Diagnosis

Some men with erectile dysfunction have a decreased sex drive (libido), particularly if the testosterone level is low. However, many men with erectile dysfunction have a normal sex drive. Regardless of sex drive, men with erectile dysfunction have difficulty engaging in sexual intercourse. Either the erect penis is not hard enough for penetration or the erection cannot be maintained. Men with severe erectile dysfunction may not be able to achieve an erection.

To diagnose erectile dysfunction, a doctor examines the man's genitals and rectum. During the examination, the doctor evaluates how the nerves and blood vessels that supply the genitals are functioning. The pulse and blood pressure in the legs are measured. Abnormalities in these measurements may indi-

---

TESTOSTERONE THERAPY: TREATMENT FOR MALE MENOPAUSE?

At about age 30, men begin to produce less testosterone (the main male sex hormone). Usually, production decreases an average of 1 to 2% a year. This decrease and its effects are less dramatic than the usually rapid, nearly universal hormonal changes that occur in women during menopause. Nonetheless, the decrease in testosterone production is sometimes called male menopause or andropause. How rapidly testosterone levels decrease varies greatly among men. Many men in their 70s have a testosterone level that matches that of the average man in his 30s.

Men with a low testosterone level may develop certain characteristics associated with aging. They may have a decreased sex drive (libido) or erectile dysfunction (impotence). They may have less muscle, more abdominal fat, porous bones that easily fracture (osteoporosis), and less energy. Complex mental tasks may take longer. The red blood cell count may be low, resulting in anemia. If the testosterone level is very low, breasts may enlarge, testicles may shrink, and pubic hair may be lost.

Many men—regardless of their testosterone level—are interested in taking testosterone to slow or reverse these effects. But testosterone is helpful only if the testosterone level is abnormally low.

The most worrisome side effect of testosterone therapy is worsening of a prostate gland disorder. Testosterone can make prostate cancers grow. Consequently, it is not given to men with prostate cancer. However, many men have undiagnosed prostate cancer. So some doctors worry that testosterone therapy may make such a cancer grow. Testosterone can also worsen benign prostatic hyperplasia.

Testosterone therapy is recommended only for men who have a low testosterone level (determined by a blood test), who have symptoms of testosterone deficiency, and who do not have a prostate disorder. Usually, testosterone is applied as a gel or a patch or is injected. Men taking testosterone should be checked frequently for prostate cancer. Such testing may detect cancers early, when they are more likely to be cured.

cate a problem with arteries in the pelvis and groin that supply blood to the penis. If a problem with the arteries or veins is suspected, ultrasonography is done to check for blockages in the arteries of the penis. A blood sample is often taken to measure the testosterone level.

Treatment

Depending on the cause, the only treatment needed may be reducing alcohol consumption, having a doctor substitute a different drug, or taking testosterone therapy. Psychologic therapy that deals with the mental and emotional factors contributing to erectile dysfunction sometimes corrects the dysfunction. In contrast, if the blood vessels or nerves supplying the penis are damaged, dysfunction usually cannot be fully corrected. However, with treatment, an erection may be possible despite the damage.

Most drugs used to treat erectile dysfunction work regardless of the cause. However, these drugs are particularly effective if erectile dysfunction results from inadequate blood flow to the penis. Most of them increase blood flow to the penis. Examples are sildenafil, tadalafil, and vardenafil. These drugs are taken by mouth. Men who take a nitrate, such as nitroglycerin, to treat a heart disorder should not take sildenafil, tadalafil, or vardenafil. If nitrates are taken within several hours of taking one of these drugs, blood pressure may become dangerously low, and occasionally, death results. Alprostadil also increases blood flow to the penis. This drug is inserted into the urethra as a pellet (suppository). Some drugs (such as alprostadil given alone or with papaverine and phentolamine) can be injected into the penis if sildenafil, tadalafil, or vardenafil does not help.

Mechanical devices can increase the amount of blood in the penis and thus help men achieve erections. For example, constriction devices, such as bands and rings made of rubber or leather, can be placed at the base of the penis to slow the flow of blood out of the penis. Constriction devices can be purchased with a doctor's prescription in a pharmacy. Inexpensive versions (often called "cock rings") can be purchased in stores that sell sexual paraphernalia.

Constriction devices should not be left on for more than 30 minutes. Occasionally, they cause bruising, particularly in men who have a blood clotting disorder or who are taking a drug that makes blood less likely to clot (anticoagulant).

Constriction devices are often used with an alprostadil suppository or a vacuum device.

A vacuum device consists of a hollow chamber attached to a source of suction. The device fits over the penis, creating a seal. When suction is applied, blood is drawn into the blood vessels in the penis. After an erection is achieved, a constriction device is used to keep blood in the penis, maintaining the erection.

When all other treatments are ineffective, a prosthesis can be surgically implanted in the penis. Several types of prostheses are available. For example, firm rods may be inserted into the penis. This prosthesis makes the penis permanently hard. Or an inflatable balloon may be inserted into the penis. Before having intercourse, the man inflates the balloon with a small pump, which may be part of the prosthesis.

DECREASED SEX DRIVE

Sex drive (libido) is considered decreased when interest in sexual activity is infrequent or apathetic.

Sex drive varies greatly among men. It tends to gradually decrease as men age. In some men, sex drive decreases substantially and remains decreased. In a few men, sex drive is decreased throughout life.

Sex drive can decrease temporarily because of fatigue. Alcohol, by suppressing social inhibitions, sometimes seems to increase sex drive. However, alcohol can temporarily decrease sex drive. Some drugs decrease sex drive as long as they are taken. They include antihypertensive drugs, antidepressants, certain sleep aids, and digoxin. A low level of testosterone can greatly decrease sex drive.

Mental or emotional factors may decrease sex drive temporarily or indefinitely.[1]

Men with a decreased sex drive lose interest in masturbation and sexual fantasies. Even sexual stimulation—by touch, sights, smells, or words—does not provoke interest. However, these

1. see box on page 894

SEXUAL ACTIVITY AND HEART DISORDERS

Heart disorders—including coronary artery disease, heart failure, abnormal heart rhythms, and heart valve disorders such as aortic stenosis—are very common among older men. A man who has a heart disorder may worry that sexual activity could be dangerously stressful to his heart.

Generally, sexual activity is safe for older men with a heart disorder. Sexual activity is no more stressful on the heart than climbing one or two flights of stairs. The risk of having a heart attack is slightly higher during sexual activity than it is during rest, but the risk is still very low. The risk appears to be highest when having sex with a new partner.

Nevertheless, a sexually active man who has a heart disorder or high blood pressure needs to take reasonable precautions. Usually, sexual activity is safe if the disorder is mild, if it causes few symptoms, and if blood pressure is controlled to a normal or near normal level. If the disorder is moderately severe or if the man has other conditions that make a heart attack likely, tests may be necessary to determine how safe sexual activity is. If the disorder is severe or interferes with blood flow from the left ventricle (as can occur in heart failure or aortic stenosis), sexual activity should be postponed until after treatment reduces the severity of the symptoms. Sexual activity should also be postponed at least 2 to 6 weeks after a heart attack.

If a man takes a nitrate, such as nitroglycerin, to treat a heart disorder, taking sildenafil or vardenafil (for erectile dysfunction) is dangerous. Nitrates can cause dangerously low blood pressure if they are taken within several hours of sildenafil.

Most often, tests to determine the safety of sexual activity are done during exercise on a treadmill. The tests involve monitoring the heart to determine whether its blood supply is adequate. If the blood supply is adequate during exercise, a heart attack during sexual activity is very unlikely.

men may still be able to function sexually. Some men continue participating in sexual activity to satisfy their partner.

The diagnosis is usually based on the man's description of his symptoms. A blood test is done to measure the level of testosterone.

Treatment of a decreased sex drive depends on the cause. Psychologic therapies that deal with mental and emotional factors may help. If the cause appears to be a drug, a doctor can often try substituting a different drug. If the testosterone level is low, testosterone therapy can be used. Testosterone is usually given as a gel or patch applied to the skin daily. It can be given as an injection, usually every 2 weeks, but injections have no advantage over daily skin application.

RETROGRADE EJACULATION

In retrograde ejaculation, semen travels backward into the bladder, rather than forward out of the penis.

Retrograde ejaculation occurs because the urinary sphincter (the band of muscle around the opening between the bladder and urethra) does not contract and close as it normally does during ejaculation. Thus, semen can travel into the bladder. Common causes include diabetes, spinal cord injuries, certain drugs (especially some used to treat high blood pressure), and some surgical procedures (such as major abdominal or pelvic surgery, particularly transurethral resection of the prostate gland, or TURP).

Symptoms and Diagnosis

The amount of fluid ejaculated from the penis is decreased. Sometimes no fluid comes out. These changes may puzzle or worry some men. Nonetheless, many men with retrograde ejaculation have orgasms and enjoy sexual activity.

Retrograde ejaculation is diagnosed when a large number of sperm are found in a urine sample.

Treatment and Outlook

Most men need no treatment. However, if the disorder is worrisome, it can be treated. Treatment is often effective.

Treatment involves taking drugs that cause the urinary sphincter to contract and close, such as pseudoephedrine, phenylephrine, chlorpheniramine, brompheniramine, or imipra-mine. However, most of these drugs can increase heart rate and blood pressure. These effects can be dangerous in men with high blood pressure or coronary artery disease.

Retrograde ejaculation is not harmful. About one third of men who are treated improve.

60

Exercise

Exercise—physical activity done regularly—is something people can and should do for a lifetime. It helps people feel and function better physically and mentally. It also helps reduce the risk of many disorders. Older age is not a reason to stop exercising. And it should not stop people from starting. In fact, doing regular exercise becomes more important as people age. Exercise can help keep older people active and living independently longer. Exercise can make even the frailest older person stronger and more fit.

Older people may have many concerns about exercising. They may think they are too old to start. They may think they have too many aches and pains. They may fear injury. They may think they have a disorder that prevents them from exercising. However, these obstacles can be overcome. In fact, exercise can reduce them. It can make people feel younger and better. It can lessen some symptoms that may be blamed on aging. And it can help people avoid or delay some disorders.

Older people may worry that they cannot do most exercises. However, almost everyone can become more active and exercise in a way that benefits health. Exercise does not have to mean a structured exercise program. It does not have to include such things as sit-ups, push-ups, or jogging. Exercise can be simple activities such as walking. Increasing the amount of time being active each day can also be a part of exercise. Classic examples are taking the stairs rather than the elevator and walking rather than driving when possible.

Exercise also does not have to involve working up a drenching sweat. Moderate exercise, preferably every day, provides significant health benefits. The key is doing enough moderately active things regularly. Exercise can also be done in small blocks of time. Less vigorous exercise can be done for a longer time. The more exercise (done more vigorously and for a longer time), the greater the benefits. But any exercise is better than none.

WHY EXERCISE?

Exercise may be the closest thing to the fountain of youth available. It improves overall health and appearance. It can maintain some of the body's functions that decline with aging. It can even restore some functions that have already declined. In addition, people who exercise—regardless of how much they weigh, whether they smoke, or whether they have a disorder—tend to live longer than those who do not exercise.

Specifically, exercise can do the following:

• Make the heart stronger. Then the heart can pump more oxygen-rich blood to the body with each heartbeat.
• Improve circulation. For example, muscles in the legs squeeze leg veins and help them return blood to the heart. Strengthening these muscles helps them do it more effectively.
• Decrease blood pressure.
• Decrease the levels of total and low density lipoprotein (LDL) cholesterol—the "bad" cholesterol—and increase the level of high density (HDL) cholesterol—the "good" cholesterol.
• Make muscles stronger and increase flexibility. As a result, people may be able to do more activities or do them more easily.
• Make bones denser and stronger if the exercise involves weight bearing. Weight bearing means that the body is supporting its entire weight. Examples are walking, stair climbing, and dancing. Swimming is not a weight-bearing exercise.
• Improve balance and coordination.
• Help prevent falls and fractures.
• Burn calories and thus help maintain a healthy weight.
• Help control the level of sugar in the blood and thus help prevent or control diabetes.
• Boost the immune system. The body is then better able to fight off infections.

- Increase the level of endorphins. Endorphins are chemicals in the brain that reduce pain and induce a sense of well-being. Thus, exercise may help improve mood and energy levels and may even lessen depression.
- Improve mental alertness and the ability to concentrate.
- Help with sleep.
- Make constipation less likely.

Exercise reduces the risk of coronary artery disease, heart attack, stroke, colon cancer, osteoporosis, and type 2 diabetes. It may reduce the risk of breast cancer. Risk factors for many of these disorders include obesity, abnormal cholesterol levels, high blood pressure, and, most obviously, physical inactivity. Exercise helps control all of them.

People benefit from exercise only as long as they continue exercising. If they stop, the benefits decrease within months.

STARTING TO EXERCISE

Most healthy people, regardless of age, can safely exercise at a moderate level without consulting a doctor first. Reasons to talk with a doctor first include having a disorder[1] or taking a prescription drug, especially one used to treat a chronic disorder. People who have risk factors for atherosclerosis (which can cause coronary artery disease or stroke) should be evaluated using an exercise stress test[2] before starting to exercise. If people do not know whether they have these risk factors, they should check with their doctor. People who have not exercised previously may benefit from talking with their doctor before starting.

How hard, how long, and how often to exercise are common questions. Starting with relatively less vigorous exercise for relatively short times is safest. How vigorous exercise is (intensity) can be determined by counting the number of heartbeats each minute (heart rate) or by observing how heavy breathing and sweating are. The intensity and length of exercise time should be comfortable. Exercise is too intense if a person cannot comfortably talk. Exercise is most beneficial when done at least 3 times a week.

1. see page 907
2. see page 662

MODERATE OR VIGOROUS?

Moderate Aerobic Exercise	Vigorous Aerobic Exercise
Bicycling	Brisk bicycling up hills
Cycling on a stationary bicycle	Climbing stairs or hills
Dancing	Cross-country skiing
Gardening, including mowing and raking	Digging holes
	Downhill skiing
Golf, without a cart	Hiking
Mopping or scrubbing the floor	Jogging
Rowing	Shoveling snow
Swimming	Swimming laps
Tennis (doubles)	Tennis (singles)
Volleyball	
Walking briskly on a level surface	

As people get used to exercising, they should gradually increase exercise time over a period of several weeks until exercise can be done for 30 minutes comfortably. As people get stronger, they may want to increase how vigorously they exercise.

Injury is one of the main reasons people stop exercising. Warming up muscles before exercising and cooling down after exercising can help prevent injury.

Warming up means doing the same movements as the exercise but doing them less vigorously. For example, a person should walk slowly first, then speed up. Or a person should gently go through the motions of hitting or serving a tennis ball before starting to play. Warming up increases the temperature of muscles by increasing blood flow. Warm muscles are more flexible and less likely to tear than cold muscles. People should warm up for about 5 minutes.

Cooling down means slowing down gradually at the end of exercise. When exercise is stopped suddenly, blood collects in the legs and not enough blood goes to the brain, causing dizziness. People should cool down for about 5 minutes.

If pain is felt during exercise, people should stop exercising immediately. The pain of injury is different from muscle soreness, which usually occurs shortly after exercise has ended.

People should choose exercise that they enjoy and will continue. Varying the types of exercise can help keep people interested and motivated. Different types of exercise also work muscles in different ways and conditions them more effectively. Exercising with another person or to music can also help keep people exercising.

TYPES OF EXERCISE

Exercise should include the three main types: endurance (aerobic), strengthening (resistive, formerly called anaerobic), and stretching or flexibility (range-of-motion) exercises. Balance exercises are also important.

Aerobic exercise requires that oxygen get from the air through the bloodstream to the muscles, where it is used to produce energy. Thus, the heart and lungs are forced to work harder than normal. Aerobic exercise strengthens the heart and lungs and supplies the body with larger amounts of oxygen-rich blood. Aerobics also burns many calories. To be aerobic, exercise must be continued for at least 20 minutes, according to many experts. Walking, running, biking, rowing, swimming, dancing, and skating are aerobic exercise. Aerobic exercise should be done three to seven times a week.

Strengthening exercise involves contracting muscles against resistance for up to 6 seconds at a time. Holding a contraction longer can increase blood pressure too much. There are two types: isotonic and isometric. Isotonic exercise involves moving the muscle against some form of resistance, such as gravity, weights, or rubber bands. (Weights may consist of cans of food or milk jugs filled with sand.) Isometric exercise involves contracting a muscle without moving a joint. The muscle is contracted and released several times. For example, in Kegel exercises, the muscles around the vagina, urethra, and rectum—the muscles used to stop the flow of urine—are contracted and then relaxed several times.

The main purpose of strengthening exercise is to make muscles stronger. Strengthening muscles is particularly important for older people because as people age, the amount of muscle tissue (muscle mass) and muscle strength tend to decrease. This type of exercise also benefits the heart and lungs but not as much as aerobic exercise. Strengthening exercise does not burn as many calories as aerobic exercise. But by increasing muscle mass, strengthening exercise eventually leads to changes in the body that make the body burn more calories. Strengthening the legs helps with balance because balance requires strong leg muscles. Strengthening exercises should be done about two or three times a week. Exercises for the same muscles should not be done 2 days in a row.

Some activities combine aerobic and strengthening exercise. For example, riding a stationary bike is aerobic (increasing endurance) and strengthens the leg muscles.

Stretching lengthens muscles and tendons and thereby improves flexibility and helps prevent injury. A person should stretch only after warming up or exercising, when the muscles are warm and less likely to tear. At first, each stretch should be held for 5 seconds, which is increased to 20 to 30 seconds as the person becomes more flexible. Then the person relaxes and does the same stretch again, stretching farther if possible. Stretching exercises should be done 5 to 7 days a week.

If a pool is available, aerobic, strengthening, and stretching exercises can often be done in water more easily than on land. Water provides resistance that improves endurance and strengthens muscles. Water takes some stress off joints. It also provides support so that people are less likely to lose their balance. Some pools are designed specifically for exercise or therapy. In these pools, the water is no deeper than midchest level. Some communities offer water aerobic classes. Walking laps in a pool can provide similar benefits.

Some exercises are designed specifically to help improve balance. An example is balancing on one foot. This exercise can be done anytime anywhere. Standing up and sitting down without using the hands also improves balance. Tai Chi may improve balance and flexibility. Tai Chi involves a series of gentle and controlled movements, which resemble a slow dance. The whole body is used, and joints are moved through their range of motion. Careful attention is paid to breathing and posture. Tai Chi also focuses on calming the mind.

EXERCISE FOR PEOPLE WITH A DISORDER

Before starting to exercise, people with a disorder should talk with their doctor. If people have several disorders, such as heart failure and arthritis, deciding on an exercise program can be more complicated. The help of a doctor or trainer who specializes in helping older people is needed. Some disorders, such as unstable angina, abnormal heart rhythms not controlled with treatment, and severe heart failure, prevent people from exercising.

When starting an exercise program, people who have a disorder that limits their physical activity need supervision and instruction, at least at first. They may work with a physical therapist or a private trainer who understands their disorder. Trainers can be located by contacting the American College of Sports Medicine or the American Council on Exercise. Such experts can help people set realistic exercise goals. Or people may join an exercise class designed for people with disorders. Some people may be able to follow a program set up by their doctor. The doctor discusses their efforts and progress periodically by phone or at visits to the doctor's office. People may be given a logbook or diary to keep track of their daily exercise.

Exercise videos for people with a specific disorder, such as arthritis or Parkinson's disease, can be useful.

Arthritis

After consulting with their doctor, people with arthritis should start with stretching and strengthening exercises. As they improve their physical condition, they can gradually add aerobic exercises. An exercise program should involve the whole body, not just the affected joints. People with arthritis should check with their doctor, a fitness instructor, or a physical therapist familiar with exercise for people with arthritis about which exercises are appropriate and how to do the exercises correctly (using the proper form). Doing each exercise correctly is particularly important for people with arthritis. For example, if people with arthritis in the knees do exercises to strengthen the leg muscles but do them incorrectly, the knee joint may be stressed too much.

Initially, physical activity can cause or worsen pain in people with arthritis or make them feel tired. However, limiting activities can result in loss of muscle mass and weight gain, which can worsen pain and joint damage. Exercise reduces pain, fatigue, and depression. It also seems to reduce inflammation. It enables people with arthritis to do their normal daily activities better.

Stretching is particularly important. People with arthritis often keep the affected joints bent because this position temporarily relieves pain. However, this tactic can result in permanent loss of mobility and can make doing daily activities more difficult. Stretching exercises help maintain a joint's flexibility and function. These exercises also stimulate cartilage to repair itself.

Stretching exercises involve gently bending and straightening the joint as far as it can go comfortably. Gradually, it is bent and straightened farther and farther until it has a normal or nearly normal range of motion. Stretching exercises for each joint should be done 5 to 7 days a week. Five repetitions one or two times a day can maintain flexibility.

Strong muscles help protect joints. Isometric exercises do not involve moving the joint and may be less painful. Thus, they are good strengthening exercises to start with. Isotonic exercises, which involve moving the joint, help improve flexibility as well as strengthen muscles.

Because the hands are affected early and severely, hand-strengthening exercises are particularly important. Crumpling pieces of paper or squeezing a ball of putty can help. (A rubber ball should not be used.) Exercises that stretch and strengthen the muscles around the hip, in the thigh, and in the abdomen are also recommended.

Aerobic exercise that does not stress the joints is recommended. Rapid, repetitive movements should be avoided. Walking or low-impact aerobics is a good choice. Shoes should be selected carefully. Shoe inserts (orthotics) may be needed to help cushion impact or to prevent the feet from turning in or out.

If walking or low-impact aerobics is too painful, swimming and water aerobics are good alternatives. Water aerobics uses the resistance of the water to improve endurance and strengthen muscles. Many people with arthritis are surprised to discover that exercise is much less painful in water. The water takes some of the stress off the joints. Finding a pool that is used for therapy can help because such pools are usually warmer than recreational pools. Warm water helps reduce stiffness and pain. Therapeutic pools may have ramps for easier access in and out.

People with arthritis should stop exercising if they become unusually tired or weak, if they feel sharp or increased pain, if joints swell more, or if range of motion decreases. They should then contact their doctor or therapist promptly.

Coronary Artery Disease

An exercise stress test, often used to diagnose coronary artery disease,[1] can help determine how well the heart and lungs tolerate exercise (exercise capacity). With this information, doctors are better able to give a person a specific program to follow.

For people who have had a heart attack, angioplasty, or coronary artery bypass graft surgery, an exercise program begins in the hospital with rehabilitation.[2] After discharge from the hospital, they continue the program in a hospital or exercise facility, where exercise is supervised. There, people are taught how to exercise safely. For example, they learn to monitor the intensity of exercise by using a heart rate counter or by counting the number of steps taken during a certain time period. After about 12 weeks, people continue a maintenance exercise program on their own or in community-based exercise classes.

Aerobic exercise is the main focus for people with coronary artery disease. Stretching and strengthening exercises may also be recommended. People who have had a heart attack may be concerned about adding resistance to strengthen muscles. However, as muscle tone and endurance improve, most people can add resistance with light weights, elastic bands, or exercise equipment. People with symptoms that vary a lot, abnormal heart rhythms, or high blood pressure that cannot be controlled should not add resistance.

1. see page 662
2. see page 179

Dementia

Before people with dementia start exercising, they or their caregiver should check with a doctor. When exercising, people with dementia must be supervised, usually by a caregiver. Supervision is necessary to make sure that they do not hurt themselves and that they exercise correctly. Caregivers may join in the exercise. Doing so can help reduce the stress of caregiving and provide the person with dementia with companionship and a sense of belonging. Alternatively, some senior centers offer exercise classes that are appropriate for people with dementia.

For people with dementia, regular exercise can provide a sense of accomplishment. Exercise can have a calming effect. It may improve sleep.

Diabetes

Before starting to exercise, people with diabetes should have a complete physical examination. A doctor or other health care practitioner can help with choosing appropriate exercises. For example, if the feet have lost feeling, swimming or bicycling may be a better choice than walking. If vision is poor, exercising indoors may be better. Regular exercise improves the body's response to insulin and helps make insulin and the drugs used to treat diabetes more effective.

Ideally, people with diabetes, especially if it is not well controlled, should exercise with a buddy. Exercise can cause the blood sugar level to become very low. A low blood sugar level can cause dizziness or fainting. To prevent the blood sugar level from becoming too low, people with diabetes should be sure to have a food or drink high in sugar with them. They should check their blood sugar level before, during, and after exercising. After an exercise program is started, the dose of any drugs taken to treat diabetes may need to be reduced.

Shoes should be chosen carefully. After exercising, people should check the skin of their feet for blisters, warm areas, redness, and tears, which could result in infection.

Disabilities

Exercise can help reduce the likelihood of problems that can result from having a disability. For example, improving strength and general fitness can prevent people from becoming tired when doing daily activities. A structured exercise program can help balance the use of muscles, which tend to be overused or misused because of a disability.

Heart Failure

People with heart failure usually need to be supervised during exercise at first. They should begin slowly and focus on exercising at a low intensity for a longer time. They may need to warm up longer (10 to 15 minutes). Alternating periods of exercise and rest is helpful. For example, people can exercise for 2 to 4 minutes, then rest 1 minute, until they can exercise for 15 minutes without resting. The time is gradually increased until they can exercise for 20 to 30 minutes without resting.

Aerobic exercise is important for people with heart failure. But exercises to strengthen the muscles used in breathing (including the diaphragm), abdomen, and legs can help lessen breathlessness and make exercise less tiring.

If chest pain occurs, breathlessness increases, or the legs swell, people should stop exercising and contact their doctor.

Lung Disorders

People with chronic lung disorders, such as chronic obstructive pulmonary disease, should start with a little exercise and build up very gradually. Gradually building up is important because these disorders make moving air in and out of the lungs with each breath take longer. So exercising can make people feel as if they have no time to breathe. With the help of a doctor, exercise can be scheduled when the effects of the drugs used to treat the disorder are greatest. Doctors can also advise people about whether taking an extra dose before exercise can help.

Exercise improves the way the body uses oxygen, so people with a lung disorder can breathe more easily and feel better. Then they can be more active. Exercise also improves mood and quality of life. Even a small amount of exercise helps.

People with a lung disorder can start by exercising their arms and legs while they are sitting. They can progress to walking from room to room, then outside, and then greater distances. Learning how to control breathing can help. When breathing in, people should relax the upper body and shoulders and push the abdomen out rather than suck it in. That way, the lungs have more room to expand and can take in more oxygen.

Low-impact aerobic exercise and exercises that target the upper body, particularly the muscles involved in breathing, are recommended.

Some people with a chronic lung disorder may benefit from using extra oxygen (oxygen therapy) when they exercise. They can use a portable oxygen system. Some medical insurance policies cover this use of oxygen therapy if the need is documented by a doctor. People who are already using oxygen therapy may need to talk with a doctor about increasing the amount of oxygen during exercise.

Parkinson's Disease

Before starting to exercise, people with Parkinson's disease should be evaluated by a doctor. Such people often have problems with blood pressure, which can affect choice of exercise. A doctor, physical therapist, or exercise class leader familiar with the disease can recommend appropriate exercises.

Exercise can help prevent the decrease in strength and stamina and the muscle rigidity that people with Parkinson's disease experience. By strengthening muscles and improving flexibility, exercise can also help maintain mobility and balance. Exercise may help people who have difficulty starting a movement. By improving blood flow, exercise can make drugs used to treat the disease more effective.

Stretching exercises are useful. Muscles should be moved through their full range of motion. Walking and yoga (because movements are slow) are good choices. Poles, similar to those used in cross-country skiing, can be used when walking to help with balance. Exercising in a warm pool may reduce stiffness and make movement easier. The pool should have a railing to help people balance.

Because controlling movement is difficult, people with Parkinson's disease may need to be very focused when they exercise. They should think about each movement they make and the best way to do it. Each movement should be done deliberately and completely.

Exercising early in the morning is recommended. People are rested and less likely to become too tired. Exercise may need to be scheduled for times when the drugs used to treat the disease are working well.

Peripheral Arterial Disease

For people with peripheral arterial disease, exercise may be supervised at first. People who are walking for exercise may be given pedometers to measure distance walked. In people with peripheral arterial disease, exercise triggers pain or discomfort (intermittent claudication) in the legs. So they may be reluctant to exercise. However, paradoxically, exercise also helps relieve the pain. It can help improve blood flow in leg arteries by causing arteries clogged by fatty deposits to widen (dilate).

If done regularly, any exercise that uses the legs—walking, climbing stairs, or riding a stationary bicycle—can help relieve the pain or discomfort of peripheral arterial disease. When pain or discomfort occurs in the legs during exercise, people should stop and rest until the pain disappears, then begin again. With this strategy, the time spent exercising without pain can be gradually increased. Walking (or doing other similar exercise) for 30 to 60 minutes a day is recommended. Most people notice improvements within 6 to 12 months.

Stroke

For many people who have had a stroke, exercise, beginning with physical therapy in the hospital,[1] is essential to being able to resume daily activities. People who have substantial disability, such as paralysis of a limb, may think exercise is beyond them. However, continuing to exercise after rehabilitation is over can help them maintain the gains made and may help them function even better. Exercise can help people who have had a stroke live as independently as possible. It also helps reduce the risk of subsequent strokes.

Strengthening exercises are important. Exercises can strengthen an affected limb, enabling it to be used more. Some people feel insecure doing strengthening and stretching exercises while they are standing. They can do most exercises effectively while sitting or lying down.

For aerobic exercise, good choices include a recumbent sta-

1. see page 180

tionary bicycle, a treadmill, and water aerobics. A recumbent stationary bicycle is secure and comfortable. It has a contoured chair that even a person who has had a stroke can sit in. Also, if one leg is paralyzed, toe clips can hold both feet in place, so that the person can pedal with one leg.

Walking on a treadmill helps people walk more efficiently and makes walking less stressful. Treadmills have bars people can hold on to for balance and support. For people who cannot increase their walking pace, treadmill walking can be made more intense by increasing the slant, so that people are walking uphill.

Water aerobics is useful because people do not have to worry about falling. Water provides support, enabling people who cannot walk without help to walk and move on their own. Water also provides resistance, which strengthens muscles efficiently.

What is more wonderful than dancing? Dancing is great for the body, heart, and emotions. It is a way to celebrate life at any age.

Now that I am 70, dancing is a greater part of my life than ever before. I learned to dance the polka at a young age and participated in ballroom dancing in high school and college. I met the love of my life in college, and we loved to swing to Big Band music, especially "In the Mood." Later, we took up "tap-ercize," joined the "Silver Top Tapper" group, and won a national tap championship. We did a simple soft shoe routine. Over 1000 people stood and applauded, including the judges. It wasn't that we were so good, it was that they were so delighted to see two "oldies" dancing. It kept us active and healthy.

After 42 years, I lost my dear husband. I was devastated. Two years ago, I collapsed on the sidewalk and was given CPR. I needed a pacemaker. So like the Energizer Bunny, I am running on batteries now. I have more energy and my life has been filled with more dancing and joy than before.

A wonderful group invited me to join them singing and dancing at Senior Centers. I got my tap shoes out again. Part of the deal was to enter the Ms. Senior Georgia Pageant. After they promised there was no bathing suit competition, I entered. I did a comical jazz dance. My goal was to make people laugh, and they did. To my surprise, I won and went to the national competition. I was fortunate to win there too.

As Ms. American Classic Woman, I speak to senior groups. My theme is to celebrate age at any age, using A G E. The A promotes staying ACTIVE, mentally and physically. The G encourages GRATITUDE for every minute of every day, for friends, family, and freedom. The E stands for ENTHUSIASM about every challenge in life.

I am grateful to be dancing, alive and well and active and helping others enjoy life and celebrate age.

Avis Fox

SECTION 4

SOCIAL, LEGAL, AND ETHICAL ISSUES

Many changes, sometimes so many that it feels like a flood, can occur when people retire or soon thereafter. These changes may affect relationships with other people or basic activities, or they may involve legal, ethical, or financial issues.

As the body ages, concerns and questions about intimacy may arise. If aging affects a fundamental activity such as driving, getting from here to there can no longer be taken for granted. A decline in health may lead to a sense of vulnerability and sometimes the potential for experiencing mistreatment—emotional, financial, or even physical—at the hands of a family member, friend, or caregiver. With aging, people may have to make decisions about unfamiliar legal and ethical matters.

Most people need to learn more about navigating the complex system that pays for health care. Information is the best aid for coping with these changes.

61

Coping With Change

Old age is a time of many changes. With aging, the ability to function declines to some degree in every person, and older people, on average, tend to have more disease and disability than do younger people. But the changes of old age are more than just changes in health. As people age, they are often faced with events that can dramatically alter their lives, such as retiring from the workforce, losing a loved one, or changing their living arrangements.

Whether the changes that accompany old age are viewed as a blessing or a curse may hinge on the older person's ability to cope with or adapt to change. Successful coping skills are often linked with how well older people stay connected with family and friends, with their community, and with their own values and sense of purpose. In general, older people are well able to cope with the many changes that occur in later life. These transitions can be substantially eased with planning and preparation as well as with assistance tailored to individual needs.

LIFE-CHANGING EVENTS

Retirement

Publisher Malcolm Forbes once remarked, "Retirement kills more people than hard work ever did." Although Forbes' words may seem grim, many people do worry about the consequences of inactivity after retirement.

On the day people leave work permanently, they lose one of the most obvious ways in which they measure their place in society. In addition, they are faced with the decision of what to do with the rest of their life. People who retire often go from a routine that fills much of their day to one in which they have much more free time.

Whether retirement is viewed as a positive or negative event often depends on the reasons for retiring. Some people choose to retire, having looked forward to quitting unpleasant work or to pursuing more fulfilling interests; others find themselves forced to retire.

About one third of retirees have difficulty coping with the consequences of retirement. People who retire unexpectedly because of illness or job loss or those who tended to work long hours and bring work home with them may be most likely to experience difficulty. Spouses may have to adjust to seeing more of one another. Some retirees have difficulty coping with reduced income. Others resent their diminished role in society, believing that they are unimportant and powerless, with little left to contribute. Still others relish the time they now have to

---

BOUNCING BACK: RESILIENCY AFTER CHANGE

Every person faces challenging changes from time to time. Many changes are welcomed and celebrated, but some are dreaded and painful. Some changes, especially the ones viewed negatively, can be shocking and abrupt (for example, the death of a loved one), whereas others can be tortuously slow (for example, experiencing the diagnosis and treatment of a chronic disease). Negative changes are a test of a person's resiliency. Resiliency is more than simply the ability to cope with change. Resiliency is the ability to "bounce back" after being "knocked down" by changes in everyday life.

People are not born with an unchangeable amount of resiliency. The thoughts, behaviors, and actions that determine how resilient a person is can be strengthened and nurtured. For most people, resiliency begins by recognizing and accepting that change is to be expected as part of everyday living. By recalling and reflecting on past stressful changes, people may be able to recognize their own strategies and approaches that were most successful and those that were not helpful. This process of self-discovery may help improve a person's resiliency when facing future changes. Learning that progress in bouncing back can be made in small steps helps people avoid the notion that tragedies and hardships must be overcome all at once. Resiliency can also be bolstered by maintaining existing relationships and establishing new ones that help ensure that someone will be there to listen and to offer support and assistance when changes need to be faced.

pursue their interests, to volunteer, and to enjoy friends and loved ones.

.   The transition from work to retirement can be eased through planning. Beginning to plan for retirement several years before retirement is anticipated is very helpful. Many employers offer retirement planning services, as do some community agencies. Retirement planning focuses on finding ways to meet financial needs and obligations and on identifying ways to fill available time through part-time employment, volunteer positions, leisure activities, or adoption of a pet. Counseling may help retirees and their families who experience difficulties despite planning or due to lack of planning.

Losing a Loved One

The death of a loved one can weigh heavily on the heart and mind of an older person. When a spouse or partner or a close family member or friend dies, a strong sense of loss is accompanied by an awareness of one's own mortality. The older person may experience a loss of companionship, less interaction with family and friends, and a decline in social standing.

The death of a spouse is perhaps the most striking loss that an older person confronts. In some cases the surviving spouse dies soon afterward, although this is more likely to occur when the survivor is the husband rather than the wife.

Dealing with multiple deaths is another difficult issue. Older people may be confronted with the death of several loved ones within a brief period of time. Many deaths occurring close together can be particularly difficult to cope with, causing the older person to feel especially lonely and isolated.

When a person is grieving over the loss of a loved one, sadness is usually apparent. Sadness, a natural response to death, is not the same as depression[1] and therefore does not necessarily indicate a need for treatment. However, some older people who are grieving find it helpful to join a support group or to discuss their feelings with a clergy member or counselor.

Feelings of intense sadness over an extended period of time or signs of declining health may indicate depression. If grief is prolonged or overwhelming, or if the person becomes unable or unwilling to perform even essential daily activities or speaks of

1. see page 442

suicide, then evaluation and treatment by a doctor are necessary. If the doctor diagnoses depression, the person often is referred to a mental health practitioner. At times, antidepressant drugs may be helpful. Some older people prefer to be counseled by a clergy member, which they may view as less stigmatizing than being counseled by a mental health practitioner. However, many clergy members do not have extensive training in mental health counseling.

Changes in Living Arrangements

Living alone is a common situation for many older people [1] and can present many challenges. Those who live alone are more likely to be poor, and this is increasingly so the longer they live alone. Many older people who live alone describe feelings of loneliness and isolation. Because eating for most people is a social activity, some older people who live alone do not prepare full, balanced meals, thus undernutrition becomes a concern.[2] Among those with health problems or difficulty seeing or hearing, it is all too easy for new or worsening symptoms of disease to go unnoticed. Many older people who live alone have problems following directions for prescribed treatments.

Despite these challenges and problems, most older people who live alone express a keen desire to maintain their independence. Many fear being overly dependent on others and wish to continue to live alone despite the challenges they face. Engaging in regular physical and mental activities and staying connected with others help older people who are living alone maintain their independence.

A person returning home from a hospital stay, particularly after surgery, may benefit from having a discussion with a social worker or health care practitioner about any extra services that will be needed. Such services, which may include home health aides[3] or visiting nurses, can help ensure that the person resumes living independently.

Alternative living arrangements may be an option when living alone is not. In some instances, someone may be willing to move into the dwelling of an increasingly dependent older per-

1. see page 24
2. see page 231
3. see page 108

son. That someone is most often an adult child, but it may be another family member or even a friend. The person moving in may be providing companionship only or may be undertaking some caregiving responsibilities. This type of living arrangement may extend the older person's time in his own home and may be quite satisfying to all involved. However, expectations of each person regarding the arrangement should be clearly expressed and agreed on.

Relocation, or moving to another residence, sometimes becomes an attractive option or even a necessity for an older person after retirement or the death of a spouse or relative. An older person may move when declining health uncovers a need for supervision or help with personal care. Alternatively, a decision to relocate may come about simply because the older person is looking for better weather, more companionship, a greater sense of safety and security, or to be closer to a family member. In other instances, an older person relocates to reduce costs or to establish a simpler lifestyle. Usually the move is from a larger to a smaller dwelling. For example, an older person might move from a family home to retirement housing and eventually to an assisted living facility or nursing home.

People who respond poorly to relocation are more likely to have been living alone, socially isolated, impoverished, and depressed. Men respond more poorly than women do. Relocation can be very stressful. Much of the stress seems to arise when people feel they lack control over the move and do not know what to expect in the new environment. For an older person who has memory loss, a move away from familiar surroundings may intensify confusion and dependence on others and lead to frustration.

In some instances, relocation involves moving into someone else's home. An older person may move into the home of an adult child. Less often, the person moves into the home of a sibling, another relative, or a friend. Even when the older person has been independent or nearly so, choosing to live with another person can produce mixed results. Problems may develop if the older person believes he is or might become a burden to others in the household. In some instances, not everyone in the household is pleased to have the older person move in; this situation may arise when an adult child asks his parent to live with him out of a sense of guilt or obligation. The older person moving into the home may be vulnerable to mistreatment[1] or other problems if others in the household feel angry and frustrated with the arrangement.

On the other hand, relocation may involve a very positive arrangement in which people provide services to one another as well as companionship and financial relief. Such relocations are most likely to go well when the older person is well prepared and when there is open discussion regarding expectations and concerns.

Many moves happen suddenly, but even a little preparation can help decrease the stress of relocating. Before a decision is made for an older person to move into someone else's home, it is important that every person already living in that home have an opportunity to participate in a discussion about what to expect and how to handle problems. This type of discussion can help everyone involved to anticipate and possibly prevent conflicts. People who are moving should be acquainted with the new setting well in advance, if possible. The opportunity to tour future surroundings and meet potential neighbors can be very helpful.

STAYING CONNECTED

Studies have shown that people who remain active and who interact with other people during old age live longer, happier, healthier lives. Volunteering, taking classes, joining social groups, engaging in hobbies, and pursuing some type of spiritual or religious practice are all ways of staying connected. Even people who are confined to their homes because of illness can stay connected by having others visit them or by communicating over the telephone or by electronic mail.

Volunteering: Volunteering allows an older person to use skills and life experiences in a way that contributes to the community and society. Hundreds of organizations across the United States welcome older volunteers. For example, the Retired and Senior Volunteer Program (RSVP) and the Foster Grandparent Program provide volunteer opportunities in many communities. Opportunities are almost limitless and include

1. see page 945

working with children, working with older adults, helping out in nonprofit organizations or municipal institutions such as libraries, and assisting small businesses.

Continuing education: Being a life-long learner can be a very enjoyable and effective way of maintaining an active mind and of meeting and interacting with others who have similar interests. Many public school systems, colleges and universities, and municipalities offer continuing education classes for people of all ages as well as classes specifically developed with older adults in mind. Classes may range from practical topics such as preparing tax returns, managing personal finances, or learning a new language to more creative or entertaining topics such as wine tasting and music appreciation.

Social groups and hobbies: For older people, hobbies can help maintain social connections as well as mental and physical fitness. People may develop new hobbies or rediscover hobbies from earlier years. Although many hobbies can be done in solitude, engaging in a hobby with another person or with a group can be more interesting and stimulating. Hobbies that involve physical activity, such as gardening or sports, can be particularly beneficial to the person's health.

Spirituality and religion: Spirituality and religion provide meaning, comfort, and a sense of belonging to many older people. Spirituality and religion are similar but not identical concepts. Religion often is associated with institutions, structure, and tradition, whereas spirituality is more associated with feelings, thoughts, and experiences. Most older people in the United States consider themselves both religious and spiritual.

Spirituality and religion may benefit older people in several ways.

• A positive and hopeful attitude about life and illness improves health.
• The social aspects of a religious community can help people feel connected to others.
• The meaning and purpose of life that religious beliefs convey and the effect of those beliefs can be steady and powerful influences, especially when a person is facing difficult changes.

A religious community is the largest source of social support for older people outside of the family, and involvement in religious organizations is the most common type of voluntary social activity—more common than all other forms of voluntary social activity combined.

Active involvement in a religious community appears to help older people maintain their ability to carry out daily activities. Older people who attend religious services are also more likely to be healthy, recover faster from illness or injury, and live longer. Many older people say that their religion provides a foundation that enables them to cope with health problems and stresses, such as loss of a spouse.

62

Driving

Driving provides a sense of freedom, independence, and involvement with the world that older people may have taken for granted in earlier adulthood. But the privilege of driving is based on a demonstrated ability to drive safely. Because drivers aged 70 and over are among those at greatest risk of traffic violations and motor vehicle crashes, old age should be viewed as a flashing yellow traffic signal—a warning that driving privileges should be reassessed.

Many factors can diminish the performance of older drivers. Among these factors are aging itself and certain disorders that become more common with aging. Certain drugs that are commonly used to treat medical disorders in older people can also impair driving performance. Some of these factors can be remedied.

CRASH RATES AND TRAFFIC VIOLATIONS

On average, older drivers actually have *fewer* crashes per year than do younger drivers. However, because they drive fewer miles than younger drivers do, older drivers average more crashes *per mile driven*. Crash rates begin to increase after about age 70, and they increase more rapidly after age 80. For every mile driven, older drivers have higher rates of traffic violations, crashes, and fatalities than do all other age groups over age 25.

Failure to yield right-of-way is one of the more common traffic violations committed by older drivers. Also, older drivers have more difficulty merging into traffic and may have problems at intersections, particularly when making left turns. And yet older drivers are often more careful than younger drivers. Older drivers have fewer crashes during the evening, early morning, and inclement weather—possibly because they tend not to drive in these conditions. Moreover, alcohol is much less likely to be a factor in crashes involving older drivers. Older drivers are also less likely to have crashes while driving on curved roads or at high speeds. For older drivers, crashes are less likely to involve a single vehicle. Multiple vehicles are more likely to be involved.

In a motor vehicle crash, older drivers are more likely than younger drivers to be injured. Crashes involving older drivers are also more likely to result in serious injuries and fatalities.

THE REASONS FOR PROBLEMS

Driving involves the precise execution of simultaneous tasks (such as braking and steering). These tasks variously require several attributes, including the following:

- A clear mind
- Attention and mental focus
- Swift reaction time
- Coordination
- Adequate strength
- Good range of motion of the upper body (upper trunk, shoulders, and neck)
- Good vision and hearing
- Good judgment

Deficits in any of these attributes can greatly affect driving performance. Such deficits can result from several causes.

Virtually all of these attributes yield to some degree to the passage of time: Aging itself usually results in a gradual and subtle decline in a person's strength, coordination, reaction time, and ability to concentrate. Vision (especially at night) and hearing also decrease with aging.

Medical disorders that are more common among older people can prove especially troublesome for older drivers. For example, the blood sugar level of drivers with diabetes may rise too high or drop too low. Such changes can interfere with thinking clearly, attention and mental focus, and vision.

Older drivers with dementia (including Alzheimer's disease) can have poor judgment and concentration, a dangerous prospect when driving. Even when dementia is in its early stages, a driver may become more easily lost or more easily confused in congested traffic.

Strokes or so-called ministrokes (transient ischemic attacks, or TIAs)[1] can slow reaction time and reduce coordination. Seizures can abruptly cause people to become unaware of their surroundings or even lose consciousness. A recent heart attack may increase a driver's risk of fainting or experiencing light-headedness.

Arthritis causes joint pain and stiffness, limiting a person's range of motion and possibly interfering with the ability to operate a car's controls. For example, pain and stiffness in the knees or hips may affect a person's ability to press the brake pedal. Arthritis can make turning the head (as is necessary when turning or reversing a car) painful and difficult.

Glaucoma and macular degeneration are eye disorders that lead to problems when driving at twilight or at night. Glaucoma can also narrow the field of vision so that cars and other objects alongside the driver are difficult to see. Cataracts, which occur almost exclusively among older people, can cause glare from oncoming headlights or street lamps.

Many older people take drugs that can have undesirable side effects. Side effects can include sleepiness, dizziness, confusion, and other symptoms that interfere with driving. Nonprescription antihistamines and sleep aids are among the drugs that produce these side effects.

For some older people, the only "deficit" in driving ability is simply a lack of driving experience. This deficit is often the case

1. see page 374

when an older person (usually a woman) learns to drive only after a spouse dies.

WAYS OF COMPENSATING

There are many strategies an older driver can adopt to compensate for factors that reduce performance and increase the risk of driving. Older drivers can use their experience from years of driving to identify and avoid hazardous situations. For example, because stamina decreases with aging, older drivers may wish to drive shorter distances between breaks. They can avoid freeways and other areas where traffic is congested or known to be dangerous. They can avoid driving at night or twilight, when glare problems are most likely. They can avoid rush hour traffic and take fewer risks in traffic.

Avoiding distractions—an important consideration for *all* drivers—is all the more essential for older drivers. Cell phones are an important safety feature for drivers who become stranded when a car unexpectedly needs repair. However, cell phone use while driving is strongly discouraged. In fact, it is illegal in some areas. Similarly, making adjustments to the stereo or another onboard system (such as climate control or seat position), eating or drinking, smoking (there are many other reasons not to smoke—at any age), applying make-up, reading maps, and even engaging in conversation with other passengers can be distracting.

New technology can help older drivers. For example, advanced vision systems for night driving include curve lighting (lighting directed around a curve) and automatic dimming of headlights (high beams convert to low beams when there is oncoming traffic). Parking aids, which use cameras or infrared systems to help with backing up, parking, and other maneuvers, are especially helpful for people who have difficulty looking over their shoulders.

Other systems that are helpful to older drivers include cruise control, antilock brakes, and electronic stability devices that improve traction and steering. Some cars offer rearview mirrors that automatically dim when hit by blinding headlights, thus reducing glare. Car manufacturers are experimenting with infrared night vision technology to enhance night driving. Many are also redesigning handles and knobs to make them easier for people who have arthritis to operate. When crashes or other urgent situations do occur, some emergency systems can automatically call and direct rescue teams to the car's location. Further innovations are anticipated in the future.

Another way that older drivers can help maintain or even improve their driving skills is through driver re-education programs. Several organizations—such as the American Association of Retired Persons (AARP) and American Automobile Association (AAA)—offer such programs to help older drivers adjust to the challenges of driving in old age. In addition, taking such programs can lower insurance rates.

What about lifestyle and medical care? There are many reasons to stay fit in older age, and the ability to continue driving is one of them, because strength and stamina affect driving performance.

Treatment of some disorders may improve driving performance. For example, cataract removal can be beneficial. Treatment of arthritis with drugs and physical therapy can improve flexibility and mobility. Good control of diabetes can prevent swings in the blood sugar level. Older drivers should review their drugs with a doctor to make sure that driving performance will not be compromised by side effects.

Many states have laws that prohibit people from driving for a specified time after certain disorders are diagnosed. This waiting period (moratorium) provides time for the disorder to be stabilized with treatment. For example, some states require a 6-month moratorium on driving after a stroke or transient ischemic attack. A 3- to 6-month moratorium may be required after a heart attack or cardiac bypass surgery. For people who have had a seizure, some states require a seizure-free period of at least 6 months before driving can be resumed.

A DRIVING DECISION

At some point, an older person may face the decision to keep or give up a driver's license. A decline in the abilities required for safe driving may make driving dangerous. Also, some people drive less and less as they get older. They may find that maintaining a car for occasional use costs more than using public transportation. But giving up a driver's license means giving up some freedom and independence.

Sometimes the family doctor or a loved one is the one who first realizes that it is time for an older driver to give up the car keys. Dealing with these issues is always difficult, but ignoring them can bring even greater misery.

One approach to the decision is to suggest that the older driver be tested by the state agency that oversees or regulates licensure. Testing can be requested by the driver, an immediate family member, or a doctor. It can include both written and on-road evaluations. In many states, doctors are required to report any driver believed to be unsafe.

Laws regulating the possession and renewal of a driver's license by older drivers vary from country to country and state to state. In the United States, renewal procedures for older drivers include the following:

• Shorter renewal intervals (ranging from 2 to 8 years) for drivers over a specified age, typically 65 or 70
• A requirement that older drivers renew their licenses in person rather than electronically or by mail
• Tests that are not routinely required of younger drivers (such as vision and road tests)

My grandfather gave me a pony when I was 4. At a race-track near home, I discovered the wonder of bigger, faster horses. The track's owner gave me a job. I would get up at 4 a.m., walk to the track, clean stalls, exercise horses, cool them down, and walk back home to get ready for school. During high school, I continued working at the track, breaking colts, racing them, and doing everything necessary to condition a racing horse. Summers were heaven. I was able to race horses I had helped train.

After graduation, I went to live with a fine couple who raced horses and had the meanest, most ornery mare I ever encountered. Her disposition and speed matched those of any stallion I ever rode. She loved to win, and we raced anywhere a woman jockey was allowed to race.

My winning record gave me a reputation. Horse racing publications wrote flattering things about me and goaded Johnny Longden, the champion jockey of the day, to challenge me to a match race. He accepted, thinking he would show that a woman could not beat a man. I won, and he was so disgusted he refused to weigh in after the match.

I loved feeling a powerful horse racing down the stretch, with wind, dirt, and mud in my face. It was especially rewarding when I won. I believe that having a goal, striving for it, and achieving it is how we all should live. Hard work, with respect, discipline, and cleanliness for body, mind, and soul is my recipe for being a winner.

After I quit racing, I continued my lifestyle of getting up early, working till sundown, getting proper nutrition, and getting to bed early.

I am 86 and live with my Jack Russell terrier. We get up early, have breakfast, and at daybreak we take our walk. We get to see neighbors out and about. I celebrate each day with the joy of having a devoted son and 3 grandchildren. I have been truly blessed.

Wantha Davis

63

Intimacy

Intimacy is a close familiarity that two people share, often with an affectionate set of feelings, thoughts, and actions. The two people may be spouses, partners, or close friends. Intimate relationships are a key source of pleasure in life.

Many people think of sex as a defining aspect of intimate relationships. But sex is only one of many aspects of intimacy. Intimate partners respect and admire each other. They find each other interesting and appealing. And they share themselves emotionally and sometimes physically in ways that may or may not include romance and sex, but that feel natural and unique to that relationship. For caring and compatible partners lucky enough to find each other, intimacy provides deep and lasting satisfaction, happiness, and security.

The desire for intimacy does not diminish with aging. However, the conditions and feelings that often accompany aging can complicate a person's ability to develop and maintain an intimate relationship. In addition, aging can change the way in which intimacy is expressed in a relationship.

INTIMACY AND LONG-TERM RELATIONSHIPS

Ideally, intimacy in any long-term relationship (which for older people may be within the context of marriage) grows as people age. Some people, however, believe that intimacy is destined to fade with time, particularly where marriage is concerned. Loss of intimacy sometimes does occur, for a variety of reasons. Some couples find it difficult to maintain closeness in the face of life's sometimes substantial challenges. Others lose their sense of need for intimacy with the mellowing of passions that comes with years of living together. Still other couples experience a loss of intimacy because one partner has decided that finding emotional and physical intimacy with a new partner is easier and more exciting than working on solving entrenched difficulties with a long-term partner.

The challenges inherent in long-term relationships, however, usually do not lead to a loss of intimacy but, rather, to changes in the way intimacy is expressed. Society idealizes older couples who, after years of being together, still dance with each other, sit together, hold hands, and kiss. For most people, physical passion and romance are the most appealing of intimacies, but they, like other fires, only rarely are sustained with unwavering strength and intensity. Romantic expressions of intimacy may diminish in importance as couples confront the ordinary stresses of daily life. In many long-term relationships, romantic expressions of intimacy may be more the exception than the rule. Partners regretting that their relationships lack romantic intimacy or who are not as romantic as they were in younger years may have unrealistic expectations or may not be expressing their needs.

Long-term partners or friends may express intimacy in less public and occasionally even contradictory ways. An older couple may not reveal outward signs of affection yet do nearly everything together in quiet companionship. A couple may unwittingly preserve a sense of intimacy, such as when an over-anxious partner or friend worries around-the-clock about the other person's health, while the relaxed partner seemingly ignores the worry and attention but does little to discourage it. Partners or friends may constantly bicker—neither conceding defeat nor settling their arguments—but their agreeing to disagree may be the very thing that sustains their relationship and helps them stay together.

Many couples—most without being aware of it—grow com-

SELF-ACCEPTANCE

Self-awareness and comfort with oneself is the foundation on which all other types of intimacy are built. A person who practices self-honesty and self-acceptance is best able to be honest with, accepting of, and loving toward another person in an intimate relationship, no matter what form that relationship takes.

fortable with alternative forms of intimacy that allow them to express familiarity, caring, or engagement with their partners in ways that are equally meaningful and more natural to their daily lives and personalities. Trust, empathy, communication, and the ability to depend on a partner usually grow in importance over time. These forms of intimacy are sometimes difficult for outsiders to detect, let alone interpret. Friends may find that intimacy and sharing experiences and thoughts increase over time.

Moreover, intimacy in long-term relationships must often be renegotiated at times of personal change. Events such as retirement, serious personal illness, or the death of a child or close friend can sometimes bring partners closer together. Other times, however, stressful life events can complicate a couple's feelings for each other, seriously challenge their ability to be intimate, change the way they are intimate, and even result in separation, divorce, or the breakup of friendships.

INTIMACY AND DATING

Dating offers single older people romance, the most exciting form of intimacy for most people regardless of their age. At its best, dating can boost an older person's self-confidence and offer the potential for happiness and companionship at a stage when, for many, the prospects for either are uncertain. At its worst, dating can obliterate self-confidence. But dating can be as thrilling, nerve-wracking, and complicated after age 65 as it was at age 25, in part because older people can be just as interesting, smart, attractive, and complex—or boring, selfish, and superficial—as younger people.

Older people are faced with unique issues surrounding dating. Single older people bring with them a longer history of past relationships than do younger people. Dating can remind an older person of the strengths and deficiencies of past relationships and can open or heal old wounds. Also, the playing field for older people is not as level as it is for younger people. Because men tend to die at a younger age, women greatly outnumber men. Older women, therefore, have greater difficulty finding partners. This imbalance in the number of men and women is further compounded when eligible older men find younger partners.

The importance of dating and romance changes as people age. Older women may not consider romantic companionship as essential for a sense of security and well-being and, therefore, may feel no need to date. A sense of loyalty to deceased partners or to other family members, issues surrounding feelings about the appropriateness of dating, and satisfaction with the independence that comes with one's later years all may contribute to this feeling. Some widows who were caregivers for their husbands avoid new relationships for fear of again needing to provide care for an ill or dying man. Some women turn toward younger men.

Care and companionship may be more essential for older men. They may want the pleasures of a serious relationship in their retirement after years of putting their career first. They may not be used to the day-to-day responsibilities involved in caring for themselves and seek a companion's help. They may fear not having a physical relationship with a woman and seek a companion for that reason, yet worry about the long-term commitment that a physical relationship implies. There are, however, many exceptions to these characterizations.

Bodily changes that accompany aging influence self-image and the sense of sexuality that women and men bring to dating, although in different ways. Older women who have seen their hair turn gray, their skin develop wrinkles, their legs develop varicose veins, and their breasts and buttocks lose their former shape may fear they are no longer attractive. They may worry about the potential embarrassment or discomfort of intercourse given these and other physical changes. These fears may inhibit them in social settings in which they could meet a potential partner, or cause them to end a promising relationship early for fear it could become physical. Older men who have lost muscle mass and strength may have similar fears but tend to focus less on their physical appearance. Instead, they tend to focus more on their physical functioning, that is, on their ability to develop and maintain an erection and to re-establish themselves as capable sexual performers in a mutually satisfying physical relationship.

The settings in which older single people meet differ from those of their youth. The social contexts of school and work, which facilitate opportunities to meet new people, are not available to most older people. Instead, social opportunities usually come from within religious and retirement communities and from shared interests, such as travel or sports and fitness. Some older people meet at school and college reunions, finding new partners among long-time acquaintances and friends. The opportunity to develop intimacy within established or familiar rather than new relationships is important to some older people. Finding such social opportunities can be difficult for older people who have relocated to be near their adult children, especially for those who live with their children.

Finally, health issues, which are rarely a factor in the younger dating population, affect nearly all older people. Health issues may inhibit older people from even imagining themselves with new partners and may affect the way in which they express intimate feelings with a partner. In general, the effects of illness on intimacy are complex and depend on the specific illness, the treatment involved, and the person's body image and attitude. Illness may weaken the bonds of intimacy, although in some cases, the limitations or needs of a person with a medical condition can be a focus of understanding, caring, and increased intimacy within a relationship.

INTIMACY AND SEX

Intimacy can occur without sex, and sex can occur without intimacy. Sex is a physical expression of intimacy that is important to many older couples. There is no age at which sexual activity is inappropriate. People who enjoyed sex in their younger years are likely to desire it no matter what their age. But sex may be dispensable to others, who may find it less of a priority or physically difficult or who found it unenjoyable or emotionally complicated in their younger years. Instead, some older people find that just having someone to sit with, converse with, hold hands with, or hug and kiss is sufficiently delightful. They may find that pleasures more lasting than sex can be had in the sharing of their daily lives with each other, including the pleasures of family, friends, and new experiences.

Some older people worry that their children might disapprove of their having a sexual relationship and thus avoid discussing the issue. Although avoiding discussion may seem to temporarily solve the problem, it can distance an older person from the very people who could be most supportive of the vigor and intensity of the growing relationship. Other older people simply conclude that they do not need the approval of their children and tell them about the change in their life without guilt or shame.

Many factors may contribute to the shift in emphasis from sex to other expressions of intimacy. Levels of sex hormones decrease in men and women as they grow older, which result in physical changes that can make sexual intercourse uncomfortable or difficult.[1] In addition, some medical conditions as well as the drugs used to treat these conditions can hamper the ability to have and enjoy sexual intercourse. Decreased hormone levels, especially testosterone, may reduce sex drive (libido) as well. Fear of being infected by microorganisms that can cause sexually transmitted diseases (STDs), including human immunodeficiency virus (HIV), chlamydia, and herpes, may inhibit older people from having sex with new or less familiar partners. Although STDs are less common in older than in younger people, age does not protect against such diseases as AIDS (caused by HIV). STDs can almost always be prevented with the use of condoms. Some older people may wish to avoid sex altogether rather than take any risk of contracting an infection.

Some older couples adjust for the physical changes that occur with aging by engaging in mutual masturbation and oral sex rather than intercourse. Masturbation and oral sex provide prolonged, direct stimulation that many older people find necessary for orgasm without the discomfort or awkwardness that they may experience with intercourse. In addition, some unmarried older people believe that masturbation or oral sex is more acceptable than sexual intercourse outside of marriage. Other older people may consider oral sex unnatural and develop satisfying alternatives to achieve intimacy.

Attraction, admiration, respect, and communication between compatible partners are the foundation for satisfying relationships at any age. Healthy physical intimacy, from hand holding to sexual intercourse, or other forms of sexual expression may follow from these key elements.

1. see pages 871 and 885

INTIMACY AND DEMENTIA

Intimacy is often unaffected by the development of very mild dementia in one partner. However, as dementia worsens, the challenges to intimacy are sometimes insurmountable. Paranoia, accusations, and aggressive demands may replace prior qualities of warmth, caring, humor, or playfulness. People with dementia often forget recent intercourse and demand sex too frequently for a frail partner, may mistake a partner for someone else, or may call a partner by a previous partner's name. In addition, people with dementia eventually forget to tend to personal hygiene matters, such as combing hair, changing clothes, brushing teeth, and bathing. When dementia reaches an advanced stage, interest in and eventually awareness of other people and the surrounding world are lost.[1]

The partner who does not have dementia carries the burden of coping with these challenges. Physical intimacy is often the first casualty of the demanding work involved in caring for an increasingly dependent partner. A shift in roles from partner to caregiver also contributes to loss of desire or comfort with physical intimacy. So does discomfort with the physical or sexual aggression or the inappropriate sexual behaviors that a partner with dementia may display. Coping with these changes is especially difficult when the partner who does not have dementia misinterprets these behaviors as deliberate attempts at antagonism or embarrassment.

The loss of memory characteristic of dementia almost always means the end of shared experiences between partners. It is no surprise that intimacy sometimes withers and dies as a result. The partner of a person with dementia can mourn the loss of the intimate relationship but cannot mourn the loss of the partner himself, as would occur in a physical death, and therefore does not have support for such private grief and loss.

Just as there is no cure for dementia, there is no easy fix for the challenges to intimacy that dementia poses. But there are strategies for coping. Acknowledging the loss of the relationship as it was, which may include feelings of depression, anger, and regret, is ultimately necessary. So is a recognition that the partner with dementia is on a journey that he did not choose to

1. see page 354

take. What is left to the surviving partner are simpler forms of expression that can still elicit responses from the partner with dementia. Touch, including hand holding, kissing, hugging, and gentle massage, is often comforting and a form of caring and communication recognized through the screen of dementia. So is gentle hair-combing and brushing. People with dementia also often recognize familiar music, even when their ability to think clearly, talk, and recognize others is seriously impaired. Singing familiar songs together may temporarily restore a sense of couple-hood. It is another way in which partners can share memories and experiences that might otherwise fade with progression of the disease.

INTIMACY AND FAMILIES

Not surprisingly, families can influence older people's relationships in both negative and positive ways.

Children can discourage and hinder an older parent's ability to form new relationships. Children stereotypically have a difficult time imagining their parents being intimate (especially sexually) under any circumstances and may be displeased and uncomfortable when an older single parent seeks or discovers a new partner. There may be many reasons for this discomfort. Children may have legitimate concerns about the character or motives of a new partner. They may equate a parent's new relationship with the betrayal of a deceased or divorced parent with whom they strongly identify. Or they may be upset that their parent is not upholding the mores that they have learned and adopted for themselves.

Sometimes, children are concerned about the financial consequences of a parent's new relationship. They worry that the money they had expected to inherit might go to a new spouse or partner. These matters are best discussed so that fears about money do not damage relationships. If need be, a lawyer can help protect assets in accordance with a person's wishes. Avoiding the issue, however, is bound to cause problems.

Children can also be a tremendous source of support to their parents. They can help parents through periods of bereavement and help them feel comfortable with finding new partners among peers. Emotional stimulation from spending time or talking with children may help parents overcome the social isolation that may result from physical frailty, depression, or other conditions. Children may also provide physical support, such as transportation, by which an older parent can get to and from social functions. Further, children can encourage older parents and their partners to move forward in a relationship. They can promote a sense of belonging and family between a parent and partner by including both in their own family's events.

Older people bring their own family-related inhibitions to relationships. Like their children, widows and widowers may remain fiercely loyal to deceased partners. They may believe strongly that their relationships with their children and grandchildren should supersede all others. They may fear that their children or other family members will react negatively to their "taking up" with someone new at their age, thus ruling out that possibility. Also, they may imitate the behavior of their own older single parents in eras when dating and intimacy among older people were not encouraged or discussed.

Sharing primary parenting responsibilities for grandchildren and other young family members is increasingly common in Western societies. This "second parenthood" brings new challenges to developing intimate relationships with new partners. Older people in these situations may feel that they have neither the time nor the energy to invest in a new relationship. In addition, they may feel that dating is irresponsible when their family requires their attention. Also, potential partners may be turned off by the older person's child-care responsibilities. Further, the presence of children may complicate attempts of willing partners to find the privacy necessary for physical intimacy.

INTIMACY AND PRIVACY

"Intimacy," by definition, requires private time. Opportunities for privacy lessen when older people no longer live alone. When living with a family member or in an assisted living community or nursing home, an older person may find that his need for intimacy is not only ignored but also discouraged and even regulated.

Whatever sense of and desire for sexual expression older people retain can be sabotaged in a long-term care facility, such as a nursing home. Shared bedrooms and bathrooms, lack of access to hair care or cosmetic services, absence of places to go or people to dress up for, and activities with ill and unhappy residents may complicate an older person's efforts to look and feel attractive. If a person does find an appealing partner, flirting may occur under the watchful eyes of staff and neighbors. In addition, sexual behaviors may be viewed as disruptive. Even masturbating as a replacement for intimacy with a partner may be difficult because of lack of privacy.

Some long-term care facilities, however, do provide private space and time for residents. Even those that do not may facilitate relationships by breaking the social isolation that threatened residents before their move. In any type of long-term care facility, older people can realize the pleasures of companionship, caring about someone else, and engaging in physical intimacies such as sitting together, holding hands, hugging, and kissing.

INTIMACY IN GAY RELATIONSHIPS

Relatively little is known about the nature of dating and intimacy as it evolves over time in the relationships of older gay (homosexual) men and women. Although older gay people experience the same bodily changes with aging and many of the same emotions as do older straight (heterosexual) people, they may also face unique challenges, such as the loss of a partner through HIV infection and a higher risk of social isolation.

The high prevalence of HIV infection among gay men increases the likelihood that many older men in gay relationships will be affected. HIV infection can alter intimacy in several ways. As the infection progresses, the healthy partner may have to assume the role of caregiver for the ill partner. Also, the healthy partner must take physical precautions against infection. The fatigue, poor health, and drug side effects that the partner with HIV infection may experience can lead to a loss of sexual desire and a change in body image. All of these stresses can be made worse when the healthy long-term partner is not even acknowledged as a legitimate guardian, caregiver, grieving partner, or beneficiary. Indeed, the stress that HIV infection places on a relationship can even drive some couples apart.

Establishing intimate relationships can be difficult for older single gay people independent of HIV-related issues. For example, although the opportunities to meet new partners may abound in larger gay communities, they are much more limited within smaller communities. Also, emotional intimacy may be more difficult to find within gay communities of any size when those communities value youth, strength, physical beauty, and sexual performance over maturity, which is often the case. Fortunately, the evolution of the gay community has created a much stronger and more integrated community for older gay men and women.

Absence of children and grandchildren means that older gay people are likely to be even more alone as they get older. Many find substitutes for these relationships in nieces, nephews, and younger men and women in their community.

Older gay people, like older straight people, may ultimately require residence in a long-term care facility. The prospects of finding adequate expression of sexual identity and intimacy in such facilities are poor, but a few gay-oriented assisted living communities do exist.

INTIMACY IN OTHER RELATIONSHIPS

Many older people find intimacy in relationships that do not involve partners. Pleasures derived from sharing time and experience with friends, grandchildren or other family members, young students or trainees, or caregivers may provide tremendous satisfaction different from but equally important to that of a partner. And despite the definition of intimacy as a close feeling shared between two people, many older people find intimacy in interactions with their dogs, cats, or other pets. Caring for a pet engenders many of the same feelings of intimacy present in human relationships but with fewer complications. And some animals are capable of giving and returning affection. Indeed, the purchase of a pet for an older person can, under proper circumstances, bring companionship and intimacy that greatly improves quality of life.

I was always crazy about music. I bought a French harp when I was too young to remember. That harp was in my pocket at all times. I got real good on it. My sister played piano. We played and sang World War I songs and had a big time.

Dad bought me a baritone horn. I got a 25-cent book from Sears and Roebuck that showed how to play. My family lived in Oklahoma and Kansas before moving to Colorado. The town there hired three brothers to form a band. I got in on that. Was I happy! The brothers soon left, and I tried to get up a high school band. I changed to trumpet. After moving again, during my 4th year of high school, I formed a band, and we played for football and basketball games and dances.

I worked my way through college, so I didn't go out for music, which I regret to this day. When I came home, I was picked up by a traveling dance band. In 1927, I went to Denver. I was picked up right away by a band. That job lasted through the winter. I played that summer at a ballroom in Phoenix. Then, I was invited to play at a ballroom in Prescott, Arizona. I also played with the city concert band, for pay. I volunteered with the American Legion drum and bugle corps. I loved Prescott and made it home.

During World War II, I worked at military camps around Arizona. Wherever I went, I played with local bands. I entered the service in 1943. I was shipped to Supreme Headquarters in London, where they were forming a band to take Glenn Miller's place. One of my duties was to play for the lowering of the flag each evening. After the war, I returned to Prescott and soon was booked into the "Pine Cone Inn," where I still play. I also play bugle with the American Legion color guard. I love to entertain and make people happy. I look forward to each gig. And that makes me happy.

Leonard Ross

64

Mistreatment

Elder mistreatment refers to harm or the threat of harm to an older person that is brought about by another person.

Older people can be mistreated by having harmful things done to them (abuse) or by having necessary things withheld from them (neglect). Elder mistreatment is a growing problem as the number of older people increases.

Each year in the United States, thousands of older people are mistreated. The perpetrator of mistreatment is often a family member, usually an adult child or spouse who is serving as the older person's caregiver. Caregivers may experience extreme stress and frustration, particularly if they are lacking in skills and resources, which may lead them to mistreat those in their care. Sometimes, professional caregivers, such as home health care workers or employees of nursing homes and other institutions, are perpetrators. Many perpetrators are financially dependent on the person they mistreat.

People who are mistreated are often frail, and many have several disabling chronic diseases. But any older person, regardless of health, can become a victim of mistreatment.

Because of their frailty and dependence, abused older people often do not seek help. They may be physically unable to seek help or may be afraid to do so. They may be afraid of further harm or of being abandoned. For all these reasons, elder mistreatment often goes unrecognized by doctors, nurses, social workers, friends, and family members.

Types of Mistreatment

Abuse: Abuse can be physical, sexual, psychologic, or financial. An older person may be subjected to one of these types of abuse or to a combination of two or more types.

Physical abuse is the use of force to harm or threaten harm. Examples of physical abuse are striking, shoving, shaking, beating, restraining, and improperly feeding. Possible indications of physical abuse include unexplained injuries or injuries that go without adequate treatment, rope burns and other rope marks, and scratches, cuts, and bruises. A caregiver's refusal to allow the older person to have time alone with visitors or health care practitioners can raise concerns about physical abuse.

Sexual abuse is sexual contact without consent or by force or threat of force. Examples are intimate touching and rape. Bruises around the breasts and genital area or unexplained bleeding from the vagina or anus may indicate sexual abuse. However, sexual abuse does not always result in physical injuries.

Psychologic abuse is the use of words or actions to cause emotional stress or anguish. Examples of psychologic abuse are issuing threats, insults, and harsh commands; remaining silent for prolonged periods; and ignoring the person. Another form of psychologic abuse is treating the older person like a child (infantilization), sometimes with the goal of encouraging the person to become dependent on the abuser. People who are psychologically abused may become passive and withdrawn, anxious, or depressed.

Financial abuse is the exploitation of a person's possessions or funds. It includes swindling, pressuring an older person to distribute assets, and managing an older person's money irresponsibly. A caregiver may spend most of an older person's income on himself, providing only minimum resources to the person for whom they were intended.

Many experts believe that restricting an older person's freedom to make important life decisions, such as whom to socialize with and how to spend money, constitutes another, more subtle, form of abuse.

Neglect: Neglect is the failure to provide food, drugs, personal care, or other necessities. In some instances, necessities are withheld intentionally; in others, they are simply forgotten or overlooked by irresponsible or inattentive caregivers. Some caregivers are unaware that their treatment of an older person has crossed the line from being less than ideal to mistreatment.

These caregivers lack a sense of what constitutes adequate and appropriate care, or they may have very different notions of what is and what is not acceptable conduct. Sometimes neglect arises out of desperate circumstances despite the caregiver's best intentions.

A person who is neglected may lose weight from malnutrition and develop dry skin and a dry mouth because of dehydration. An unpleasant odor may emanate from a person who is poorly cleaned. Pressure sores may develop on the buttocks or heels from sitting or lying in one position for prolonged periods.

SELF-NEGLECT

The perpetrator and the victim of self-neglect are one and the same.

Self-neglect occurs more often than mistreatment. Self-neglect is most likely to occur among older people who live alone and who isolate themselves. People who neglect themselves may have a disorder that impairs their judgment and memory or may have several chronic diseases. Some people, however, have no particular medical problems: It is unclear why such people engage in self-neglect.

The effects of self-neglect can range from poor personal hygiene to failure to seek care for a life-threatening condition. For example, a person may eat too little, which may lead to dehydration and malnourishment. He may refuse to seek treatment for a medical disorder or skip follow-up visits. He may lack the necessary clothing or other means with which to protect against extremes of hot and cold weather, yet choose not to seek help from others. The person's dwelling may be hazardous because of lack of basic maintenance or infestation by animal or insect pests.

Knowing where to draw the line between self-neglect and a person's right to autonomy and privacy can be very difficult for family, friends, and health care practitioners alike. The person may be making completely informed and capable choices. He may simply have elected to live in a way that others might find undesirable. Often, a social worker is in the best position to make such a determination and can intervene if alerted by the person's family or friends.

When the decision is made to intervene, help can be just a phone call away. Reporting self-neglect and seeking help for an affected person are done in much the same way as reporting elder mistreatment. The older person's primary care doctor should be contacted. Adult Protective Services or the state unit on aging (whose numbers are available through the Eldercare Locator at 800-677-1116) can be contacted as well.

Prevention of Mistreatment

An older person who fears being vulnerable to mistreatment can take steps to decrease its likelihood. Living with someone who has a history of violent behavior or substance abuse should be avoided. Keeping in touch with friends and former neighbors is helpful if an older person has to relocate to a caregiver's house. Likewise, family members and friends can help prevent mistreatment by maintaining close ties with the person. Staying connected with social and community organizations reduces the chances that mistreatment will go unnoticed.

Older people can also avoid mistreatment by insisting on legal advice before signing any documents related to where they will live or who controls their finances. The local Area Agency on Aging can refer people for legal help.

Responding to Mistreatment

An older person should never think that mistreatment is part of being old or being dependent. At the very least, being mistreated threatens a person's dignity and sense of well-being. At the very worst, it can cost him his life.

Detecting mistreatment of an older person can be difficult. The person may isolate himself, hiding mistreatment because of shame, fear of retaliation, or a desire to protect the perpetrator. The person may fear being abandoned or forced into a nursing home if he tells others about the mistreatment. Further, the perpetrator often increases this sense of isolation by limiting phone calls or access to visitors and health care practitioners.

If an older person who is being mistreated believes he is in danger, he can call an elder abuse hotline for immediate help. Such hotlines are listed in the local phone book, usually in the Blue Pages, or can be provided by a phone operator. The local Area Agency on Aging is another good source of information and referral. If the person does not feel endangered but is still seeking help, he can try to convey word of his situation to his doctor or other health care practitioner. However, many health care practitioners are unfamiliar with addressing problems of elder mistreatment because the topic has not been a traditional part of medical training and education.

In general, because mistreatment and its effects can vary greatly, interventions need to be tailored to each person's situation. Interventions may include medical assistance, education (such as information about mistreatment and available options as well as help with devising safety plans), and psychologic support (such as psychotherapy and support groups). Law enforcement and legal intervention (such as arrest of the perpetrator, orders of protection, and legal advocacy) may be called in. Alternative housing options (such as housing that provides safe shelter, with protection from the perpetrator) may be needed.

Relatives, friends, and acquaintances have a responsibility to help if they know of or strongly suspect mistreatment. Health care practitioners who become aware of or suspect mistreatment have the same responsibility. The reporting of suspected or confirmed abuse or neglect is mandatory in all states if the mistreatment occurs in an institution and in most states if it occurs in a home. Indeed, every state has laws protecting and providing services for vulnerable, incapacitated, or disabled adults. In most states, the agency designated to receive abuse reports is the state social service department (Adult Protective Services). In a few states, the designated agency is the state unit on aging. For abuse within an institution, the local long-term care ombudsman's office or the state department of health should be contacted. Telephone numbers for these agencies and offices in any part of the United States can be found by calling the Eldercare Locator (800-677-1116) or the National Center on Elder Abuse (202-682-2470) and giving the person's county and city of residence or zip code.

65

Understanding Legal and Ethical Issues

The last thing people want to be faced with in old age is a legal and ethical quagmire. Older people may be confronted with questions involving:

- Their ability to make health care decisions
- Their selection of people who can make health and financial decisions for them
- Their medical care preferences when near death
- Their living arrangements

Such questions may become legal issues when the answers are determined in part by laws. Such questions always become ethical issues because the answers involve principles and personal preferences that guide decision making without the authority of a formal law.

Having to make decisions about health care when near death and having to fight for the right to make those decisions can bring on anxiety and stress, increased costs, and a feeling of loss of control. With some careful planning, however, older people can use the legal system to their advantage.

The legal and ethical issues that older people most commonly encounter are not unique to this age group. However, many older people face these issues with fewer family members and fewer financial resources with which to seek legal counsel. And they often face these issues when they are sick and frail. Additional resources and support are usually welcomed but should not indiscriminately be offered to a person based on age alone. Rather, older people benefit most when these resources and services are tailored to meet specific needs.

INFORMED CONSENT

Informed consent is a voluntary decision to go forward on a health-related matter. Consent may be an agreement to undergo a diagnostic test or a treatment. Consent becomes informed when the person has the ability to understand and ultimately does understand the potential benefits and risks of his decision and the alternatives to the choice he is making. When a person gives consent, the doctor and all other health care practitioners are then legally and ethically obligated to abide by the conditions of the consent agreement. Their obligation ends only if the person later withdraws or modifies consent.

Underpinning informed consent is a person's right to self-determination. "Self-determination" means, in the language of one judge, that "every human being of adult years and sound mind has the right to decide what shall be done with his own body." Doctors are legally and ethically obligated to respect a person's right of self-determination, or autonomy. However, self-determination and consent do not mean that a person can dictate health care services. The doctor is obligated to provide choices among medically appropriate options. The person cannot demand diagnostic tests or treatments that the doctor determines are unsafe or unnecessary.

The right of informed consent has a partner of sorts: the right of informed refusal. In other words, doctors have the same legal and ethical obligation to respect "no" as they do "yes." However, if a person declines a recommended diagnostic test or treatment, then doctors must continue the discussion to ensure that the person fully understands the choices at hand. Although doctors may encourage acceptance of a choice judged to be in a person's best interests, they cannot resort to coercion or deception.

Informed consent and informed refusal sometimes require time for full consideration. They arise from an appropriately thorough discussion between doctor and patient. The doctor is responsible for sharing information along with support and advice. The person making the decision is responsible for listening carefully and asking questions until the choices are understood.

Family members need to be aware that older people who cannot easily understand or evaluate alternatives may be treated as if they can, simply because they quietly go along with a plan proposed by a doctor. Also, older people may have vision or hearing loss or other disorders or may experience drug side effects that impair their ability to comprehend and communicate. They also may have family members who for whatever reason want to influence their decision making.

CONFIDENTIALITY

Confidentiality laws and ethical principles protect the privacy of communication between a person and his doctor and what is written in his medical record. Even a well-intentioned family member who accompanies an older person on doctor's visits is not privy to private health information without the person's consent. Such information requires the person's permission for disclosure, unless the person lacks the capacity to grant permission. Almost all managed care and health insurance plans require information from the medical record to authorize payment. But under a new law, the Health Insurance Portability and Accountability Act (HIPAA), every person is informed of his right to limit how much of and with whom his private health information can be shared.

CAPACITY

Capacity is a medical judgment regarding the ability to make decisions about health-related matters. An older person faced with a health care decision is presumed capable of making that decision unless or until proven otherwise.

Capacity may come into question if an older person exhibits memory problems or has difficulty thinking clearly. In such a case, doctors may be asked to evaluate the person's capacity. Doctors determine whether the person understands the condition of his health and the good and harm that might come from each decision he is asked to make. They also determine if the person can weigh the consequences of treatment or a refusal of treatment against personal preferences and values. Doctors are more confident in a person's capacity to make decisions if the person has a consistent pattern of choices over time that reflect values that have been discussed with others.

Ideally, doctors apply the results of the evaluation only to the specific matter at hand. A person who experiences difficulty making choices in one situation may not experience difficulty in every situation. Capacity is decision-specific, and some decisions are far more complex than others.

When an older person already has some loss of mental function, a sudden illness may further undercut his ability to make decisions about health-related matters. This abrupt decrease in capacity often happens during a hospitalization, when the change in surroundings and daily routine adds to any confusion caused by the illness. If the person becomes incapacitated, health care practitioners must rely on family members, unless the incapacitated person has made his wishes known before becoming incapacitated. If the person has no family (or, in some cases, even if the person does), the local court can appoint someone to make decisions.

COMPETENCY

Competency is a legal presumption applied to people when they become adults. Competency gives adults the right to negotiate certain legal tasks, such as make a will or enter into a contract. In most states, a person is considered competent at age 18, unless there is evidence to the contrary that persuades a court to declare the person incompetent. Once presumed to be competent, people are presumed to remain competent until they die, unless a court determines that a person is no longer competent based on evidence, often provided by a doctor.

A person who has lost abilities—for example, the ability to manage financial affairs or make health care decisions—may be declared incompetent by a court of law. The court looks at what the person needs to do and what he can actually do. When asked to make such a declaration, the court usually relies on information gathered from a medical evaluation of a person's specific abilities. Only a court can declare a person incompetent. Old age used to be but no longer is sufficient cause to declare a person incompetent. The court must consider a person's disabilities along with his remaining abilities and craft an order that addresses the person's individual needs.

When the court declares someone incompetent, it appoints a guardian, who assumes responsibility for some or all of the decisions for the incompetent person.

ADVANCE DIRECTIVES

In some states in the United States, to create an advance directive, it may suffice for a person to have a conversation with a doctor. The specific information from such a conversation, sometimes referred to as an oral advance directive, should be placed in the person's medical records.

More often, an advance directive takes the form of one of two documents.

• A living will enables a person to specify his choices for medical care in advance of when such decisions might have to be made.

• A durable power of attorney for health care (sometimes referred to as a proxy) appoints another person (referred to as the health care agent) to make decisions on behalf of the person should he become incapacitated.

With advance directives, an older person informs family, friends, and health care practitioners on how to care for him when he can no longer speak for himself. Being able to follow plans that reflect a person's values and preferences can comfort family members in the event of serious illness and death.

A person should give copies of his living will or durable power of attorney for health care to his doctors. A copy of the durable power of attorney for health care should also be given to the person appointed to carry out the wishes discussed and another copy placed with important papers. The person's lawyer should hold a copy of all documents, and the person should keep copies at home.

Living Will

A living will expresses a person's preferences for medical care in the event that he becomes incapacitated and can no longer communicate his decisions. In some states, the document is called a medical directive to doctors. To be valid, a living will must comply with state law. Some states require that living wills be written in a standardized way. Other states are more flexible, permitting any language as long as the document is appropriately signed and witnessed. Examples of living wills and kits for creating living wills are available from community organizations and government agencies, such as the state department of health and the local Area Agency on Aging, and such kits are also sold in many bookstores. Legal professionals can also provide examples and offer specific advice, but completion of these documents does not require a lawyer.

Most people use living wills to refuse life-sustaining treatment when there is little hope of recovery. Specific issues that may be addressed include:

• Undergoing cardiopulmonary resuscitation (CPR) when the heart stops beating
• Receiving assistance from a ventilator when breathing stops
• Using antibiotics to treat infections

  • Allowing blood transfusions to replace blood that has been lost

Some people request in their living will that food and fluids be withheld or withdrawn if their medical condition is likely to permanently prevent them from recognizing or relating to loved ones or friends.

Living wills need not serve only as a "menu" listing all unwanted types of care. They can also serve to request certain types of care. For example, a living will might specify that the person wants to be evaluated for hospice care if he is diagnosed with advanced cancer and unable to understand further discussions about options for treating the cancer. It may also request certain measures intended to keep the person as comfortable as possible, such as pain relief. In some cases, a living will is even used to request resuscitation under certain circumstances.

Vague statements are a pitfall to avoid in making a living will. Different doctors may take very different meanings from statements like, "I do not want any heroic measures to be used if my doctors say that I will not recover" or "I want every reasonable kind of care to be offered regardless of how ill I am." However, no matter how specific a person tries to be when preparing a living will, it is impossible to anticipate every possible set of circumstances that might arise.

Reviewing a living will with the doctor at the time it is written helps ensure that it will work the way in which it is intended. Periodic reviews of the document with the doctor allow the person to ask questions and to consider adding or removing certain requests as health status changes and preferences evolve.

Durable Power of Attorney for Health Care

A durable power of attorney for health care (proxy) enables an older person to appoint someone to make health care decisions in the event that he becomes temporarily or permanently incapacitated. The person sought to fill this role is most often a trusted family member or friend. The older person should first establish the person's willingness to serve as health care agent. It is important to make those wishes clear and to ensure that the agent is willing to represent those wishes. A living will can be a valuable tool for structuring the discussion between a person and the health care agent. When a living will is used for this purpose, to avoid confusion, the living will should not be signed, but merely used as a guide.

A durable power of attorney for health care is sometimes prepared by a legal professional, but such preparation is not required. However, some states do require that signatures be notarized. The decisions made by the agent may be guided by specific written or spoken instructions from the older person. A durable power of attorney for health care may include a living will provision—a description of health care choices—but the living will in such cases serves as guidance for the agent rather than as a binding directive. To ensure this, the living will should state that in the event of any differences between the living will and the agent, the agent should have final say in decisions.

The older person should review instructions periodically with the agent to ensure that the appointed person's understanding remains current. If the older person has not given the agent any instructions, the agent makes decisions based on what he believes the person would have wanted under the circumstances or on what he believes to be in the person's best interests.

When an older person with a durable power of attorney for health care becomes incapacitated, the agent discusses treatment alternatives and outlook for recovery with the health care team. The agent then makes decisions based on current circumstances and on what is known about the older person's preferences and values. The agent is also an advocate for the person and can argue for aggressive care or for withholding care as the person's diagnosis, condition, and outlook change. The agent's flexibility while making decisions makes a durable power of attorney preferable to a living will for many people.

A person who is competent can cancel a durable power of attorney at any time. The appointment of an agent does not have to be permanent. If circumstances change, the person can create a new durable power of attorney appointing a new health care agent.

SURROGATES

When a person is incapable of making health care decisions, another person may act as an informal substitute (surrogate). In the absence of a court-appointed guardian, a living will, or a durable power of attorney for health care, the health care team must turn elsewhere. Some states have regulations or statutes that direct the choice of who should fill this role. When this is not the case, the team generally accepts a person, agreed upon by everyone involved (such as family members), who has a relationship that might provide insight into the older person's values and preferences. This person, who becomes a surrogate without formal legal empowerment, may be a spouse, an adult child, a sibling, or, in some cases, even a parent.

A surrogate may be asked to provide consent to treat the incapacitated older person. However, a surrogate who refuses treatment on behalf of the older person, when members of the health care team feel that treatment is in the person's best interest, is likely to be challenged. This is especially so if the surrogate is a distant relative or a friend. If health care practitioners have reason to doubt the surrogate's ability to make decisions based on the person's preferences and values, they are more likely to seek court involvement to name a guardian. But this process is rarely invoked because it is cumbersome, costly, and slow, often leaving the person in a decision-making limbo.

66

Paying for Health Care

Dealing with the costs of a serious or chronic disorder can be as distressing as dealing with the disorder itself. The costs are often beyond the personal resources of most people. For older people, most health care expenses are paid for by Medicare, Medicaid, or other government programs such as the Department of Veterans Affairs (VA). Medicare was set up to help people who are old. Medicaid was set up to help people who are disabled or poor. The VA provides health care for honorably discharged veterans. These programs are supplemented by private insurance or personal funds, including those of family members.

Understanding how Medicare, Medicaid, or other government programs work is complicated. What is completely paid for, what is partly paid for, who pays for how much of what, and how the payments are arranged are hard to figure out. Part of the problem is that regulations vary from state to state and that they change frequently. The government and health care foundations provide current information about these programs on the Internet and in booklets available by mail. But part of the problem is the complexity and fragmented nature of the health care system (lack of continuity of care)[1] and of the payment system for health care.

Health care can be paid for in two ways: as fee for service or as part of managed care.

• With the fee-for-service approach, each hospital stay, each visit to a health care practitioner, each test, and each treatment is paid for as it happens. The fee may be paid by the person, Medicare, Medicaid, or private insurance.

• In managed care, a fee is paid regularly to a managed care organization, such as a health maintenance organization (HMO).[2] The fee may be paid by Medicare, Medicaid, the person, or by the person's employer as a benefit. When care is received, the person may pay only a small part of the charge for that care (as a deductible or copayment). The managed care organization pays the rest. In some cases, the managed care organization pays all of the costs for care received.

MEDICARE

Medicare helps older people pay for health care services. But it pays only for services it considers appropriate. These services are called covered services. Costs for covered services are called allowable charges. However, Medicare does not pay for all of the costs for covered services. The first time a certain service is needed, people must usually pay a small fixed amount (called a deductible) before Medicare pays anything. If people need the same service again after a specified time has passed, they have to pay another deductible. After the deductible has

1. see page 101
2. see page 970

been paid, people usually also have to pay a certain percentage of the costs (called a copayment) each time they use a service. For example, the deductible for outpatient services (such as a doctor's visit) may be $100 each calendar year, and the copayment for each use of outpatient service may be 20% of the allowable charges. This arrangement means that people pay the first $100 of their outpatient bills. Then, for the next year, they pay 20% of the allowable charges each time they use a service, and Medicare pays the rest. When the calendar year is over, they must pay another deductible for services used in the next year.

Medicare offers two types of health care plans: the original Medicare plan and Medicare + Choice. Medicare + Choice offers alternative plans for health care, including managed care and fee-for-service care.

Original Medicare plan: Available nationwide, this plan operates on a fee-for-service basis. It has two parts, Part A and Part B.

• Part A (often referred to as hospital insurance) covers hospital services and some outpatient services commonly needed for a short time after a hospital stay.
• Part B (often referred to as medical insurance) covers outpatient services, including doctors' fees.

With the original Medicare plan, choice of doctor and hospital is not limited. However, some doctors require that the person pay the bill and fill out the paperwork (file the claim) for reimbursement by Medicare. Other doctors file the claim themselves and receive payment directly from Medicare.

Some doctors do not accept Medicare payments as full payment (that is, they do not accept "assignment" from Medicare). They may charge more for a service than Medicare pays. (Medicare pays a set amount—what it considers a usual, customary, and reasonable amount—for each service it covers.) These doctors charge up to an extra 15% of the Medicare-approved amount. Paying any extra charges is the person's responsibility. So a person should ask doctors in advance if they accept Medicare as full payment.

CHANGES IN MEDICARE

Medicare often changes. Late in 2003, Congress approved perhaps the most dramatic change since Medicare began in the early 1960s. This change is called the Medicare Prescription Drug, Improvement, and Modernization Act. This act adds prescription drug coverage, to be called Medicare Part D, to Medicare's benefits. The new benefit does not begin until January 1, 2006, and changes may be made before then. It is voluntary. That is, people have to sign up for it (enroll). For this benefit, a person pays a premium each month, probably $35 in 2006.

Each year, before receiving any reimbursement, the person must pay the first $250 of drug costs (the deductible). Then, Medicare pays 75% of costs up to a total of $2,250. The person must pay the other 25%

of costs (the copayment) for each prescription out of pocket. After the total of $2,250 is reached, the person must pay for all drug costs until the total reaches $5,100. Then, Medicare pays 95% of any additional drug costs for the rest of the year. Each year, the process starts over, with the person having to pay another deductible.

People will continue to have a choice between the original Medicare plan (Parts A and B) or Medicare + Choice (to be called Medicare Advantage). Under Medicare + Choice, an HMO may manage care. Under an HMO, the premiums, deductibles, and copayments for the drug benefit may vary somewhat from those under original Medicare. Insurance companies will not be allowed to sell Medigap plans that pay all or part of drug costs not covered by the new Medicare plan.

The premiums, deductibles, and copayments vary depending on income level. For people with a very low annual income and few assets, these costs may be lower or be nothing. Premiums for all types of Medicare plans will increase for people with an annual income of more than $80,000.

During 2004 and 2005, Medicare recipients will have the option of purchasing a drug discount card, which may reduce their cost for prescriptions, typically by 10 to 15%.

The new drug benefit will not remain the same from year to year. Premiums, deductibles, and copayments are expected to increase annually through at least 2013.

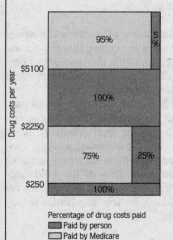

Percentage of drug costs paid

▨ Paid by person
☐ Paid by Medicare

Part A is automatic for most people when they reach age 65. Anyone who is eligible for Social Security, Railroad Retirement, or Civil Service Retirement benefits has Part A. Such people are sent their Medicare card about 3 months before their 65th birthday. Part A is paid for by a federal tax that is automatically deducted each month from payroll checks (as for Social Security). Thus, people who are enrolled in Part A do not have to pay monthly fees for it. People who continue to work after age 65 should enroll in Part A during open enrollment (the 6-month period starting 3 months before their 65th birthday and ending 3 months after). Enrolling after this period often costs more. People who are not eligible may be able to purchase Part A.

WHO PAYS FOR WHAT?

Type of Care	Services	Covered by
Hospital care	Inpatient care, including mental health care General nursing and other hospital services and supplies Semiprivate room (private room only if medically necessary) Meals	Medicare Part A Medicare + Choice Medicaid Department of Veterans Affairs (VA)*
Short-term care in a certified skilled nursing facility (nursing home)	Skilled nursing care Social services Drugs Medical supplies and equipment used in facility Dietary counseling Physical, occupational, and speech therapy (if needed) to meet patient's health goals Transportation by ambulance (when other transportation endangers health) to the nearest facility providing needed	Medicare Part A if a person needs it temporarily after a hospital stay Medicare + Choice if a person needs it temporarily after a hospital stay Medicaid VA*

Table continues on the following page.

Type of Care	Services	Covered by
	services unavailable at the skilled nursing facility	
	Semiprivate room	
	Meals	
Outpatient care	Doctor's fees	Medicare Part B
	Emergency department visits	Medicare + Choice
		Medicaid
	Transportation by ambulance (when other transportation endangers health)	VA*
	Outpatient surgery (with no overnight stay in the hospital)	
	Rehabilitation (physical, occupational, and speech therapy)	
	Diagnostic tests	
	Outpatient mental health care	
	A second opinion if surgery is recommended and a third opinion if opinions differ	
	For people with diabetes, part of the costs of monitoring sugar (glucose) levels in the blood	
Home health care	Personal care, including help with eating, bathing, going to the bathroom, dressing	Medicare Part A if a person is homebound and needs part-time skilled nursing care or rehabilitation on a daily basis
	Part-time skilled nursing care	
	Physical, occupational, and speech therapy	
	Home health aide services	Medicare Part B
	Social services	Medicare + Choice
		Medicaid
	Durable medical equipment, such as	VA

Type of Care	Services	Covered by
	wheelchairs, hospital beds, oxygen, and walkers Medical supplies, such as wound dressings, but not prescription drugs	
Preventive care	Screening tests for prostate and colorectal cancer Mammography Papanicolaou (Pap) test Bone density measurements	Medicare Part B Medicare + Choice Medicaid VA*
Extra benefits	Prescription drugs Eyeglasses Hearing aids	Medicare + Choice Medicaid in some states VA*
Long-term care in an assisted living community	Varies greatly from community to community Meals Help with daily activities Some social and recreational activities Some health care	Medicaid in a few states (partial coverage) VA* in some situations
Long-term care in a certified skilled nursing facility (nursing home)	Varies from state to state	Medicaid VA*
Hospice care	Physical care and counseling Room and meals only during inpatient respite care and short-term hospital stays	Medicare Part A Medicare + Choice

*For the Veterans Administration, the rules of eligibility vary for different services and change frequently.

Part A helps pay for hospital care, care in a skilled nursing facility (if services are needed daily after a related 3-day stay in a hospital), and hospice care.[1] Hospice care is available only for people with a life expectancy of no more than 6 months. When hospice care is selected, the hospice organization manages all benefits from Medicare (and Medicaid).

For people who are homebound and need part-time skilled nursing care or rehabilitation, Part A helps pay for home health care, including help with personal care (such as bathing, going to the bathroom, and dressing).

Part A pays for care on the basis of benefit periods. A benefit period begins when a person is admitted to a hospital or skilled nursing facility and ends when the person has been out of the facility for 60 days in a row. If a person is readmitted after the 60 days, a new deductible must be paid. There is no limit to the number of benefit periods.

Part B is optional. If people are eligible for Part A, they are eligible for Part B. People who choose to enroll can purchase Part B insurance for a fee paid each month. The fee is usually deducted from their Social Security, Railroad Retirement, or Civil Service Retirement check. The best time to sign up for Part B is during open enrollment. Otherwise, the rates may be higher. At age 65, some people are still working, or their spouse is still working. Many of these people have health insurance through their or their spouse's employer. These people have a delayed enrollment option, which enables them to enroll in Part B later but at the open-enrollment rate. The open-enrollment rate for Part B changes every year. In 2003, the rate was $58.70 a month for most people.

Part B helps pay for many services and supplies that are used on an outpatient basis and that are medically necessary. For example, it helps pay for doctors' fees, emergency department visits, and outpatient surgery (with no overnight stay in the hospital). It also helps pay for transportation by ambulance when other types of transportation are likely to be unsafe, rehabilitation, diagnostic tests, outpatient mental health care, and reusable (durable) medical equipment for home use such as wheelchairs. Part B may pay for home health care for homebound people when Part A does not. If surgery is recommended, Part B helps pay for a second opinion and, if opinions differ, a third opinion.

Part B helps pay for some preventive care. Examples are an

1. see page 112

annual influenza (flu) vaccine and screening tests such as mammography, Papanicolaou (Pap) tests, bone density measurements, and tests for prostate cancer and colorectal cancer. It helps pay for glaucoma tests for people who are at increased risk because they are black and over 50, have diabetes, or have a family history of glaucoma. For people with diabetes, Part B pays for some costs of monitoring sugar (glucose) levels in the blood.

Neither part A nor part B covers the following:

- Private-duty nursing
- Telephone and television in the hospital
- A private hospital room (unless medically necessary)
- Most prescription drugs and all nonprescription drugs
- Personal care at home or in a nursing home unless people also need skilled nursing care or rehabilitation
- Hearing aids
- Vision care
- Dental care
- Care outside the United States, except in certain circumstances
- Experimental procedures
- Some preventive care
- Cosmetic surgery
- Most chiropractic services
- Acupuncture

Medicare + Choice: For this plan, Medicare makes arrangements with other organizations, such as insurance companies, hospital systems, or managed care organizations, to provide care. This plan is available in many areas of the United States.

Medicare + Choice may be a fee-for-service or managed care plan. In fee-for-service plans, a person can choose any doctor or hospital, and the plan pays for a share of the cost. However, a private company, not Medicare, decides how much a service costs, so costs may be higher.

Medicare managed care is handled by a health maintenance organization (HMO) or preferred provider organization (PPO). In HMOs, a person chooses a primary care doctor within the HMO's network. (The network includes doctors, medical clinics, and hospitals that the HMO or other managed care organization has selected and contracted with to care for its members.) The primary care doctor may refer the person to other health care practitioners as needed. Practitioners must be part of the HMO network for the HMO to cover care. Emergency care when a person is out of the area is an exception. In PPOs, a person can, within some limits, choose doctors outside the PPO's network. But the monthly fee for PPOs is higher than that for HMOs. Some HMOs offer a point-of-service option for an additional monthly fee. As in PPOs, a person with this option can choose some doctors outside the HMO's network, and the HMO pays for part of the costs.

Some Medicare + Choice plans offer coordination of care, lower or no deductibles and copayments, and extra benefits. For example, the plans may help pay for prescription drugs, eyeglasses, hearing aids, and preventive care. Some plans cover services not usually covered by the original Medicare plan. An example is an assessment by an interdisciplinary team that specializes in caring for older people. Medicare + Choice requires people to pay the same fee (sometimes less) as that for Part B. Often, there is an additional monthly fee. Medicare + Choice plans vary from state to state.

When deciding about Medicare options, people should consider what they want in terms of out-of-pocket costs, extra benefits, choice of doctors, convenience, and quality.

Another Medicare Option

Programs are being designed to provide more comprehensive, better-integrated health care for older people. An example is the Program of All-Inclusive Care for the Elderly (PACE). This program is an optional benefit of Medicare and uses funds from Medicare and Medicaid. As a type of managed care, it may require a monthly fee. PACE is designed for older people frail enough to need care in a nursing home. However, the goal of the PACE program is to enable older people to live at home as long as possible. In PACE, an interdisciplinary team assesses the participant's needs, develops a care plan, and provides all necessary health care. It includes medical and dental care, adult day care (including transportation to and from the facility), health and personal care at home, prescription drugs, social services, rehabilitation, meals, nutritional counseling, and hospital and long-term care when needed. PACE is available in 13 states.

MEDICAID

Medicaid helps pay for health care for people of all ages who have a very low income and few assets. For older people, Medicaid often pays for nursing home care.

If people have a very low income but have assets such as a home or stock investments, they may not qualify for Medicaid. To qualify, they may have to "spend down." That is, they may have to sell their stocks and other assets and use the money to pay for health care until their income plus assets is low enough to qualify. In some states, people may be able to keep their home so that certain family members can remain there. However, when the family members leave, the government can sell the home to recover the money it has spent on care. Eligibility requirements for Medicaid vary from state to state. If people qualify for Medicaid and Medicare, most health care costs are covered.

Medicaid, which is funded by the federal and state governments, is the main public payer for long-term care, such as skilled nursing care (including that in a nursing home).[1] Medicaid is required to offer long-term care to eligible people who are 21 years or older and who participate in the Medicaid program. Medicaid also helps pay for hospital care, laboratory tests (such as blood and urine tests), diagnostic tests (such as x-rays), visits to the doctor, and home health care. Because each state manages its own Medicaid program, the services covered vary from state to state. In some states, Medicaid helps pay for other items, such as prescription drugs, dental care, eyeglasses, and intermediate-level nursing care. Intermediate-level nursing care involves less care than skilled nursing care but more care than personal care. Its purpose is to maintain a person's condition and, if possible, to improve it.

PRIVATE INSURANCE

Many older people buy supplemental health insurance from private companies. Some insurance companies offer long-term

1. see page 190

care insurance, paid for with monthly fees. The decision to buy long-term care insurance depends partly on whether a person would need help paying for long-term care and on whether the person can afford long-term care insurance. Some states have special private insurance programs in which a person can qualify for Medicare reimbursement of long-term care expenses without the usual spend-down requirement. To qualify, the person must have received benefits from the private insurance policy for a specified period.

Medigap: Medigap is supplemental insurance designed to pay for medical care not covered by Medicare, including the deductibles and copayments required by Medicare and extra charges by doctors who do not accept Medicare as full payment for a service. Medigap policies do not duplicate payment for services covered by Medicare Parts A and B. However, Medigap policies may duplicate payment for many services covered by Medicare + Choice plans. The best time to purchase Medigap insurance is during an enrollment period that begins when Medicare Part B is purchased and ends 6 months later. At other times, Medigap may be unavailable or more expensive. Many insurance companies offer Medigap insurance.

There are 10 types of Medigap policies, labeled A through J. Each type offers a different set of benefits. But the benefits of a specific type are the same no matter which insurance company offers it. No Medigap policy covers payment for long-term personal care (at home or in a nursing home), vision or dental care, hearing aids, private-duty nursing, or all prescription drugs. However, additional insurance policies that cover such services can be purchased.

UNDERSTANDING MANAGED CARE

Managed care means that health care is paid for in advance. Funds come from payments made regularly into an account by all members in the managed care plan, members' employers, Medicare, or Medicaid. When care is received, the person pays only a small part of the cost (as a deductible or copayment). Managed care organizations manage health care using a fixed budget. They also have set amounts that they will pay for each service.

WHO NEEDS LONG-TERM CARE INSURANCE?

Because people are living longer, more people are likely to need long-term care. Long-term care involves helping people function as well as possible. It includes help with daily activities, such as preparing meals, bathing, and dressing, as well as with health care. Long-term care may be provided in the home or a long-term care facility, such as a nursing home.

Because long-term care is needed for a long time, it is likely to be expensive. Many people need help paying for it. Many people mistakenly think that Medicare covers long-term care.

Whether to buy long-term care insurance depends on several things:

Need: Is long-term care insurance needed? People who do *not* need this insurance include those

• Whose only income comes from Social Security and who have limited assets
• Who qualify for Medicaid or will qualify soon after they enter a nursing home
• Who have large financial reserves

People who should consider this insurance include those who are neither rich nor poor and

• Who want to protect their assets or those of a family member
• Who do not want to depend on a family member for care
• Who want to make sure they receive high-quality care
• Who want to have more control over when, how, and where they receive care—for example, in their home rather than in a nursing home

Costs: Will buying long-term care insurance cause financial hardship? People should consider whether they can pay the premiums over the long term, even if their income decreases. They should find out how often and how much premiums increase and how many days a person has to pay for before the insurance pays (the elimination period).

Timing: Is it better to buy long-term care insurance now or later? The younger people are, the more cheaply they can buy long-term care insurance. On the other hand, the younger people are when they start paying for it, the longer they are likely to pay before they need to use it. However, if people wait too long, they may develop disorders that make long-term care insurance difficult or impossible to obtain.

Coverage: People who have decided to buy long-term care insurance have to decide how many years of coverage they want (the benefit period). The average stay in a nursing home is 2 to 3 years, so most people choose a slightly longer time: 4 to 6 years. They must decide what maximum amount is needed to pay for each day of care (the daily benefit). Most people choose $100 to $150 a day. The amount should be close to the average cost of care at local nursing homes. They must choose what options they want. Examples are built-in inflation protection and a well-defined trigger for the start of benefits—for example, when a person can no longer do a basic daily activity, such as bathing and dressing.

Managed care has many variations. So one explanation of managed care does not fit all. For example, a person can choose a health maintenance organization (HMO) or preferred provider organization (PPO).[1] There are many more HMOs than PPOs. When people are choosing a managed care organization or switching from one to another, information about preexisting health problems cannot be used to deny them access to health care insurance. Doing so is against the law.

Different types of managed care plans are available. Anyone who has a managed care insurance plan should keep a copy of the description of the plan handy for easy reference.

Managed care has several advantages, particularly for older people. Some managed care plans are designed specifically for older people. These plans coordinate the services of the needed health care practitioners at the appropriate sites of care (such as hospital, rehabilitation facility, or long-term care facility).[2] Managed care organizations encourage access to health care services in the home so that older people may be able to avoid a stay in a hospital or long-term care facility.

Managed care may emphasize prevention. For example, in some plans, people are notified when they need a particular screening test, such as mammography to check for breast cancer. Managed care organizations provide information about care that can help prevent problems in older people. For example, practitioners and members may be sent information about the benefit of annual influenza (flu) vaccination. The information includes specific steps to follow so that members know how to get vaccinated. Practitioners may be sent guidelines about which tests and treatments are helpful to older people and which are unnecessary or may do more harm than good.

Managed care organizations may try to identify members who have specific needs, who need complex health care, or who are likely to develop a disorder. To identify such people, these organizations may periodically send members health appraisals to fill out. Information is also collected from doctors' visits, insurance claims, and pharmacies. This information is used to tailor a managed care plan to fit individual health care needs. Then

1. see page 965
2. see page 101

these organizations distribute guidelines for managing specific needs. For example, members who use many prescriptions within a short time may be sent a letter describing the risks of taking many drugs. They are advised to bring all their drugs (prescription and nonprescription) to their primary care doctor. The doctor can then check to make sure the drugs the person is taking are appropriate and not likely to interact harmfully with one another. The doctor can also sometimes simplify the drug schedule or recommend strategies for remembering to take drugs as prescribed.[1]

Information about a member may be available to health care practitioners. Such information is kept in a central database and can be accessed from different places of care. With accessible and complete health care information in one place, a person's practitioners can know about all of the person's medical problems, avoid duplicating treatments and tests, and take steps to prevent harmful interactions among drugs.

Managed care has some disadvantages. HMOs cover care provided only at specific facilities and by certain health care practitioners. People must choose from a list of approved facilities and practitioners. If a person receives health care at another facility or from another practitioner without prior authorization, the HMO often refuses to pay for any of the costs. However, true emergencies handled through the closest hospital are usually partly or fully covered. Some HMOs have a point-of-service option. With it, people may choose facilities or practitioners outside the network, but the copayment is higher. PPOs allow some choice of facilities or practitioners but are more expensive than HMOs. Managed care does not usually include long-term care.

A formal referral approved by the primary care doctor is usually required before a person can see a specialist or undergo certain diagnostic tests. In such cases, the specialist or testing facility usually refuses to see the person without the referral or requires the person to pay directly for the service. Each person is responsible for having the correct referral form.

Most managed care plans limit coverage of some types of health care. For example, certain procedures, such as cosmetic surgery, may not be covered. Sometimes the total number of

1. see page 61

treatments (for example, the number of physical therapy treatments or visits for mental health problems) is limited during a year or over a lifetime. People can talk to their doctor about what types of care are covered. Managed care organizations also provide a list of tests, treatments, and other resources that are covered.

Every day when I awake, I give thanks to my God. Immediately I begin to plan my routine activities for the day. In these activities I include a variety of exercises according to the state of my health that day, organize craft activities (such as bobbing lace and crocheting) and domestic activities, and visit nursing homes and hospices.

I feel very happy to share my knowledge of crafts with people of different ages, especially those who are 45 years or older.

In general, crafts have been for me a medicine, a therapy, because they help me to be alert so that my physical, emotional, and mental health can be at their best. For this reason, I recommend that older people, no matter what their age, interest themselves in doing any craft in order to keep their minds busy. Sharing my crafts and emotions with older people and having conversations with them help me feel useful, and this is beneficial to my health.

Some of these crafts, such as crocheting, bobbing lace, embroidering collars, sewing, and doing fancy stitching, are all great therapy for a sound mind and a healthy body. This is because these tasks require that I move my wrists and fingers in specific ways and that, above all, I maintain a high level of concentration. When I exercise my mind and body in this way, I can only think positively about myself.

Through the crafts that I create and the instruction that I provide to older people, I maintain a very good state of mental, physical, and emotional health. Although I am 77 years old, I don't feel or look so, and I'm very happy. My experiences with older people have made me stronger, and I have done the same for them. Many of these people were in a state of depression and managed to conquer it. The same is true for people with cancer.

Eduvina Colón Ferrer

Appendix I

Drug Names:
Generic and Trade

Most prescription drugs placed on the market are given trade names (also called proprietary, brand, or specialty names) to distinguish them as being produced and marketed exclusively by a particular manufacturer. In the United States, these names are usually registered as trademarks with the Patent Office; this gives the registrant certain legal rights with respect to the use of the name. A trade name may be registered for a product containing a single active ingredient, with or without additives, or for one containing two or more active ingredients.

A drug marketed by several companies may have several trade names. A drug manufactured in one country and marketed in many countries may have different trade names in each country.

Throughout this book, generic (nonproprietary) names have been used whenever possible. However, because trade names are used commonly and may be more readily recognized, the generic drugs mentioned in this book are listed below in alphabetic order along with many of their trade names. A second table follows, listing the trade names in alphabetic order along with their generic name.

With few exceptions, the trade names in these tables are limited to those marketed in the United States. These tables are by no means all-inclusive, and no effort has been made to list every trade name in current use for each drug. The inclusion of a drug in these tables does not indicate approval of a drug's use, nor does it imply that a drug is effective or safe. Many drugs are marketed almost exclusively under their generic name. Including a trade name of such a drug in these tables does not indicate an endorsement or preference for the trade name version over the generic version.

Whether it is best to use a trade or a generic version of a drug may be a complex decision. It is best to discuss such matters with a doctor or pharmacist.

℞ SOME TRADE NAMES OF GENERIC DRUGS

Generic	Trade	Generic	Trade
Abciximab	REOPRO	Bimatoprost	LUMIGAN
Acarbose	PRECOSE	Bisacodyl	DULCOLAX
Acebutolol	SECTRAL	Bisoprolol	ZEBETA
Acetaminophen	TYLENOL	Bretylium	BRETYLOL
Acetylcholine	MIOCHOL, MIOCHOL-E	Brimonidine	ALPHAGAN
		Brinzolamide	AZOPT
Albuterol	PROVENTIL, VENTOLIN	Bromocriptine	PARLODEL
		Bumetanide	BUMEX
Alemtuzumab	CAMPATH	Bupropion	WELLBUTRIN, ZYBAN
Alendronate	FOSAMAX		
Alfuzosin	UROXATRAL	Buspirone	BUSPAR
Allopurinol	LOPURIN, ZYLOPRIM	Calcitonin	MIACALCIN, CALCIMAR
Alteplase	ACTIVASE	Candesartan	ATACAND
Amantadine	SYMMETREL	Capsaicin	ZOSTRIX, CAPSIN, CAPZASIN
Amiloride	MIDAMOR		
Amiodarone	CORDARONE, PACERONE	Captopril	CAPOTEN
		Carbachol	MIOSTAT, CARBASTAT
Amitriptyline	ELAVIL		
Amlodipine	NORVASC	Carbamazepine	TEGRETOL, EPITOL
Amoxicillin	AMOXIL, TRIMOX, LAROTID		
		Carbidopa	LODOSYN
Amoxicillin-clavulanate	AUGMENTIN	Carisoprodol	SOMA
		Carteolol	CARTROL, OCUPRESS
Ampicillin-sulbactam	UNASYN		
		Carvedilol	COREG
Anastrozole	ARIMIDEX	Celecoxib	CELEBREX
Anistreplase	EMINASE	Cephalexin	KEFLEX
Apraclonidine	IOPIDINE	Cetirizine	ZYRTEC
Argatroban	ARGATROBAN	Cevimeline	EVOXAC
Aripiprazole	ABILIFY	Chlorambucil	LEUKERAN
Aspirin	ECOTRIN, ASPERGUM	Chloramphenicol	CHLOROMYCETIN
		Chlordiazepoxide	LIBRIUM
Atenolol	TENORMIN	Chlorothiazide	DIURIL
Atorvastatin	LIPITOR	Chlorphenira-mine	CHLOR-TRIMETON
Azithromycin	ZITHROMAX		
Baclofen	LIORESAL		
Benazepril	LOTENSIN	Chlorpromazine	THORAZINE, SONAZINE
Bendroflume-thiazide	NATURETIN-5		
		Chlorpropamide	DIABINESE
		Chlorthalidone	HYGROTON
Benztropine	COGENTIN	Chlorzoxazone	PARAFON FORTE, STRIFON FORTE
Betaxolol	BETOPTIC, KERLONE		
		Cholestyramine	QUESTRAN
Bethanechol	URECHOLINE	Cimetidine	TAGAMET
Bicalutamide	CASODEX	Ciprofloxacin	CILOXAN, CIPRO

Rx SOME TRADE NAMES OF GENERIC DRUGS

Generic	Trade	Generic	Trade
Cisplatin	PLATINOL	Docetaxel	TAXOTERE
Citalopram	CELEXA	Docusate	COLACE, CORRECTOL, SURFAK
Clarithromycin	BIAXIN		
Clindamycin	CLEOCIN		
Clonazepam	KLONOPIN	Dofetilide	TIKOSYN
Clopidogrel	PLAVIX	Donepezil	ARICEPT
Clozapine	CLOZARIL	Dopamine	INTROPIN
Codeine	CODEINE	Dorzolamide	TRUSOPT
Colchicine-probenecid	COL-PROBENECID	Doxazosin	CARDURA
		Doxepin	SINEQUAN, ZONALON
Colesevelam	WELCHOL		
Colestipol	COLESTID	Doxorubicin	ADRIAMYCIN, RUBEX
Cyclobenzaprine	FLEXERIL		
Cyclophospha-mide	CYTOXAN, NEOSAR	Doxycycline	VIBRAMYCIN, VIBRA-TABS, DORYX
Cyclosporine	SANDIMMUNE, NEORAL, GENGRAF		
		Dronabinol	MARINOL
Cyproheptadine	PERIACTIN	Edrophonium	TENSILON, ENLON
Dalteparin	FRAGMIN	Enalapril	VASOTEC
Darbepoietin	ARANESP	Enoxaparin	LOVENOX
Desipramine	NORPRAMIN	Entacapone	COMTAN
Dextroampheta-mine	DEXEDRINE	Entacapone plus levodopa/carbidopa	STALEVO
Diazepam	VALIUM, DIASTAT	Epirubicin	ELLENCE
Dicyclomine	BENTYL	Eplerenone	INSPRA
Digitoxin (not available in US)	DIGITALINE	Eprosartan	TEVETEN
		Eptifibatide	INTEGRILIN
Digoxin	LANOXIN, LANOXICAPS	Ergoloid mesylates	HYDERGINE
Diltiazem	CARDIZEM, DILACOR XR, TIAZAC	Erythromycin	E-MYCIN, ERYTHROCIN, ILOSONE
Dimethyl sulfoxide	RIMSO-50	Erythropoietin [also Epoetin alfa]	EPOGEN, PROCRIT
Diphenhydra-mine	BENADRYL, NYTOL, SOMINEX		
		Escitalopram	LEXAPRO
		Estazolam	PROSOM
Diphenoxylate plus atropine sulfate	LOMOTIL, LONOX	Ethacrynic acid	EDECRIN
		Etidronate	DIDRONEL
		Ezetimibe	ZETIA
Dipyridamole	PERSANTINE	Famotidine	PEPCID
Disopyramide	NORPACE	Felodipine	PLENDIL, LEXXEL
Divalproex	DEPAKOTE		
Dobutamine	DOBUTREX	Fenofibrate	TRICOR

℞ SOME TRADE NAMES OF GENERIC DRUGS

Generic	Trade	Generic	Trade
Fentanyl	SUBLIMAZE, DURAGESIC, ACTIQ	Hydroxyzine	ATARAX, VISTARIL
		Hyoscyamine	LEVSIN, ANASPAZ, LEVBID
Fexofenadine	ALLEGRA	Ibuprofen	ADVIL, MOTRIN, MOTRIN IB, IBU
Flecainide	TAMBOCOR		
5-fluorouracil	EFUDEX	Ibutilide	CORVERT
Fluconazole	DIFLUCAN	Imipenem	PRIMAXIN
Fludarabine	FLUDARA	Indapamide	LOZOL
Fludrocortisone	FLORINEF	Indinavir	CRIXIVAN
Fluorouracil	ADRUCIL	Indomethacin	INDOCIN
Fluoxetine	PROZAC, SARAFEM	Infliximab	REMICADE
		Insulin	HUMULIN, NOVOLIN, HUMALOG
Fluphenazine	PERMITIL, PROLIXIN		
Flurazepam	DALMANE	Ipratropium	ATROVENT
Flutamide	EULEXIN	Irbesartan	AVAPRO
Fluvastatin	LESCOL	Irinotecan	CAMPTOSAR
Fluvoxamine	FLUVOXAMINE	Isosorbide dinitrate	ISORDIL, SORBITRATE, DILATRATE-SR
Fosinopril	MONOPRIL		
Furosemide	LASIX		
Gabapentin	NEURONTIN	Isosorbide mononitrate	IMDUR, ISMO, MONOKET
Galantamine	REMINYL		
Gatifloxacin	TEQUIN, ZYMAR	Isradipine	DYNACIRC
Gemfibrozil	LOPID	Itraconazole	SPORANOX
Glimepiride	AMARYL	Labetalol	NORMODYNE, TRANDATE
Glipizide	GLUCOTROL, GLUCOTROL XL		
		Lactulose	CONSTULOSE, CONSTILAC, HEPTALAC
Glyburide	DIABETA, MICRONASE, GLYNASE		
		Lansoprazole	PREVACID
Glycerol [also Glycerin]	OSMOGLYN	Latanoprost	XALATAN
		Lepirudin	REFLUDAN
Goserelin	ZOLADEX	Leuprolide	LUPRON, ELIGARD, VIADUR
Guaifenesin	FENESIN, ROBITUSSIN		
		Levodopa with carbidopa	SINEMET, SINEMET CR
Haloperidol	HALDOL		
Heparin	CALCIPARINE, LIQUAEMIN	Levofloxacin	QUIXIN, LEVAQUIN
		Levorphanol	LEVO-DROMORAN
Hyaluronate	HYALGAN		
Hydralazine	APRESOLINE	Lidocaine	XYLOCAINE, LIDOPEN, LIDODERM
Hydrochloro-thiazide	ESIDRIX, ORETIC		
Hydroflume-thiazide	SALURON		
Hydromorphone	DILAUDID	Lisinopril	PRINIVIL, ZESTRIL

℞ SOME TRADE NAMES OF GENERIC DRUGS

Generic	Trade	Generic	Trade
Lithium	ESKALITH, ESKALITH CR, LITHOBID	Milrinone	PRIMACOR
		Mirtazapine	REMERON
		Misoprostol	CYTOTEC
Loratadine	CLARITIN, ALAVERT	Mitomycin	MUTAMYCIN, MYTOZYTREX
Lorazepam	ATIVAN	Modafinil	PROVIGIL
Losartan	COZAAR	Moexipril	UNIVASC
Lovastatin	MEVACOR, ALTOCOR	Molindone	MOBAN
		Moricizine	ETHMOZINE
Loxapine	LOXITANE	Morphine	MS CONTIN, ORAMORPH, KADIAN
Mannitol	OSMITROL		
Megestrol	MEGACE		
Melphalan	ALKERAN	Moxifloxacin	AVELOX, VIGAMOX
Memantine	NAMENDA		
Meperidine	DEMEROL	Nadolol	CORGARD
Meprobamate	MILTOWN, TRANMEP	Nafcillin	NALLPEN
		Naloxone	NARCAN
Mesoridazine	SERENTIL	Naproxen	ALEVE, ANAPROX, NAPRELAN
Metaxalone	SKELAXIN		
Metformin	GLUCOPHAGE, GLUCOPHAGE XR		
		Nateglinide	STARLIX
		Nefazodone	SERZONE
Methadone	DOLOPHINE, METHADOSE	Nesiritide	NATRECOR
		Niacin	NIASPAN, NICOLAR
Methocarbamol	ROBAXIN		
Methotrexate	RHEUMATREX, FOLEX, TREXALL	Nicardipine	CARDENE
		Nifedipine	ADALAT CC, PROCARDIA
Methyclothiazide	ENDURON	Nilutamide	NILANDRON
Methyldopa	ALDOMET	Nisoldipine	SULAR
Methylphenidate	RITALIN, CONCERTA, METHYLIN	Nitrazepam (not available in US)	MOGADON
		Nitrofurantoin	FURADANTIN, MACRODANTIN
Metoclopramide	REGLAN		
Metolazone	MYKROX, ZAROXOLYN	Nitroglycerin	NITRO-BID, NITROSTAT, NITRO-DUR
Metoprolol	LOPRESSOR, TOPROL-XL		
		Nitroprusside	NITROPRESS
Metronidazole	FLAGYL, METROGEL, METROMIDOL	Nizatidine	AXID
		Nortriptyline	AVENTYL, PAMELOR
Mexiletine	MEXITIL	Nystatin	MYCOSTATIN, NILSTAT
Midazolam	MIDAZOLAM		
Midodrine	PROAMATINE	Olanzapine	ZYPREXA
Miglitol	GLYSET	Olmesartan	BENICAR

℞ SOME TRADE NAMES OF GENERIC DRUGS

Generic	Trade	Generic	Trade
Omeprazole	PRILOSEC	Prazosin	MINIPRESS
Ondansetron	ZOFRAN	Prednisone	DELTASONE
Orlistat	XENICAL	Primidone	MYSOLINE
Oseltamivir	TAMIFLU	Probenecid	PROBALAN
Oxacillin	BACTOCILL	Procainamide	PROCANBID,
Oxazepam	SERAX		PRONESTYL,
Oxycodone	OXYCONTIN,		PRONESTYL-SR
	ROXICODONE	Prochlorperazine	COMPAZINE,
Oxymorphone	NUMORPHAN		COMPRO
Paclitaxel	TAXOL	Promethazine	PHENERGAN
Pamidronate	AREDIA	Propafenone	RYTHMOL
Pantoprazole	PROTONIX	Propantheline	PRO-BANTHINE
Paroxetine	PAXIL	Propoxyphene	DARVON,
Penbutolol	LEVATOL		KESSO-GESIC
Penicillin	PENICILLIN-VK,	Propranolol	INDERAL
	BEEPEN-VK,	Quetiapine	SEROQUEL
	VEETIDS	Quinapril	ACCUPRIL
Pentazocine	TALWIN	Quinidine	QUINAGLUTE
Pentosan	ELMIRON		DURA-TABS,
polysulfate			QUINIDEX
Pergolide	PERMAX		EXTENTABS
Perindopril	ACEON	Raloxifene	EVISTA
Perphenazine	TRILAFON	Ramipril	ALTACE
Phenazopyridine	PYRIDIUM,	Ranitidine	ZANTAC
	URISTAT	Repaglinide	PRANDIN
Phenelzine	NARDIL	Reserpine	SERPALAN
Phenobarbital	LUMINAL,	Reteplase	RETAVASE
	PHENOBARBI-	Rimantadine	FLUMADINE
	TONE	Risedronate	ACTONEL
Phenytoin	DILANTIN,	Risperidone	RISPERDAL
	PHENYTEK	Ritonavir	NORVIR
Pilocarpine	ISOPTOCARPINE,	Rivastigmine	EXELON
	PILOCAR,	Ropinirole	REQUIP
	PILOPINE HS	Rosiglitazone	AVANDIA
Pimozide	ORAP	Rosuvastatin	CRESTOR
Pindolol	VISKEN	Salmeterol	SEREVENT
Pioglitazone	ACTOS	Scopolamine	ISOPTO
Polycarbophil	EQUALACTIN,	[also Hyoscine]	HYOSCINE,
	FIBERCON		TRANSDERM
	CAPLETS,		SCOP, SCOPACE
	FIBER-LAX,	Secobarbital	SECONAL
	FIBERNORM	Selegiline	ELDEPRYL
Pramipexole	MIRAPEX	Sertraline	ZOLOFT
Pravastatin	PRAVACHOL	Simvastatin	ZOCOR
		Sorbitol	SORBITOL

Rx SOME TRADE NAMES OF GENERIC DRUGS

Generic	Trade	Generic	Trade
Sotalol	BETAPACE, BETAPACE AF, SORINE	Tolcapone	TASMAR
		Topiramate	TOPAMAX
Spironolactone	ALDACTONE	Torsemide	DEMADEX
Streptokinase	STREPTASE, KABIKINASE	Trandolapril	MAVIK
		Trastuzumab	HERCEPTIN
Sulfinpyrazone	ANTURANE	Trazodone	DESYREL
Tacrine	COGNEX	Triamterene	DYRENIUM
Tadalafil	CIALIS	Trifluoperazine	STELAZINE
Tamoxifen	NOLVADEX	Trihexyphenidyl	TRIHEXY-PHENIDYL
Tamsulosin	FLOMAX		
Telmisartan	MICARDIS	Trimethobenza-mide	TIGAN
Temazepam	RESTORIL		
Tenecteplase	TNKASE	Trimethoprim	PROLOPRIM, PRIMSOL
Terazosin	HYTRIN		
Terbinafine	LAMISIL	Trimethoprim-sulfame-thoxazole	BACTRIM, SEPTRA, SULFATRIM
Teriparatide	FORTEO		
Thalidomide	THALOMID		
Theophylline	THEOLAIR, SLO-BID, THEO-24, UNIPHYL	Tripelennamine	PBZ
		Urokinase	ABBOKINASE
		Valproate	DEPAKENE, DEPACON
Thioridazine	THIORIDAZINE		
Thiothixene	NAVANE	Valsartan	DIOVAN
Thyroxine	SYNTHROID, LEVO-T, NOVOTHYROX	Vancomycin	VANCOCIN, VANCOLED
		Vardenafil	LEVITRA
Ticlopidine	TICLID	Venlafaxine	EFFEXOR
Timolol	BLOCADREN, TIMOPTIC, BETIMOL	Verapamil	CALAN, ISOPTIN, VERELAN
		Vincristine	ONCOVIN
		Vinorelbine	NAVELBINE
Tinzaparin	INNOHEP	Warfarin	COUMADIN
Tirofiban	AGGRASTAT	Zaleplon	SONATA
Tocainide	TONOCARD	Zanamivir	RELENZA
Tolazamide	TOLINASE	Ziprasidone	GEODON
Tolbutamide	ORINASE DIAGNOSTIC, TOL-TAB	Zoledronic acid	ZOMETA
		Zolpidem	AMBIEN

℞ GENERIC NAMES OF SOME TRADE NAME DRUGS

Trade	Generic	Trade	Generic
ABBOKINASE	Urokinase	AXID	Nizatidine
ABILIFY	Aripiprazole	AZOPT	Brinzolamide
ACCUPRIL	Quinapril	BACTOCILL	Oxacillin
ACEON	Perindopril	BACTRIM	Trimethoprim-sulfame-thoxazole
ACTIQ	Fentanyl		
ACTIVASE	Alteplase		
ACTONEL	Risedronate	BEEPEN-VK	Penicillin
ACTOS	Pioglitazone	BENADRYL	Diphenhydramine
ADALAT CC	Nifedipine	BENICAR	Olmesartan
ADRIAMYCIN	Doxorubicin	BENTYL	Dicyclomine
ADRUCIL	Fluorouracil	BETAPACE, BETAPACE AF	Sotalol
ADVIL	Ibuprofen		
AGGRASTAT	Tirofiban	BETIMOL	Timolol
ALAVERT	Loratadine	BETOPTIC	Betaxolol
ALDACTONE	Spironolactone	BIAXIN	Clarithromycin
ALDOMET	Methyldopa	BLOCADREN	Timolol
ALEVE	Naproxen	BRETYLOL	Bretylium
ALKERAN	Melphalan	BUMEX	Bumetanide
ALLEGRA	Fexofenadine	BUSPAR	Buspirone
ALPHAGAN	Brimonidine	CALAN	Verapamil
ALTACE	Ramipril	CALCIMAR	Calcitonin
ALTOCOR	Lovastatin	CALCIPARINE	Heparin
AMARYL	Glimepiride	CAMPATH	Alemtuzumab
AMBIEN	Zolpidem	CAMPTOSAR	Irinotecan
AMOXIL	Amoxicillin	CAPOTEN	Captopril
ANAPROX	Naproxen	CAPSIN	Capsaicin
ANASPAZ	Hyoscyamine	CAPZASIN	Capsaicin
ANTURANE	Sulfinpyrazone	CARBASTAT	Carbachol
APRESOLINE	Hydralazine	CARDENE	Nicardipine
ARANESP	Darbepoietin	CARDIZEM	Diltiazem
AREDIA	Pamidronate	CARDURA	Doxazosin
ARGATROBAN	Argatroban	CARTROL	Carteolol
ARICEPT	Donepezil	CASODEX	Bicalutamide
ARIMIDEX	Anastrozole	CELEBREX	Celecoxib
ASPERGUM	Aspirin	CELEXA	Citalopram
ATACAND	Candesartan	CHLORO-MYCETIN	Chloramphenicol
ATARAX	Hydroxyzine		
ATIVAN	Lorazepam	CHLOR-TRIMETON	Chlorpheniramine
ATROVENT	Ipratropium		
AUGMENTIN	Amoxicillin-clavulanate	CIALIS	Tadalafil
		CILOXAN	Ciprofloxacin
AVANDIA	Rosiglitazone	CIPRO	Ciprofloxacin
AVAPRO	Irbesartan	CLARITIN	Loratadine
AVELOX	Moxifloxacin	CLEOCIN	Clindamycin
AVENTYL	Nortriptyline	CLOZARIL	Clozapine

℞ GENERIC NAMES OF SOME TRADE NAME DRUGS

Trade	Generic	Trade	Generic
CODEINE	Codeine	DILATRATE-SR	Isosorbide dinitrate
COGENTIN	Benztropine		
COGNEX	Tacrine	DILAUDID	Hydromorphone
COLACE	Docusate	DIOVAN	Valsartan
COLESTID	Colestipol	DIURIL	Chlorothiazide
COL-PROBENECID	Colchicine-probenecid	DOBUTREX	Dobutamine
		DOLOPHINE	Methadone
COMPAZINE	Prochlorperazine	DORYX	Doxycycline
COMPRO	Prochlorperazine	DULCOLAX	Bisacodyl
COMTAN	Entacapone	DURAGESIC	Fentanyl
CONCERTA	Methylphenidate	DYNACIRC	Isradipine
CONSTILAC	Lactulose	DYRENIUM	Triamterene
CONSTULOSE	Lactulose	ECOTRIN	Aspirin
CORDARONE	Amiodarone	EDECRIN	Ethacrynic acid
COREG	Carvedilol	EFFEXOR	Venlafaxine
CORGARD	Nadolol	EFUDEX	5-fluorouracil
CORRECTOL	Docusate	ELAVIL	Amitriptyline
CORVERT	Ibutilide	ELDEPRYL	Selegiline
COUMADIN	Warfarin	ELIGARD	Leuprolide
COZAAR	Losartan	ELLENCE	Epirubicin
CRESTOR	Rosuvastatin	ELMIRON	Pentosan polysulfate
CRIXIVAN	Indinavir		
CYTOTEC	Misoprostol	EMINASE	Anistreplase
CYTOXAN	Cyclophos-phamide	E-MYCIN	Erythromycin
		ENDURON	Methyclothiazide
DALMANE	Flurazepam	ENLON	Edrophonium
DARVON	Propoxyphene	EPITOL	Carbamazepine
DELTASONE	Prednisone	EPOGEN	Erythropoietin [also epoetin alfa]
DEMADEX	Torsemide		
DEMEROL	Meperidine		
DEPACON	Valproate	EQUALACTIN	Polycarbophil
DEPAKENE	Valproate	ERYTHROCIN	Erythromycin
DEPAKOTE	Divalproex	ESIDRIX	Hydrochloro-thiazide
DESYREL	Trazodone		
DEXEDRINE	Dextroampheta-mine	ESKALITH, ESKALITH CR	Lithium
DIABETA	Glyburide	ETHMOZINE	Moricizine
DIABINESE	Chlorpropamide	EULEXIN	Flutamide
DIASTAT	Diazepam	EVISTA	Raloxifene
DIDRONEL	Etidronate	EVOXAC	Cevimeline
DIFLUCAN	Fluconazole	EXELON	Rivastigmine
DIGITALINE	Digitoxin (not available in US)	FENESIN	Guaifenesin
		FIBERCON CAPLETS	Polycarbophil
DILACOR XR	Diltiazem		
DILANTIN	Phenytoin	FIBERLAX	Polycarbophil

℞ GENERIC NAMES OF SOME TRADE NAME DRUGS

Trade	Generic	Trade	Generic
FIBERNORM	Polycarbophil	ISORDIL	Isosorbide dinitrate
FLAGYL	Metronidazole	KABIKINASE	Streptokinase
FLEXERIL	Cyclobenzaprine	KADIAN	Morphine
FLOMAX	Tamsulosin	KEFLEX	Cephalexin
FLORINEF	Fludrocortisone	KERLONE	Betaxolol
FLUDARA	Fludarabine	KESSO-GESIC	Propoxyphene
FLUMADINE	Rimantadine	KLONOPIN	Clonazepam
FLUVOXAMINE	Fluvoxamine	LAMISIL	Terbinafine
FOLEX	Methotrexate	LANOXICAPS	Digoxin
FORTEO	Teriparatide	LANOXIN	Digoxin
FOSAMAX	Alendronate	LAROTID	Amoxicillin
FRAGMIN	Dalteparin	LASIX	Furosemide
FURADANTIN	Nitrofurantoin	LESCOL	Fluvastatin
GENGRAF	Cyclosporine	LEUKERAN	Chlorambucil
GEODON	Ziprasidone	LEVAQUIN	Levofloxacin
GLUCOPHAGE	Metformin	LEVATOL	Penbutolol
GLUCOTROL	Glipizide	LEVBID	Hyoscyamine
GLYNASE	Glyburide	LEVITRA	Vardenafil
GLYSET	Miglitol	LEVO-DROMORAN	Levorphanol
HALDOL	Haloperidol		
HEPTALAC	Lactulose	LEVO-T	Thyroxine
HERCEPTIN	Trastuzumab	LEVSIN	Hyoscyamine
HUMALOG	Insulin	LEXAPRO	Escitalopram
HUMULIN	Insulin	LEXXEL	Felodipine
HYALGAN	Hyaluronate	LIBRIUM	Chlordiazepoxide
HYDERGINE	Ergoloid mesylates	LIDODERM	Lidocaine
		LIDOPEN	Lidocaine
HYGROTON	Chlorthalidone	LIORESAL	Baclofen
HYTRIN	Terazosin	LIPITOR	Atorvastatin
ILOSENE	Erythromycin	LIQUAEMIN	Heparin
IMDUR	Isosorbide mononitrate	LITHOBID	Lithium
		LODOSYN	Carbidopa
INDOCIN	Indomethacin	LOMOTIL	Diphenoxylate plus atropine sulfate
INNOHEP	Tinzaparin		
INSPRA	Eplerenone		
INTEGRILIN	Eptifibatide	LONOX	Diphenoxylate plus atropine sulfate
INTROPIN	Dopamine		
IOPIDINE	Apraclonidine		
ISMO	Isosorbide mononitrate	LOPID	Gemfibrozil
		LOPRESSOR	Metoprolol
ISOPTIN	Verapamil	LOPURIN	Allopurinol
ISOPTO HYOSCINE	Scopolamine [also Hyoscine]	LOTENSIN	Benazepril
		LOVENOX	Enoxaparin
ISOPTOCARPINE	Pilocarpine	LOXITANE	Loxapine

℞ GENERIC NAMES OF SOME TRADE NAME DRUGS

Trade	Generic	Trade	Generic
LOZOL	Indapamide	NAVANE	Thiothixene
LUMIGAN	Bimatoprost	NAVELBINE	Vinorelbine
LUMINAL	Phenobarbital	NEORAL	Cyclosporine
LUPRON	Leuprolide	NEOSAR	Cyclophos-phamide
MACRODANTIN	Nitrofurantoin		
MARINOL	Dronabinol	NEURONTIN	Gabapentin
MAVIK	Trandolapril	NIASPAN	Niacin
MEGACE	Megestrol	NICOLAR	Niacin
METHADOSE	Methadone	NILANDRON	Nilutamide
METHYLIN	Methylphenidate	NILSTAT	Nystatin
METROGEL	Metronidazole	NITRO-BID	Nitroglycerin
METROMIDOL	Metronidazole	NITRO-DUR	Nitroglycerin
MEVACOR	Lovastatin	NITROPRESS	Nitroprusside
MEXITIL	Mexiletine	NITROSTAT	Nitroglycerin
MIACALCIN	Calcitonin	NOLVADEX	Tamoxifen
MICARDIS	Telmisartan	NORMODYNE	Labetalol
MICRONASE	Glyburide	NORPACE	Disopyramide
MIDAMOR	Amiloride	NORPRAMIN	Desipramine
MIDAZOLAM	Midazolam	NORVASC	Amlodipine
MILTOWN	Meprobamate	NORVIR	Ritonavir
MINIPRESS	Prazosin	NOVOLIN	Insulin
MIOCHOL	Acetylcholine	NOVOTHYROX	Thyroxine
MIOSTAT	Carbachol	NUMORPHAN	Oxymorphone
MIRAPEX	Pramipexole	NYTOL	Diphenhydramine
MOBAN	Molindone	OCUPRESS	Carteolol
MOGADON	Nitrazepam (not available in US)	ONCOVIN	Vincristine
		ORAMORPH	Morphine
MONOKET	Isosorbide mononitrate	ORAP	Pimozide
		ORETIC	Hydrochloro-thiazide
MONOPRIL	Fosinopril		
MOTRIN	Ibuprofen	ORINASE DIAGNOSTIC	Tolbutamide
MS CONTIN	Morphine		
MUTAMYCIN	Mitomycin	OSMITROL	Mannitol
MYCOSTATIN	Nystatin	OSMOGLYN	Glycerol [also Glycerin]
MYKROX	Metolazone		
MYSOLINE	Primidone	OXYCONTIN	Oxycodone
MYTOZYTREX	Mitomycin	PACERONE	Amiodarone
NALLPEN	Nafcillin	PAMELOR	Nortriptyline
NAMENDA	Memantine	PARAFON FORTE	Chlorzoxazone
NAPRELAN	Naproxen	PARLODEL	Bromocriptine
NARCAN	Naloxone	PAXIL	Paroxetine
NARDIL	Phenelzine	PBZ	Tripelennamine
NATRECOR	Nesiritide	PENICILLIN-VK	Penicillin
NATURETIN-5	Bendroflume-thiazide	PEPCID	Famotidine
		PERIACTIN	Cyproheptadine

℞ GENERIC NAMES OF SOME TRADE NAME DRUGS

Trade	Generic	Trade	Generic
PERMAX	Pergolide	REGLAN	Metoclopramide
PERMITIL	Fluphenazine	RELENZA	Zanamivir
PERSANTINE	Dipyridamole	REMERON	Mirtazapine
PHENERGAN	Promethazine	REMICADE	Infliximab
PHENOBARBI-TONE	Phenobarbital	REMINYL	Galantamine
		REOPRO	Abciximab
PHENYTEK	Phenytoin	REQUIP	Ropinirole
PILOCAR	Pilocarpine	RESTORIL	Temazepam
PILOPINE HS	Pilocarpine	RETAVASE	Reteplase
PLATINOL	Cisplatin	RHEUMATREX	Methotrexate
PLAVIX	Clopidogrel	RIMSO-50	Dimethyl sulfoxide
PLENDIL	Felodipine		
PRANDIN	Repaglinide	RISPERDAL	Risperidone
PRAVACHOL	Pravastatin	RITALIN	Methylphenidate
PRECOSE	Acarbose	ROBAXIN	Methocarbamol
PREVACID	Lansoprazole	ROBITUSSIN	Guaifenesin
PRILOSEC	Omeprazole	ROXICODONE	Oxycodone
PRIMACOR	Milrinone	RUBEX	Doxorubicin
PRIMAXIN	Imipenem	RYTHMOL	Propafenone
PRIMSOL	Trimethoprim	SALURON	Hydroflume-thiazide
PRINIVIL	Lisinopril		
PROAMATINE	Midodrine	SANDIMMUNE	Cyclosporine
PROBALAN	Probenecid	SARAFEM	Fluoxetine
PRO-BANTHINE	Propantheline	SCOPACE	Scopolamine [also Hyoscine]
PROCANBID	Procainamide		
PROCARDIA	Nifedipine	SECONAL	Secobarbital
PROCRIT	Erythropoietin [also Epoetin alfa]	SECTRAL	Acebutolol
		SEPTRA	Trimethoprim-sulfame-thoxazole
PROLIXIN	Fluphenazine		
PROLOPRIM	Trimethoprim	SERAX	Oxazepam
PRONESTYL	Procainamide	SERENTIL	Mesoridazine
PROSOM	Estazolam	SEREVENT	Salmeterol
PROTONIX	Pantoprazole	SEROQUEL	Quetiapine
PROVENTIL	Albuterol	SERPALAN	Reserpine
PROVIGIL	Modafinil	SERZONE	Nefazodone
PROZAC	Fluoxetine	SINEMET	Levodopa with carbidopa
PYRIDIUM	Phenazopyridine		
QUESTRAN	Cholestyramine	SINEQUAN	Doxepin
QUINAGLUTE DURA-TABS	Quinidine	SKELAXIN	Metaxalone
		SLO-BID	Theophylline
QUINIDEX EXTENTABS	Quinidine	SOMA	Carisoprodol
		SOMINEX	Diphenhydramine
QUIXIN	Levofloxacin	SONATA	Zaleplon
REFLUDAN	Lepirudin	SONAZINE	Chlorpromazine

℞ GENERIC NAMES OF SOME TRADE NAME DRUGS

Trade	Generic	Trade	Generic
SORBITOL	Sorbitol	TOL-TAB	Tolbutamide
SORBITRATE	Isosorbide dinitrate	TONOCARD	Tocainide
SORINE	Sotalol	TOPAMAX	Topiramate
SPORANOX	Itraconazole	TOPROL-XL	Metoprolol
STALEVO	Entacapone plus levodopa/ carbidopa	TRANDATE	Labetalol
		TRANMEP	Meprobamate
		TRANSDERM SCOP	Scopolamine [also Hyoscine]
STARLIX	Nateglinide	TREXALL	Methotrexate
STELAZINE	Trifluoperazine	TRICOR	Fenofibrate
STREPTASE	Streptokinase	TRIHEXYPHEN-IDYL	Trihexyphenidyl
STRIFON FORTE	Chlorzoxazone		
SUBLIMAZE	Fentanyl	TRILAFON	Perphenazine
SULAR	Nisoldipine	TRIMOX	Amoxicillin
SULFATRIM	Trimethoprim-sulfame thoxazole	TRUSOPT	Dorzolamide
		TYLENOL	Acetaminophen
		UNASYN	Ampicillin-sulbactam
SURFAK	Docusate		
SYMMETREL	Amantadine	UNIPHYL	Theophylline
SYNTHROID	Thyroxine	UNIVASC	Moexipril
TAGAMET	Cimetidine	URECHOLINE	Bethanechol
TALWIN	Pentazocine	URISTAT	Phenazopyridine
TAMBOCOR	Flecainide	UROXATRAL	Alfuzosin
TAMIFLU	Oseltamivir	VALIUM	Diazepam
TASMAR	Tolcapone	VANCOCIN	Vancomycin
TAXOL	Paclitaxel	VANCOLED	Vancomycin
TAXOTERE	Docetaxel	VASOTEC	Enalapril
TEGRETOL	Carbamazepine	VEETIDS	Penicillin
TENORMIN	Atenolol	VENTOLIN	Albuterol
TENSILON	Edrophonium	VERELAN	Verapamil
TEQUIN	Gatifloxacin	VIADUR	Leuprolide
TEVETEN	Eprosartan	VIBRAMYCIN	Doxycycline
THALOMID	Thalidomide	VIBRA-TABS	Doxycycline
THEO-24	Theophylline	VIGAMOX	Moxifloxacin
THEOLAIR	Theophylline	VISKEN	Pindolol
THIORIDAZINE	Thioridazine	VISTARIL	Hydroxyzine
THORAZINE	Chlorpromazine	WELCHOL	Colesevelam
TIAZAC	Diltiazem	WELLBUTRIN	Bupropion
TICLID	Ticlopidine	XALATAN	Latanoprost
TIGAN	Trimethobenza mide	XENICAL	Orlistat
		XYLOCAINE	Lidocaine
TIKOSYN	Dofetilide	ZANTAC	Ranitidine
TIMOPTIC	Timolol	ZAROXOLYN	Metolazone
TNKASE	Tenecteplase	ZEBETA	Bisoprolol
TOLINASE	Tolazamide	ZESTRIL	Lisinopril

R GENERIC NAMES OF SOME TRADE NAME DRUGS

Trade	Generic	Trade	Generic
ZETIA	Ezetimibe	ZONALON	Doxepin
ZITHROMAX	Azithromycin	ZOSTRIX	Capsaicin
ZOCOR	Simvastatin	ZYBAN	Bupropion
ZOFRAN	Ondansetron	ZYLOPRIM	Allopurinol
ZOLADEX	Goserelin	ZYMAR	Gatifloxacin
ZOLOFT	Sertraline	ZYPREXA	Olanzapine
ZOMETA	Zoledronic acid	ZYRTEC	Cetirizine

Appendix II

Resources for Help and Information

The following list is selective and restricted largely to national organizations in the United States, many of which have local chapters. Sites chosen are generally not-for-profit and usually offer information or support rather than advocacy. Telephone numbers and web sites are included as appropriate; however, such information changes frequently. Additional information is available through health care professionals, local libraries, telephone listings, and the Internet.

AGING
Administration on Aging
Washington, DC
800-677-1116 (Eldercare Locator)
800-877-8339 (TTY)
www.aoa.gov

Regional Support Centers:

Region I: CT, MA, ME, NH, RI, VT
Boston, MA
617-565-1158

Region II & III: DC, DE, MD, NJ, NY, PA, VA, WV, PR, VI
New York, NY
212-264-2976

Region IV: AL, FL, GA, KY, MS, NC, SC, TN
Atlanta, GA
404-562-7600

Region V: IL, IN, MI, MN, OH, WI
Chicago, IL
312-353-3141

Region VI: AR, LA, NM, OK, TX
Dallas, TX
214-767-2971

Region VII: IA, KS, MO, NE
Kansas City, MO
816-426-3511

Region VIII: CO, MT, ND, SD, UT
Denver, CO
303-844-2951

Region IX: AZ, CA, HI, NV, AS, GU, TTPI, CNMI
San Francisco, CA
415-437-8782

Region X: AK, ID, OR, WA
Seattle, WA
206-615-2298

American Association of Retired People
Washington, DC
800-424-3410
www.aarp.org

Benefits Check Up
The National Council on the Aging
www.benefitscheckup.org

Health and Age
Novartis Foundation for Gerontology
www.healthandage.com

Infoaging.org (AFAR)
New York, NY
212-703-9977
www.infoaging.org

National Association of Area Agencies on Aging
Washington, DC
202-296-8130
www.n4a.org

National Council on the Aging
Washington, DC
202-479-1200
202-479-6674 (TDD)
www.ncoa.org

National Institute on Aging
Bethesda, MD
800-222-2225
800-222-4225 (TTY)
301-496-1752
www.nia.nih.gov

National Institutes of Health SeniorHealth
Bethesda, MD
301-496-4000
www.nihseniorhealth.gov

Older Women's League
Washington, DC
800-825-3695
202-783-6686
www.owl-national.org

ALCOHOLISM
Al-Anon Family Group Headquarters
Virginia Beach, VA
800-356-9996
757-563-1600
www.al-anon.org

Alcoholics Anonymous
New York, NY
212-870-3400
www.alcoholics-anonymous.org

Hazelden
Center City, MN
800-257-7810
651-213-4000
www.hazelden.org

National Council on Alcoholism & Drug Dependence
New York, NY
800-622-2255
212-269-7797
www.ncadd.org

ALZHEIMER'S DISEASE & OTHER DEMENTIAS
Alzheimer's Association
Chicago, IL
800-272-3900
312-335-8700
www.alz.org

Alzheimer's Disease Education & Referral Center
Silver Spring, MD
800-438-4380
www.alzheimers.org

The Alzheimer's Society
London, UK
020 7306 0606
www.alzheimers.org.uk

The Alzheimer's Society CJD Support Group
London, UK
www.alzheimers.org.uk/cjd

AMPUTATION
(see also Disabilities & Rehabilitation)

The American Amputee Foundation, Inc.
Little Rock, AR
501-666-2523

National Amputation Foundation
Malverne, NY
516-887-3600
www.nationalamputation.org

ARTHRITIS
Arthritis Foundation
Atlanta, GA
800-283-7800
www.arthritis.org

BEREAVEMENT
(see Death & Bereavement)

BLINDNESS & VISION PROBLEMS
American Council of the Blind
Washington, DC
800-424-8666
202-467-5081
www.acb.org

American Foundation for the Blind
New York, NY
800-232-5463
212-502-7600
www.afb.org

Association for Macular Diseases
New York, NY
212-605-3719
www.macula.org

Fight for Sight
New York, NY
212-679-6060
www.fightforsight.com

The Foundation Fighting Blindness
Owing Mills, MD
888-394-3937
800-683-5551 (TDD)
410-568-0150
www.blindness.org

Glaucoma Research Foundation
San Francisco, CA
800-826-6693
415-986-3162
www.glaucoma.org

Helen Keller Services for the Blind
Sands Point, NY
516-944-8900 (TTY)
718-522-2122 (Brooklyn Senior Center)
516-485-1234 (Hempstead Senior Center)
631-424-0022 (Huntington Senior Center)
www.helenkeller.org/national

National Association for Visually Handicapped
New York, NY
212-255-2804
212-889-3141
www.navh.org

Prevent Blindness America
Schaumburg, IL
800-331-2020
847-843-2020
www.preventblindness.org

BLOOD DISORDERS
Leukemia Society of America
White Plains, NY
800-955-4572
914-949-5213
www.leukemia.org

BRAIN DISORDERS
(see also Cancer & Other Tumors; Alzheimer's Disease & Other Dementias; Epilepsy)

National Institute of Neurological Disorders & Stroke
Bethesda, MD
800-352-9424
301-468-5981 (TTY)
www.ninds.nih.gov

CANCER & OTHER TUMORS
American Cancer Society
Atlanta, GA
800-227-2345
www.cancer.org

Cancer Care, Inc.
New York, NY
800-813-4673
212-712-8080
www.cancercare.org

National Cancer Institute
Bethesda, MD
800-422-6237
800-332-8615 (TTY)
www.cancer.gov

National Coalition for Cancer Survivorship
Silver Spring, MD
301-650-9127
www.canceradvocacy.org

BREAST
National Alliance of Breast Cancer Organizations
New York, NY
888-806-2226
www.nabco.org

The Susan G. Komen Breast Cancer Foundation
Dallas, TX
800-462-9273
972-855-1600
www.komen.org

Y-ME: National Breast Cancer Organization
Chicago, IL
800-221-2141
312-986-8338
www.y-me.org

PROSTATE
US-TOO International
Downers Grove, IL
800-808-7866
630-795-1002
www.ustoo.com

SKIN
The Skin Cancer Foundation
New York, NY
800-754-6490
www.skincancer.org

CARDIOVASCULAR DISORDERS
American Heart Association
Dallas, TX
800-242-8721
214-373-6300
www.americanheart.org

National Heart, Lung, and Blood Institute
Bethesda, MD
301-251-1222
www.nhlbi.nih.gov

National Stroke Association
Englewood, CO
800-787-6537
303-649-9299
www.stroke.org

Sister Kenny Institute
Minneapolis, MN
612-863-4457
www.sisterkennyinstitute.com

Vascular Disease Foundation
Lakewood, CO
866-723-4636
303-949-8337
www.vdf.org

CONTINUING EDUCATION
Elderhostel
Boston, MA
877-426-8056
877-426-2167 (TTY)
www.elderhostel.org

DEAFNESS & HEARING DISORDERS
American Tinnitus Association
Portland, OR
800-634-8978
503-248-9985
www.ata.org

Deafness Research Foundation
Washington, DC
800-829-5934
202-289-5850
www.drf.org

The Ear Foundation
Nashville, TN
800-545-4327
615-284-7807
www.earfoundation.org

Helen Keller National Center
Sands Point, NY
800-255-0411
516-944-8637 (TTY)
www.helenkeller.org/national

National Association of the Deaf
Silver Spring, MD
301-587-1788
301-587-1789 (TTY)
www.nad.org

DEATH & BEREAVEMENT
Compassion in Dying Federation
Portland, OR
503-221-9556
www.compassionindying.org

The Compassionate Friends
Oak Brook, IL
877-969-0010
630-990-0010
www.compassionatefriends.org

Hospice Education Institute
Machiasport, ME
800-331-1620
207-255-8800
www.hospiceworld.org

National Hospice Foundation
Alexandria, VA
703-516-4928
www.hospiceinfo.org

Partnership for Caring
Washington, DC
800-989-9455
202-296-8071
www.partnershipforcaring.org

DEMENTIA
(see Alzheimer's Disease &
Other Dementias)

DEPRESSION
Depression and Related Affective Disorders Association (DRADA)
Baltimore, MD
410-955-4647
www.drada.org

National Depressive and Manic-Depressive Association
Chicago, IL
800-826-3632
312-642-0049
www.ndmda.org

Recovery, Inc.
Chicago, IL
312-337-5661
www.recovery-inc.com

DIABETES
American Diabetes Association
Alexandria, VA
800-342-2383
www.diabetes.org

National Institute of Diabetes & Digestive & Kidney Diseases
Bethesda, MD
301-654-3327
301-435-0714
www.niddk.nih.gov

DIGESTIVE DISORDERS
Digestive Disease National Coalition
Washington, DC
202-544-7497
www.ddnc.org

International Foundation for Functional Gastrointestinal Disorders
Milwaukee, WI
888-964-2001
414-964-1799
www.iffgd.org

Intestinal Disease Foundation
Pittsburgh, PA
877-587-9606
412-261-5888
www.intestinalfoundation.org

National Digestive Diseases Information Clearinghouse
Bethesda, MD
800-891-5389
301-654-3810
www.digestive.niddk.nih.gov

United Ostomy Association
Irvine, CA
800-826-0826
949-660-8624
www.uoa.org

DISABILITIES & REHABILITATION
(see also Amputation)

Disabled American Veterans
Cold Springs, KY
877-726-2838
859-441-7300
www.dav.org

Easter Seals
Chicago, IL
800-221-6827
312-726-6200
312-726-4258 (TTY)
www.easter-seals.org

National Organization on Disability
Washington, DC
202-293-5960
www.nod.org

National Rehabilitation Association
Alexandria, VA
888-258-4295
703-836-0850
www.nationalrehab.org

National Rehabilitation Information Center
Lanham, MD
800-346-2742
www.naric.com

Paralyzed Veterans of America
Washington, DC
800-424-8200
202-872-1300
www.pva.org

DRIVING
AAA Foundation for Traffic Safety
Senior Drivers
Washington, DC
202-638-5944
www.seniordrivers.org

Drivers.com
Toronto, Canada
416-767-4885
www.drivers.com/topic/10

EAR
(see Deafness & Hearing Disorders)

EATING DISORDERS
Overeaters Anonymous
Rio Rancho, NM
505-891-2664
www.overeatersanonymous.org

ENDOCRINE DISORDERS
(see also Diabetes)

Thyroid Foundation of America
Boston, MA
800-832-8321
617-726-8500
www.tsh.org

ERECTILE DYSFUNCTION (IMPOTENCE)
Impotents Anonymous
Maryville, TN
615-983-6064

EYE
(see Blindness & Vision Problems)

GENERAL

American Academy of Family Physicians
Leawood, KS
www.familydoctor.org

American Academy of Neurology
Saint Paul, MN 55116
800-879-1960
www.aan.com

American Medical Association
Chicago, IL
312-464-5000
www.ama-assn.org

Centers for Disease Control and Prevention
Atlanta, GA
800-311-3435
404-639-3311
www.cdc.gov

Electronic Orange Book
Approved Drug Products With Therapeutic Equivalence Evaluations
www.fda.gov/cder/ob

The Merck Manuals
Merck & Co., Inc.
West Point, PA
800-819-9456
www.merck.com

National Institutes of Health
Bethesda, MD
301-496-4000
www.nih.gov

University of Medicine and Dentistry of New Jersey
www.healthynj.org

US Department of Health and Human Services
Washington, DC
877-696-6775
202-619-0257
www.os.dhhs.gov

US Food and Drug Administration
Office of Consumer Affairs
Inquiry Information Line
Rockville, MD
888-463-6332
www.fda.gov

Virtual Hospital (University of Iowa)
Iowa City, IA
www.vh.org

HEAD INJURY
(see Brain Disorders)

HEARING
(see Deafness & Hearing Disorders)

HEART DISORDERS
(see Cardiovascular Disorders)

HOME CARE
National Association for Home Care
Washington, DC
202-547-7424
www.nahc.org

HOSPICES
(see Death & Bereavement)

IMPOTENCE
(see Erectile Dysfunction)

INCONTINENCE
National Association for Continence
Spartanburg, SC
800-252-3337
864-579-7900
www.nafc.org

The Simon Foundation for Continence
Wilmette, IL
800-237-4666
www.simonfoundation.org

KIDNEY DISORDERS
American Association of Kidney Patients
Tampa, FL
800-749-2257
www.aakp.org

American Kidney Fund
Rockville, MD
800-638-8299
www.akfinc.org

National Kidney and Urologic Diseases Information Clearinghouse
Bethesda, MD
800-891-5390
301-654-4415
www.kidney.niddk.nih.gov

National Kidney Foundation
New York, NY
800-622-9010
212-889-2210
www.kidney.org

LUNG DISORDERS
(see Respiratory Disorders)

MEDIC ALERT
MedicAlert Foundation
Turlock, CA
888-633-4298
209-668-3333
www.medicalert.org

MENTAL HEALTH
(see Depression and Psychiatric Disease)

MOVEMENT DISORDERS
We Move
New York, NY
800-437-6682
www.wemove.org

NUTRITION
American Dietetic Association
Chicago, IL
800-877-1600
312-899-0040
www.eatright.org

OSTEOPOROSIS
National Osteoporosis Foundation
Washington, DC
202-223-2226
www.nof.org

PAGET'S DISEASE
The Paget Foundation
New York, NY
800-237-2438
212-509-5335
www.paget.org

PAIN RELIEF
American Chronic Pain Association
Baltimore, MD
888-615-7246
www.painfoundation.org

PARKINSON'S DISEASE
American Parkinson Disease Association
Staten Island, NY
800-223-2732
718-981-8001
www.apdaparkinson.com

National Parkinson Foundation
Miami, FL
800-327-4545
800-433-7022 (in FL)
www.parkinson.org

Parkinson's Action Network
Alexandria, VA
800-850-4726
703-518-8877
www.parkinsonsaction.org

Parkinson's Disease Foundation
New York, NY
800-457-6676
212-923-4700
www.pdf.org

PAYING FOR HEALTH CARE
Centers for Medicare and Medicaid Services
Washington, DC
800-633-4227
www.medicare.gov

The Henry J. Kaiser Family Foundation
Washington, DC
202-347-5270
www.kff.org

PROSTATE DISORDERS
(see also Cancer & Other Tumors)

The Prostatitis Foundation
Smithshire, IL
888-891-4200
www.prostatitis.org

PSYCHIATRIC DISEASE
(see also Depression)

National Alliance for the Mentally Ill
Arlington, VA
800-950-6264
703-524-7600
www.nami.org

National Institute of Mental Health
Bethesda, MD
301-443-4513
www.nimh.nih.gov

National Mental Health Association
Alexandria, VA
800-969-6642
800-443-5959 (TTY)
703-684-7722
www.nmha.org

Survivors of Suicide
www.survivorsofsuicide.com

RESPIRATORY (LUNG) DISORDERS
American Lung Association
New York, NY
800-586-4872
212-315-8700
www.lungusa.org

SJÖGREN'S SYNDROME
National Sjögren's Syndrome Association
Bethesda, MD
800-475-6473
www.sjogrens.org

SLEEP DISORDERS
American Sleep Apnea Association
Washington, DC
202-293-3650
www.sleepapnea.org

American Academy of Sleep Medicine
Rochester, MN
708-492-0930
www.aasmnet.org

TRAVEL HEALTH
CDC National Center for Infectious Diseases
Travelers' Health
888-394-8747
www.cdc.gov/travel

Federal Aviation Administration
Information for the Air Traveler
   With a Disability
www.faa.gov

International Association for Medical Assistance to Travelers
Lewiston, NY
716-754-4883
www.iamat.org

International SOS
Trevose, PA
800-523-8930
215-244-1500
www.internationalsos.org

Travel Health Online
www.tripprep.com

US State Department
Help for Americans Abroad
www.travel.state.gov/acs

World Health Organization
International Travel and Health
www.who.int/ith

VOLUNTEERING ORGANIZATIONS
Senior Corps (Retired and Senior Volunteer Program [RSVP], The Foster Grandparent Program [FGP], The Senior Companion Program [SCP])
Washington, DC
202-606-5000
202-565-2799 (TTY)
www.seniorcorps.org

WOMEN'S HEALTH
(see also Aging)

American College of Obstetricians and Gynecologists
Washington, DC
202-638-5577
202-863-2518
www.acog.org

National Women's Health Network
Washington, DC
202-347-1140
www.womenshealthnetwork.org

Index